Hormone Therapy and Castration Resistance of Prostate Cancer

Yoichi Arai • Osamu Ogawa
Editors

Hormone Therapy and Castration Resistance of Prostate Cancer

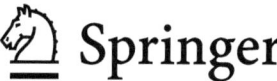

Editors
Yoichi Arai
Department of Urology
Tohoku University School of Medicine
Sendai
Japan

Osamu Ogawa
Department of Urology
Kyoto University Graduate School
of Medicine
Kyoto
Japan

ISBN 978-981-10-7012-9   ISBN 978-981-10-7013-6 (eBook)
https://doi.org/10.1007/978-981-10-7013-6

Library of Congress Control Number: 2018941209

© Springer Nature Singapore Pte Ltd. 2018
This work is subject to copyright. All rights are reserved by the Publisher, whether the whole or part of the material is concerned, specifically the rights of translation, reprinting, reuse of illustrations, recitation, broadcasting, reproduction on microfilms or in any other physical way, and transmission or information storage and retrieval, electronic adaptation, computer software, or by similar or dissimilar methodology now known or hereafter developed.
The use of general descriptive names, registered names, trademarks, service marks, etc. in this publication does not imply, even in the absence of a specific statement, that such names are exempt from the relevant protective laws and regulations and therefore free for general use.
The publisher, the authors and the editors are safe to assume that the advice and information in this book are believed to be true and accurate at the date of publication. Neither the publisher nor the authors or the editors give a warranty, express or implied, with respect to the material contained herein or for any errors or omissions that may have been made. The publisher remains neutral with regard to jurisdictional claims in published maps and institutional affiliations.

Printed on acid-free paper

This Springer imprint is published by the registered company Springer Nature Singapore Pte Ltd. part of Springer Nature.
The registered company address is: 152 Beach Road, #21-01/04 Gateway East, Singapore 189721, Singapore

Contents

1. Introduction.. 1
   Yoichi Arai and Osamu Ogawa

2. Recent Trends in Hormone Therapy for Prostate Cancer in Japan.. 3
   Mizuki Onozawa and Hideyuki Akaza

3. Risk Assessment Among Patients Receiving Primary ADT for Prostate Cancer.. 13
   Shiro Hinotsu

4. Patient-Derived Xenografts for Research on Hormonal Therapy of Prostate Cancer.. 19
   Takahiro Inoue

5. Impact of GnRH Antagonist and LHRH Agonist on the Gonadal Axis... 31
   Yoshiyuki Miyazawa, Yoshitaka Sekine, and Kazuhiro Suzuki

6. Controversies on Combined Androgen Blockade for Prostate Cancer.. 41
   Atsushi Mizokami

7. Adrenal Androgen in Prostate Cancer 51
   Yasuhiro Shibata

8. Intermittent ADT for Prostate Cancer 59
   Koichiro Akakura

9. Prognostic Significance of Monitoring Serum Testosterone in Primary ADT for Prostate Cancer 69
   Shinichi Sakamoto

10. Ethnic Variation in Clinical Outcomes of Hormone Therapy for Prostate Cancer.. 77
    Takashi Fukagai, Masashi Morita, Robert G. Carlile, John L. Lederer, and Thomas Namiki

11	**Androgen Deprivation Therapy in Combination with Radical Prostatectomy**................................. Takuya Koie and Chikara Ohyama	89
12	**ADT in Combination with Radiation Therapy for Clinically Localized Prostate Cancer** .... Takashi Mizowaki	99
13	**ADT as Salvage Therapy After Definitive Treatment for Clinically Localized Prostate Cancer** .... Akira Yokomizo	113
14	**Androgen Deprivation Therapy for Clinically Localized Prostate Cancer**... Yoichi Arai and Koji Mitsuzuka	121
15	**Complications of ADT for Prostate Cancer: Hot Flashes**.......... Hideki Sakai and Tomoaki Hakariya	133
16	**Complications of ADT for Prostate Cancer: Osteoporosis and the Risk of Fracture.**.................................. Hiroji Uemura	141
17	**Metabolic Health for Patients with Prostate Cancer During Androgen Deprivation Therapy** .... Koji Mitsuzuka and Yoichi Arai	151
18	**Bone Scan Index as a Biomarker of Bone Metastasis**.............. Kenichi Nakajima and Lars Edenbrandt	165
19	**Genetic Polymorphism Analysis in Predicting Prognosis of Advanced Prostate Cancer.**...................... Norihiko Tsuchiya	175
20	**Local Therapy in Combination with Androgen Deprivation Therapy for Metastatic Prostate Cancer**............. Hideyasu Tsumura, Ken-Ichi Tabata, and Masatsugu Iwamura	189
21	**Oxidative Stress and Castration-Resistant Prostate Cancer** .... Masaki Shiota	201
22	**Alternative Antiandrogen Therapy for CRPC**.................... Takanobu Utsumi, Naoto Kamiya, Masashi Yano, Takumi Endo, and Hiroyoshi Suzuki	215
23	**Optimization of Sequential AR Targeted Therapy for CRPC** ...... Naoki Terada	225
24	**Enzalutamide Therapy for mCRPC in Japanese Men** .... Go Kimura	231

25	**Abiraterone Acetate Therapy for mCRPC in Japanese Men** Masaomi Ikeda and Takefumi Satoh	241
26	**Role of Estramustine Phosphate and Other Estrogens for Castration-Resistant Prostate Cancer** Takahiro Inoue	249
27	**Corticosteroid Therapy for CRPC** Kazuo Nishimura	257
28	**microRNA Analysis in Prostate Cancer** Hideki Enokida	267
29	**AR Splice Variant in Prostate Cancer** Shinichi Yamashita and Yoichi Arai	293
30	**Detection of Circulating Tumor Cells in Castration-Resistant Prostate Cancer** Takatsugu Okegawa	299
31	**New Biomarker for Castration-Resistant Prostate Cancer: A Glycobiological Perspective** Shingo Hatakeyama, Tohru Yoneyama, Hayato Yamamoto, Yuki Tobisawa, Shin-Ichiro Nishimura, and Chikara Ohyama	307
32	**Bone-Targeted Treatment in CRPC Management** Tomomi Kamba	317
33	**Skeletal Complications in Patients with CRPC** Takamitsu Inoue and Tomonori Habuchi	327
34	**Urological Complications in Men Dying from Prostate Cancer** Takashi Kobayashi	339
35	**Prediction of Optimal Number of Cycles in Docetaxel Regimen for Patients with mCRPC** Hideyasu Matsuyama, Tomoyuki Shimabukuro, Isao Hara, Kazuhiro Suzuki, Hirotsugu Uemura, Munehisa Ueno, Yoshihiko Tomita, and Nobuaki Shimizu	345
36	**Intermittent Chemotherapy with Docetaxel for Metastatic Castration-Resistant Prostate Cancer** Shintaro Narita and Tomonori Habuchi	357
37	**Chemotherapy with Cabazitaxel for mCRPC in Japanese Men** Masahiro Nozawa and Hirotsugu Uemura	369
38	**New Targeted Approach to CRPC** Takeo Kosaka and Mototsugu Oya	375

39	**Molecular Basis of Neuroendocrine Prostate Cancer** 387
	Shusuke Akamatsu

40	**Gene Therapy for Prostate Cancer: Current Status and Future Prospects** 397
	Yasutomo Nasu and Masami Watanabe

41	**Immune Therapy for Castration-Resistant Prostate Cancer** 407
	Kazuhiro Yoshimura, Takafumi Minami, Masahiro Nozawa, and Hirotsugu Uemura

42	**A New Approach to Castration-Resistant Prostate Cancer Using Inactivated Virus** 419
	Kazutoshi Fujita, Yasufumi Kaneda, and Norio Nonomura

43	**Patient-Reported Outcome in the Management of CRPC** 427
	Nobuaki Matsubara

Introduction

Yoichi Arai and Osamu Ogawa

Abstract

This comprehensive reference expounds the current state of hormone therapy and castration resistance of prostate cancer. Prostate cancer is the most commonly diagnosed malignancy in men of Western countries. Previously, its incidence in Northeast Asia including Japan had been considered to be relatively low, but it has been dramatically increasing in recent years. Based on the Cancer Information Service of the National Cancer Center, there were 98,400 estimated new cases of prostate cancer in 2015, making the disease the leading cancer in Japanese men. Although most of the new cases are diagnosed in early stages, a significant proportion of patients receive hormone therapy for metastatic disease or for relapse after local treatment. Thus the situation has gradually changed toward earlier and longer use of hormone therapy. The malignancy will finally form castration-resistant prostate cancer (CRPC) despite the lack of testicular androgen.

This comprehensive reference expounds the current state of hormone therapy and castration resistance of prostate cancer. Prostate cancer is the most commonly diagnosed malignancy in men of Western countries. Previously, its incidence in Northeast Asia including Japan had been considered to be relatively low, but it has been dramatically increasing in recent years. Based on the Cancer Information Service of the National Cancer Center, there were 98,400 estimated new cases of prostate cancer in 2015, making the disease the leading cancer in Japanese men. Although most of the new cases are diagnosed in early stages, a significant proportion of patients receive hormone therapy for metastatic disease or for relapse after local treatment.

Y. Arai
Department of Urology, Tohoku University Graduate School of Medicine, Sendai, Japan

O. Ogawa (✉)
Department of Urology, Kyoto University Graduate School of Medicine, Kyoto, Japan
e-mail: ogawao@kuhp.kyoto-u.ac.jp

© Springer Nature Singapore Pte Ltd. 2018
Y. Arai, O. Ogawa (eds.), *Hormone Therapy and Castration Resistance of Prostate Cancer*, https://doi.org/10.1007/978-981-10-7013-6_1

Thus the situation has gradually changed toward earlier and longer use of hormone therapy. The malignancy will finally form castration-resistant prostate cancer (CRPC) despite the lack of testicular androgen.

With advance in understanding on the molecular basis of hormone dependence and castration-resistant prostate cancer, many new androgen receptor-targeted agents have emerged. During the last decade, many evidences on hormone therapy have been accumulated from Japan. Interestingly some of these findings seem to be different from those reported from Western countries, suggesting the ethnic variation of outcome of hormone therapy. In this context, further accumulation of evidence from Asian countries is warranted in this research field. In the chapters of this book, expert authors provide exhaustive interpretations of the evidence recently reported from Japan and provide important Asian perspectives on hormone therapy for PCa. In addition, some novel concepts of the treatment for CRPC are introduced. This work benefits not only Asian urologists but also their Western counterparts and all physicians and medical personnel who are involved in the treatment of PCa.

Recent Trends in Hormone Therapy for Prostate Cancer in Japan

Mizuki Onozawa and Hideyuki Akaza

Abstract

Advanced prostate cancer is usually treated by hormonal therapy. In contrast, localized disease can be treated by various approaches including radical prostatectomy, radiation, hormonal therapy, and active surveillance. Wide variation in the treatment selection by era and country is a characteristic of prostate cancer. In this chapter, we review four large-scale observational studies across Japan conducted during different time periods. In Japan, the proportion of hormonal therapy as the treatment selection for newly diagnosed prostate cancer has decreased from 57% in 2000 to 40% in 2010, but it remains the most frequently selected treatment. During the same period, the proportion of metastatic disease for which hormonal therapy was the first treatment choice decreased from 21% to 11%, and that of patients with non-metastatic disease who selected hormonal therapy decreased from 46% to 32%. This lowered stage migration and shift toward radical treatment were the reasons for decrease in hormonal therapy in Japan. Regarding the type of hormonal therapy, the use of combined androgen blockade (CAB) increased from 59% in 2001–2003 to 74% in 2010.

Keywords

Prostate cancer · Hormonal therapy · Combined androgen blockade · Trend in treatment · Database study

---

M. Onozawa (✉)
Department of Urology, International University of Health and Welfare, School of Medicine, Tokyo, Japan
e-mail: onozawa-jua@umin.ac.jp

H. Akaza
Strategic Investigation on Comprehensive Cancer Network, Interfaculty Initiative in Information Studies/Graduate School of Interdisciplinary Information Studies, The University of Tokyo, Tokyo, Japan
e-mail: akazah@med.rcast.u-tokyo.ac.jp

© Springer Nature Singapore Pte Ltd. 2018
Y. Arai, O. Ogawa (eds.), *Hormone Therapy and Castration Resistance of Prostate Cancer*, https://doi.org/10.1007/978-981-10-7013-6_2

2.1 Introduction

Since Huggins and Hodges' 1941 paper demonstrating the usefulness of hormonal therapy for prostate cancer [1], hormonal therapy has long played the central role in prostate cancer treatment. In Japan, Akakura et al. reported the results of their survey of 565 prostate cancer patients from nine institutions in 1988 [2]. According to that paper, about half of the patients were stage D, and the initial treatment was hormonal therapy in 62.6% of the patients [2]. However, clinical practice patterns of prostate cancer have dramatically changed since that era. Prostate-specific antigen (PSA) was introduced around 1990, enabling the early detection of prostate cancer [3], which resulted in lowered stage migration. The median patient age also fell.

At the same time, many new approaches were introduced that provide radical treatment with less invasiveness and a higher success rate. Regarding drug-based treatments for prostate cancer, luteinizing hormone-releasing hormone (LH-RH) agonist and nonsteroidal antiandrogens became available in the mid-1990s. It is thus important to assess how hormonal therapy has changed in the treatment of prostate cancer. In this chapter, with the use of data from a large observational study, we present recent trends in hormonal therapy for prostate cancer in Japan and compared them with the trends in the USA. Only the trends observed over time regarding hormonal therapy used as the main treatment for prostate cancer will be covered.

2.2 Source of Data

Several studies have examined the initial prostate cancer treatment pattern in Japan. Tables 2.1 and 2.2 summarize the four large-scale real-world database studies conducted across Japan that we review herein. The characteristics of these studies (referred to here as Japanese Urological Association [JUA] "JUA2000," the Japan Study Group of Prostate Cancer [J-CaP] "JCaP2001-3," "JUA2004," and "JCaP2010") and their background databases are summarized as follows.

1. JUA2000
    The subjects were 4529 prostate cancer patients diagnosed in 2000 from 173 institutions across Japan [4]. The clinicopathological characteristics, initial treatment pattern, and outcomes were determined. The study was managed by the Cancer Registration Committee of the Japanese Urological Association (JUA).
2. JCaP2001-3
    The database consists of 26,272 prostate cancer patients from 395 institutions across Japan for whom hormonal therapy was initiated between 2001 and 2003 [5, 6]. In contrast to the other three studies discussed herein, this database included only patients treated with hormonal therapy. Thus, patients who received hormonal therapy as neoadjuvant or adjuvant therapy were included, but those treated by only radical treatment were not included. The study was managed by the nonprofit organization (NPO) Japan Study Group of Prostate Cancer (J-CaP), and it examined clinicopathological characteristics, treatment patterns, and outcomes.

Table 2.1 Background characteristics and initial treatment pattern in Japanese database study

Study name in this chapter No. of patients No. of institutions	Distribution of Age	T stage	N stage	M stage	Initial treatment
JUA2000 4529 patients 173 institutions	<70: nm (32.5) <75: nm (26.8) 75≤: nm (40.7)	T0: 12 (0.3) T1: 1145 (25.3) T2: 1739 (38.4) T3: 1193 (26.3) T4: 358 (7.9)	N0: 3569 (78.8) N1: 501 (11.1) Nx: 459 (10.1)	M0: 3243 (71.6) M1: 964 (21.3) Mx: 322 (7.1)	HT: nm (56.9) Ope: 1240 (27.4) Radiation: nm (8.1) AS/WW: nm (5.6)
JCaP2001-3 395 institutions	See Table 2.2	See Table 2.2	See Table 2.2	See Table 2.2	See Table 2.2
JUA2004 10,280 patients 239 institutions		T0: 5 (0.0) T1: 4082 (39.7) T2: 3533 (34.4) T3: 2130 (20.7) T4: 451 (4.4) Tx: 77 (0.7)	N0: 9237 (89.9) N1: 684 (6.7) Nx: 358 (3.5)	M0: 8746 (85.1) M1: 1195 (11.6) Mx: 339 (3.3)	HT: 4934 (48.0) Ope: 3212 (31.2) Radiation: 1625 (15.8) AS/WW: 485 (4.7) Other: 44 (0.4)
JCaP2010 8291 patients 140 institutions	<70: 3532 (42.6) <75: 2029 (24.5) 75≤: 2729 (32.9)	T1: 3442 (41.5) T2: 2957 (35.7) T3: 1516 (18.3) T4: 355 (4.3) Unknown: 21 (0.3)	N0: 7563 (91.2) N1: 640 (7.7) Nx: 88 (1.1)	M0: 7425 (89.6) M1: 865 (10.5) Mx: 1 (0.0)	HT: 3337 (40.2) Ope: 2657 (32.0) Radiation: 1741 (21.0) AS/WW: 527 (6.4)

Number represents patient number. Number in parenthesis represents percent
Abbreviation: *AS/WW* active surveillance or watch and wait, *HT* hormonal therapy, *nm* not mentioned, *Ope* prostatectomy

3. JUA2004

   A total of 11,385 prostate cancer patients diagnosed in 2004 from 239 institutions across Japan were included [3]. The patients' clinicopathological characteristics, treatment patterns, and outcomes were identified. The study, managed by the JUA, was the first large population report of survival data in Japanese prostate cancer patients [3].

4. JCaP2010

   This study was of 8291 prostate cancer patients from 140 institutions across Japan started treatment in 2010 [7]. Their clinicopathological background characteristics and initial treatments were analyzed. Follow-up patient status was not included. The study was managed by the J-CaP.

Table 2.2 Hormonal therapy in Japanese database study

Study name in this chapter No. of patients treated by hormonal therapy	Distribution of Age	T stage	N stage	M stage	Type of hormonal therapy	Type of castration
JUA2000 (No. of patients not described)	Not described	Not described	Not described	Not described	Not described	Not described
JCaP2001-3 19,409 patients	<70: 3954 (20.4) <75: 4811 (24.8) 75≤: 10,644 (54.8)	T1: 4020 (20.8) T2: 6288 (32.4) T3: 7053 (16.3) T4: 1944 (16.1)	N0: 15,206 (78.3) N1: 2875 (14.8) Nx: 1224 (6.3)	M0: 13,244 (68.2) M1: 5288 (27.3) Mx: 773 (4.0)	Castration mono: 5628 (29.0) CAB: 11,435 (58.9) AA mono: 1513 (7.8) Others: 833 (4.3)	Surgical: 1956 (11.5) Medical: 15,107 (88.5)
JUA2004 4934 patients	Not described	Not described	Not described	M0: 3582 (72.6) M1b: 1061 (21.5)	Castration mono: 1084 (22.0) CAB: 3313 (67.1) AA mono: 223 (4.5) CAB + other: 209 (4.2) AA + other: 12 (0.2) Others: 93 (1.9)	Surgical: 323 (6.9) Medical: 4364 (93.1)
JCaP2010 3337 patients	<70: 651 (19.5) <80: 1706 (51.1) 80≤: 980 (29.4)	T1: 861 (25.8) T2: 1055 (31.6) T3: 1078 (32.3) T4: 329 (9.9)	N0: 2671 (80.0) N1: 610 (18.3)	M0: 2495 (74.8) M1: 841 (25.2)	Castration mono: 700 (21.0) CAB: 2477 (74.2) AA mono: 156 (4.7) Others: 4 (0.1)	Surgical: 151 (4.7) Medical: 3045 (95.3)

Number represents patient number. Number in parenthesis represents percent
Abbreviations: *AA* antiandrogen, *CAB* combined androgen blockade, *Castration* castration, *mono* monotherapy

2.3 Trend in Hormonal Therapy as Main Treatment

2.3.1 Initial Treatment Patterns in Japan

Overall, the proportion of patients treated by hormonal therapy as the main treatment has been decreasing over time (Fig. 2.1). In Japan, the proportion of prostate cancer patients treated by primary hormonal therapy was 57% of 4529 patients in JUA2000, 4934 (48.0%) of 10,280 patients in JUA2004, and 3337 (40.2%) of 8291 patients in JCaP2010 [3, 4, 7]. In a study that was not nationwide, the practice pattern in the mid-1980s in Japan revealed that as many as 62.6% of all patients and approx. 50% of stage B patients were treated by hormonal therapy [2]. It is thus clear that the proportion of hormonal therapy has markedly decreased in Japan, but hormonal therapy remains the most frequently chosen treatment for prostate cancer in Japan.

There are some explanations for the decrease in hormonal therapy use. Since primary hormonal therapy is used for various conditions, the possible explanations should be considered separately. These include the following:

Case 1: Definitive treatment for advanced disease

Case 2: Alternative treatment for aged or morbid patients with localized disease for which radical treatment can be applicable

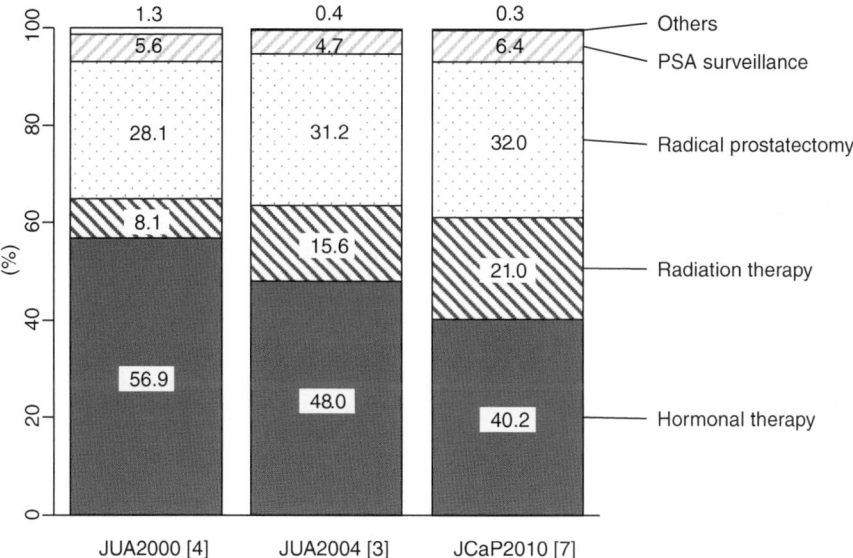

Fig. 2.1 Time trend in initial therapy in Japan. Numbers in the graph represent percentages within each group. As the initial therapy for newly diagnosed prostate cancer in Japan, hormonal therapy made up a decreased proportion but it made up still a high proportion

Case 3: Preferred treatment for healthy non-aged patients with localized disease for which radical treatment can be applicable

Case 1 is an absolute indication for hormonal therapy, whereas Cases 2 and 3 are relative indications.

The proportion of metastatic disease is also decreasing over time. The proportion of M1 disease was 21.3%, 11.6%, and 10.5% in JUA2000, JUA2004, and JCaP2010, respectively [3, 4, 7]. As patients with M1 disease are usually treated by hormonal therapy (absolute indication), this lowered stage migration is one of the reasons for the decrease in hormonal therapy use. Over the past two decades, radical treatment for localized disease has progressed. For example, the use of anatomical prostatectomy spread all over the world, and less-invasive to minimally invasive prostatectomy became possible. Radiation therapy also became safe and effective. Therefore, more patients including aged and morbid patients can be successfully treated by these methods.

Regarding relative indications for hormonal therapy (Cases 2 and 3), 45.9% of approx. 2700 T1c-T3N0M0 patients in JUA2000, 39.8% of approx. 8400 T1-4N0M0 patients in JUA2004, and 31.6% of over 7000 T1-3N0M0 patients in JCaP2010 [3, 4, 7] were treated by hormonal therapy. The decrease in the use of hormonal therapy under relative indications is thus another reason contributing to the decrease in hormonal therapy use.

2.3.2 Treatment Pattern Difference Between Japan and the USA

As mentioned above, the continuing high percentage of hormonal therapy use in non-metastatic disease in Japan appears to be a unique feature in contrast to what is seen in the American practice pattern [8, 9]. The University of California, San Francisco (UCSF) Cancer of the Prostate Strategic Urologic Research Endeavor (CaPSURE) study demonstrated that among prostate cancer patients with T1-3a,Nx/N0, and Mx/M0 disease whose treatment was initiated between 1989 and 2002, 50% were treated by prostatectomy, 26% by radiation (13% externally and 13% internally), and only 14% by hormonal therapy [10].

However, there seems to have been a shift toward conservative management in the USA; data from the American Urological Association (AUA) Quality (AQUA) Registry in the USA revealed an increase in the use of hormonal therapy in that country. In the low-risk group, the proportion of hormonal therapy was 11.2% in 2014, 19.0% in 2015, and 22.8% in 2016; in the high-risk group, the proportion of hormonal therapy was 31.1% in 2014, 41.2% in 2015, and 43.3% in 2016 [11].

Several research groups have observed a racial difference in the effect of hormonal therapy and have reported that outcomes after hormonal therapy have been better in Japanese compared to Caucasian men [12–14]. With regard to adverse events, many studies conducted in Western countries that include clinical guidelines have emphasized the side effects of hormonal therapy such as cardiovascular and cerebrovascular events, diabetes mellitus, loss of bone mineral density, and more [15]. In Japan, such side effects associated with hormonal therapy are not often encountered; for example, a 2008 study demonstrated that hormonal therapy did not significantly increase the prevalence of osteoporosis in the Japanese population [16]. With regard to cardiovascular events, the incidence of cardiovascular death in patients treated by hormonal therapy was no greater than that expected in the general Japanese population [17]. In light of these findings, it seems that Japanese urologists consider hormonal therapy appropriate for Japanese patients.

2.3.3 Types of Hormonal Therapy in Japan

With regard to the type of hormonal therapy used in Japan, more patients were treated by combined androgen blockade (CAB) in the JCaP2001-3, JUA2004, and JCaP2010 studies, 58.7%, 71.4%, and 74.2%, respectively, and the type of hormonal therapy used was related to the extent of disease in all three studies [3, 6, 7]. In JCaP2001-3, the proportions of CAB used for stage II, III, and IV patients were roughly 55%, 60%, and 70%, respectively [6]. In JUA2004, 69.1% of 3490 patients with M0 disease and 84.1% of 941 patients with M1 disease received CAB [3]. In JCaP2010, 69.7% and 87.6% in M0 and M1 patients, respectively, and 67.4%, 80.7%, and 86.9% of stage II, III, and IV disease, respectively, received CAB [7]. Thus, CAB use was positively associated with disease extent, and this has contributed to the increase in CAB use despite the lowered stage migration. Guidelines issued by the JUA reflect CAB's superior effect on overall survival in locally advanced disease and metastatic disease [18, 19]. Japanese urologists may thus accept CAB as safe and reliable, which would contribute to the increased use of CAB at all stages of prostate cancer.

2.3.4 Types of Castration

In Japan, the LH-RH agonists goserelin and leuprolide became available in 1991 and 1994, respectively; the LH-RH antagonist degarelix became available in 2012. In the Akakura et al. report from Japan (1988), surgical castration had been used in approx. one-half of the patients that received hormonal therapy [2], whereas surgical castration had been used in 11.5% of over 17,000 patients who received medical or surgical castration in JCaP2001-3 [6], in 6.9% of approx. 4300 patients in JUA2004 [3], and 4.7% of approx. 3200 patients in JCaP2010 [7]. In JCaP2010, surgical castration was performed significantly more often in the patients with high-risk disease as evaluated by the J-CAPRA risk assessment tool [20]: 33 vs. 1372, 43 vs. 1023, and 66 vs. 584 in the low-, intermediate- and high-risk groups, respectively; Cochran-Armitage trend test, $p < 0.001$ [7], indicates that disease risk was a trigger for the selection of surgical castration.

2.3.5 Types of Antiandrogen

In Japan, the steroidal antiandrogen chlormadinone acetate and the nonsteroidal antiandrogens flutamide and bicalutamide became available in 1983, 1994, and 1999, respectively. In JUA2004, a steroidal antiandrogen was used in 433 patients, accounting for 15.6% of all antiandrogen use in the study's patient series [3]. Although it is difficult to know the exact current prescription pattern of antiandrogens from the published literature, it appears that a nonsteroidal antiandrogen is being used in almost all of the prostate cancer patients in Japan at this time.

Conclusion

Although hormonal therapy is not a curative treatment for advanced metastatic prostate cancer, it is reliable in terms of its very high response rate and its convenience for patients. Hormonal therapy as a treatment for prostate cancer is well accepted in Japan, and, except for changes in the procedure such as the increase in CAB use and the decreases in orchiectomy and steroidal antiandrogen use, hormonal therapy has long been playing the central position in treatment. The proportion of hormonal therapy has been decreasing in Japan, but numerous patients are still treated with this hormonal therapy for prostate cancer in part because this cancer is one of the most frequently diagnosed male cancers in recent years [21]. In this sense, further observational studies designed to follow the changes in prostate cancer treatment patterns are necessary.

Reference

1. Huggins C, Hodges CV. Studies on prostatic cancer. I. The effect of castration, of estrogen and of androgen injection on serum phosphatases in metastatic carcinoma of the prostate. Cancer Res. 1941;1:293–7.
2. Akakura K, Isaka S, Fuse H, Akimoto S, Imai K, Yamanaka H, et al. Trends in patterns of care for prostatic cancer in Japan: statistics of 9 institutions for 5 years. Hinyokika kiyo Acta urologica Japonica. 1988;34:123–9.
3. Fujimoto H, Nakanishi H, Miki T, Kubota Y, Takahashi S, Suzuki K, et al. Oncological outcomes of the prostate cancer patients registered in 2004: report from the Cancer Registration Committee of the JUA. Int J Urol. 2011;18:876–81.
4. Cancer Registration Committee of the Japanese Urological Association. Clinicopathological statistics on registered prostate cancer patients in Japan: 2000 report from the Japanese Urological Association. Int J Urol. 2005;12:46–61.
5. Akaza H, Usami M, Hinotsu S, Ogawa O, Kagawa S, Kitamura T, et al. Characteristics of patients with prostate cancer who have initially been treated by hormone therapy in Japan: J-CaP surveillance. Jpn J Clin Oncol. 2004;34:329–36.
6. Hinotsu S, Akaza H, Usami M, Ogawa O, Kagawa S, Kitamura T, et al. Current status of endocrine therapy for prostate cancer in Japan—analysis of primary androgen deprivation therapy on the basis of data collected by J-CaP. Jpn J Clin Oncol. 2007;37:775–81.
7. Onozawa M, Hinotsu S, Tsukamoto T, Oya M, Ogawa O, Kitamura T, et al. Recent trends in the initial therapy for newly diagnosed prostate cancer in Japan. Jpn J Clin Oncol. 2014;44:969–81.
8. Cooperberg MR, Broering JM, Carroll PR. Time trends and local variation in primary treatment of localized prostate cancer. J Clin Oncol. 2010;28:1117–23.

9. Cary KC, Punnen S, Odisho AY, Litwin MS, Saigal CS, Cooperberg MR. Nationally representative trends and geographic variation in treatment of localized prostate cancer: the Urologic Diseases in America project. Prostate Cancer Prostatic Dis. 2015;18:149–54.
10. Kawakami J, Cowan JE, Elkin EP, Latini DM, DuChane J, Carroll PR. Androgen-deprivation therapy as primary treatment for localized prostate cancer. Cancer. 2006;106:1708–14.
11. Cooperberg MR, Fang R, Wolf Jr JS, Hubbard H, Pendharkar S, Gupte S et al. The Current Management of Prostate Cancer in the United States: Data from the AQUA Registry. AUA Annual Meeting. 2017, Abstract no. PNFBA-07.
12. Fukagai T, Namiki TS, Carlile RG, Yoshida H, Namiki M. Comparison of the clinical outcome after hormonal therapy for prostate cancer between Japanese and Caucasian men. BJU Int. 2006;97:1190–3.
13. Chao GF, Krishna N, Aizer AA, Dalela D, Hanske J, Li H, et al. Asian Americans and prostate cancer: a nationwide population-based analysis. Urol Oncol. 2016;34:233.e7–15.
14. Cooperberg MR, Hinotsu S, Namiki M, Carroll PR, Akaza H. Trans-Pacific variation in outcomes for men treated with primary androgen-deprivation therapy (ADT) for prostate cancer. BJU Int. 2016;117:102–9.
15. Cornford P, Bellmunt J, Bolla M, Briers E, De Santis M, Gross T, et al. EAU-ESTRO-SIOG guidelines on prostate cancer. Part II: treatment of relapsing, metastatic, and castration-resistant prostate cancer. Eur Urol. 2017;71:630–42.
16. Wang W, Yuasa T, Tsuchiya N, Maita S, Kumazawa T, Inoue T, et al. Bone mineral density in Japanese prostate cancer patients under androgen-deprivation therapy. Endocr Relat Cancer. 2008;15:943–52.
17. Akaza H. Future prospects for luteinizing hormone-releasing hormone analogues in prostate cancer treatment. Pharmacology. 2010;85:110–20.
18. The Japanese Urological Association: Clinical practice guideline for prostate cancer 2012. 1st ed. Tokyo: Kanehara Shuppan; 2012. P. 178–179.
19. The Japanese Urological Association: Clinical practice guideline for prostate cancer 2016. 1st ed. Osaka: Medical Review; 2016. P. 202–204.
20. Cooperberg MR, Hinotsu S, Namiki M, Ito K, Broering J, Carroll PR, Akaza H. Risk assessment among prostate cancer patients receiving primary androgen deprivation therapy. J Clin Oncol. 2009;27:4306–13.
21. Hori M, Matsuda T, Shibata A, Katanoda K, Sobue T, Nishimoto H. Cancer incidence and incidence rates in Japan in 2009: a study of 32 population-based cancer registries for the monitoring of cancer incidence in Japan (MCIJ) project. Jpn J Clin Oncol. 2015;45:884–91.

Risk Assessment Among Patients Receiving Primary ADT for Prostate Cancer

Shiro Hinotsu

Abstract

Many risk assessment tools have been developed for prostate cancer patients. The risk classifications, for example, the D'Amico classification and NCCN classification, are widely used. In addition, a nomogram to predict pathological stage and prognosis has also been developed. In this chapter, J-CAPRA score for all stage of patients treated by androgen depletion therapy is explained in detail.

Keywords

Risk assessment · Nomogram · Risk score · Prognosis · Survival

Urologists and medical oncologists perform risk assessments of each patient and use the risk assessment tools in the situation of medical decision-making for selecting treatment options for urogenital cancers.

Many risk assessment tools have been developed for prostate cancer patients and are widely used (Table 3.1). The risk classification is based on the clinical practice guidelines used in each country. For example, the D'Amico classification [1] and NCCN classification [2] are presented in the Clinical Practice Guideline for Prostate Cancer prepared by the Japanese Urological Association [3]. In addition, a nomogram to predict endpoints, such as the probability of a positive margin, has also been developed. Among the nomograms, Partin's nomogram [4] is widely known. Since this nomogram was developed for patients in the USA, a study to verify Partin's nomogram for Japanese patients [5] has been performed and is well known. Also, Kattan nomogram is also a well-known nomogram [6], validated by the Japanese patient data [7] and Chinese data [8]. Some nomograms present the probability of

S. Hinotsu, M.D.
Center for Innovative Clinical Medicine, Okayama University Hospital, Okayama, Japan
e-mail: hinotsus@okayama-u.ac.jp

© Springer Nature Singapore Pte Ltd. 2018
Y. Arai, O. Ogawa (eds.), *Hormone Therapy and Castration Resistance of Prostate Cancer*, https://doi.org/10.1007/978-981-10-7013-6_3

Table 3.1 Risk assessment tools

Name of tool	Population	Factors	Reference no.
D'Amico classification	No metastasis	PSA, Gleason score, T stage	[1]
NCCN classification	No metastasis	PSA, Gleason score, T stage, (no. of positive core, % of positive core, PSA density for very low risk evaluation)	[2]
Partin's nomogram	Prostatectomy	Clinical stage, PSA, biopsy Gleason score	[4]
Japanese nomogram	Prostatectomy	Clinical stage, PSA, biopsy Gleason score	[5]
Kattan nomogram	Localized	Preoperative PSA, no. of positive cores, no. of negative cores, clinical stage, biopsy Gleason score	[6]
TNM classification (7th ed) Prognostic grouping	All stages	T, N, M, Gleason, PSA	[9]
CAPRA	Prostatectomy	Age at diagnosis, PSA, biopsy Gleason score, T stage, % of positive core	[12]
J-CAPRA	All stages Treated by ADT	PSA, Gleason score, T stage, N stage, M stage	[11]

observing the endpoint of each factor as a percentage, and others calculate the score of each factor and determine the probability from the total score.

Nomogram data are periodically updated in consideration of the changes in both the patient factors and improvements in diagnostic technology. Therefore, accurate assessment cannot be performed unless attention is paid to both the patients' cohort and the results of the risk assessment based on the risk assessment tool. For example, the D'Amico classification was developed targeting prostate cancer patients without metastasis, so that it cannot be employed for patients with metastasis. Risk classifications developed using the data of patients in Western countries cannot accurately predict the outcome of all Japanese patients. Therefore, when using a risk assessment tool developed in the other country, it requires validation study involving patients from their own country and with various disease stages. In this chapter, the prognostic grouping in the TNM classification and J-CAPRA score are explained taking into account that androgen depletion therapy (ADT) is administered for all stages.

3.1 TNM Classification

In the TNM classification for prostate cancer, the prognostic grouping using the PSA level, the Gleason score, and disease stage was introduced in the 7th edition [9]. The details of this prognostic grouping are shown in Table 3.2. Since this classification was developed using data collected in Western countries, it is not

Table 3.2 Prognostic grouping of TNM classification

Prognostic group	Factors and criteria
Group I	T1a–c N0 M0 PSA < 10 Gleason <= 6
	T2a N0 M0 PSA < 10 Gleason <= 6
Group IIA	T1a–c N0 M0 PSA < 20 Gleason = 7
	T1a–c N0 M0 PSA >= 10 < 20 Gleason <= 6
	T2a,b N0 M0 PSA < 20 Gleason <= 7
Group IIB	T2c N0 M0 any PSA any Gleason
	T1–2 N0 M0 PSA >= 20 any Gleason
	T1–2 N0 M0 any PSA Gleason >= 8
Group III	T3a,b N0 M0 any PSA any Gleason
Group IV	T4 N0 M0 any PSA any Gleason
	Any T N1 M0 any PSA any Gleason
	Any T any N M1 any PSA any Gleason

necessarily accurate in predicting the outcomes of all patients worldwide. Moreover, although the categories are presented, the outcome of each category (e.g., 5-year survival rate) is not presented, so that the differences of prognosis among the risk classifications are unclear. Considering these points, the validation study was needed to identify the outcomes predicted using the TNM classification of prognostic grouping. Kimura et al. performed a validation study [10] using the database of the J-CaP study, a large-scale and over 10 years cohort study conducted in Japan. They predicted the outcomes of 15,259 patients treated with ADT by applying their data to the prognostic grouping of the TNM classification. The validation study clarified that the accuracy of prediction for Japanese prostate cancer patients was improved by partially reclassifying the prognostic grouping and taking the one more factor of age at diagnosis of the patient into consideration. As noted in this study, a risk classification developed for a specific outcome may require validation using another patient population.

3.2 J-CAPRA Score

The J-CAPRA score was developed based on a joint study using both the database of the Japanese J-CaP Study Group and the US database of prostate cancer patients, CaPSURE, and was published in the Journal of Clinical Oncology in 2009 [11]. A risk classification, the CAPRA score, had already been developed in CaPSURE [12]. The variables used in the CAPRA score were the age at diagnosis, PSA at diagnosis, Gleason score of the biopsy, T stage, and percent of positive biopsy cores containing cancer. There were two problems with applying the CAPRA score directly to the J-CaP Study Group database of Japan. One was a marked difference in the age distribution between the Japanese and US patients, and the age score was added to the majority of Japanese patients. In that situation, including the age factor biased toward high risk for Japanese patients. The other was that the J-CaP Study Group database did not collect the data on the percent of positive biopsy cores containing cancer, and

Table 3.3 J-CAPRA score

Factor	Point
Gleason 2–6	0
Gleason 7	1
Gleason 8–10	2
PSA 0–20	0
PSA >20–100	1
PSA >100–500	2
PSA >500	3
T1a–T2a	0
T2b, T3a	1
T3b	2
T4	3
N0	0
N1	1
M0	0
M1	3

when including the factor, this variable is missing in all Japanese cases. Therefore, it was decided to develop a new risk assessment tool without applying the CAPRA score to the Japanese data. Factors influencing the outcome were extracted from the data present in both J-CaP and CaPSURE database and included the Gleason score, PSA, T stage, N stage, and M stage. Each variable was scored from 0 to 3 corresponding to the degree of the influence on the outcome considering the hazard ratio in the multivariate analysis (Table 3.3). Using this risk assessment tool, the J-CAPRA score is calculated from 0 to 12 in each patient. When progression-free survival was estimated using the scores from the Japanese and US patient databases, the outcomes were determined to be appropriately classified. In addition, the scores with close survival rates could be categorized. Scores of 0–2, 3–7, and 8 or higher were evaluated as low, intermediate, and high risk, respectively.

A validation study [13] using the J-CAPRA score was performed by Kitamura et al. and included 319 ADT-treated prostate cancer patients not registered in the J-CaP Study Group. These patients were evaluated for risk using the J-CAPRA score, and all of the patients could be classified into low-, intermediate-, and high-risk groups with regard to progression-free survival, cause-specific survival, and overall survival. This finding clarified the usefulness of the J-CAPRA score for Japanese patients generally.

Using the J-CAPRA score, it is now possible to compare patients in the same risk category between Japan and the USA. Cooperberg et al. [14] compared prostate cancer-specific survival, which was the outcome that eliminated the effect of the death from other causes, between the CaPSURE and J-CaP data, and showed that the outcomes of Japanese patients were favorable in all low-, intermediate-, and high-risk groups. Taking the age and the methods of ADT into consideration in a multivariate analysis, the hazard ratio was 0.52 (95% CI: 0.40–0.68). This study clarified the difference of prognosis treated with ADT between Japanese patients and patients in the USA applying the same risk assessment tool. Thus, the J-CAPRA score was a one of useful risk assessment tools for international comparisons.

3.3 Risk Assessment in the Next Generation

A sufficient observation period is necessary to prepare a risk assessment tool, because preparation of a database requires a prolonged time. Especially, prostate cancer patients have relatively favorable prognosis; survival data collection may require nearly 10 years. For example, the JCAPRA score was prepared using data of prostate cancer patients diagnosed between 2001 and 2003, and thus all patients' risk using J-CAPRA score of overall survival were the risk of patients treated without novel drugs introduced into clinical practice around 5 years. A research organization or system is necessary to construct a database with periodic data updates and should develop a method of data collection that is not a burden for urologists. There are some challenges to make a system of data transfer from hospital information system to the electric data capture system. However, the data transfer system is not completed now. In addition, once a risk assessment tool is prepared, the accuracy of the predicted risk has to be verified by a validation study. High-quality risk assessments will be made possible by the efforts of many researchers and clinicians.

References

1. D'Amico AV, Whittington R, Malkowicz BS, et al. Biochemical outcome after radical prostatectomy, external beam radiation therapy, or internal radiation therapy for clinically localized prostate cancer. JAMA. 1998;280:969–74.
2. https://www.nccn.org/professionals/physician_gls/pdf/prostate.pdf
3. Japanese Urological Association Edit. Clinical practice guideline for prostate cancer. Tokyo: Medical Review Co., Ltd.; 2016.
4. Partin AW, Kattan MW, Subong EN, et al. Combination of prostate-specific antigen, clinical stage, and Gleason score to predict pathological stage of localized prostate cancer. A multi-institutional update. JAMA. 1997;227:1445–51.
5. Naito S, Kuroiwa K, Kinukawa N, et al. Validation of Partin tables and development of a preoperative nomogram for Japanese patients with clinically localized prostate cancer using 2005 International Society of Urological Pathology consensus on Gleason grading: data from the Clinicopathological Research Group for Localized Prostate Cancer. J Urol. 2008;180:904–9.
6. Stephenson AJ, Scardino PT, Eastham JA, Bianco FJ Jr, Dotan ZA, Fearn PA, Kattan MW. Preoperative nomogram predicting the 10-year probability of prostate cancer recurrence after radical prostatectomy. J Natl Cancer Inst. 2006;98(10):715–7.
7. Tanaka A, Ohori M, Paul L, Yu C, Kattan MW, Ohno Y, Tachibana M. External validation of preoperative nomograms predicting biochemical recurrence after radical prostatectomy. Jpn J Clin Oncol. 2013;43(12):1255–60.
8. Yeung VH, Chiu Y, SS Y, WH A, Chan SW. Are preoperative Kattan and Stephenson nomograms predicting biochemical recurrence after radical prostatectomy applicable in the Chinese population? ScientificWorldJournal. 2013;2013:506062. https://doi.org/10.1155/2013/506062.
9. Sobin LH, Gospodarowicz MK, Wittekind C, editors. TNM classification of malignant tumours. 7th ed. New York, NY: Wiley-Blackwell; 2011. ISBN: 978-1-4443-5896-4.
10. Kimura T, Onozawa M, Miyazaki J, Kawai K, Nishiyama H, Hinotsu S, Akaza H. Validation of the prognostic grouping of the seventh edition of the tumor-nodes-metastasis classification using a large-scale prospective cohort study database of prostate cancer treated with primary androgen deprivation therapy. Int J Urol. 2013;20(9):880–8.

11. Cooperberg MR, Hinotsu S, Namiki M, Ito K, Broering J, Carroll PR, Akaza H. Risk assessment among prostate cancer patients receiving primary androgen deprivation therapy. J Clin Oncol. 2009;27(26):4306–13.
12. Cooperberg MR, Pasta DJ, Elkin EP, et al. The University of California, San Francisco cancer of the prostate risk assessment score: a straightforward and reliable preoperative predictor of disease recurrence after radical prostatectomy. J Urol. 2005;173:1938–42.
13. Kitagawa Y, Hinotsu S, Shigehara K, Nakashima K, Kawaguchi S, Yaegashi H, Mizokami A, Akaza H, Namiki M. Japan cancer of the prostate risk assessment for combined androgen blockade including bicalutamide: clinical application and validation. Int J Urol. 2013;20(7):708–14.
14. Cooperberg MR, Hinotsu S, Namiki M, Carroll PR, Akaza H. Trans-Pacific variation in outcomes for men treated with primary androgen-deprivation therapy (ADT) for prostate cancer. BJU Int. 2016;117(1):102–9.

Patient-Derived Xenografts for Research on Hormonal Therapy of Prostate Cancer

Takahiro Inoue

Abstract

Patient-derived xenograft (PDX) models are characterized by direct transplantation of human tissues into immunocompromised mice. PDXs can highly preserve the original histology, as well as the molecular and genetic characteristics of the original tumors. Recently, there are studies describing a large number of PDX models, representing a wide range of human cancers. PDX models have great potential to be used for both basic and clinical research and have resulted in an increase in the use for the analysis of tumor biology and for drug development. However, establishment of prostate cancer PDX models is still limited, and existing PDX repositories, such as Jackson Laboratories, contain very few prostate cancer PDX models, which cannot represent the molecular diversity of human prostate cancer. Herein, we will introduce representative prostate cancer PDX models, including our established models, and discuss potential usefulness together with future perspectives.

Keywords

Patient-derived xenograft · Prostate cancer · Hormonal therapy · Research · Basic Clinical

4.1 Introduction

Cancer cell lines or cell-line-derived xenograft (CDX) models have provided valuable information that has improved our understanding of cancer development and the mechanisms of drug actions. But majority of them have certain homogenous

---

T. Inoue, M.D., Ph.D.
Department of Urology, Kyoto University Graduate School of Medicine, Kyoto, Japan
e-mail: takahi@kuhp.kyoto-u.ac.jp

morphology after long-term in vitro culturing that is quite different from human malignancies. Therefore, CDXs are not particularly predictive of human response to pharmaceutical agents. Additionally, limited availability of tissue for molecular studies and human prostate cancer cell lines that harbor both intact androgen receptor (AR) expression and androgen dependency, which are hallmarks of PCa, have interfered PCa research. Patient-derived xenograft (PDX) models, surgically derived clinical tumor samples that are implanted in immunocompromised mice, more accurately reflect underlying tumor biology and heterogeneity of individual human cancers than CDXs [1, 2]. PDX models of PCa are also expected to recapitulate the complexity of human cancer with preserved cellular lineage hierarchy and tumor-stroma interaction [3–5]. Although some engraftment pressure is observed, PDX models seemingly preserve most of the genetic alterations as well as the histological characteristics of the original patient tumors in prostate cancer (PCa) at least for three to six passages [3]. They can be propagated for long periods of time *in vivo*, enabling the study of tumor progression. Indeed, treatment of PDXs reproduces clinical outcomes observed in the individual patient donors [6, 7]. Thus, PDXs have emerged as an important platform to elucidate new treatments and biomarkers in PCa research [8].

4.2 Establishment of Prostate Cancer Patient-Derived Xenograft Models

Schroeder et al. have first reported that PCa tissue can be transplanted on nude mice [9]. PDX models of PCa from fresh primary or metastatic human prostate tissue have been extensively described in the literature (Table 4.1) [3, 8, 10–28]. KUCaP-1 was the first PDX model established in our department. It had W742C mutant AR, showed androgen dependency, and could grow with bicalutamide stimulation. This model is appropriate for studying antiandrogen withdrawal syndrome. Additionally, flutamide treatment regresses its growth, showing that it could replicate clinical situation of alternative androgen therapy [26, 30]. KUCaP-2 is an androgen-sensitive model of PCa and expressed wild-type AR [27]. KUCaP-2 tumors can regress soon after castration of the host mice, and they restore their ability to proliferate within a few months. This mode is mimicking clinical castration-resistant progression, and it is suitable for revealing mechanisms of progression to castration-resistant PCa (CRPC). Our recent reported PDX model, KUCaP-3, is an androgen-dependent tumor with H875Y AR mutation. KUCaP-3 is unique as these cells grew into cystic feature, which contained extremely high level of PSA. Therefore, it is a potential model for identifying secreted molecules for diagnostic and therapeutic markers in serum or other body fluids [28].

Obtaining fresh tumor tissue is difficult from primary localized prostate cancer, since tumor lesions are not easily macroscopically detected at the time of radical prostatectomy. Metastatic CRPC tissues are also difficult to obtain, and when acquired, they are often limited quantity. Most of the PDX models of PCa reported were derived and established from locally recurrent or metastatic

Table 4.1 Characteristics of representative PDX models of prostate cancer (Modified from Inoue T et al. Nature Reviews Urology 2017)

Name	Origin	Host mouse	Sites	Androgen response	AR expression	PSA expression	AR sequence	References
PC-EW	LN	Nude	Subcutaneous	AD	Yes	Yes	Wt	Hoehn et al. Prostate (1984) [10]
PC82	Primary	Nude	Subcutaneous	AD	Yes	Yes	Wt	Hoehn et al. Prostate (1980) [29]
PC295	LN	Nude	Subcutaneous	AD	Yes	Yes	Wt	van Weerden et al. Am J Pathol (1996) [11]
PC310	Primary	Nude	Subcutaneous	AD	Yes	Yes	Wt	
PC324	Primary	Nude	Subcutaneous	AI	No	No	n/a	
PC374	Skin	Nude	Subcutaneous	AI	No	No	n/a	
PC346P	Primary	Nude	Subcutaneous	AS	Yes	Yes	Wt	
PC346B	Primary	Nude	Subcutaneous	AS	Yes	Yes	Wt	van Weerden et al. Prostate (2000) [12]
CWR21	Primary	SCID	Subcutaneous	n/a	n/a	n/a	n/a	Pretlow et al. J Natl Cancer Inst (1993) [13]
CWR22	Primary	SCID	Subcutaneous	AS	Yes	Yes	H875Y	
CWR31	Primary	SCID	Subcutaneous	n/a	n/a	n/a	n/a	
CWR91	Primary	SCID	Subcutaneous	n/a	n/a	n/a	n/a	
LuCaP23.1	LN	Nude	Subcutaneous	AS	Yes	Yes	n/a	Ellis et al. Clin Cancer Res (1996) [14]
LuCaP23.8	LN	Nude	Subcutaneous	AS	Yes	Yes	n/a	
LuCaP23.12	Liver	Nude	Subcutaneous	AS	Yes	Yes	n/a	
LuCaP35	LN	Nude	Subcutaneous	AS	Yes	Yes	Wt	Corey et al. Prostate (2003) [15]
LuCaP41	Primary	Nude	Subcutaneous	AS	Yes	Yes	n/a	Laitinen et al. Genes Chromosomes Cancer (2002) [16]
LuCaP58	LN	Nude	Subcutaneous	AS	Yes	Yes	Wt	
LuCaP69	Bowel	Nude	Subcutaneous	n/a	Yes	Yes	n/a	
LuCaP70	Liver	Nude	Subcutaneous	n/a	Yes	Yes	n/a	
LuCaP73	Pelvis	Nude	Subcutaneous	AS	Yes	Yes	n/a	
LuCaP49	LN(NE)	Nude	Subcutaneous	AI	No	No	n/a	True et al. Am J Pathol (2002) [17]
LAPC-3	Primary	SCID	Subcutaneous	AI	Yes	Yes	Wt	Klein et al. Nat Med (1997) [18]
LAPC-4	LN	SCID	Subcutaneous	AS	Yes	Yes	Wt	

(continued)

Table 4.1 (continued)

Name	Origin	Host mouse	Sites	Androgen response	AR expression	PSA expression	AR sequence	References
LAPC-9	Bone	SCID	Subcutaneous	AS	Yes	Yes	Wt	Craft et al. Cancer Res (1999) [19]
TEN12	Primary	Nude	Subcutaneous	AS	Yes	Yes	Wt	Harper, Prostate (2004) [20]
BM18	Bone	SCID	Subcutaneous	AD	Yes	Yes	n/a	McCulloch, Prostate (2005) [21]
JDCaP	Skin	SCID	Subcutaneous	AD	Yes	Yes	Wt	Kimura et al. Prostate (2009) [22]
LTL310	Primary	NOD-SCID-SRC	Renal capsule	AD	Yes	Yes	n/a	Lin et al. Cancer Res (2014) [3]
LTL311	Primary	NOD-SCID-SRC	Renal capsule	AD	Yes	Yes	n/a	
LTL331	Primary	NOD-SCID-SRC	Renal capsule	AS	Yes	Yes	n/a	
LTL412	LN	NOD-SCID-SRC	Renal capsule	AD	Yes	Yes	n/a	
LTL418	Primary	NOD-SCID-SRC	Renal capsule	AD	Yes	Yes	n/a	
LTL313	Primary	NOD-SCID-SRC	Renal capsule	AS	Yes	Yes	n/a	
LTL352	Urethra(NE)	NOD-SCID-SRC	Renal capsule	AI	No	No	n/a	
LTL370	Penile(NE)	NOD-SCID-SRC	Renal capsule	AI	No	No	n/a	
MDA-PCa-118a	Bone	SCID	Subcutaneous	AI	No	No	n/a	Li et al. J Clin Invest (2008) [23]
MDA-PCa-118b	Bone	SCID	Subcutaneous	AI	No	No	n/a	
MDA-PCa-79	Rectum	SCID	Subcutaneous	n/a	Yes	Yes	n/a	Tzelepi et al. Clin Cancer Res (2012) [25]
MDA-PCa-117-9	Primary	SCID	Subcutaneous	n/a	Yes	Yes	n/a	
MDA-PCa-130	Primary	SCID	Subcutaneous	n/a	Yes	Yes	n/a	

MDA-PCa-144-13	Bladder(NE)	SCID	Subcutaneous	AI	No	No	n/a	Aparicio et al. Prostate (2011) [24]
MDA-PCa-144-4	Primary(NE)	SCID	Subcutaneous	AI	Yes	No	n/a	Tzelepi et al. Clin Cancer Res (2012) [25]
MDA-PCa-146-10	Bladder(NE)	SCID	Subcutaneous	n/a	No	No	n/a	
MDA-PCa-146-17	Bladder(NE)	SCID	Subcutaneous	n/a	No	No	n/a	
MDA-PCa-146-20	Bladder(NE)	SCID	Subcutaneous	n/a	No	No	n/a	
MDA-PCa-155-2	Bladder(NE)	SCID	Subcutaneous	n/a	No	No	n/a	
MDA-PCa-155-9	Bladder(NE)	SCID	Subcutaneous	n/a	No	No	n/a	
MDA-PCa-155-12	Bladder(NE)	SCID	Subcutaneous	n/a	No	No	n/a	
MDA-PCa-155-16	Primary(NE)	SCID	Subcutaneous	n/a	No	No	n/a	
MDA-PCa-170-1	Primary	SCID	Subcutaneous	n/a	Yes	Yes	n/a	
MDA-PCa-170-4	Primary	SCID	Subcutaneous	n/a	Yes	Yes	n/a	
MDA-PCa-180-11	Bladder	SCID	Subcutaneous	n/a	Yes	No	n/a	
MDA-PCa-180-14	Bladder	SCID	Subcutaneous	n/a	Yes	No	n/a	
MDA-PCa-180-18	Bladder	SCID	Subcutaneous	n/a	Yes	Yes	n/a	
MDA-PCa-180-21	Bladder	SCID	Subcutaneous	n/a	Yes	Yes	n/a	
MDA-PCa-180-30	Seminal vesicle	SCID	Subcutaneous	n/a	Yes	Yes	n/a	

(continued)

Table 4.1 (continued)

Name	Origin	Host mouse	Sites	Androgen response	AR expression	PSA expression	AR sequence	References
KUCaP1	Liver	SCID	Subcutaneous	AD	Yes	Yes	W742C	Yoshida et al. Cancer Res (2005) [11]
KUCaP2	Primary	Nude	Subcutaneous	AS	Yes	Yes	Wt	Terada et al. Cancer Res (2010) [10]
KUCaP3	Primary	SCID	Subcutaneous	AS	Yes	Yes	H875Y	Yoshikawa et al. Prostate (2016) [13]

NE neuroendocrine cell, *SRC* subrenal capsule transplantation, *AD* androgen dependent, *AS* androgen sensitive, *AI* androgen independent

castration-resistant PCa tumors, because PDX engraftment rates are positively correlated with the clinical aggressiveness and metastatic potential of the original tumors. Localized tumors are intermediate- to low-grade malignancies in most cases, so the cells derived from the localized cancers seldom survive and grow both *in vitro* and *in vivo*. Therefore, it is difficult to study the transition mechanisms of truly hormone-naïve PCa to aggressive disease such as CRPC. However, Toivanen et al. and Lawrence et al. reported sophisticated methods for effectively xenografting localized prostate cancer tissue [31, 32]. They presented recombination of prostate cancer tissues together with mouse seminal vesicle mesenchymes and xenotransplantation under renal capsule of the host mice. Not only the tissues maintained their original tumor characters including Gleason score and other pathological features, but also they expressed AR and PSA. Moreover, the tumors can be grown for several months enabling us to evaluate the effectiveness of new therapeutic drugs.

Several types of immunocompromised mice are available for xenografting human cancer tissues. The athymic (*nude*) mouse is most commonly used for PDX establishment, since it is less expensive to use than others and is hairless so it does not require shaving to evaluate the growth of a tumor in subcutaneous site. However, the presence of intact B cells and an intact innate immune system, including natural killer cells, inhibit efficient engraftment of human prostate cancer tissues. Severe combined immunodeficiency (*Scid*) mice are impaired in the development of mature T cells and B cells so they are more suitable for engraftment of prostate cancer tissues than *nude* mice. But mature T cells and B cells develop in some *scid* mice when they get old and they have an intact innate immunity, including moderate NK cell activity. The nonobese diabetic (NOD) *scid* mice defects in both humoral and innate immunity, and are more receptive of prostate cancer tissues, but the shortcomings of this strain include the development of thymic lymphomas by 8–9 months old and a short life span [8].

The most commonly used site for engraftment is the subcutaneous space of the dorsal side of immunocompromised mice, since it is technically easier to handle, to monitor, and to evaluate compared to other methods below. But the subcutaneous implantation made the development of PCa PDX difficult with low success rates, partly owing to poor vascularization at the graft site. In contrast to the subcutaneous graft site, the subrenal capsule site is highly vascularized and associated with impressive tumor take rates [3]. Additionally, xenografts transplanted into the subrenal capsule preserve the characteristics of the parent tumor in terms of histopathology, genetic changes, and biology [3]. Orthotopic engraftment models more accurately reconstitute an organ microenvironment preserving original tumor phenotypes [33]. However, this method is still technically challenging. Engraftment success of prostate tumors can also be affected by testosterone supplementation, since the hormonal microenvironment of mice is quite different from that of humans, which is particularly important when xenografting prostate tumors. In immunodeficient adult male mice, total testosterone levels vary >100-fold in the same mouse measured longitudinally, which is quite different from total testosterone variation in the same eugonadal aging men, showing less than tenfold difference when measured longitudinally. Only one-quarter of the intact mice had total testosterone values that reached the 95% reference range for eugonadal 40–80-year-old men, and one-quarter of the mice had total testosterone level in men with prostate cancer receiving androgen deprivation therapy [34, 35]. Moreover, values of biologically active free testosterone in 70% of the mice were below the International Society for the Study of the Aging Male value of 74 pg/mL, which is used as criterion for the diagnosis of hypogonadism in human males [34, 36].

4.3 Basic and Clinical Application of PDX Models for Understanding Resistance to Hormonal Therapy

Toivanen R et al. established a protocol in which co-grafting of primary tumors with mouse neonatal stroma under the kidney capsule of host NOD *scid* or NOD. Cg-*Prkdc^{scid} Il2rg^{tm1Wjl}* (NSG) mice resulted in increased engraftment rate and growth *in vivo* [8, 31]. They engrafted 12 localized prostate cancer specimens from men who were naïve for hormonal therapy using their protocol and evaluate responses to androgen withdrawal by castrating host mice. They found that, after castration of host mice, residual populations of quiescent, stemlike tumor cells remained and these cells can regenerate by readministration of testosterone. These results show that residual populations of stemlike tumor cells preexist in localized PCa tissues before the onset of CRPC and characterization of these populations might bring us novel seeds for successful eradication of potential precursors to lethal CRPC disease.

Advances in next-generation sequence technology, including increased sequencing speed with high data accuracy and reduced cost per sample, enable the characterization of the cancer genome in a time frame that is compatible with treatment decisions. Within many mutations detected in cancer samples, it is difficult and complicated to interpret this genomic information including evaluation of the actionability of each detected mutation, determination of the meaning of the action, and prioritization among multiple detected alterations. One way to resolve these difficulties is to combine genomic information gained from a patient's tumor and PDX models to identify suitable treatments and to assess mechanisms of resistance to drugs and to develop biomarkers predictive of treatment outcome [8]. Indeed, drug studies involving panels of PDX models have identified molecular characteristics of PDXs which are concordance between the response of the model and the response clinically against the same drug [7, 37]. However, the paucity of PCa PDX models hampered clinical application of the PCa PDX models, as avatar mouse models. From 2002 our laboratory has started xenografting prostate cancer tissues and collected 28 samples from 28 patients and implanted them subcutaneously into immunocompromised male intact mice. Of these, seven were successfully propagated beyond three passages for an overall take rate of 28% (unpublished data). Nguyen H et al. recently summarized LuCaP series and reported that among 261 samples derived from 156 PCa patients, 26 were successfully propagated beyond three passages for an overall take rate of less than 10%, almost comparable to our series [38]. They identified that LuCaP series represent the major genomic and phenotypic features of PCa in humans, including amplification of androgen receptor, *PTEN* deletion, *TP53* deletion and mutation, *RB1* loss, TMPRSS2-ERG rearrangements, *SPOP* mutation, hypermutations due to MSH2/MSH6 aberrations, and *BRCA2* loss. They evaluated responses of LuCaP series to androgen deprivation and docetaxel treatment and showed their heterogeneities of response to the treatments. Notably, AR amplification/activity and AR splice variants were detected as important mechanisms of resistance to ADT using LuCaP PDXs, supporting the usefulness of enzalutamide and the needs to develop new AR *N*-terminal-targeting drugs.

Neuroendocrine prostate cancer (NEPC) is an aggressive variant of prostate cancer, also termed anaplastic or small-cell carcinoma of the prostate due to the morphological resemblance to small-cell lung carcinoma, that is often observed in biopsies of metastatic sites in patients with progressive CRPC after AR signaling targeting drugs and has been reported that incidence of this variant is rising [39, 40]. Thus, an improved understanding of the mechanisms of progression to prostatic NEPC is required. A unique PDX model of NEPC transdifferentiation, LTL331/LTL331R model, has been reported [3, 41]. They found that the placental gene *PEG 10* is derepressed during the adaptive response to AR interference and subsequently upregulated in clinical NEPC. They also revealed that the AR and the E2F/RB pathway dynamically regulate distinct posttranslational isoforms of PEG 10 at distinct stage of NEPC development and demonstrate that distinct PEG 10 isoforms promote cell proliferation and invasion of NEPC cells. The details of molecular pathogenesis of NEPC are described elsewhere in this textbook.

4.4 Future Perspectives

The failure rate of engraftment of PCa tissues derived from human is still very high. For application in clinical practice as avatar models, tumor take rates need to be improved to 60–70%, which is one of the main issues that needs addressing [8]. Subrenal capsule may be an appropriate engraftment site since it is highly vascularized [3]. However, the generation, propagation of PCa PDX tumors, and subsequent drug testing usually take 4–6 months or more, which is usually not a feasible time frame for immediate application in decision-making at clinical practice. Collaboration between research groups to investigate the best way to apply existing models and to continuously establish new ones is very important. It will enable the establishment and housing of an abundance of models with well-annotated biological and genetic data, which can provide a preclinical data that accurately predicts which drugs and drug combinations should be assessed clinically for precision medicine. The need for reliable and optimal preservation methods for prostate cancer PDXs is indispensable. Lin et al. discussed that their LTL series of PDXs were frozen at early generations with 10% DMSO and might be able to be recovered with high tumor take rates in immunocompromised mice [3]. However, the precise procedures have not been described, and we should evaluate and establish more reliable methods for prostate cancer PDX cryopreservation.

References

1. Hidalgo M, Amant F, Biankin AV, Budinska E, Byrne AT, Caldas C, et al. Patient-derived xenograft models: an emerging platform for translational cancer research. Cancer Discov. 2014;4(9):998–1013.
2. Tentler JJ, Tan AC, Weekes CD, Jimeno A, Leong S, Pitts TM, et al. Patient-derived tumour xenografts as models for oncology drug development. Nat Rev Clin Oncol. 2012;9(6):338–50.
3. Lin D, Wyatt AW, Xue H, Wang Y, Dong X, Haegert A, et al. High fidelity patient-derived xenografts for accelerating prostate cancer discovery and drug development. Cancer Res. 2014;74(4):1272–83.
4. Priolo C, Agostini M, Vena N, Ligon AH, Fiorentino M, Shin E, et al. Establishment and genomic characterization of mouse xenografts of human primary prostate tumors. Am J Pathol. 2010;176(4):1901–13.
5. Wang Y, Revelo MP, Sudilovsky D, Cao M, Chen WG, Goetz L, et al. Development and characterization of efficient xenograft models for benign and malignant human prostate tissue. Prostate. 2005;64(2):149–59.
6. Malaney P, Nicosia SV, Dave V. One mouse, one patient paradigm: new avatars of personalized cancer therapy. Cancer Lett. 2014;344(1):1–12.
7. Gao H, Korn JM, Ferretti S, Monahan JE, Wang Y, Singh M, et al. High-throughput screening using patient-derived tumor xenografts to predict clinical trial drug response. Nat Med. 2015;21(11):1318–25.
8. Inoue T, Terada N, Kobayashi T, Ogawa O. Patient-derived xenografts as in vivo models for research in urological malignancies. Nat Rev Urol. 2017;14(5):267–83.
9. Schroeder FH, Okada K, Jellinghaus W, Wullstein HK, Heinemeyer HM. Human prostatic adenoma and carcinoma. Transplantation of cultured cells and primary tissue fragments in "nude" mice. Invest Urol. 1976;13(6):395–403.
10. Hoehn W, Wagner M, Riemann JF, Hermanek P, Williams E, Walther R, et al. Prostatic adenocarcinoma PC EW, a new human tumor line transplantable in nude mice. Prostate. 1984;5(4):445–52.
11. van Weerden WM, de Ridder CM, Verdaasdonk CL, Romijn JC, van der Kwast TH, Schroder FH, et al. Development of seven new human prostate tumor xenograft models and their histopathological characterization. Am J Pathol. 1996;149(3):1055–62.
12. van Weerden WM, Romijn JC. Use of nude mouse xenograft models in prostate cancer research. Prostate. 2000;43(4):263–71.
13. Pretlow TG, Wolman SR, Micale MA, Pelley RJ, Kursh ED, Resnick MI, et al. Xenografts of primary human prostatic carcinoma. J Natl Cancer Inst. 1993;85(5):394–8.
14. Ellis WJ, Vessella RL, Buhler KR, Bladou F, True LD, Bigler SA, et al. Characterization of a novel androgen-sensitive, prostate-specific antigen-producing prostatic carcinoma xenograft: LuCaP 23. Clin Cancer Res. 1996;2(6):1039–48.
15. Corey E, Quinn JE, Buhler KR, Nelson PS, Macoska JA, True LD, et al. LuCaP 35: a new model of prostate cancer progression to androgen independence. Prostate. 2003;55(4):239–46.
16. Laitinen S, Karhu R, Sawyers CL, Vessella RL, Visakorpi T. Chromosomal aberrations in prostate cancer xenografts detected by comparative genomic hybridization. Genes Chromosomes Cancer. 2002;35(1):66–73.
17. True LD, Buhler K, Quinn J, Williams E, Nelson PS, Clegg N, et al. A neuroendocrine/small cell prostate carcinoma xenograft-LuCaP 49. Am J Pathol. 2002;161(2):705–15.
18. Klein KA, Reiter RE, Redula J, Moradi H, Zhu XL, Brothman AR, et al. Progression of metastatic human prostate cancer to androgen independence in immunodeficient SCID mice. Nat Med. 1997;3(4):402–8.
19. Craft N, Chhor C, Tran C, Belldegrun A, DeKernion J, Witte ON, et al. Evidence for clonal outgrowth of androgen-independent prostate cancer cells from androgen-dependent tumors through a two-step process. Cancer Res. 1999;59(19):5030–6.

20. Harper ME, Goddard L, Smith C, Nicholson RI. Characterization of a transplantable hormone-responsive human prostatic cancer xenograft TEN12 and its androgen-resistant sublines. Prostate. 2004;58(1):13–22.
21. McCulloch DR, Opeskin K, Thompson EW, Williams ED. BM18: A novel androgen-dependent human prostate cancer xenograft model derived from a bone metastasis. Prostate. 2005;65(1):35–43.
22. Kimura T, Kiyota H, Nakata D, Masaki T, Kusaka M, Egawa S. A novel androgen-dependent prostate cancer xenograft model derived from skin metastasis of a Japanese patient. Prostate. 2009;69(15):1660–7.
23. Li ZG, Mathew P, Yang J, Starbuck MW, Zurita AJ, Liu J, et al. Androgen receptor-negative human prostate cancer cells induce osteogenesis in mice through FGF9-mediated mechanisms. J Clin Invest. 2008;118(8):2697–710.
24. Aparicio A, Tzelepi V, Araujo JC, Guo CC, Liang S, Troncoso P, et al. Neuroendocrine prostate cancer xenografts with large-cell and small-cell features derived from a single patient's tumor: morphological, immunohistochemical, and gene expression profiles. Prostate. 2011;71(8):846–56.
25. Tzelepi V, Zhang J, Lu JF, Kleb B, Wu G, Wan X, et al. Modeling a lethal prostate cancer variant with small-cell carcinoma features. Clin Cancer Res. 2012;18(3):666–77.
26. Yoshida T, Kinoshita H, Segawa T, Nakamura E, Inoue T, Shimizu Y, et al. Antiandrogen bicalutamide promotes tumor growth in a novel androgen-dependent prostate cancer xenograft model derived from a bicalutamide-treated patient. Cancer Res. 2005;65(21):9611–6.
27. Terada N, Shimizu Y, Kamba T, Inoue T, Maeno A, Kobayashi T, et al. Identification of EP4 as a potential target for the treatment of castration-resistant prostate cancer using a novel xenograft model. Cancer Res. 2010;70(4):1606–15.
28. Yoshikawa T, Kobori G, Goto T, Akamatsu S, Terada N, Kobayashi T, et al. An original patient-derived xenograft of prostate cancer with cyst formation. Prostate. 2016;76(11):994–1003.
29. Hoehn W, Schroeder FH, Reimann JF, Joebsis AC, Hermanek P. Human prostatic adenocarcinoma: some characteristics of a serially transplantable line in nude mice (PC 82). Prostate. 1980;1(1):95–104.
30. Terada N, Shimizu Y, Yoshida T, Maeno A, Kamba T, Inoue T, et al. Antiandrogen withdrawal syndrome and alternative antiandrogen therapy associated with the W741C mutant androgen receptor in a novel prostate cancer xenograft. Prostate. 2010;70(3):252–61.
31. Toivanen R, Frydenberg M, Murphy D, Pedersen J, Ryan A, Pook D, et al. A preclinical xenograft model identifies castration-tolerant cancer-repopulating cells in localized prostate tumors. Sci Transl Med. 2013;5(187):187ra71.
32. Lawrence MG, Taylor RA, Toivanen R, Pedersen J, Norden S, Pook DW, et al. A preclinical xenograft model of prostate cancer using human tumors. Nat Protoc. 2013;8(5):836–48.
33. Saar M, Korbel C, Linxweiler J, Jung V, Kamradt J, Hasenfus A, et al. Orthotopic tumorgrafts in nude mice: a new method to study human prostate cancer. Prostate. 2015;75(14):1526–37.
34. Michiel Sedelaar JP, Dalrymple SS, Isaacs JT. Of mice and menDOUBLEHYPHENwarning: intact versus castrated adult male mice as xenograft hosts are equivalent to hypogonadal versus abiraterone treated aging human males, respectively. Prostate. 2013;73(12):1316–25.
35. Morote J, Orsola A, Planas J, Trilla E, Raventos CX, Cecchini L, et al. Redefining clinically significant castration levels in patients with prostate cancer receiving continuous androgen deprivation therapy. J Urol. 2007;178(4 Pt 1):1290–5.
36. Mohr BA, Guay AT, O'Donnell AB, McKinlay JB. Normal, bound and nonbound testosterone levels in normally ageing men: results from the Massachusetts Male Ageing Study. Clin Endocrinol (Oxf). 2005;62(1):64–73.
37. Bertotti A, Migliardi G, Galimi F, Sassi F, Torti D, Isella C, et al. A molecularly annotated platform of patient-derived xenografts ("xenopatients") identifies HER2 as an effective therapeutic target in cetuximab-resistant colorectal cancer. Cancer Discov. 2011;1(6):508–23.
38. Nguyen HM, Vessella RL, Morrissey C, Brown LG, Coleman IM, Higano CS, et al. LuCaP prostate cancer patient-derived xenografts reflect the molecular heterogeneity of advanced

disease an‑d serve as models for evaluating cancer therapeutics. Prostate. 2017;77(6):654–71.
39. Hirano D, Okada Y, Minei S, Takimoto Y, Nemoto N. Neuroendocrine differentiation in hormone refractory prostate cancer following androgen deprivation therapy. Eur Urol. 2004;45(5):586–92. discussion 92
40. Beltran H, Prandi D, Mosquera JM, Benelli M, Puca L, Cyrta J, et al. Divergent clonal evolution of castration-resistant neuroendocrine prostate cancer. Nat Med. 2016;22(3):298–305.
41. Akamatsu S, Wyatt AW, Lin D, Lysakowski S, Zhang F, Kim S, et al. The placental gene PEG10 promotes progression of neuroendocrine prostate cancer. Cell Rep. 2015;12(6):922–36.

Impact of GnRH Antagonist and LHRH Agonist on the Gonadal Axis

Yoshiyuki Miyazawa, Yoshitaka Sekine, and Kazuhiro Suzuki

Abstract

Androgens deprivation therapy for prostate cancer (PCa) has been widely established for the treatment of metastatic PCa cases and some localized PCa cases. With the discovery of LHRH agonists, it became possible to perform medical castration, and the range of options further expanded, but flare-up in progressive cases has been considered as a problem. As GnRH antagonists became available, we were able to begin the treatment without flare-up in advanced cases. In this chapter, we discuss the topics on LHRH agonists and antagonists and the relationships with adrenal androgens examined in our laboratory.

Keywords

Prostate cancer · LHRH agonist · GnRH antagonist · Adrenal androgen

5.1 Impact of GnRH Antagonist and LHRH Agonist on the Gonadal Axis

5.1.1 First Impact: Discovery of LHRH Agonist

Since Huggins et al. reported in 1941 [1], the androgen sensitivity of prostate cancer (PCa) has been well established. Androgen deprivation therapy (ADT) has been the mainstay of therapy of PCa. Surgical castration and estrogen preparations were used early in the development of ADT, but estrogen preparations had been avoided to side effects such as cardiovascular event or thrombosis. Surgical castration is still in progress, but it is a problem that the effect of surgical castration is permanent,

Y. Miyazawa · Y. Sekine · K. Suzuki (✉)
Department of Urology, Gunma University Graduate School of Medicine, Gunma, Japan
e-mail: kazu@gunma-u.ac.jp

continuous, and irreversible [2]. Schally's achievement has resulted in a major turning point in hormonal therapy. Elucidation of the structure of luteinizing hormone-releasing hormone (LHRH) by Schally et al. at 1971 developed LHRH agonist [3]. LHRH agonist changed the mainstay of ADT. With the advent of LHRH agonist, it could be possible to perform medical castration to patients with limited administration period. LHRH agonist made it possible to combine radiation therapy and hormone therapy for curative treatment. ADT by LHRH agonist has been widely spread afterward; Labrie et al. reported that surgical or medical castration alone had insufficient effect and effectiveness of combination therapy with antiandrogen agent [4]. In current, it is widely used for primary treatment of metastatic prostate cancer and relapse after radical therapy with the name combined androgen blockade (CAB). In the comparative study of CAB therapy and castration monotherapy conducted in Japan, the overall survival rate of CAB therapy using bicalutamide was significantly higher than that of castration monotherapy (hazard ratio: 0.78) [5, 6]. Whether or not to perform CAB for all cases of prostate cancer is considered to be controversial [7], leuprolide and goserelin have been used as LHRH agonists and have long played a major role of ADT for prostate cancer continues to be widely used today in Japan.

5.1.2 Second Impact: New Hope, GnRH Antagonist

With LHRH agonists, medical castration is as effective as bilateral orchiectomy, but main concern with the use of LHRH agonists for ADT is the clinical worsening of symptoms such as spinal cord compression, bone pain, and urethral obstruction due to a testosterone surge upon initiation of LHRH agonist treatment. Therefore, antiandrogens are often used to reduce the risk of flare-up. However, the additional administration of an antiandrogen agent couldn't inhibit flare-up of testosterone in the early stage of agonist administration, so clinical use of the gonadotropin-releasing hormone (GnRH) antagonist has been desired [8]. Abarelix, the first GnRH antagonist available clinically for treatment of PCa, showed safety profile comparable to that of the LHRH agonist, leuprolide, with or without bicalutamide [9]. However, abarelix had systemic allergic reactions [10]; the manufacturer withdrew abarelix from the US market for related commercial reasons.

The next generation GnRH antagonist degarelix is a newly discovered agent that blocks GnRH receptors immediately and testosterone production rapidly, preventing a testosterone surge. Klotz et al. evaluated the efficacy and safety of degarelix vs. leuprolide for achieving and maintaining testosterone suppression in a 1-year phase III trial involving patients with prostate cancer in CS21 study. They showed that treatment with degarelix resulted in a rapid suppression of testosterone levels; by day 3, the median testosterone levels were ≤ 0.5 ng/mL in 96.1% and 95.5% of patients in the degarelix 240/80 and 240/160 mg groups, respectively (median testosterone levels 0.24 and 0.26 ng/mL, respectively) [8]. In the results of exploratory analyses of CS21 study, Thombal et al. showed patients with PSA >20 ng/mL had a significantly longer time to PSA recurrence with degarelix compared to leuprolide

(p = 0.04) [11]. From these research results, There are two major advantages of degarelix compared to LHRH agonist. Degarelix causes rapid suppression of testosterone, and there is no flare-up. Although degarelix seems to be suitable for introduction of ADT for all PCa patients, it seems particularly that degarelix is suitable for safely introducing therapy in case of advanced PCa patients such as bone metastasis is concerned for spinal cord compression or symptoms like dysuria or urinary retention accompanying from local PCa are strong. In CS21, overall frequency of adverse events was similar for degarelix and leuprolide. Injection site reactions were more frequent with degarelix 240/80 mg (35%) than with leuprolide (<1%), predominantly occurring after the first injection. Frequency of injection site reactions decreased after the second time [8].

Various reports about secondary objectives in research of degarelix have been shown. There were fewer joint-related signs and symptoms, musculoskeletal events, and urinary tract events in the degarelix group compared to the leuprolide group [12]. One of the serious complications of ADT is the occurrence of cardiovascular events. Among men with pre-existing cardiovascular disease, the risk of cardiac events within 1 year of initiating therapy was significantly lower among men treated with degarelix compared with LHRH agonists (hazard ratio: 0.44; 95% confidence interval, 0.26–0.74; p = 0.002) [13]. Degarelix has a profound and persistent FSH declining tendency, whereas agonist has a partial FSH lowering effect [8]. The clinical advantage of FSH suppression with GnRH antagonists is not fully studied. However, several studies on the relationship between FSH and PCa have been reported. Thus, FSH stimulates PCa cell growth in vitro [14]. FSH receptors occur on prostate tumors and the surface of tumor blood vessels and are expressed at higher levels on prostate versus normal tissue [15–17]. Also, FSH may affect the pathogenesis and progression of castration-resistant PCa [18]. Further studies are expected on the effect caused by the antagonist other than testosterone suppression.

5.1.3 Relationship Between LHRH Agonist and Adrenal Androgen

In the treatment of prostate cancer, we have already mentioned that suppression of pituitary-testicular axis testosterone is the main axis by LHRH agonist or antagonist. Suppression of adrenal androgens is also important as a target of therapy. Adrenal androgens account for about 10% of androgens in the physiologic state in males, and they are the main source of androgens after medical or surgical castration [19, 20]. Various drugs that interact with androgen receptors (ARs) have been developed and used clinically. In addition to "conventional" AR inhibitors, such as flutamide [21] and bicalutamide [22], enzalutamide prolongs survival time before and after chemotherapy [23, 24]. Abiraterone, an androgen biosynthetic enzyme inhibitor, also improves patient prognosis [25]. Adrenal androgens have been targeted as key hormones for developing castration-resistant prostate cancer therapeutics. Although circulating adrenal androgens mainly originate from the adrenal glands, the testes supply about 10% [26]. In addition, the role of aberrant expression

Table 5.1 Clinical characteristics of the patients

Characteristic		
No. of patients	47	
Age (year, mean ± SD)	67.7 ± 3.5	
Initial PSA (median ± SD)	12.8 ± 10.3 ng/mL	
Stage	No. of patients	
T1cN0M0	13	27.7%
T2N0M0	15	31.9%
T3N0M0	19	40.4%
Gleason score		
GS 6	1	2.1%
GS 7	29	61.7%
GS ≥ 8	17	36.2%
Risk classification[a]		
Intermediate	16	34.0%
High	31	66.0%

Abbreviations: *PSA* prostate specific antigen
[a]D'Amico classification

of the luteinizing hormone (LH) receptor in adrenal glands has been studied in patients with adrenocorticotropic hormone (ACTH)-independent Cushing's syndrome [27–29]. However, the roles of LH and the presence of LH receptors in normal adrenal glands have not been fully studied. We examined the effect of LHRH agonist on changes in serum adrenal androgen levels [30]. Further, LH receptor localization was investigated in adrenal glands. This study included 47 prostate cancer patients. Table 5.1 shows the clinical characteristics of the enrolled patients. Testosterone (T), dihydrotestosterone (DHT), estradiol (E2), dehydroepiandrosterone (DHEA), and androstenedione (A-dione) were measured by liquid chromatography-mass spectrometry (LC-MS/MS). Dehydroepiandrosterone-sulfate (DHEA-S) and ACTH were measured by the chemiluminescence enzymatic immunity assay (CLIA) and electrochemiluminescence immunity assay (ECLIA), respectively. A significant reduction in testosterone levels (97.5% reduction) was observed in LH-RH agonist-treated patients 6 months after the initiation of treatment. In addition, levels of DHT, E2, adrenal androgen, DHEA-S, DHEA, and A-dione were reduced 6 months after the initiation of treatment (95.0%, 92.5%, 26.4%, 26.5%, 26.5%, and 40.6% reduction, respectively). Twelve months after the initiation of treatment, a significant suppressive state was maintained, as measured by levels of T, DHT, E2, DHE-S, DHAS, and A-dione (98.0%, 95.1%, 91.3%, 29%, 30.7%, and 41.6% reduction, respectively). Adrenal androgen levels 6 and 12 months after the initiation of treatment were significantly lower than those during the pretreatment period. ACTH levels showed an increasing trend at 6 months but were significantly increased at 12 months (126.3%). The changes in hormone levels during the treatment are shown in Table 5.2. Serum adrenal androgen levels significantly decreased after 6 and 12 months of treatment with LH-RH agonist. We also identified LH receptors in the adrenal cortex cells in the reticular layer by immunohistochemistry.

5 Impact of GnRH Antagonist and LHRH Agonist on the Gonadal Axis

Table 5.2 Changes of hormone levels in prostate cancer patients treated with GnRH agonist

	Pre	6 mo	12 mo	Statistics
T Measurement, ng/dL Percentile change	387.0 ± 157.0	10.0 ± 5.0 −97.5%	8.0 ± 5.0 −98.0%	$p < 0.01$ Pre vs. 6 mo, 12 mo
DHT Measurement, pg/mL Percentile change	426.3 ± 199.6	21.4 ± 12.0 −95.0%	20.9 ± 11.1 −95.1%	$p < 0.01$ Pre vs. 6 mo, 12 mo
E2 Measurement, pg/mL Percentile change	16.3 ± 5.5	1.2 ± 1.0 −92.5%	1.4 ± 1.0 −91.3%	$p < 0.01$ Pre vs. 6 mo, 12 mo
DHEA-S Measurement, μg/dL Percentile change	146.0 ± 67.0	107.5 ± 47.6 −26.4%	103.6 ± 53.7 −29.0%	$p < 0.01$ Pre vs. 6 mo, 12 mo
DHEA Measurement, ng/mL Percentile change	1.89 ± 0.92	1.39 ± 0.67 −26.5%	1.31 ± 0.64 −30.7%	$p < 0.01$ Pre vs. 6 mo, 12 mo
A-dione Measurement, ng/mL Percentile change	0.390 ± 0.135	0.232 ± 0.109 −40.6%	0.228 ± 0.118 −41.6%	$p < 0.01$ Pre vs. 6 mo, 12 mo

Abbreviations: *T* testosterone, *DHT* dihydrotestosterone, *E2* estradiol, *DHEA* dehydroepiandrosterone, *DHEA-S* dehydroepiandrosterone-sulfate, *A-dione* androstenedione, *Pre* Pre treatment of GnRH antagonist, *6 mo, 12 mo*, 6, 12 months after initiation of GnRH antagonist treatment
Percentile change indicates changes in comparison with pretreatment levels. Values are expressed as mean ± SD

5.1.4 The Effect of Antagonist on Adrenal Androgen

We also examined the effects of a GnRH antagonist on changes in serum adrenal androgen levels [31]. This study included 47 prostate cancer patients. Pretreatment blood samples were collected from all of the patients, and posttreatment samples were taken at 1, 3, 6, and 12 months after starting the treatment. Serum was stored at −80 °C until measurements. T, DHT, E2, DHEA, and A-dione were measured by LC-MS/MS. DHEA-S was measured by ECLIA. Table 5.3 shows the clinical characteristics of the enrolled patients. T levels decreased significantly (97.3% reduction) in GnRH antagonist-treated patients 1 month after initiating treatment compared to those at baseline. In addition, the lower T level was maintained until 12 months after initiating treatment (97.1% reduction). DHT and E2 decreased 1 month after initiating treatment (DHT, 93.2%; E2, 84.9% reduction, respectively), and these levels were maintained until 12 months after initiating treatment. DHEA-S and A-dione levels significantly decreased 1, 3, 6, and 12 months after initiating treatment and remained low until 12 months after the start of treatment (DHEA-S, 23.9%; A-dione, 40.5% reduction, respectively). We did not observe a decrease in DHEA levels 1, 3, or 6 months after initiating treatment, but DHEA level was significantly lower 12 months after treatment compared to baseline (15.4% reduction) (Table 5.4).

Table 5.3 Clinical characteristics of the patients

Characteristic		
No. of patients	47	
Age (year, mean ± SD)	73.6 ± 7.02	
Initial PSA (median ± SD)	11.1 ± 489.1 ng/mL	
Stage	No. of patients	
T1cN0M0	8	17%
T2N0M0	14	29.8%
T3N0M0	9	19.1%
T4N0M0	2	4.3%
TanyN1M0	4	8.5%
TanyN0M1	5	10.6%
TanyN1M1	5	10.6%
Metastasis		
All distant metastasis	10	21.2%
Bone metastasis	7	14.9%
Visceral metastasis	3	6.4%
Gleason score		
GS 6	4	9%
GS 7	15	32%
GS≥8	28	59%

Abbreviations: *PSA* prostate specific antigen

Cases of ACTH-independent adrenal hyperplasia have been reported [26, 27], and functional LH receptors have been discovered in patients with ACTH-independent Cushing's syndrome [27, 28]. Those studies have shown that LH-RH agonist treatment reduces serum cortisol levels and demonstrated an association between cortisol production and the presence of LH receptors in the adrenal glands. Pabon et al. [32] identified LH receptors on the reticular layer of adrenal cortex cells and demonstrated the presence of the cytochrome P450 side-chain cleavage enzyme in the same cells. These findings suggest that LH-positive adrenal cortex cells are steroidogenic. Rao et al. [33] showed that in DHEA-S is produced in H295R adrenal cortical cells by LH via functional LH receptors. These findings suggest that LH may affect adrenal gland function and regulate the secretion of adrenal hormones.

We discovered that the adrenal cortex cells in the reticular layer were positive for LH receptors in patients treated with a LH-RH agonist (Fig. 5.1) [30]. Furthermore, we found that the correlation between ACTH and DHEA-S levels shifted to an inverse relationship during the treatment period. These findings suggest that reduced adrenal synthesis of androgens stimulates ACTH secretion through a feedback mechanism. Therefore, long-term GnRH antagonist treatment may reduce serum adrenal androgen levels via LH receptors. We speculated the existence of another mechanism by which GnRH antagonists inhibit adrenal androgen production directly via GnRH receptor protein in the adrenal glands. In addition to its expression in the pituitary gland, GnRH receptor is expressed in lymphocytes and many extra-pituitary tissues, including breast, ovary, and prostate [34]. Ziegler et al. [35] demonstrated that GnRH receptor is present in the adrenal glands at the mRNA and

Table 5.4 Changes of hormone levels in prostate cancer patients treated with GnRH antagonist

	Pre	1 mo	3 mo	6 mo	12 mo	Statistics
T	376.66 ± 161.71	10.23 ± 5.09	10.09 ± 3.98	10.49 ± 4.52	10.81 ± 5.36	$p < 0.05$
Measurement, ng/dL						Pre vs. 1 mo, 3 mo, 6 mo, 12 mo
Percentile change		−97.3%	−97.3%	−97.2%	−97.1%	
DHT	442.76 ± 256.68	29.95 ± 15.89	27.09 ± 15.28	25.30 ± 14.48	24.12 ± 14.01	$p < 0.05$
Measurement, pg/mL						Pre vs. 1 mo, 3 mo, 6 mo, 12 mo
Percentile change		−93.2%	−93.9%	−94.3%	−94.6%	
E2	23.58 ± 12.81	3.56 ± 2.58	3.25 ± 2.21	3.32 ± 2.01	3.46 ± 2.37	$p < 0.05$
Measurement, pg/mL						Pre vs. 1 mo, 3 mo, 6 mo, 12 mo
Percentile change		−84.9%	−86.2%	−85.9%	−85.3%	
DHEA-S	125.47 ± 62.48	104.38 ± 56.03	103.7 ± 52.52	104.17 ± 57.03	95.47 ± 58.23	$p < 0.05$
Measurement, μg/dL						Pre vs. 1 mo, 3 mo, 6 mo, 12 mo
Percentile change		−16.8%	−17.3%	−17.0%	−23.9%	
DHEA	2.50 ± 1.46	2.19 ± 1.52	2.27 ± 1.45	2.23 ± 1.57	2.11 ± 1.69	$p < 0.05$
Measurement, ng/mL						Pre vs. 12 mo
Percentile change		−12.0%	−8.7%	−10.8%	−15.4%	
A-dione	0.715 ± 0.348	0.458 ± 0.278	0.472 ± 0.231	0.448 ± 0.230	0.426 ± 0.220	$p < 0.05$
Measurement, ng/mL						Pre vs. 1 mo, 3 mo, 6 mo, 12 mo
Percentile change		−35.5%	−33.9%	−37.4%	−40.5%	
LH	7.20 ± 7.31	0.285 ± 0.385	0.255 ± 0.306	0.303 ± 0.355	0.453 ± 0.479	$p < 0.05$
Measurement, mIU/mL						Pre vs. 1 mo, 3 mo, 6 mo, 12 mo
Percentile change		−96.0%	−96.5%	−95.8%	−93.7%	
FSH	14.56 ± 14.47	0.889 ± 1.100	0.993 ± 0.100	1.224 ± 1.135	1.83 ± 1.424	$p < 0.05$
Measurement, mIU/mL						Pre vs. 1 mo, 3 mo, 6 mo, 12 mo
Percentile change		−93.9%	−93.2%	−91.6%	−87.4%	

Abbreviations: *T* testosterone, *DHT* dihydrotestosterone; *E2* estradiol; *DHEA* dehydroepiandrosterone, *DHEA-S* dehydroepiandrosterone-sulfate, *A-dione* androstenedione, *LH* luteinizing hormone, *FSH* follicle stimulating hormone, *Pre* pretreatment, *1, 3, 6, 12 mo*, 1, 3, 6, 12 months after initiation of GnRH antagonist treatment.
Percentile change indicates changes in comparison with pretreatment levels. Values are expressed as mean ± SD

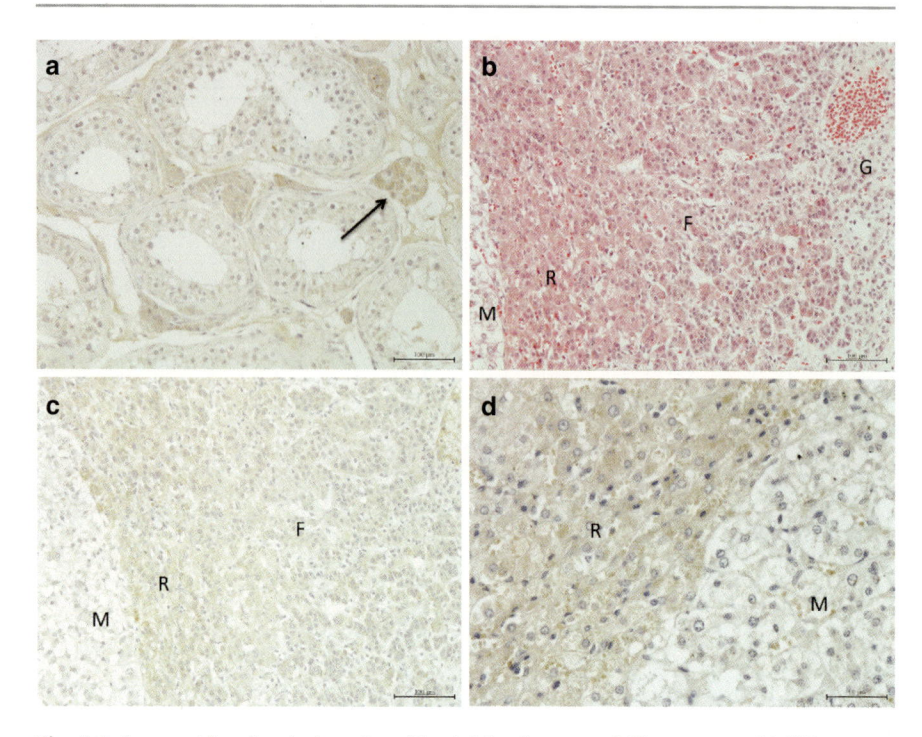

Fig. 5.1 Immunohistochemical results of luteinizing hormone (LH) receptors. (**a**) LH receptor staining, testes, Leydig cells (arrow), intensity 2+. (**b**) Adrenal gland, hematoxylin-eosin staining. (**c**) LH receptor staining (LH staining of the same sample as in **b**), adrenal gland, intensity 1+. (**d**) LH receptor staining, adrenal gland, intensity 2+. Paraffin-embedded testes or adrenal glands were immunohistochemically stained by the enzyme-labeled polymer method using a 1:100 dilution of polyclonal LH receptor antibody (H-50:sc25828; Santa Cruz Biotechnology). *M* indicates adrenal medulla, *R* reticular layer, *F* fascicular layer, *G* glomerular layer

protein levels in normal human adrenal tissues, adrenocortical and adrenomedullary tumors, and adrenal cell lines. Although the presence of GnRH receptor in the adrenal glands suggests that adrenal androgen production was suppressed via GnRH receptor, it is unclear how the receptor works in the adrenal glands. In summary, we found a significant decrease in adrenal androgen levels in patients treated with a GnRH agonist and antagonist for 12 months. Considering the existence of functional LH receptors in cases of ACTH-independent Cushing's syndrome or in human adrenal cortex cells, long-term GnRH antagonist administration may reduce serum adrenal androgen levels via LH receptors.

References

1. Huggins C, Hodges CV. Studies on prostatic cancer. I. The effect of castration, of estrogen and of androgen injection on serum phosphatases in metastatic carcinoma of the prostate. Cancer Res. 1941;1:293–7.

2. Mottet N, Bellmunt N, Briers E, et al. European Association of Urology Guidelines on Prostate Cancer. 2015. http://uroweb.org/wp-content/uploads/EAU-Guidelines-Prostate-Cancer-2015-v2.pdf. Accessed 17 Aug 2015.
3. Schally AV, Arimura A, Kastin AJ, et al. Gonadotropin-releasing hormone: one polypeptide regulates secretion of luteinizing and follicle-stimulating hormones. Science. 1971;173:1036–8.
4. Labrie F, Dupont A, Belanger A, et al. New hormonal therapy in prostatic carcinoma: combined treatment with an LHRH agonist and an antiandrogen. Clin Invest Med. 1982;5:267–75.
5. Akaza H, Hinotsu S, Usami M, Study Group for the Combined Androgen Blockade Therapy of Prostate Cancer, et al. Combined androgen blockade with bicalutamide for advanced prostate cancer: long-term follow-up of a phase 3, double-blind, randomized study for survival. Cancer. 2009;115:3437–45.
6. Akaza H, Yamaguchi A, Matsuda T, et al. Superior anti-tumor efficacy of bicalutamide 80mg in combination with a leuteinizing hormone-releasing hormone(LHRH)agonist versus LHRH agonist monotherapy as first-line treatment for advanced prostate cancer:interim results of a randomized study in Japanese patients. Jpn J Clin Oncol. 2004;34:20–8.
7. Japanese Urological Association. Clinical Practice Guideline for Prostate cancer in Japan. 2016:202–204.
8. Klotz L, Boccon-Gibod L, Shore ND, et al. The efficacy and safety of degarelix: a 12-month, comparative, randomized, open-label, parallel-group phase III studies in patients with prostate cancer. BJU Int. 2008;102(11):1531–8.
9. Debruyne F, Bhat G, Garnick MB. Abarelix for injectable suspension: first-in-class gonadotropin-releasing hormone antagonist for prostate cancer. Future Oncol. 2006;2(6):677–96.
10. Shore ND, Abrahamsson PA, Anderson J, Crawford ED, Lange P. New considerations for ADT in advanced prostate cancer and the emerging role of GnRH antagonists. Prostate Cancer Prostatic Dis. 2013;16(1):7–15.
11. Tombal B, Miller K, Boccon-Gibod L, et al. Additional analysis of the secondary end point of biochemical recurrence rate in a phase 3 trial (CS21) comparing degarelix 80 mg versus leuprolide in prostate cancer patients segmented by baseline characteristics. Eur Urol. 2010;57(5):836–42.
12. Klotz L, Miller K, Crawford ED, et al. Disease control outcomes from analysis of pooled individual patient data from five comparative randomised clinical trials of degarelix versus luteinising hormone-releasing hormone agonists. Eur Urol. 2014;66(6):1101–8.
13. Albertsen PC, Klotz L, Tombal B, et al. Cardiovascular morbidity associated with gonadotropin releasing hormone agonists and an antagonist. Eur Urol. 2014;65:565–73.
14. Ben-Josef E, Yang SY, Ji TH, Bidart JM, Garde SV, Chopra DP, et al. Hormone- refractory prostate cancer cells express functional follicle-stimulating hormone receptor (FSHR). J Urol. 1999;161:970–6.
15. Huhtaniemi I. Are gonadotrophins tumorigenic a critical review of clinical and experimental data. Mol Cell Endocrinol. 2010;329:56–61.
16. Radu A, Pichon C, Camparo P, Antoine M, Allory Y, Couvelard A, et al. Expression of follicle-stimulating hormone receptor in tumor blood vessels. N Engl J Med. 2010;363:1621–30.
17. Mariani S, Salvatori L, Basciani S, Arizzi M, Franco G, Petrangeli E, et al. Expression and cellular localization of follicle-stimulating hormone receptor in normal human prostate, benign prostatic hyperplasia and prostate cancer. J Urol. 2006;175:2072–7.
18. Porter AT, Ben-Josef E. Humoral mechanisms in prostate cancer: a role for FSH. Urol Oncol. 2001;6:131–8.
19. Vermeulen A, Schelfout W, Sy W. Plasma androgen levels after subcapsular orchiectomy or oestrogen treatment for prostatic carcinoma. Prostate. 1982;3:115–21.
20. Belanger A, Dupont A, Labrie F. Inhibition of basal and adrenocor- ticotropin-stimulated plasma levels of adrenal androgens after treatment with an antiandrogen in castrated patients with prostate cancer. J Clin Endocrinol Metab. 1984;59:422–6.
21. Crawford ED, Eisenberger MA, McLeod DG, et al. A controlled trial leuprolide with and without flutamide in prostatic carcinoma. N Engl J Med. 1989;321:419–24.

22. Schellhammer PF, Sharifi R, Block NL, et al. A controlled trial of bicalutamide versus flutamide, each in combination with luteinizing hormone-releasing hormone analogue therapy, in patients with advanced prostate carcinoma. Analysis of time to progression. CASODEX Combination Study Group. Cancer. 1996;78(10):2164–9.
23. Scher HI, Fizzazi K, Saad F, et al. Increased survival with enzalutamide in prostate cancer after chemotherapy. N Engl J Med. 2012;367:1187–97.
24. Beer TM, Armstrong AJ, Rathkopf DE, et al. Enzalutamide in metastatic prostate cancer before chemotherapy. N Engl J Med. 2014;371:424–33.
25. Ryan CJ, Smith MR, Fizazi K, et al. Abiraterone acetate plus prednisone versus placebo plus prednisone in chemotherapy-naive men with metastatic castration-resistant prostate cancer (COU-AA-302): final overall survival analysis of a randomised, double-blind, placebo-controlled phase 3 study. Lancet Oncol. 2015;16:152–60.
26. Braunstein DG. Testes. In: Greenspan FS, editor. Basic and clinical endocrinology. 3rd ed. Englewood Cliffs, NJ: Prentice Hall; 1991. p. 407–41.
27. Lacroix A, Mamet P, Boutin JM. Leuprolide acetate therapy in luteinizing hormone-dependent Cushing's syndrome. N Engl J Med. 1999;341:1577–81.
28. Feelders RA, Lamberts WJ, Hofland LJ, et al. Luteinizing hormone (LH)- responsive Cushing's syndrome: the demonstration of LH receptor messenger ribonucleic acid in hyperplastic adrenal cells, which respond to chorionic gonadotropin and serotonin agonists in vitro. J Clin Endocrinol Metab. 2003;88:230–7.
29. de Groot JWB, Links TP, Themmen APN, et al. Aberrant expression of multiple hormone receptors in ACTH-independent macronodular adrenal hyperplasia causing Cushing's syndrome. Eur J Endocrinol. 2010;163:293–9.
30. Nishii M, Nomura M, Sekine Y, et al. Luteinizing hormone (LH)-releasing hormone agonist reduces serum adrenal androgen levels in prostate cancer patients: implications for the effect of LH on the adrenal glands. J Androl. 2012;33:1233–8.
31. Miyazawa Y, Sekine Y, Syuto T, et al. A gonadotropin-releasing hormone antagonist reduces serum adrenal androgen levels in prostate cancer patients. BMC Urol. 2017;17:70. https://doi.org/10.1186/s12894-017-0261-z.
32. Pabon JE, Li X, Lei ZM, et al. Novel presence of luteinizing hormone/chorionic gonadotropin receptors in human adrenal glands. J Clin Endocrinol Metab. 1996;81:2397–400.
33. Rao CV, Zhou XL, Lei ZM. Functional luteinizing hormone/chorionic gonadotropin receptors in human adrenal cortical H295R cells. Biol Reprod. 2004;71:579–87.
34. Cheng CK, Leung PC. Molecular biology of gonadotropin-releasing hormone (GnRH)-I, GnRH-II, and their receptors in humans. Endocr Rev. 2005;26:283–306.
35. Ziegler CG, Brown JW, Schally AV, et al. Expression of neuropeptide hormone receptors in human adrenal tumors and cell lines: antiproliferative effects of peptide analogues. PNAS. 2009;106:15879–84.

Controversies on Combined Androgen Blockade for Prostate Cancer

Atsushi Mizokami

Abstract

The key factor which is very important in order that prostate cancer proliferates is androgen. More than 90% of androgen is of testicular origin, and the remainder is of adrenal origin. Because much more androgen remained in prostate cancer tissue than in serum after castration, it was expected that combined androgen blockade (CAB) (castration plus antiandrogen) had a better prognosis than castration monotherapy. As a result, although it was suggested that CAB had better prognosis, the extreme superiority was not observed in CAB. However, this significant difference was clear in Asia. CAB was superior to castration monotherapy. The difference between Asia and Western countries may be due to the difference in dose of bicalutamide or race. Clinical trials to examine superiority of complete androgen blockade using adrenal androgen synthesis inhibitor or more powerful new antiandrogen instead of CAB as an initial treatment is ongoing for advanced prostate cancer.

Keywords

Combined androgen blockade · Complete androgen blockade · Castration Prostate cancer

Hormone therapy for prostate cancer was first proposed by C. Huggins in 1941; the effectiveness of which has been confirmed, and Huggins was awarded the Nobel Prize.

Thereafter, the initial treatment for advanced prostate cancer has been primarily castration-based androgen deprivation therapy (ADT). The reason that ADT is

---

A. Mizokami, M.D., Ph.D.
Department of Integrative Cancer Therapy and Urology, Kanazawa University Graduate School of Medical Science, Kanazawa, Japan
e-mail: mizokami@staff.kanazawa-u.ac.jp

© Springer Nature Singapore Pte Ltd. 2018
Y. Arai, O. Ogawa (eds.), *Hormone Therapy and Castration Resistance of Prostate Cancer*, https://doi.org/10.1007/978-981-10-7013-6_6

effective for prostate cancer is attributed to the presence of androgen receptors (AR) in the cytoplasm of prostate cancer cells. When the active androgen, dihydrotestosterone, binds to AR, AR becomes activated and translocates into the nucleus. AR causes the target gene to activate by binding to the target gene associated with growth, and ultimately dihydrotestosterone (DHT) acts as a growth factor. That is, contrarily, upon performing castration, androgen is depleted, which prevents the activation of and impedes the growth of AR, thereby producing an antitumor effect.

Hormone therapy has primarily been conducted on the basis of surgical castration up to the early 1990s; however, in the 1980s, luteinizing hormone-releasing hormone (LH-RH) agonists (such as leuprolide and goserelin) were developed (Fig. 6.1) [2–4]. Excessive administration of LH-RH agonists bind to LH-RH receptors located in the pituitary gland then subsequently inhibit the expression of LH-RH receptors entirely, after which LH-RH cannot bind to the receptor, thereby inhibiting the secretion of luteinizing hormone (LH) from the pituitary and lowering serum testosterone to levels comparable to surgical castration. Therefore, to date, chemical castration using LH-RH agonists has become common practice. Furthermore, in recent years, degarelix, an LH-RH antagonist with relatively a little inflammatory response and allergic reaction, has also been developed [5]. Upon administration of degarelix, LH-RH cannot bind to LH-RH receptors, thereby impeding LH secretion from the pituitary gland and reducing serum testosterone to levels similar to surgical castration.

When castration is performed, serum testosterone is reduced to below 10%; however, a small amount of testosterone remains. It is believed that more than 90% of serum testosterone is derived from the testis, while the remaining testosterone is

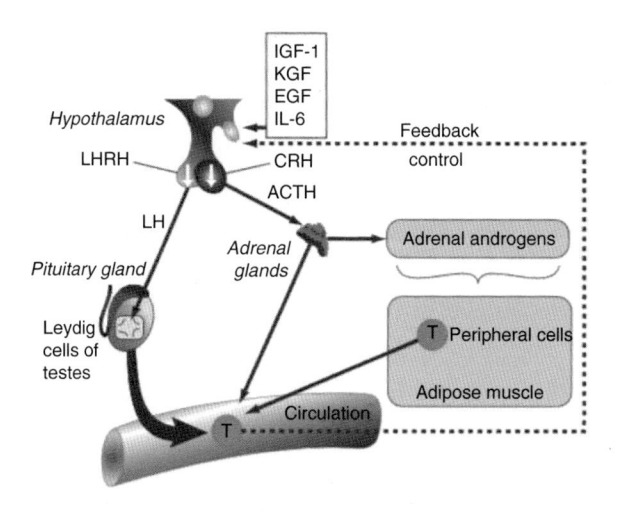

Fig. 6.1 The rationale for combination therapy consisting of castration plus an antiandrogen. ACTH Adrenocorticotropic hormone, CRH Corticotropin-releasing hormone, EGF Epidermal growth factor, IGF-1 Insulin-like growth factor-1, IL-6 Interleukin-6, KGF Keratinocyte growth factor, T Testosterone. Klotz L, A re-assessment of the role of combined androgen blockade for advanced prostate cancer. BJU Int (2004) [1]

derived from the adrenal gland. It is believed that even small amounts of testosterone have an adverse effect on the growth of prostate cancer. Labrie et al. noted that following castration, there remains sufficient adrenal androgens DHEA and DHEA-S, and therefore not only the action of testosterone from the testis should be blocked, but adrenal androgen should be inhibited also; thus, they proposed the theory that maximal androgen blockade (MAB) should be performed [6]. Furthermore, Labrie et al. reported that in prostate cancer tissue following castration, androgen is only decreased to 60% and testosterone accounts for the remaining 40%. In other words, it was suggested that even after castration, androgen is biosynthesized in the prostate cancer tissue and peripheral tissue [7]. In other studies also, it is reported that even following castration, dihydrotestosterone (DHT) levels remained at 20–25% in the prostate cancer tissue [8, 9]. It is possible that even with less than 10% adrenal androgen, biosynthesis to DHT is promoted such as in prostate cancer tissue and bones, and as a result, DHT levels greater than the serum level could have contribute to the growth of prostate cancer. In fact, one reason that hormone-naïve prostate cancer progresses to castration-resistant prostate cancer (CRPC) is attributed to the involvement of adrenal androgen, and therefore as the treatment for CRPC, abiraterone acetate, an inhibitor of adrenal androgen synthesis, is used, and the effectiveness of which has been confirmed [10].

However, in the 1980s, there were no drugs capable of sufficiently inhibiting the production of adrenal androgen, and therefore physicians believed that MAB should be performed by using antiandrogens that block DHT synthesized from adrenal androgen in prostate cancer tissue. Consequently, several clinical trials were performed to confirm the effectiveness of MAB combining castration and antiandrogen therapy. In these trials, castration was performed by surgical castration or LH-RH agonists. Furthermore, as the antiandrogen, the steroid cyproterone acetate or nonsteroids nilutamide or flutamide were used (Fig. 6.2) [11]. In a meta-analysis summarizing the data of these 27 studies (of 8275 patients, 88% had metastatic prostate cancer, and 12% had localized advanced prostate cancer), the 5-year survival rate was 23.6% for castration monotherapy, in contrast to 25.4% for MAB, and while negligible, MAB had a better survival rate; however, there was no significant difference ([SE 1.3], log-rank 2p = 0·11) [11]. This meta-analysis revealed that upon analyzing according to each antiandrogen agent, in MAB using cyproterone acetate, the 5-year survival rate for MAB was significantly poorer (MAB: 15.4% vs. castration 18.1%, [SE 2·4], log-rank 2p = 0.04). On the other hand, in MAB using nilutamide or flutamide, the 5-year survival rate was significantly improved (MAB: 27.6% vs. castration: 24.7%, [SE 1·3], log-rank 2p = 0.005). Furthermore, in a single-center trial comparing leuprolide monotherapy against MAB combining leuprolide and flutamide in 603 patients with stage D2 prostate cancer, compared to leuprolide monotherapy, MAB showed improved progression-free survival (PFS) (16.5 vs. 13.9 months, p = 0.039) and median survival (35.6 vs. 28.3 months, p = 0.035) [12]. Moreover, in this clinical trial, the rate of improvement in symptoms at 12 weeks after the start of treatment was superior for MAB. Thereafter, bicalutamide was developed, which is a nonsteroidal antiandrogen that has affinity to AR that is four times more potent than hydroxyflutamide [13]. A trial was

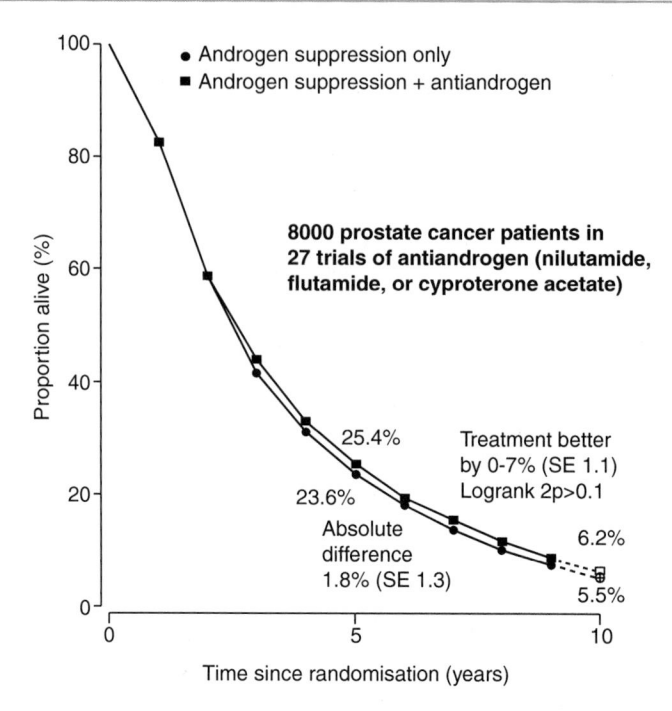

Fig. 6.2 10-year survival in the 27 randomised trials of MSB vs. AS alone. Maximum androgen blockade in advanced prostate cancer: an overview of the randomised trials. The Lancet (2000) [11]

conducted comparing MAB combining LH-RH agonist and bicalutamide against MAB combining LH-RH agonist and flutamide in 813 patients with stage D2 prostate cancer [14]. As a result, the PFS and hazard ratio for survival in the bicalutamide combination group were 0.93 (95% confidence interval [CI] 0.79–1.10, $p = 0.41$) and 0.87 (95% CI 0.72–1.05, $p = 0.15$), respectively. While there was no significant difference concluded for the bicalutamide combination group, the results were good. Furthermore, on the basis of the results consolidating the PCTCG meta-analysis results [11] and the data from Schellhammer et al. [14], it was reported that MAB combining bicalutamide and castration for stage D2 prostate cancer was more effective than castration monotherapy with a hazard ratio of 0.8 (95% CI of 0.66–0.98) (Fig. 6.3) [1]. However, in Western countries, trials to directly compare MAB using bicalutamide against castration monotherapy have not been conducted for ethical reasons. In the results of these meta-analyses, while MAB using nonsteroidal antiandrogens was 3–5% superior to castration monotherapy, the difference was not so great. Given the side effects, at present MAB is rarely administered in Western countries [16].

On the other hand, MAB has a different status in Japan compared to Western countries. Bicalutamide became available in Japan in 1998. A Japanese phase II study using bicalutamide compared the effectiveness and safety of bicalutamide at 50 mg/day, 80 mg/day, and 100 mg/day, with the best results obtained for 80 mg/

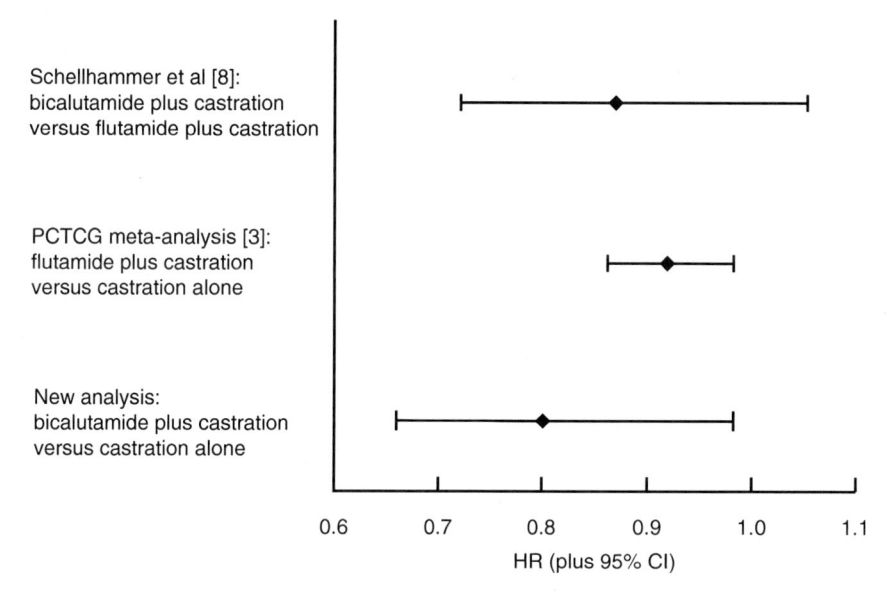

Fig. 6.3 HRs and 95% CI for overall survival for bicalutamide plus castration vs. flutamide plus castration, flutamide plus castration vs. castration alone, and for bicalutamide plus castration vs. castration alone. Schellhammer et al. [14]: bicalutaimide plus castration vs. flutamide plus castration. PCTCG meta-analysis [15]: flutamide plus castration vs. castration alone. New analysis: bicalutamide plus castration vs. castration alone. Klotz L, A re-assessment of the role of combined androgen blockade for advanced prostate cancer. BJU Int (2004) [1]

day, and thus in Japan, the administered dose of bicalutamide is set at 80 mg/day [17]. Thereafter, a prospective clinical trial was conducted for LH-RH agonist monotherapy, in contrast to combination therapy using LH-RH agonist and bicalutamide (combined androgen blockade, CAB, or MAB) (Fig. 6.4) [18]. The results of this clinical trial revealed that overall survival was predominantly improved in the CAB group than with monotherapy (hazard ratio, 0.78; 95% CI, 0.60–0.99; $p = 0.0498$; log-rank test: $p = 0.0425$). Upon performing a subgroup analysis, overall survival for stage C/D1 patients was predominantly improved more with CAB than with LH-RH agonist monotherapy ($p = 0.0041$), and for stage D2, there was no particular difference observed. On the basis of the results of this clinical trial and that Japanese people have a high incidence of liver function impairment due to flutamide, as the initial treatment for advanced prostate cancer, in Japan CAB using bicalutamide has gained popularity.

Furthermore, in the Japanese Study Group of Prostate Cancer (J-CaP) study, follow-up observation of 10 years or more after the initial treatment was performed for 26,272 patients with prostate cancer enrolled at 385 institutions from 2001 to 2003. Among these patients, 5618 patients with metastatic prostate cancer were examined, and as a result, for stages N1 M0, M1a, M1b, and M1c, the CAB group had significantly better overall survival than then non-CAB group (Table 6.1) [19]. Why does the response to hormone therapy for prostate cancer differ in Japan compared to

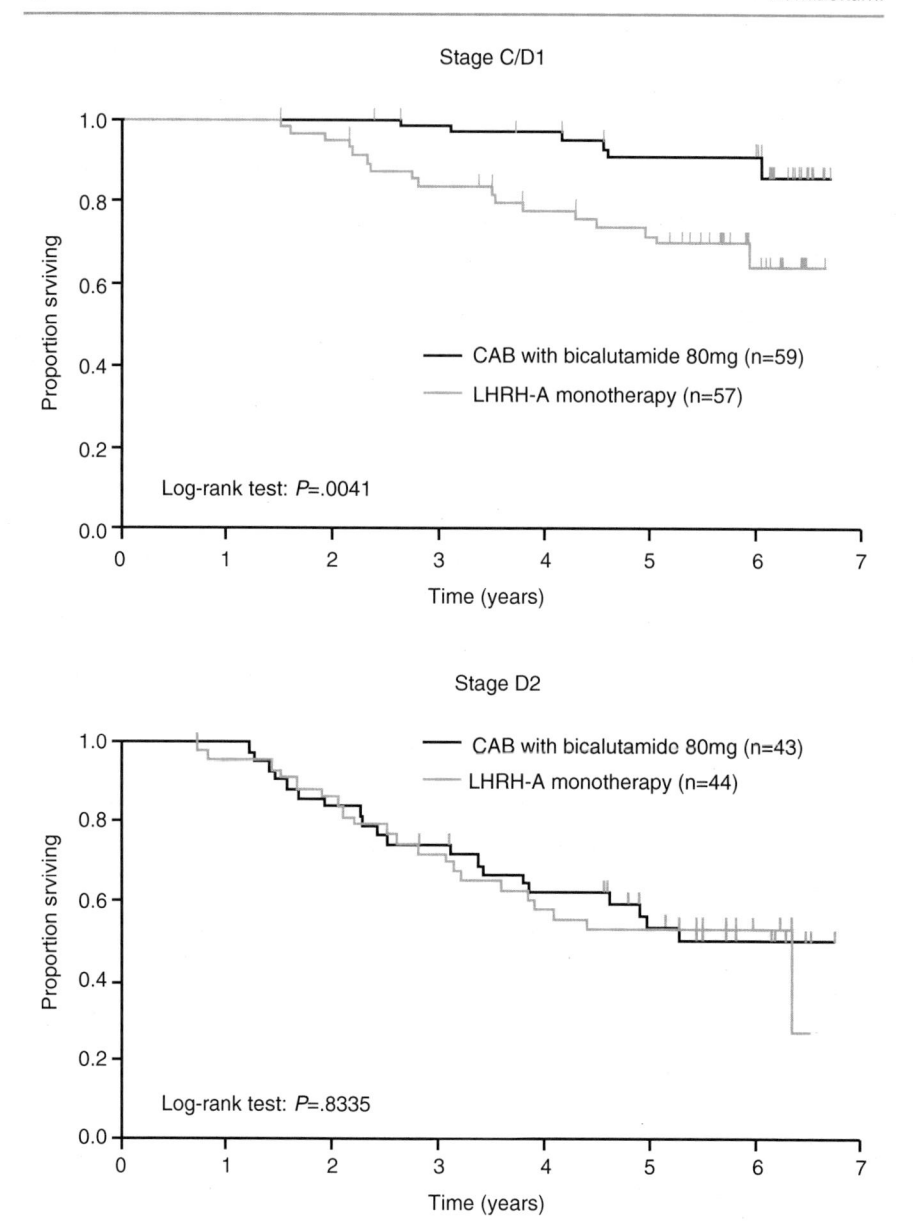

Fig. 6.4 Akaza et al. Cancer (2009) [18]

Western countries? Bicalutamide is administered at a dose of 50 mg/day in Western countries, in contrast to 80 mg/day in Japan, which is a higher dose of 1.6-fold. In the results of the phase II study of bicalutamide in Japan, effectiveness was higher for 80 mg/day than 50 mg/day [17]. The fact that bicalutamide is administered at a higher dose in Japan could explain the effectiveness of MAB in Japan.

Table 6.1 Multivariate analysis of factors that impact on overall survival in patients at different stages

Factor	N1M0 n (%)	HR	95 % CI	p value	M1a n (%)	HR	95 % CI	p value	M1b n (%)	HR	95 % CI	p value	M1c n (%)	HR	95 % CI	p value
Age.				0.046				0.524				<0.001				0.007
<75	364 (57.5)	Ref.			123(63.0)	Ref.			1980 (53.1)	Ref.			146 (60.0)	Ref.		
≥75	269 (42.5)	1.41	1.007–1.981		72 (37.0)	1.17	0.718–1.919		1748 (46.9)	1.27	1.138–1.414		97 (40.0)	1.72	1.162–2.542	
GS				0.026				0.003				<0.001				0.003
≤7	287 (45.3)	Ref.			60 (30.8)	Ref.			1612 (43.2)	Ref.			100(41.2)	Ref.		
≥8	346(54.7)	1.5	1.050–2.132		135(69.2)	2.5	1.361–4.586		2116 (56.8)	1.53	1.369–1.718		143(58.8)	1.85	1.226–2.788	
PSA				0.782				0.03				<0.001				0.789
<100	356 (56.2)	Ref.			68 (34.9)	Ref.			1325 (35.5)	Ref			80 (32.8)	Ref.		
≥100	277 (43.8)	1.05	0.747–1.472		127 (65.1)	0.57	0.348–0.947		2403 (64.5)	1.47	1.306–1.662		163(67.1)	0.95	0.625–1.430	
Treatment				0.016				0.12				<0.001				0.023
Non-CAB	222(35.1)	Ref.			131 (67.2)	Ref.			1124 (30.2)	Ref.			87(35.8)	Ref.		
CAB	411 (64.9)	0.66	0.469–0.925		64 (32.8)	0.82	0.644–1.052		2604(69.8)	0.75	0.666–0.837		156(64.2)	0.63	0.423–0.937	

HR Hazard ratio, *CI* Confidence interval, *GS* Gleason score, *PSA* Prostate-specific antigen, *CAB* Combined androgen blockade (Kadono et al., WJU [19])

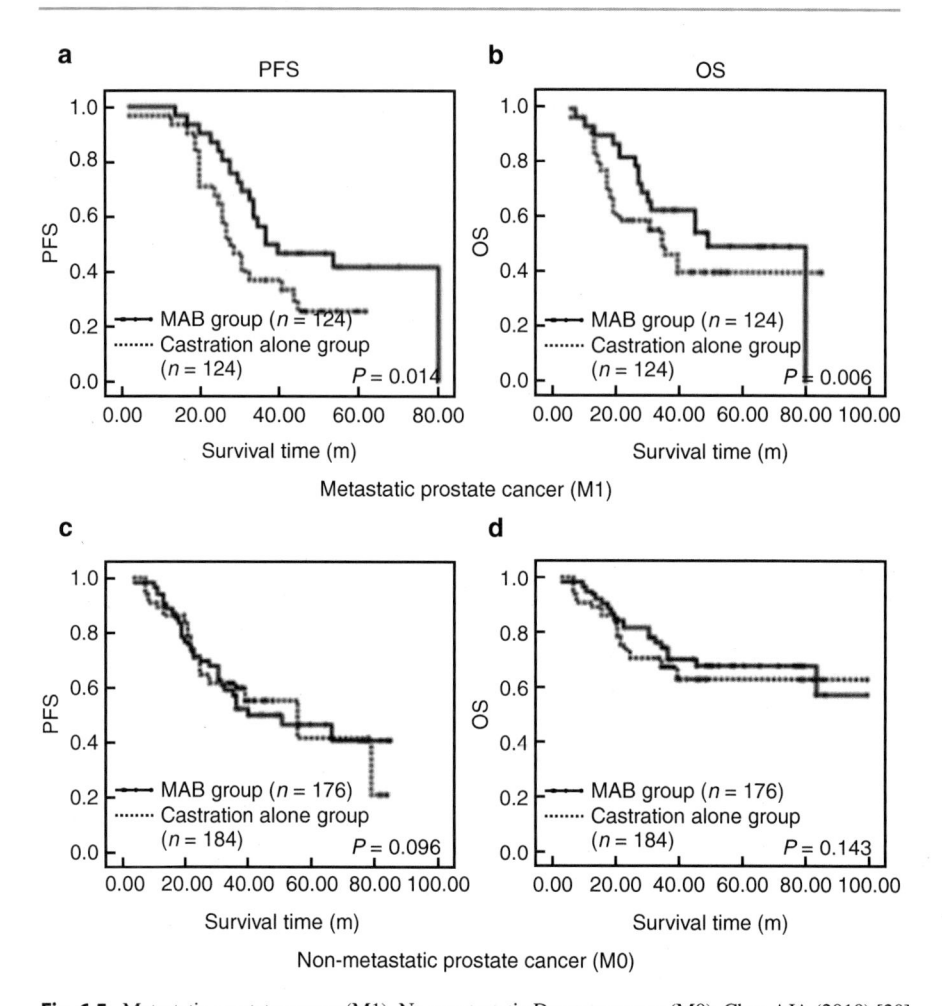

Fig. 6.5 Metastatic prostate cancer (M1). Non-metastatic Drostate cancer (M0), Chen AJA (2010) [20]

On the other hand, in a retrospective analysis conducted in China, for nonmetastatic prostate cancer, there was no significant difference observed in the overall survival between MAB (castration + bicalutamide or flutamide) and castration monotherapy. However, for metastatic prostate cancer, overall survival was clearly superior for MAB than for castration monotherapy (51.49 ± 16.83 vs. 45.26 ± 17.15 months, respectively; hazard ratio 0.794; 95% CI 0.627–0.954; $p = 0.006$) (Fig. 6.5) [20]. Taking this report also into account, responsiveness to hormone therapy appears better compared to that in Western countries. Thus, why does responsiveness to hormone therapy for prostate cancer differ between Western and Asian countries? This could possibly be attributed to ethnic differences. The overall survival and cancer-specific survival in prostate cancer patients who received hormone therapy for prostate cancer was better for Japanese-American men than Caucasian men living in Hawaii ($p = 0.001$ and 0.036) [21]. Furthermore, in an analysis using the Surveillance, Epidemiology, and End Results (SEER) registry, the median overall survival of patients who received hormone therapy was better for Asian patients than for other ethnic groups (30 months vs. 24–25 months, $p < 0.001$) [22]. Sensitivity to hormone therapy differs according to different ethnic groups, and therefore depending on ethnicity, the question of whether monotherapy or CAB is better might need to be considered.

In an effort to achieve a more reliable complete androgen blockade in CAB (MAB), some clinical studies are currently underway of the use of abiraterone acetate, which inhibits adrenal androgen synthesis completely, and LH-RH agonist, rather than antiandrogens. One clinical study showed the addition of abiraterone acetate and prednisone to castration in patients with newly diagnosed high-risk, metastatic, castration-sensitive prostate cancer significantly increased overall survival compared to the placebo group (castration only) (not reached vs. 34.7 months) (hazard ratio for death, 0.62; 95% CI, 0.51–0.76; $p < 0.001$) [23]. This clinical trial indicates that complete androgen blockade from the initial treatment might prolong overall survival. Physicians, however, must consider adverse effects of complete androgen blockade as an initial treatment and also the sequential treatment when castration-sensitive prostate cancer becomes CRPC after complete androgen blockade.

References

1. Klotz L, Schellhammer P, Carroll K. A re-assessment of the role of combined androgen blockade for advanced prostate cancer. BJU Int. 2004;93(9):1177–82.
2. Allen JM, O'Shea JP, Mashiter K, Williams G, Bloom SR. Advanced carcinoma of the prostate: treatment with a gonadotrophin releasing hormone agonist. Br Med J. 1983;286(6378):1607–9.
3. Warner B, Worgul TJ, Drago J, Demers L, Dufau M, Max D, Santen RJ. Effect of very high dose D-leucine6-gonadotropin-releasing hormone proethylamide on the hypothalamic-pituitary testicular axis in patients with prostatic cancer. J Clin Invest. 1983;71(6):1842–53.
4. Nicholson RI, Walker KJ, Turkes A, Turkes AO, Dyas J, Blamey RW, Campbell FC, Robinson MR, Griffiths K. Therapeutic significance and the mechanism of action of the LH-RH agonist ICI 118630 in breast and prostate cancer. J Steroid Biochem. 1984;20(1):129–35.
5. Jiang G, Stalewski J, Galyean R, Dykert J, Schteingart C, Broqua P, Aebi A, Aubert ML, Semple G, Robson P, Akinsanya K, Haigh R, Riviere P, Trojnar J, Junien JL, Rivier JE. GnRH antagonists: a new generation of long acting analogues incorporating p-ureido-phenylalanines at positions 5 and 6. J Med Chem. 2001;44(3):453–67.
6. Belanger A, Dupont A, Labrie F. Inhibition of basal and adrenocorticotropin-stimulated plasma levels of adrenal androgens after treatment with an antiandrogen in castrated patients with prostatic cancer. J Clin Endocrinol Metab. 1984;59(3):422–6.
7. Labrie F. Endocrine therapy for prostate cancer. Endocrinol Metab Clin N Am. 1991;20(4):845–72.
8. Nishiyama T, Hashimoto Y, Takahashi K. The influence of androgen deprivation therapy on dihydrotestosterone levels in the prostatic tissue of patients with prostate cancer. Clin Cancer Res. 2004;10(21):7121–6.
9. Mizokami A, Koh E, Fujita H, Maeda Y, Egawa M, Koshida K, Honma S, Keller ET, Namiki M. The adrenal androgen androstenediol is present in prostate cancer tissue after androgen deprivation therapy and activates mutated androgen receptor. Cancer Res. 2004;64(2):765–71.
10. Fizazi K, Scher HI, Molina A, Logothetis CJ, Chi KN, Jones RJ, Staffurth JN, North S, Vogelzang NJ, Saad F, Mainwaring P, Harland S, Goodman OB Jr, Sternberg CN, Li JH,

Kheoh T, Haqq CM, de Bono JS. Abiraterone acetate for treatment of metastatic castration-resistant prostate cancer: final overall survival analysis of the COU-AA-301 randomised, double-blind, placebo-controlled phase 3 study. Lancet Oncol. 2012;13(10):983–92.
11. Maximum androgen blockade in advanced prostate cancer: an overview of the randomised trials. Prostate Cancer Trialists' Collaborative Group. Lancet. 2000;355(9214):1491–8.
12. Crawford ED, Eisenberger MA, McLeod DG, Spaulding JT, Benson R, Dorr FA, Blumenstein BA, Davis MA, Goodman PJ. A controlled trial of leuprolide with and without flutamide in prostatic carcinoma. N Engl J Med. 1989;321(7):419–24.
13. Furr BJ, Valcaccia B, Curry B, Woodburn JR, Chesterson G, Tucker H. ICI 176,334: a novel non-steroidal, peripherally selective antiandrogen. J Endocrinol. 1987;113(3):R7–9.
14. Schellhammer PF, Sharifi R, Block NL, Soloway MS, Venner PM, Patterson AL, Sarosdy MF, Vogelzang NJ, Schellenger JJ, Kolvenbag GJ. Clinical benefits of bicalutamide compared with flutamide in combined androgen blockade for patients with advanced prostatic carcinoma: final report of a doubleblind, randomized, multicenter trial. Casodex Combination Study Group. Urology. 1997;50(3):330–6.
15. Caubet JF, Tosteson TD, Dong EW, Naylon EM, Whiting GW, Ernstoff MS, Ross SD. Maximum androgen blockade in advanced prostate cancer: a meta-analysis of published randomized controlled trials using nonsteroidal antiandrogens. Urology. 1997;49(1):71–8.
16. Gillessen S, Omlin A, Attard G, de Bono JS, Efstathiou E, Fizazi K, Halabi S, Nelson PS, Sartor O, Smith MR, Soule HR, Akaza H, Beer TM, Beltran H, Chinnaiyan AM, Daugaard G, Davis ID, de Santis M, Drake CG, Eeles RA, Fanti S, Gleave ME, Heidenreich A, Hussain M, James ND, Lecouvet FE, Logothetis CJ, Mastris K, Nilsson S, WK O, Olmos D, Padhani AR, Parker C, Rubin MA, Schalken JA, Scher HI, Sella A, Shore ND, Small EJ, Sternberg CN, Suzuki H, Sweeney CJ, Tannock IF, Tombal B. Management of patients with advanced prostate cancer: recommendations of the St Gallen advanced prostate cancer consensus conference (APCCC) 2015. Ann Oncol. 2015;26(8):1589–604.
17. Kotake T, Usami M, Isaka S, Shimazaki J, Nakano E, Okuyama A, Okajima E, Kanetake H, Saitoh Y, Kumamoto Y, Orikasa S, Sakata Y, Hosaka M, Akaza H, Koiso K, Honma Y, Aso Y, Oishi K, Yoshida O, Naitoh S, Kumazawa J, Koyanagi T, Yachiku S, Shiraiwa Y, Tsukagoshi S. Clinical early phase II study of bicalutamide (Casodex) in patients with prostatic cancer. Hinyokika Kiyo. 1996;42(2):157–68.
18. Akaza H, Hinotsu S, Usami M, Arai Y, Kanetake H, Naito S, Hirao Y. Combined androgen blockade with bicalutamide for advanced prostate cancer: long-term follow-up of a phase 3, double-blind, randomized study for survival. Cancer. 2009;115(15):3437–45.
19. Kadono Y, Nohara T, Ueno S, Izumi K, Kitagawa Y, Konaka H, Mizokami A, Onozawa M, Hinotsu S, Akaza H, Namiki M. Validation of TNM classification for metastatic prostate cancer treated using primary androgen deprivation therapy. World J Urol. 2016;34(2):261–7.
20. Chen XQ, Huang Y, Li X, Zhang P, Huang R, Xia J, Chen N, Wei Q, Zhu YC, Yang YR, Zeng H. Efficacy of maximal androgen blockade versus castration alone in the treatment of advanced prostate cancer: a retrospective clinical experience from a Chinese medical centre. Asian J Androl. 2010;12(5):718–27.
21. Fukagai T, Namiki TS, Carlile RG, Yoshida H, Namiki M. Comparison of the clinical outcome after hormonal therapy for prostate cancer between Japanese and Caucasian men. BJU Int. 2006;97(6):1190–3.
22. Bernard B, Muralidhar V, Chen YH, Sridhar SS, Mitchell EP, Pettaway CA, Carducci MA, Nguyen PL, Sweeney CJ. Impact of ethnicity on the outcome of men with metastatic, hormone-sensitive prostate cancer. Cancer. 2017;123(9):1536–44.
23. Fizazi K, Tran NP, Fein L, Matsubara N, Rodriguez-Antolin A, Alekseev BY, Özgüroğlu M, Ye D, Feyerabend S, Protheroe A, De Porre P, Kheoh T, Park YC, Todd MB, Chi KN, for the LATITUDE Investigators. Abiraterone plus prednisone in metastatic, castration-sensitive prostate cancer. N Engl J Med. 2017;377(4):352–60.

Adrenal Androgen in Prostate Cancer

7

Yasuhiro Shibata

Abstract

Recent progress in hormone determination method in prostate tissue had revealed that adrenal androgen exists abundantly in the prostate even after androgen deprivation therapy (ADT) for the treatment of prostate cancer. Dehydroepiandrosterone (DHEA) is the most existing adrenal androgen in prostate after ADT that serves as the substrate for the production of more active androgens by steroidal metabolism enzymes. Production of active androgens participates in cancer proliferation to become castration-resistant Pca (CRPC).

Keywords

Prostate cancer · Adrenal androgen · Metabolism · Enzyme · Castration resistant

7.1 Introduction

Since the prostate is an androgen-dependent organ, androgen is deeply involved in the development and progression of prostate cancer (PCa). Therefore, since Dr. Huggins, who received the Nobel Prize in 1966, discovered the effect of castration on PCa [1], androgen deprivation therapy (ADT) has been used widely as a standard treatment for advanced PCa. PCa regresses in almost all cases after initial ADT, but most patients have PCa relapse while continuing treatment and develop castration-resistant PCa (CRPC). There are various theories such as elevated expression and sensitivity of the androgen receptor (AR), activation of the coactivator, phosphorylation of the ligand-independent AR, and transmission of the proliferation signal without AR intervention [2]. The

Y. Shibata
Department of Urology, Gunma University Graduate School of Medicine, Maebashi, Gunma, Japan
e-mail: yash@gunma-u.ac.jp

Y. Arai, O. Ogawa (eds.), *Hormone Therapy and Castration Resistance of Prostate Cancer*, https://doi.org/10.1007/978-981-10-7013-6_7

involvement of adrenal androgen is another theory. More than 90% of testosterone, the main active androgen in adult men, is derived from the testes, while the remaining 5% is said to originate from adrenal-derived androgens. Since testis-derived androgens are almost completely suppressed when ADT is administered, adrenal-derived androgens are involved in the proliferation of PCa after ADT.

Early studies reported that bilateral adrenalectomy or hypophysectomy results in pain relief in the majority of patients with CRPC and objective improvements in one-third of them [3]. Medical adrenalectomy with aminoglutethimide or ketoconazole also showed similar responses in patients with CRPC [4, 5]. In clinical practice, combined androgen blockade (CAB), which uses an oral antiandrogen in addition to surgical or medical castration, was developed to suppress the action of adrenal androgens and is reported to improve the survival rate [6, 7]. In addition, the effectiveness of abiraterone acetate, an inhibitor of the steroid metabolizing enzyme CYP17A1 that is involved in the synthesis of dehydroepiandrosterone (DHEA) in the adrenal gland, has been confirmed [8]. These facts suggest that adrenal-derived androgens are involved in the proliferation of PCa, especially CRPC.

7.2 Evaluation of Prostate Androgen Concentration by Highly Sensitive Quantitative Analysis

Regarding adrenal-derived androgens and PCa, it is important to establish the accurate quantification method for prostate tissue steroid hormones. It is difficult to precisely evaluate tissue hormones, but recent advances in analytical methods using liquid chromatography–tandem mass spectrometry (LC-MS/MS) with chemical derivatization and purification of the target hormones have enabled prostate hormone quantification from a small amount of tissue with high sensitivity and reliability. Using this method, it is possible to quantify multiple hormones simultaneously in a very small amount of tissue such as a needle biopsy specimen.

A brief explanation of the actual quantification is as follows. After tissue homogenization, internal standards labeled with an isotope were added, and the steroidal fraction was extracted. The fraction was purified as shown in Fig. 7.1.

This highly sensitive quantitative method was validated, and the lower analytical limit was 2 pg for dehydroepiandrosterone (DHEA) and 1 pg for androstenedione (Adione), androstenediol (Adiol), testosterone (T), and dihydrotestosterone (DHT). Details of the quantification method were reported previously [9].

Figure 7.2 shows the results of the prostate tissue androgen analysis of PCa patients, PCa patients after ADT, and patients with benign prostatic hypertrophy, using the quantification method. After ADT, blood T level rapidly decreased to 5–10% of the normal level, followed by a decrease in prostate T and DHT levels. In contrast, DHEA, an adrenal-derived androgen, is invariant and exists at a considerably higher concentration than other androgens. Adione and Adiol are also unaffected by ADT, suggesting the conversion from substrate DHEA. Furthermore, even after ADT, T and DHT in the prostate existed at 29% and 8% of the pretreatment levels, respectively [9].

Fig. 7.1 Flow sheet of the analytical method (quotation from Ref. no. [9])

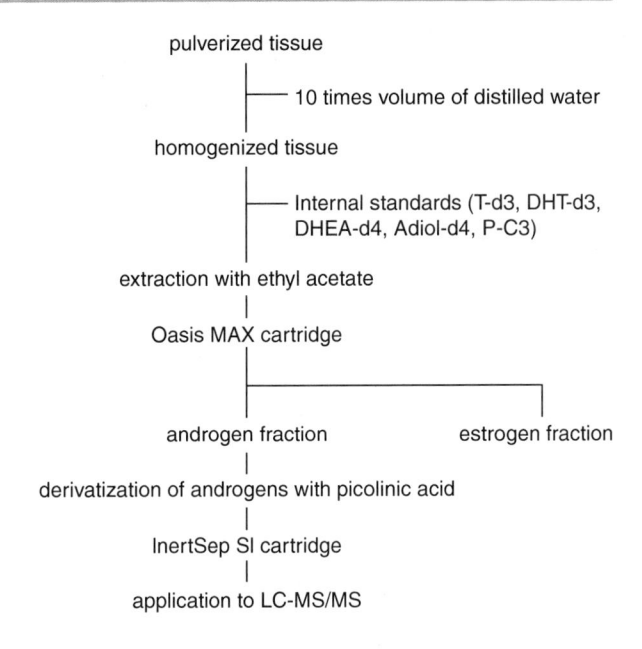

```
                    pulverized tissue
                           |
                           ├── 10 times volume of distilled water
                           |
                    homogenized tissue
                           |
                           ├── Internal standards (T-d3, DHT-d3,
                           |    DHEA-d4, Adiol-d4, P-C3)
                           |
                  extraction with ethyl acetate
                           |
                    Oasis MAX cartridge
                    ┌──────┴──────┐
              androgen fraction   estrogen fraction
                    |
       derivatization of androgens with picolinic acid
                    |
             InertSep SI cartridge
                    |
            application to LC-MS/MS
```

7.3 Hormone Metabolism in the Prostate

Steroid hormones are metabolized by the metabolic enzyme shown in Fig. 7.3, and active androgens are produced in the tissue. Hormonal treatments alter the hormone compositions in the prostate that may affect the enzymatic activity in the tissue.

For example, in clinical practice, when a 5α-reductase inhibitor is administered to a patient with benign prostatic hyperplasia, T accumulates due to the suppression of metabolism of T to DHT, while the reverse metabolism from T to Adione is enhanced. In the metabolic analysis of tissues using isotope label substrates, metabolism from T to Adione is enhanced 42 times the normal level. The accumulation of substrate T and metabolism of T to Adione results in increased concentrations of T and Adione to 70 and 11 times the normal level, respectively [10]. This finding indicates that metabolism is enhanced by an increase in converting enzyme activity, mainly HSD17B2, which is responsible for the metabolism of T to Adione (Fig. 7.4). In this manner, when the hormone composition in the tissue is changed by hormone treatment, a subsequent change in enzyme activity occurs.

7.4 Role of Adrenal-Derived Androgens in PCa

As described above, when ADT is administered, T and DHT levels in the prostate rapidly decrease, and the hormone composition changes. DHEA derived from the adrenal gland exists abundantly in the prostate even after ADT. The androgen receptor in CRPC is thought to be hypersensitive, so although the androgenic activity of DHEA is low, it contributes to PCa progression [11].

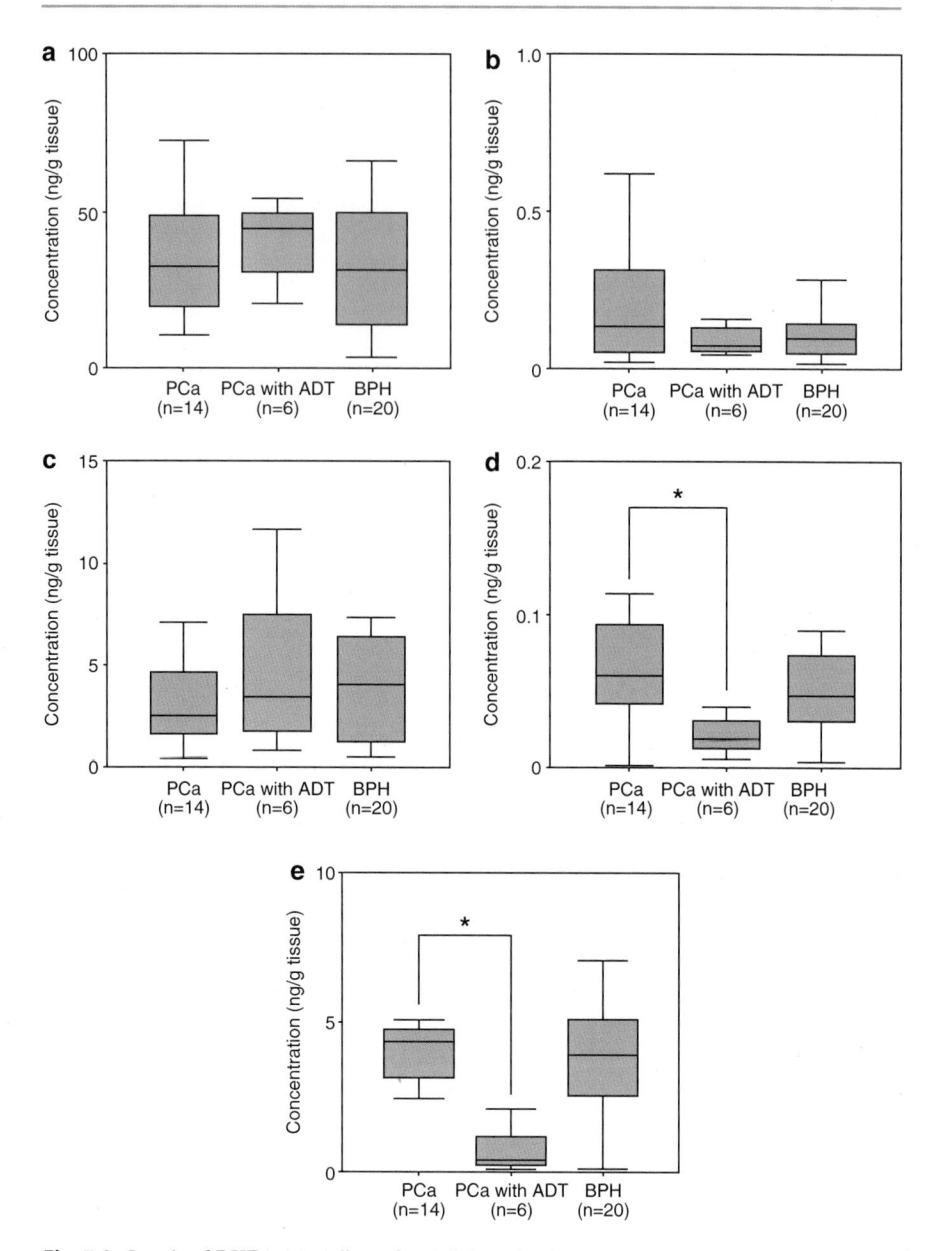

Fig. 7.2 Levels of DHEA (**a**), Adione (**b**), Adiol (**c**), T (**d**), and DHT (**e**) in PCa, PCa with ADT, and BPH (quotation from Ref. no. [9]). The gray-shaded areas represent the upper and lower quartiles, with the black bar representing the median intensity of the samples within each group. *$p < 0.05$

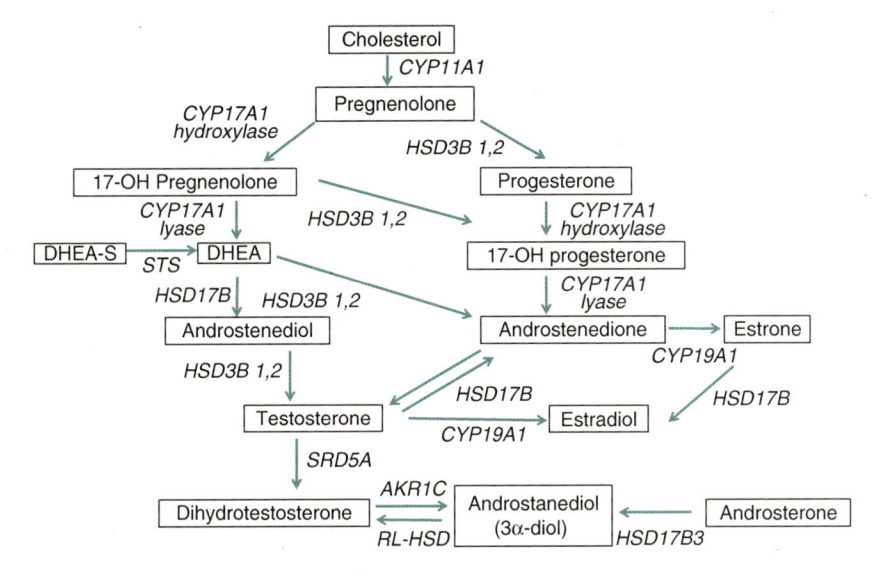

Fig. 7.3 Steroid pathway and metabolic enzymes

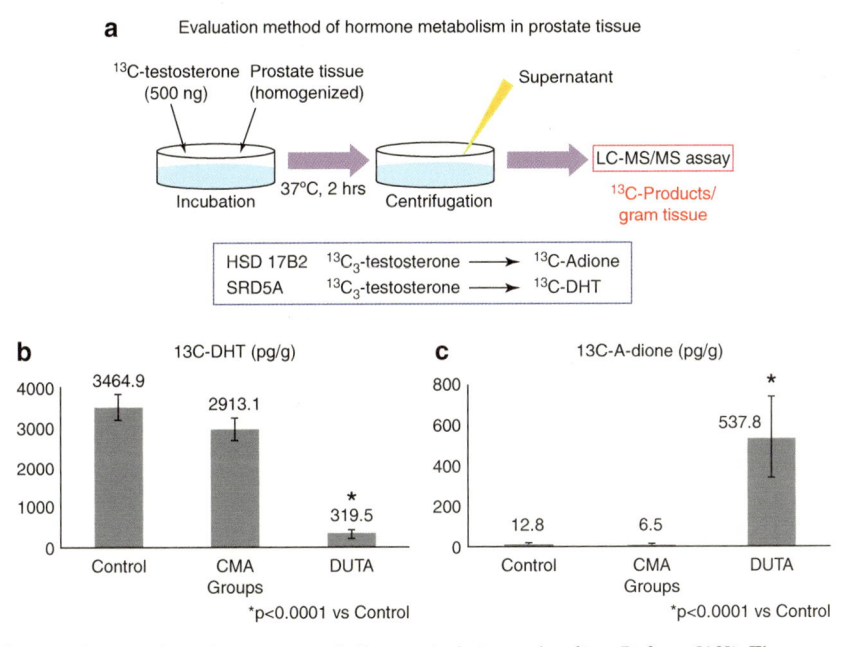

Fig. 7.4 Prostate tissue hormone metabolism analysis (quotation from Ref. no. [10]). The conversion of T to 4-androstene-3,17-dione and DHT in the prostate tissue was analyzed using ^{13}C-labeled T combined with LC-MS/MS hormone determination (**a**). The conversion of ^{13}C-T to ^{13}C-DHT was significantly suppressed in the DUTA group (**b**, $p < 0.0001$). Conversion of ^{13}C-T to ^{13}C-4-androstene-3,17-dione was significantly accelerated in the DUTA group (**c**, $p < 0.0001$). *LC-MS/MS* liquid chromatography–tandem mass spectrometry, *HSD17B2* hydroxysteroid 17-beta dehydrogenase 2, *SRD5A* steroid 5-alpha reductase, *CMA* chlormadinone acetate, *DUTA* dutasteride, *DHT* dihydrotestosterone, *Adione* 4-androstene-3,17-dione, *T* testosterone

All of the enzymes required for the production of DHT from DHEA exist in the prostate gland, and produced T and DHT may contribute to PCa progression. El-Alfy et al. demonstrated that 3-hydroxysteroid dehydrogenase (3-HSD), which catalyzes conversion of DHEA into Adione, and type 5 17-HSD, which catalyzes conversion of Adione into T, are expressed in the stromal fibroblasts in the prostate [12]. Nakamura et al. have revealed that types 5 17-HSD and 5-reductase, which catalyze conversion of T to DHT, are expressed in the majority of PCa [13]. Mizokami et al. demonstrated that PCa stromal cells and LNCaP cells coordinately activate AR via the synthesis of T and DHT from DHEA [14]. Stanbrough et al. reported that the expressions of metabolic enzymes such as HSD3B2, AKR1C3, SRD5A1, and AKR1C2 involved in androgen production are elevated in relapsed PCa and its metastatic bone marrow. As a result of increased activity of these enzymes involved in androgen synthesis, metabolism to Adiol, Adione, T, and DHT occurs in an intracrine manner in the PCa tissue even after ADT [15]. Montgomery et al. revealed that tissue T levels in metastases of PCa from anorchid men were significantly higher than those in primary PCa from untreated eugonadal men [16]. Locke et al. used the LNCaP xenograft model to show that the expression of enzymes involved in androgen synthesis was partly increased during the course of CRPC development [17]. Since DHEA was the most existing androgen precursor in PCa tissues after ADT, these findings suggested that the enhanced intraprostatic synthesis of T and DHT from adrenal androgens, especially DHEA, might account for the development of CRPC from androgen-dependent PCa after ADT.

DHT produced in the prostate is thought to activate the AR of PCa cells, which are androgen hypersensitive. To suppress the action of this androgen, abiraterone acetate, a CYP17A1 inhibitor that inhibits the synthesis of adrenal androgens, or MDV 3100, an AR antagonist that has high antagonistic activity against various affinity and mutant androgen receptors, has been clinically applied and demonstrated useful. Accordingly, trace amounts of active androgens produced in the prostate are becoming increasingly important to treatment strategies for PCa.

Conclusion

The importance of adrenal-derived androgens in PCa proliferation is obvious from the effectiveness of clinical application of abiraterone acetate, a CYP17A1 inhibitor involved in DHEA synthesis in the adrenal gland. This adrenal-derived androgen is abundant even after ADT and metabolized in the PCa tissue to T and DHT, activates the AR, and then affects PCa proliferation and progression. This is particularly true in cases of PCa that become CRPC.

Furthermore, in recent years, it has been reported that the tumor itself in CRPC tissues expresses the enzymes involved in androgen synthesis from cholesterol, enabling de novo production of active androgens. The development of further new treatment strategies targeting the control of steroid metabolism in the tissues is eagerly awaited.

References

1. Huggins C, Hodges CV. Studies on prostatic cancer: I. The effect of castration, of estrogen and of androgen injection on serum phosphatases in metastatic carcinoma of the prostate. Cancer Res. 1941;1:293–7.
2. Azzouni F, Mohler J. Biology of castration-recurrent prostate cancer. Urol Clin North Am. 2012;39:435–52.
3. Mahoney EM, Harrison JH. Bilateral adrenalectomy for palliative treatment of prostatic cancer. J Urol. 1972;108:936–8.
4. Drago JR, Santen RJ, Lipton A, Worgul TJ, Harvey HA, Boucher A, Manni A, Rohner TJ. Clinical effect of aminoglutethimide, medical adrenalectomy, in treatment of 43 patients with advanced prostatic carcinoma. Cancer. 1984;53:1447–50.
5. Small EJ, Halabi S, Dawson NA, Stadler WM, Rini BI, Picus J, Gable P, Torti FM, Kaplan E, Vogelzang NJ. Antiandrogen withdrawal alone or in combination with ketoconazole in androgen-independent prostate cancer patients: a phase III trial (CALGB 9583). J Clin Oncol. 2004;22:1025–33.
6. Prostate Cancer Trialists' Collaborative Group. Maximum androgen blockade in advanced prostate cancer: an overview of the randomised trials. Lancet. 2000;355:1491–8.
7. Akaza H, Hinotsu S, Usami M, Arai Y, Kanetake H, Naito S, Hirao Y, Study Group for the Combined Androgen Blockade Therapy of Prostate Cancer. Combined androgen blockade with bicalutamide for advanced prostate cancer: long-term follow-up of a phase 3, double-blind, randomized study for survival. Cancer. 2009;115:3437–45.
8. de Bono JS, Logothetis CJ, Molina A, Fizazi K, North S, Chu L, Chi KN, Jones RJ, Goodman OB Jr, Saad F, Staffurth JN, Mainwaring P, Harland S, Flaig TW, Hutson TE, Cheng T, Patterson H, Hainsworth JD, Ryan CJ, Sternberg CN, Ellard SL, Fléchon A, Saleh M, Scholz M, Efstathiou E, Zivi A, Bianchini D, Loriot Y, Chieffo N, Kheoh T, Haqq CM, Scher HI, COU-AA-301 Investigators. Abiraterone and increased survival in metastatic prostate cancer. N Engl J Med. 2011;364:1995–2005.
9. Arai S, Miyashiro Y, Shibata Y, Tomaru Y, Kobayashi M, Honma S, Suzuki K. Effect of castration monotherapy on the levels of adrenal androgens in cancerous prostatic tissues. Steroids. 2011;76:301–8.
10. Shibata Y, Arai S, Miyazawa Y, Shuto T, Nomura M, Sekine Y, Koike H, Matsui H, Ito K, Suzuki K. Effects of steroidal antiandrogen or 5-alpha-reductase inhibitor on prostate tissue hormone content. Prostate. 2017;77:672–80.
11. Tan J, Sharief Y, Hamil KG, Gregory CW, Zang DY, Sar M, Gumerlock PH, deVere White RW, Pretlow TG, Harris SE, Wilson EM, Mohler JL, French FS. Dehydroepiandrosterone activates mutant androgen receptors expressed in the androgen-dependent human prostate cancer xenograft CWR22 and LNCaP cells. Mol Endocrinol. 1997;11:450–9.
12. El-Alfy M, Luu-The V, Huang XF, Berger L, Labrie F, Pelletier G. Localization of type 5 17beta-hydroxysteroid dehydrogenase, 3beta-hydroxysteroid dehydrogenase, and androgen receptor in the human prostate by in situ hybridization and immunocytochemistry. Endocrinology. 1999;140:1481–91.
13. Nakamura Y, Suzuki T, Nakabayashi M, Endoh M, Sakamoto K, Mikami Y, Moriya T, Ito A, Takahashi S, Yamada S, Arai Y, Sasano H. In situ androgen producing enzymes in human prostate cancer. Endocr Relat Cancer. 2005;12:101–7.
14. Mizokami A, Koh E, Izumi K, Narimoto K, Takeda M, Honma S, Dai J, Keller ET, Namiki M. Prostate cancer stromal cells and LNCaP cells coordinately activate the androgen receptor through synthesis of testosterone and dihydrotestosterone from dehydroepiandrosterone. Endocr Relat Cancer. 2009;16:1139–55.
15. Stanbrough M, Bubley GJ, Ross K, Golub TR, Rubin MA, Penning TM, Febbo PG, Balk SP. Increased expression of genes converting adrenal androgens to testosterone in androgen-independent prostate cancer. Cancer Res. 2006;66:2815–25.

16. Montgomery RB, Mostaghel EA, Vessella R, Hess DL, Kalhorn TF, Higano CS, True LD, Nelson PS. Maintenance of intratumoral androgens in metastatic prostate cancer: a mechanism for castration-resistant tumor growth. Cancer Res. 2008;68:4447–54.
17. Locke JA, Guns ES, Lubik AA, Adomat HH, Hendy SC, Wood CA, Ettinger SL, Gleave ME, Nelson CC. Androgen levels increase by intratumoral de novo steroidogenesis during progression of castration-resistant prostate cancer. Cancer Res. 2008;68:6407–15.

Intermittent ADT for Prostate Cancer

Koichiro Akakura

Abstract

Intermittent ADT (androgen deprivation therapy) was proposed to prolong androgen dependency of prostate cancer and was found to possess potential benefits of reduced toxicities during the off-treatment period. For application of intermittent ADT, ADT with LHRH agonist or antagonist is introduced, and those who show PSA response are candidates of intermittent ADT. Then ADT is terminated, and serum PSA and testosterone are measured every 3–6 months. When PSA reaches a certain level, ADT is resumed. This cycle of on- and off-treatment is repeated. According to systematic reviews and meta-analyses comparisons between intermittent versus continuous ADT, no significant difference was revealed in terms of overall survival, time to progression, and cancer-specific survival. There was a tendency favor of intermittent ADT for adverse effects and QOL. Therefore, intermittent ADT is considered as one of the standards of care for prostate cancer patients who show PSA failure after curative therapy or have advanced disease. Tasks to be resolved are to establish selection of good candidates and to determine an optimal and personalized method of intermittent ADT.

Keywords

Prostate cancer · Androgen deprivation therapy · Intermittent · Testosterone PSA

K. Akakura
Department of Urology, Japan Community Health-care Organization (JCHO) Tokyo Shinjuku Medical Center, Tokyo, Japan
e-mail: akakurak@ae.auone-net.jp

8.1 Introduction

For the management of advanced prostate cancer, hormone therapy has been utilized as a principal modality of treatment. Since surgical castration was introduced, hormone therapy continues to be one of the most common strategies effected by means of androgen deprivation therapy (ADT). Although the initial effect of ADT is prominent, progression to androgen-independent status (castration-resistant prostate cancer) often occurs within a few years. Therefore, several attempts have been made to maintain the androgen-dependent status of the tumor for as long as possible. In addition, a variety of adverse effects may be associated with ADT, which include hot flush, sexual dysfunction, metabolic disorders, and osteoporosis. The long-term use of ADT would contribute to the development of those adverse effects. Intermittent ADT was proposed to prolong androgen dependency of prostate cancer [1] and was found to possess potential benefits of reduced toxicities during the off-treatment period.

8.2 Concept of Intermittent ADT

In general, adenocarcinoma of the prostate shows androgen dependency; the tumor develops and grows in the presence of androgen and regresses through apoptosis by deprivation of androgen. However, the regressed tumor progresses after a while and becomes androgen independent. In in vitro and in vivo experiments using androgen-dependent tumor models, androgen dependency can be maintained in the presence of androgen; androgen-dependent cancer cell lines can be serially cultured in the physiological concentration of androgen in the medium, and androgen-dependent xenografts are successfully transplanted into the male hosts. However, long-term deprivation of androgen causes these cancer cells to become androgen independent. Androgen deprivation could be a trigger for progression to an androgen-independent status. Therefore, it is hypothesized that when the androgen-dependent tumor regresses following androgen deprivation, if androgen is replaced again, the tumor might recover the potency of apoptosis induced by androgen deprivation. Accordingly, it is expected that, by repeated cycles of androgen deprivation and replacement, androgen dependency of the tumor could be maintained for a longer time period (Fig. 8.1) [1].

8.3 Intermittent ADT in Animal Models

Shionogi carcinoma is an androgen-dependent mouse mammary tumor; surgical castration of a tumor-bearing male mouse results in regression of the tumor through induction of apoptosis. Using the Shionogi model, four to five cycles of tumor regression and regrowth were obtained by repeated androgen deprivation and replacement [1]. In a human prostate cancer cell line, LNCaP, which is transplanted into nude mice, serum PSA level was maintained in an androgen-dependent manner for a longer period by intermittent ADT, compared with continuous ADT [2]. On the

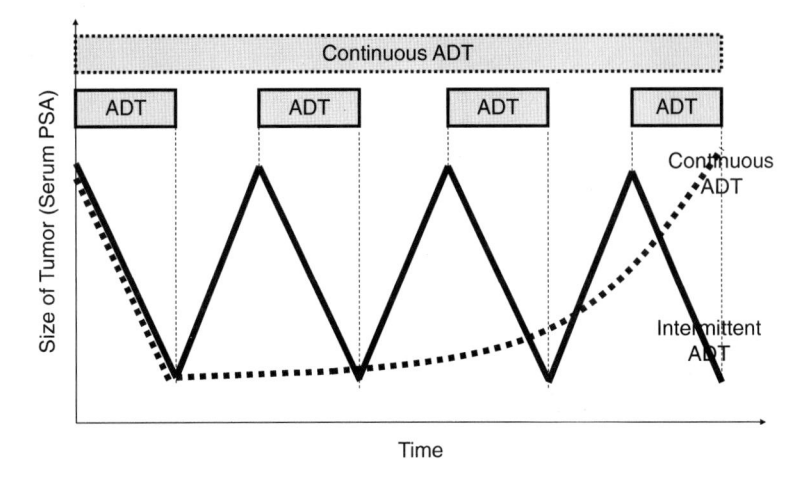

Fig. 8.1 Schematic of the course of intermittent versus continuous ADT

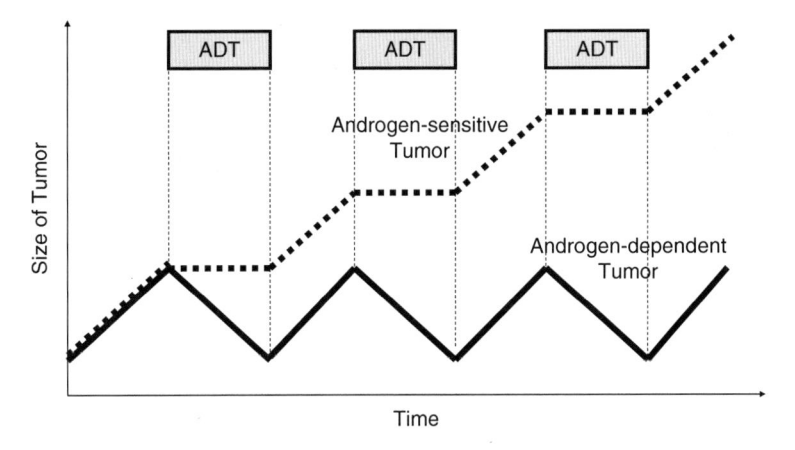

Fig. 8.2 Schematic of the course of intermittent ADT for androgen-dependent or androgen-sensitive tumor

contrary, in an androgen-sensitive but -independent rat prostate cancer xenograft, the Dunning R3327H tumor, intermittent ADT was inferior to continuous ADT. Intermittent ADT in the Dunning tumor demonstrated cycles of stabilization and growth of the tumor during on- and off-treatment periods, respectively (Fig. 8.2) [3]. Therefore, to obtain the benefits of intermittent ADT, the tumor must be strictly androgen dependent; the tumor regresses by androgen deprivation.

8.4 Clinical Experiences of Intermittent ADT

The development of reversible hormonal agents such as LHRH agonists/antagonists or antiandrogens and prevalence of serum prostate-specific antigen (PSA) as a reliable and feasible tool for monitoring made it possible to apply ADT intermittently.

Based on the promising results of investigational research using an androgen-dependent animal model, our group in Vancouver reported 47 cases of prostate cancer treated with intermittent ADT [4]. Thereafter, a number of clinical experiences of intermittent ADT have been published for various stages of prostate cancer by different methods and for different durations of ADT [5]. Most of the studies demonstrated promising results and emphasized improved QOL by intermittent ADT [6]. Moreover, a recent report described a lower risk of heart failure and fracture in intermittent ADT than in continuous ADT [7].

8.5 Randomized Controlled Trials and Meta-analyses/Systematic Reviews Comparing Intermittent Versus Continuous ADT

Several randomized controlled trials (RCT) have been conducted to compare the efficacy of intermittent and continuous ADT (Table 8.1) [8–16]. All trials except for the SWOG 9346 trial [13] showed similar or non-inferior outcomes with intermittent ADT than those with continuous ADT. On the other hand, most trials pointed out the benefits of intermittent ADT with regard to adverse effects and QOL.

In the SWOG 9346 trial [13], overall survivals had been compared between intermittent versus continuous ADT in the metastatic prostate cancer patients. The median overall survivals were 5.1 years in intermittent ADT and 5.8 years in continuous ADT, and the hazard ratio was estimated to be 1.09 (90% confidence interval, 0.95–1.24). Since the obtained 90% confidence interval exceeded 1.20 (the upper boundary for non-inferiority), non-inferiority of intermittent ADT was not supported compared to continuous ADT. In this study, the included cases consisted of metastatic patients only, and the PSA level to resume ADT was set at 20 ng/mL. Thus, it is suggested that intermittent ADT would not be suitable for the far-advanced prostate cancer patients with systemic metastasis.

Crook et al. reported the result of RCT in a patient who demonstrated PSA failure after definitive radiotherapy for prostate cancer [11]. The hazard ratio of overall survival was estimated to be 1.03 (95% confidence interval, 0.87–1.22), showing non-inferiority of intermittent ADT compared to continuous ADT.

The comparisons between intermittent and continuous ADT in several systematic reviews and meta-analyses of RCTs were published [17–22]. No significant difference was revealed in terms of overall survival, time to progression, and cancer-specific survival. There was a tendency favor of intermittent ADT for adverse effects and QOL.

A recently reported randomized controlled trial showed that in patients with a rising PSA after curative therapy, immediate ADT significantly improved overall survival compared with delayed ADT [23]. In this trial, the majority of patients had been treated with intermittent ADT in both arms (immediate ADT arm, 67%; delayed ADT arm, 65%). Therefore, for patients with PSA failure after curative therapy, if systemic therapy is considered, immediate initiation of intermittent ADT would be recommended.

Table 8.1 Randomized controlled trials comparisons of intermittent versus continuous ADT

Year	Author	Randomized patients	Subjects	PSA for stop	PSA for restart
2002	de Leval	68	Locally adv/met/rec	<4	>10
2009	Calais da Silva	626	Locally adv/met	<4/<80%	>10/>20%
2012	Salonen	554	Locally adv/met	<10/<50%	>20
2012	Crook	690	PSA failure after RTx	<4	>10
2012	Mottet	173	Met	<4	>10/symptom
2013	Hussain	1535	Met	<4	>20
2013	Langenhuijsen	193	Met	<4	>10 or 20
2014	Calais da Silva	918	Locally adv/met	<4	>20/symptom
2016	Schulman	701	Locally adv/rec	<1	>2.5
Author	**Time to progression**	**Cancer-specific survival**	**Overall survival**		
de Leval	7.0% vs. 38.9% (3-year rate, $p = 0.0052$)				
Calais da Silva	HR 0.81 (0.63–1.05)		HR 0.99 (0.80–1.23)		
Salonen	HR 1.08 (0.90–1.29)	HR 1.17 (0.91–1.51)	HR 1.15 (0.94–1.40)		
Crook		HR 1.23 (0.94–1.66)			
Mottet	20.7 vs. 15.1 (months, $p = 0.74$)		42 vs. 52 (months, $p = 0.75$)		
Hussain			HR 1.10 (0.99–1.23*)		
Langenhuijsen	18.0 vs. 24.1 (months)				
Calais da Silva			HR 0.90 (0.76–1.07)		
Schulman	30 vs. 34 (events, $p = 0.718$)		42 vs. 44 (events, $p = 0.969$)		

Adv, advanced; *met*, metastatic; *rec*, recurrent; *RTx*, radiation therapy; *HR*, hazard ratio (95% confidence interval); *90% confidence interval

8.6 Clinical Guidelines Concerning Intermittent ADT

Although intermittent ADT has been previously classified as an experimental method of treatment, the latest guidelines strongly recommend intermittent ADT especially for patients who demonstrate PSA failure after treatment with curative intent. Guidelines on prostate cancer by the European Association of Urology recommend that if salvage ADT (postprimary radiotherapy) is started, intermittent ADT is offered to responding patients, and that in asymptomatic M1 patients, intermittent ADT is offered to highly motivated men. According to NCCN Guidelines Version 2.2017 on prostate cancer, in ADT for biochemical failure without metastasis, men who choose ADT should consider intermittent ADT.

8.7 Methods of Intermittent ADT

Generally, ADT with LHRH agonist or antagonist is utilized for intermittent hormone therapy, and the majority of guidelines recommend suppression of testosterone for application of intermittent hormone therapy. Although a few attempts have been made to use antiandrogen or estrogen intermittently [24, 25] and such method of intermittent hormone therapy has potential benefits of less adverse effects and cost, there has been no confirmed evidence to demonstrate the usefulness of intermittent administration of antiandrogen or estrogen. There is no consensus on the use of combined androgen blockade (LHRH agonist/antagonist plus antiandrogen) for intermittent ADT. However, it may be advised to add antiandrogen at induction of LHRH agonist of each cycle of ADT to prevent the flare-up phenomenon by a transient increase in serum testosterone.

For monitoring, serial (every 3–6 months) measurements of serum PSA are recommended along with assessment of symptoms. When consecutive increase in serum PSA is observed during the ADT period, or clinical evidence of disease progression is demonstrated, intermittent ADT should be considered as failure for the patient and they should be moved to continuous ADT.

8.8 Advantages and Disadvantages of Intermittent ADT

With intermittent ADT, it is possible to achieve several benefits. The incidence and degree of adverse effects of ADT decrease or improve by intermittent ADT. Most of the adverse effects, including sexual dysfunction, hot flush, and fatigue, cease during the off-treatment period, and the risk of cardiovascular events and osteoporosis may be reduced by intermittent ADT [7]. Several domains of the quality of life are improved by stopping ADT [6]. From the economical point of view, cost of treatment is reduced by intermittent ADT, compared to continuous ADT as far as the same agent is used. Finally, it may be expected that intermittent ADT will achieve prolonged progression-free and overall survival.

As for the disadvantages of intermittent ADT, during its application, frequent measurements of serum PSA and testosterone are required. Although there is no certainty whether the prostate cancer will be cured by ADT, chances of cure might be missed by stopping the therapy. Although serum PSA is thought to be a useful marker for monitoring the disease status, there is a risk of developing progression without elevation of serum PSA during intermittent ADT.

8.9 Future Directions for Intermittent ADT

Intermittent ADT was initially used for patients with metastatic or advanced prostate cancer. However, recently observed stage shift to early disease, probably due to the prevalence of serum PSA measurements, resulted in a dramatic increase in the number of curative therapies used, such as radical prostatectomy and radiotherapy. In recent times, a number of patients develop PSA failure after curative therapy. Some of these patients are treated with ADT and may be under control for a long time period. Therefore, adverse effects of ADT will be serious problems for those patients, and intermittent ADT could be an option for the long-term management of prostate cancer patients without metastasis. In general, it is supposed that intermittent ADT has been widely used in localized, locally advanced, metastatic, or recurrent prostate cancer patients for the purpose of QOL improvement and cost reduction [26].

Meta-analysis studies demonstrated significant factors for progression-free survival for patients treated with intermittent ADT [27]. However, good candidates for intermittent ADT are still unknown. Moreover, a number of questions are still to be answered: Which is the appropriate method of ADT for each patient, LHRH agonist, LHRH antagonist, antiandrogen alone, or combined androgen blockade? At which PSA levels should therapy be terminated and restarted? To resolve these, accumulation of clinical data is crucial. Recent studies of mathematical models of intermittent ADT may be able to determine the future course of each patient by a precise analysis of PSA kinetics [28–30]. This model will be extremely useful for the establishment of personalization of intermittent ADT, selection of good candidates, and optimization of the method and duration of ADT for each patient.

References

1. Akakura K, Bruchovsky N, Goldenberg SL, Rennie PS, Buckley AR, Sullivan LD. Effects of intermittent androgen suppression on androgen-dependent tumors: apoptosis and serum prostate-specific antigen. Cancer. 1993;71:2782–90.
2. Sato N, Gleave ME, Bruchovsky N, Rennie PS, Goldenberg SL, Lange PH, Sullivan LD. Intermittent androgen suppression delays progression to androgen-independent regulation of prostate-specific antigen gene in the LNCaP prostate tumour model. J Steroid Biochem Mol Biol. 1996;58:139–46.
3. Trachtenberg J. Experimental treatment of prostatic cancer by intermittent hormonal therapy. J Urol. 1987;137:785–8.

4. Goldenberg SL, Bruchovsky N, Gleave ME, Sullivan LD, Akakura K. Intermittent androgen suppression in the treatment of prostate cancer: a preliminary report. Urology. 1995;45:839–44.
5. Abrahamsson PA. Potential benefits of intermittent androgen suppression therapy in the treatment of prostate cancer: a systematic review of the literature. Eur Urol. 2010;57:49–59.
6. Sato N, Akakura K, Isaka S, Nakatsu H, Tanaka M, Ito H, Masai M, Chiba Prostate Study Group. Intermittent androgen suppression for locally advanced and metastatic prostate cancer: preliminary report of a prospective multicenter study. Urology. 2004;64:341–5.
7. Tsai HT, Pfeiffer RM, Philips GK, Barac A, AZ F, Penson DF, Zhou Y, Potosky AL. Risks of serious toxicities from intermittent versus continuous androgen deprivation therapy for advanced prostate cancer: a population based study. J Urol. 2017;197:1251–7.
8. de Leval J, Boca P, Yousef E, Nicolas H, Jeukenne M, Seidel L, Bouffioux C, Coppens L, Bonnet P, Andrianne R, Wlatregny D. Intermittent versus continuous total androgen blockade in the treatment of patients with advanced hormone-naïve prostate cancer: results of a prospective randomized multicenter trial. Clin Prostate Cancer. 2002;1:163–71.
9. Calais da Silva FE, Bono AV, Whelan P, Brausi M, Marques Queimadelos A, Martin JA, Kirkali Z, Calais da Silva FM, Robertson C. Intermittent androgen deprivation for locally advanced and metastatic prostate cancer: results from a randomised phase 3 study of the South European Uroncological Group. Eur Urol. 2009;55:1269–77.
10. Salonen AJ, Taari K, Ala-Opas M, Viitanen J, Lundstedt S, Tammela TL, FinnProstate Group. The FinnProstate Study VII: intermittent versus continuous androgen deprivation in patients with advanced prostate cancer. J Urol. 2012;187:2074–81.
11. Crook JM, O'Callaghan CJ, Duncan G, Dearnaley DP, Higano CS, Horwitz EM, Frymire E, Malone S, Chin J, Nabid A, Warde P, Corbett T, Angyalfi S, Goldenberg SL, Gospodarowicz MK, Saad F, Logue JP, Hall E, Schellhammer PF, Ding K, Klotz L. Intermittent androgen suppression for rising PSA level after radiotherapy. N Engl J Med. 2012;367:895–903.
12. Mottet N, Van Damme J, Loulidi S, Russel C, Leitenberger A, Wolff JM, TAP22 Investigators Group. Intermittent hormonal therapy in the treatment of metastatic prostate cancer: a randomized trial. BJU Int. 2012;110:1262–9.
13. Hussain M, Tangen CM, Berry DL, Higano CS, Crawford ED, Liu G, Wilding G, Prescott S, Kanaga Sundaram S, Small EJ, Dawson NA, Donnelly BJ, Venner PM, Vaishampayan UN, Schellhammer PF, Quinn DI, Raghavan D, Ely B, Moinpour CM, Vogelzang NJ, Thompson IM Jr. Intermittent versus continuous androgen deprivation in prostate cancer. N Engl J Med. 2013;368:1314–25.
14. Langenhuijsen JF, Badhauser D, Schaaf B, Kiemeney LA, Witjes JA, Mulders PF. Continuous vs. intermittent androgen deprivation therapy for metastatic prostate cancer. Urol Oncol. 2013;31:549–56.
15. Calais da Silva F, Calais da Silva FM, Gonçalves F, Santos A, Kliment J, Whelan P, Oliver T, Antoniou N, Pastidis S, Marques Queimadelos A, Robertson C. Locally advanced and metastatic prostate cancer treated with intermittent androgen monotherapy or maximal androgen blockade: results from a randomised phase 3 study by the South European Uroncological Group. Eur Urol. 2014;66:232–9.
16. Schulman C, Cornel E, Matveev V, Tammela TL, Schraml J, Bensadoun H, Warnack W, Persad R, Salagierski M, Gómez Veiga F, Baskin-Bey E, López B, Tombal B. Intermittent versus continuous androgen deprivation therapy in patients with relapsing or locally advanced prostate cancer: a phase 3b randomised study (ICELAND). Eur Urol. 2016;69:720–7.
17. Niraula S, Le LW, Tannock IF. Treatment of prostate cancer with intermittent versus continuous androgen deprivation: a systematic review of randomized trials. J Clin Oncol. 2013;31:2029–36.
18. Tsai HT, Penson DF, Makambi KH, Lynch JH, Van Den Eeden SK, Potosky AL. Efficacy of intermittent androgen deprivation therapy vs conventional continuous androgen deprivation therapy for advanced prostate cancer: a meta-analysis. Urology. 2013;82:327–33.
19. Sciarra A, Abrahamsson PA, Brausi M, Galsky M, Mottet N, Sartor O, Tammela TL, Calais da Silva F. Intermittent androgen-deprivation therapy in prostate cancer: a critical review focused on phase 3 trials. Eur Urol. 2013;64:722–30.

20. Botrel TE, Clark O, dos Reis RB, Pompeo AC, Ferreira U, Sadi MV, Bretas FF. Intermittent versus continuous androgen deprivation for locally advanced, recurrent or metastatic prostate cancer: a systematic review and meta-analysis. BMC Urol. 2014;14:9.
21. Brungs D, Chen J, Masson P, Epstein RJ. Intermittent androgen deprivation is a rational standard-of-care treatment for all stages of progressive prostate cancer: results from a systematic review and meta-analysis. Prostate Cancer Prostatic Dis. 2014;17:105–11.
22. Magnan S, Zarychanski R, Pilote L, Bernier L, Shemilt M, Vigneault E, Fradet V, Turgeon AF. Intermittent vs continuous androgen deprivation therapy for prostate cancer: a systematic review and meta-analysis. JAMA Oncol. 2015;1(9):1261.
23. Duchesne GM, Woo HH, Bassett JK, Bowe SJ, D'Este C, Frydenberg M, King M, Ledwich L, Loblaw A, Malone S, Millar J, Milne R, Smith RG, Spry N, Stockler M, Syme RA, Tai KH, Turner S. Timing of androgen-deprivation therapy in patients with prostate cancer with a rising PSA (TROG 03.06 and VCOG PR 01-03 [TOAD]): a randomised, multicentre, non-blinded, phase 3 trial. Lancet Oncol. 2016;17:727–37.
24. Latz S, Fisang C, Ebert W, Orth S, Engehausen DG, Müller SC, Anding R. Long term progression-free survival in a patient with locally advanced prostate cancer under low dose intermittent androgen deprivation therapy with bicalutamide only. Case Rep Urol. 2015;2015:928787.
25. Klotz LH, Herr HW, Morse MJ, Whitmore WF Jr. Intermittent endocrine therapy for advanced prostate cancer. Cancer. 1986;58:2546–50.
26. Salomon L, Ploussard G, Coloby P, Kouri G, Lebret T, Méjean A, Prunet D, Soulié M. Observational survey of the French Urological Association evaluating intermittent hormonal modalities treatment in prostate cancer in France. Prog Urol. 2014;24:367–73.
27. Shaw GL, Wilson P, Cuzick J, et al. International study into the use of intermittent hormone therapy in the treatment of carcinoma of the prostate: a meta-analysis of 1446 patients. BJU Int. 2007;99:1056–65.
28. Ideta AM, Tanaka G, Takeuchi T, Aihara K. A mathematical model of intermittent androgen suppression for prostate cancer. J Nonlinear Sci. 2008;18:593–641.
29. Hirata Y, Morino K, Akakura K, Higano CS, Bruchovsky N, Gambol T, Hall S, Tanaka G, Aihara K. Intermittent androgen suppression: estimating parameters for individual patients based on initial psa data in response to androgen deprivation therapy. PLoS One. 2015;10:e0130372.
30. Hirata Y, Akakura K, Higano CS, Bruchovsky N, Aihara K. Quantitative mathematical modeling of PSA dynamics of prostate cancer patients treated with intermittent androgen suppression. J Mol Cell Biol. 2012;4:127–32.

Prognostic Significance of Monitoring Serum Testosterone in Primary ADT for Prostate Cancer

Shinichi Sakamoto

Abstract

In the 1940s, Charles Huggins et al. published a paper describing the clinical benefits of surgical castration and estrogen administration in prostate cancer patients. Later, Huggins was awarded the Nobel Prize to acknowledge the importance of his findings in this field. Since that time, androgen deprivation therapy (ADT) remains a standard therapy for metastatic prostate cancer. Although the main aim of ADT is the control of the serum testosterone (TST) level below the castration level, a series of evidences indicated the clinical significance of controlling the serum TST level even below the standard castration level. In terms of TST production, multiple pathways exist, such as "classical pathway" and "backdoor pathway." Upregulation of such pathways, even inside the tumor, contributes to the acquisition of castration resistance. Thus, monitoring serum TST levels provides us further understanding of tumor behavior in individual patients. In this chapter, we will discuss the prognostic significance of monitoring serum TST levels in primary ADT for prostate cancer.

Keywords

Androgen deprivation therapy · Testosterone · Prostate cancer · LHRH analog GnRH antagonist

S. Sakamoto
Chiba University Graduate School of Medicine, Chiba, Japan
e-mail: rbatbat1@chiba-u.jp

9.1 Introduction

The serum testosterone (TST) level was a significant factor associated with other clinical variables in prostate cancer. In earlier pieces of evidence, pretreatment TST levels were related to the Gleason score [1–4], pathological stage [5–7], and risk of biochemical failure after radical prostatectomy [8]. In the case of metastatic prostate cancer, androgen deprivation therapy (ADT) is the mainstay of treatment [3, 9, 10]. According to current clinical guidelines, the castrated TST level during androgen deprivation therapy for prostate cancer is defined as TST <50 ng/dL [11]. However, this was established more than 40 years ago, when the TST tests were limited [10].

9.2 The Significance of Lower Testosterone Level Below 50 ng/dL

A recent advance in chemiluminescence has made it possible to accurately measure serum TST levels even below 50 ng/dL. The nadir serum TST level below 20 ng/dL has been reported whether it is surgically or medically castrated. Van et al. indicated that medically castrated men had significantly lower TST levels (median 4.0 ng/dL) than those surgically castrated (median 9.2 ng/dL) [12]. Several studies provided evidence about the correlation between castration level and prognosis [9, 10, 13]. The most clinically significant castration level during ADT remains controversial. Morote et al. reported the clinical significance of breakthrough TST increases of 20 ng/dL and 50 ng/dL (Table 9.1) [10]. They argued that absence of breakthrough below TST 20 ng/dL is a good predictive factor for survival free of androgen-independent progression [10]. They also mentioned patients who achieved nadir TST below 32 ng/dL showed favorable prognosis. They reported the clinical significance of the lower castration level for the first time. Perachino et al. revealed a direct correlation between the risk of death and TST at 6 months (29 ng/dL; median) during ADT ($p < 0.05$) [13] (Table 9.1). Bertaglia et al. reported the clinical significance of TST levels after 6 months of ADT, and they concluded that a TST level <30 ng/dL was a favorable prognostic factor for survival [9] (Table 9.1). In the case of evidence with regard to the combined androgen blockade (CAB), Yasuda et al. reported that the mean TST levels did not show a significant relationship with time to PSA progression, cancer-specific survival, and overall survival (OS) [14] (Table 9.1). On the other hand, Kamada et al. reported nadir TST <20 ng/dL was the best predictor for OS in patients on CAB. Furthermore, it takes about 1 year (median, 11.3 months) to reach the nadir TST level on CAB [15]. These results were in accordance with the result of Klotz et al. reporting the clinical significance of minimum (nadir) testosterone levels within the first year of ADT. It also supported the prognostic impact of lower TST levels below 20 ng/dL [16].

Table 9.1 Levels of serum TST and prognosis in patients treated with androgen deprivation therapy

Authors	Morote [10]	Perachino [13]	Bertaglia [9]	Yasuda [14]	Kamada [15]	Klotz [18]
Year	2007	2010	2013	2014	2015	2015
n	73	129	153	69	225	626
Age	70.7	75	71	70	73	73.2
cT ≥3	13.7	–	67.3	–	65.2	–
GS ≥8	31.5	37.2	37.8	–	57.0	–
Metastatic ca. (%)	0.0	100.0	35.3	–	60.3	0.0
Pretreatment (%)	31.5	–	64.9	0.0	0.0	–
CAB (%)	38.4	0.0	0.0	100.0	100.0	–
TST evaluation	Breakthrough	At 6 months	Lower in two tests	Mean	Nadir	Nadir/median/max at 12 months
PFS						
50 ng/dL	○	NE	X	NE	NE	Nadir/median/maximum
32 ng/dL	○	NE	NE	X	X	NE
20 ng/dL	○	NE	X	X	X	Nadir/median
OS/CSS						
50 ng/dL	NE	NE	X	NE	NE	Nadir/maximum
40 ng/dL	NE	○	NE	NE	NE	NE
30 ng/dL	NE	NE	○	X	○	NE
20 ng/dL	NE	NE	○	X	○	Nadir
15 ng/dL	NE	NE	NE	X	NE	NE
8 ng/dL	NE	NE	NE	NE	X	NE

○: $p < 0.05$; X: $p \geq 0.05$
NE no related evidence

9.3 The Difference in Clinical Outcome Between GnRH Antagonist and LHRH Agonist

The gonadotropin-releasing hormone (GnRH) antagonist degarelix was noninferior to the luteinizing hormone-releasing hormone (LHRH) agonist for the proportion of the patients to achieve castration levels [17]. However, based on the meta-analysis of the current five randomized control trials, degarelix seems to have a clinical advantage over the LHRH agonist. Prostate-specific antigen (PSA) progression-free survival (PFS) and OS were improved in the degarelix group (HR: 0.71, $p = 0.017$; HR: 0.47, $p = 0.023$, respectively). OS was particularly improved with degarelix in patients with baseline TST levels >2 ng/mL (HR: 0.36, $p = 0.006$) [18]. Degarelix also seems to have an advantage over the LHRH agonist concerning disease-related adverse events overall, including joint-related signs and symptoms, musculoskeletal events, and urinary tract symptoms [18]. The difference may be explained by the distinct mode of action of degarelix compared with LHRH agonists. First, degarelix causes rapid and consistent TST suppression. Micro-surges of TST mediated by the re-administration of the LHRH agonist may potentially have an adverse effect on the prognosis. Second, although the precise role of extra-pituitary GnRH receptor expressions is not yet clear, a number of extra-pituitary tissues including peripheral blood mononuclear cells and prostate cancer cells express GnRH receptors [18]. Third, degarelix provides consistent follicle-stimulating hormone (FSH) suppression compared with LHRH agonists [17]. Inhibition of FSH is considered to have significance with regard to tumor growth, bone resorption, and control of adipocytes and obesity. A number of mechanistic differences may affect the prognostic advantage of the GnRH antagonist over the LHRH agonists.

9.4 Intratumoral Androgen Synthesis

In spite of maintenance under the castration level, the majority of prostate cancer patients will develop castration resistance. One of the critical factors of castration resistance is the development of a compensatory TST production mechanism during androgen deprivation therapy, proposed as an intratumoral androgen synthesis. It has shown in mouse xenograft models that TST levels within metastasis cancer under castrated conditions are even higher than the TST levels within primary cancer under noncastrated conditions [19]. The TST level within the metastatic tumor was sufficient to activate the androgen receptor-mediated pathway to further promote the tumor growth even under castrated conditions. The reason behind this seems to be mediated by alteration in genes encoding steroidogenesis which mediates intratumoral steroidogenesis. The castration-resistant metastatic tumor showed a significant increase in the expression of *FASN, CYP17A1, HSD3B1, HSD3B2, CYP17A1, SDKR1C3*, and *HSD17B3*, key enzymes required for the metabolism of progestins to adrenal androgens and subsequent conversion to TST. Another mechanism is the increased production of dihydrotestosterone (DHT) without the usage of TST as a substrate, called alternate "backdoor pathway." Classically, DHT is created as a result of the metabolism of TST; however, in the case of the backdoor pathway, DHT is created by the progesterone metabolism mediated through the upregulation of *SRD5A1* and *RDH5* in the metastatic tumor (Fig. 9.1) [20]. Although not statistically significant, the patients with high nadir TST (≥ 20 ng/dL) had more bone metastatic lesion compared to those with low nadir TST (<20 ng/dL) [15]. The nadir TST level during androgen deprivation therapy may potentially indicate the amount of intratumoral TST production mediated by primary and metastatic cancer lesions.

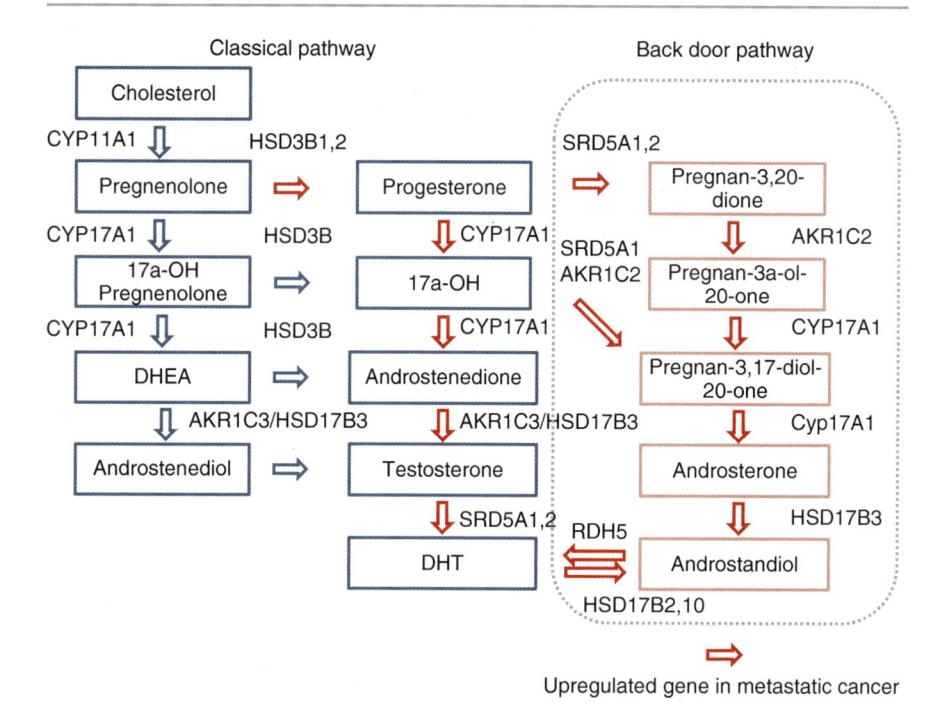

Fig. 9.1 Schematic outline of the steroidogenic pathway from cholesterol to dihydrotestosterone, including classical and backdoor pathways. Inside the prostate cancer cells, genes such as *HSD3B1*, *CYP17A1*, *AKR1C3*, *SRD5A1*, and *SRD5A2* were upregulated and activate the TST/DHT synthesis in the classical pathway. Upregulation of *SRD5A1*, *SRD5A2*, and *RDH5* contributes to DHT production, independent of TST, through the backdoor pathway

9.5 Significance of TST Suppression at Early Stage of Prostate Cancer

A series of evidence indicated that reduced serum TST levels under primary ADT in castration-sensitive prostate cancer (CSPC) patients result in favorable prognosis [15, 16]. However, there has been a controversy concerning TST suppression, whether (1) the reduction of serum TST itself has a therapeutic significance or (2) the cases reduced serum TST is the one to have prolonged survival.

An essential mechanism to escape from cancer control by androgen ablation therapy includes the intracellular steroid precursors to androgen by prostate cancer cells. Abiraterone acetate is a selective, irreversible *CYP17* inhibitor that is critical in the production of androgen in the testis, adrenal gland, and tumor cells. The recent two reports based on the therapeutic utility of abiraterone acetate as the primary treatment may provide a practical answer. Fizazi et al. reported that abiraterone acetate with 5 mg of prednisolone prolonged OS compared to control (HR 0.62, $p < 0.001$) in high-risk metastatic CSPC patients (having at least two of the following: Gleason score of 8 or more, three bone metastases, and the presence of visceral metastasis) [21]. James et al. also reported a clinical advantage of primary treatment with abiraterone acetate in various stages of CSPC patients even includes 28% of nonmetastatic status. Abiraterone prolonged OS in all the patients (HR0.63, $p < 0.001$). The prognostic advantage of abiraterone acetate seems to be regardless of metastatic status, with an HR of 0.75 in nonmetastatic and 0.61 in metastatic patients [22]. These data indicated clinical significance of complete TST suppression at the early stage of prostate cancer treatment. Furthermore, these data may as well provide the evidence that reduction of TST comes first to extend the survival of prostate cancer patients.

9.6 Future Directions

Current pieces of evidence indicating control of low serum TST levels seem to be the key to mediate favorable prognosis in patients treated with ADT. On the other hand, in prostate cancer, adrenal and intratumoral sources of androgen stimulate tumor growth, which cannot be controlled by LHRH analogs and GnRH antagonists. Although the mechanisms are quite different, novel androgen receptor (AR)-targeted agents such as abiraterone acetate and enzalutamide are potentially able to suppress extragonadal TST-mediated activation of AR. As the early use of abiraterone showed survival advantage [21, 22], treatment with intensive blockade of TST-AR axis during the primary treatment of CSPC may become the standard therapy in future. On the other hand, treatment with novel AR-targeted drugs is known to create AR splicing variants in over 95% of patients when detected with circulating tumor cells (CTCs) in the patients' blood [23]. The early use of novel AR-targeted drugs may potentially induce rapid development of castration resistance in some patients. It may be ideal to establish a marker to identify those who will benefit or not benefit from the primary intensive treatment among prostate cancer patients.

References

1. Regis L, Iztueta I, Servian P, Kosntantinidis C, Planas J, Celma A, et al. Free serum testosterone versus total testosterone as surrogate marker for the clinical benefit of androgen suppression in prostate cancer patients. J Urol. 2014;191(4):E856-E.
2. Hoffman MA, DeWolf WC, Morgentaler A. Is low serum free testosterone a marker for high grade prostate cancer? J Urol. 2000;163(3):824–7.
3. Schatzl G, Madersbacher S, Thurridl T, Waldmuller J, Kramer G, Haitel A, et al. High-grade prostate cancer is associated with low serum testosterone levels. Prostate. 2001;47(1):52–8.
4. Neuzillet Y, Pichon A, Ghoneim T, Lebret T, Radulescu C, Molinie V, et al. High incidence of predominant gleason pattern 4 is associated with low testosterone serum level in localized prostate cancer: an update with 937 patients. J Urol. 2014;191(4):E412-E.
5. Isom-Batz G, Bianco FJ, Kattan MW, Mulhall JP, Lilja H, Eastham JA. Testosterone as a predictor of pathological stage in clinically localized prostate cancer. J Urol. 2005;173(6):1935–7.
6. Suzuki H, Yano M, Imamoto T, Kato T, Komiya A, Naya Y, et al. Pretreatment serum testosterone level can improve the efficiency of prostate cancer screening. J. Urology. 2007;177(4):573.

7. Massengill JC, Sun L, Moul JW, HY W, McLeod DG, Amling C, et al. Pretreatment total testosterone level predicts pathological stage in patients with localized prostate cancer treated with radical prostatectomy. J Urol. 2003;169(5):1670–5.
8. Yamamoto S, Yonese J, Kawakami S, Ohkubo Y, Tatokoro M, Komai Y, et al. Preoperative serum testosterone level as an independent predictor of treatment failure following radical prostatectomy. Eur Urol. 2007;52(3):696–701.
9. Bertaglia V, Tucci M, Fiori C, Aroasio E, Poggio M, Buttigliero C, et al. Effects of serum testosterone levels after 6 months of androgen deprivation therapy on the outcome of patients with prostate cancer. Clin Genitourin Cancer. 2013;11(3):325–30. e1
10. Morote J, Orsola A, Planas J, Trilla E, Raventos CX, Cecchini L, et al. Redefining clinically significant castration levels in patients with prostate cancer receiving continuous androgen deprivation therapy. J Urol. 2007;178(4 Pt 1):1290–5.
11. Tombal B. The importance of testosterone control in prostate cancer. Eur Urol Suppl. 2007;6(15):834–9.
12. van der Sluis TM, Bui HN, Meuleman EJ, Heijboer AC, Hartman JF, van Adrichem N, et al. Lower testosterone levels with luteinizing hormone-releasing hormone agonist therapy than with surgical castration: new insights attained by mass spectrometry. J Urol. 2012;187(5):1601–6.
13. Perachino M, Cavalli V, Bravi F. Testosterone levels in patients with metastatic prostate cancer treated with luteinizing hormone-releasing hormone therapy: prognostic significance? BJU Int. 2010;105(5):648–51.
14. Yasuda Y, Fujii Y, Yuasa T, Yamamoto S, Yonese J, Fukui I. Do testosterone levels have prognostic significance in patients with metastatic prostate cancer treated with combined androgen blockade? Int J Urol. 2015;22(1):132–3.
15. Kamada S, Sakamoto S, Ando K, Muroi A, Fuse M, Kawamura K, et al. Nadir testosterone after long-term follow-up predicts prognosis of prostate cancer patients treated with combined androgen blockade. J Urol. 2015;193(4):E1086-E.
16. Klotz L, O'Callaghan C, Ding K, Toren P, Dearnaley D, Higano CS. Nadir testosterone within first year of androgen-deprivation therapy (ADT) predicts for time to castration-resistant progression: a secondary analysis of the PR-7 trial of intermittent versus continuous ADT (vol 33, pg 1151, 2015). J Clin Oncol. 2016;34(16):1965.
17. Klotz L, Boccon-Gibod L, Shore ND, Andreou C, Persson BE, Cantor P, et al. The efficacy and safety of degarelix: a 12-month, comparative, randomized, open-label, parallel-group phase III study in patients with prostate cancer. BJU Int. 2008;102(11):1531–8.
18. Klotz L, Miller K, Crawford ED, Shore N, Tombal B, Karup C, et al. Disease control outcomes from analysis of pooled individual patient data from five comparative randomised clinical trials of degarelix versus luteinising hormone-releasing hormone agonists. Eur Urol. 2014;66(6):1101–8.
19. Montgomery RB, Mostaghel EA, Vessella R, Hess DL, Kalhorn TF, Higano CS, et al. Maintenance of intratumoral androgens in metastatic prostate cancer: a mechanism for castration-resistant tumor growth. Cancer Res. 2008;68(11):4447–54.
20. Locke JA, Guns ES, Lubik AA, Adomat HH, Hendy SC, Wood CA, et al. Androgen levels increase by intratumoral de novo steroidogenesis during progression of castration-resistant prostate cancer. Cancer Res. 2008;68(15):6407–15.
21. Fizazi K, Tran N, Fein L, Matsubara N, Rodriguez-Antolin A, Alekseev BY, et al. Abiraterone plus prednisone in metastatic, castration-sensitive prostate cancer. N Engl J Med. 2017;377:352–60.
22. James ND, de Bono JS, Spears MR, Clarke NW, Mason MD, Dearnaley DP, et al. Abiraterone for prostate cancer not previously treated with hormone therapy. N Engl J Med. 2017;377:338–51.
23. Qu F, Xie W, Nakabayashi M, Zhang H, Jeong SH, Wang X, et al. Association of AR-V7 and prostate-specific antigen RNA levels in blood with efficacy of abiraterone acetate and enzalutamide treatment in men with prostate cancer. Clin Cancer Res. 2017;23(3):726–34.

Ethnic Variation in Clinical Outcomes of Hormone Therapy for Prostate Cancer

Takashi Fukagai, Masashi Morita, Robert G. Carlile, John L. Lederer, and Thomas Namiki

Abstract

The racial differences in clinical outcome after hormone therapy for prostate cancer, especially between Caucasians and Japanese, are discussed in this chapter. Several studies reported better survival in Asians than Caucasians, after hormonal therapy, in the United States. A marked racial difference in clinical outcome after hormonal therapy was observed in our study between Japanese and Caucasians in Hawaii. The efficacy of hormone therapy is not uniform with regard to different countries or races. These findings support both existing guidelines endorsing hormone therapy in Asia and those which caution its use in Western countries.

Keywords

Prostate cancer · Clinical outcome · Racial differences · Hormone therapy

---

T. Fukagai, M.D., Ph.D. (✉) · M. Morita, M.D., Ph.D.
Department of Urology, Showa University Koto Toyosu Hospital, Tokyo, Japan
e-mail: fukagai@med.showa-u.ac.jp

R. G. Carlile, M.D.
Department of Surgery, University of Hawaii School of Medicine, Honolulu, HI, USA

J. L. Lederer, M.D.
Department of Radiation Oncology, University of Hawaii School of Medicine, Honolulu, HI, USA

T. Namiki, M.D.
Department of Pathology, University of Hawaii School of Medicine, Honolulu, HI, USA

© Springer Nature Singapore Pte Ltd. 2018
Y. Arai, O. Ogawa (eds.), *Hormone Therapy and Castration Resistance of Prostate Cancer*, https://doi.org/10.1007/978-981-10-7013-6_10

10.1 Introduction

The incidence of prostate cancer is increasing worldwide. It is well known that the incidence of prostate cancer is markedly different among various races and countries. Prostate cancer is the most commonly diagnosed cancer in Western countries [1]. Asians, especially, Japanese and Chinese, have prostate cancer incidences lower than Caucasians [2]. Interestingly, the prostate cancer incidence in Japanese Americans is intermediate between Japanese living in Japan and Caucasians in the United States [3] (Fig. 10.1). The reasons for the risk differential are unknown. The lower incidence among Japanese born in the United States compared with US whites may mean that Japanese immigrant's descendants retain some genetic and/or lifestyle characteristics that make their risk for prostate cancer less than that of US whites. If the prostate cancer's behavior is due to any genetic differences related to race, this may result in different clinical responses to treatment. Also, prostate cancer is well known as an androgen-dependent cancer, and some studies indicate that the different character of prostate cancer in each race might be associated with the different hormonal environments [4, 5]. This may influence the effectiveness of hormone therapy in different races. Only few publications have compared prostate cancer treatment and patient survival among different ethnic groups. Several studies indicate that race is a prognostic factor for African-American and White men. But the differences in survival between Asian and White men are not well known.

In this chapter, we will discuss the racial differences in clinical outcome after hormone therapy for prostate cancer, especially between Caucasians and Japanese.

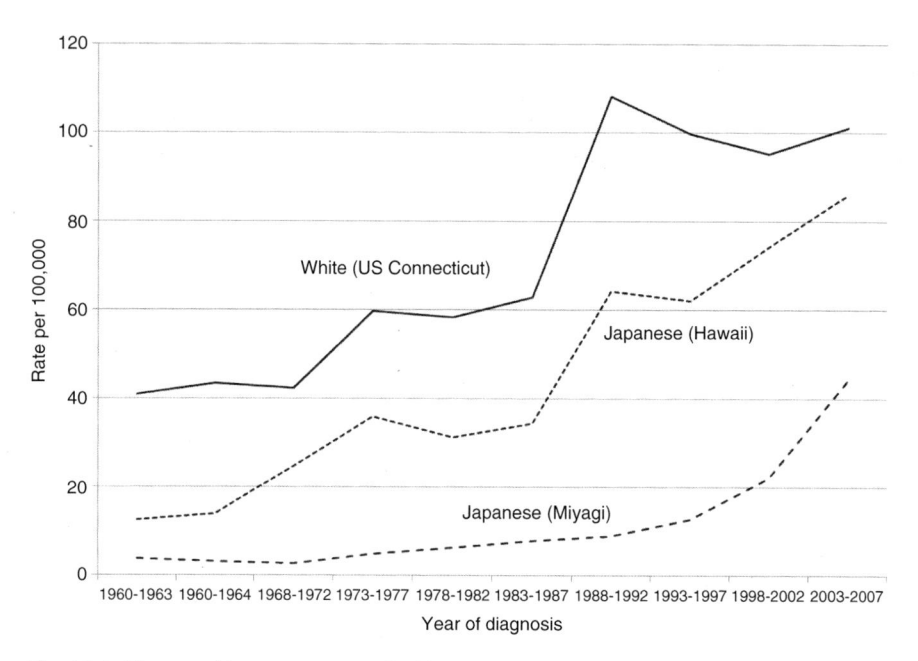

Fig. 10.1 Time trend in prostate cancer incidence

10.2 Impact of Ethnicity on the Survival of Men with Prostate Cancer in the United States

Several studies reported different clinical outcomes among various ethnicities in the United States. Many studies reported the higher mortality and poor prognosis of African-American men with prostate cancer after various treatment modalities. There have been just a few studies reporting the clinical outcome of prostate cancer in Asian ethnic groups in the United States. A study in the 1970s reported better 5-year- relative survival rates for prostate cancer in Japanese and Chinese American men than Caucasian men in the United States [6]. McCracken et al. investigated cancer incidence and mortality for five Asian-American ethnic groups in California in order of population size (Chinese, Filipino, Vietnamese, Korean, and Japanese). In this study, all Asian ethnic groups showed lower mortality than non-Hispanic whites in California. These studies indicate Asian-Americans with prostate cancer had longer life expectancies than Caucasians in the United States [7]. The report from the National Cancer Institute (NCI) introduced 5-year relative survival by race/ethnicity and stage in 1983–1993. This monograph showed similar 5-year relative survival in Japanese Americans and whites with localized prostate cancer. But interestingly, Japanese Americans showed higher 5-year relative survivals (about 50%) than whites (about 30%) with prostate cancer with distant metastasis [8]. Recently, Bernard investigated the impact of ethnicity on the outcome of men with metastatic, hormone-sensitive prostate cancer [9]. This study showed that Asian men have superior median overall survival (OS) and prostate cancer-specific mortality for distant, de novo, metastatic PCa than men of other races in the SEER data. The superior survival of Asians in the SEER results from this study suggests a possible biologic difference between the races with respect to the risk of relapse after therapy for localized disease and responsiveness to therapy given potentially similar environmental exposures in this US population. One large cohort study of patients with prostate cancer who received androgen deprivation therapy (ADT) demonstrated better survival among Asians and Hispanics than among whites or African Americans [10]. The best survival rates were observed among Asians, who had a 37% lower risk of mortality than whites, after adjusting for prognostic factors such as tumor characteristics, treatments, and sociodemographic data.

10.3 Comparison of Clinical Outcome of Prostate Cancer Among Various Ethnics in Hawaii

10.3.1 Comparison of Clinical Outcome Between Caucasians and Japanese

As previously stated, few publications have compared prostate cancer treatment and patient survival between Caucasian and Asian men. Young et al. reported with SEER program data that Japanese had higher survival for prostate cancer [6]. But the reason for this was not established, and survival was not examined by the type of treatment received. We have investigated racial differences in clinical outcome after treatment for prostate cancer in Hawaii [11]. The findings of our research are as follows.

During 1992–2001, 2074 prostate cancer patients were registered in Tumor Oncology Registry, of The Queen's Medical Center, Honolulu, Hawaii, USA. Of these prostate cancer patients, 642 Japanese men and 465 Caucasian men were included. We divided these patients according to race and treatment methods, prostatectomy, radiation therapy, hormone therapy, or no treatment (watchful waiting), and compared the clinical outcomes between Caucasians and Japanese. Clinical information was obtained from the hospital tumor registry. All living patients were followed to the end of 2001, and none were lost to follow-up. Age, stage, Gleason score, race, and pretreatment PSA values were abstracted. The Caucasian and Japanese patient groups were similar in terms of age, clinical stage, pretreatment PSA levels, and Gleason scores. We could not find any significant differences in clinical outcome after treatment with prostatectomy or watchful waiting (Fig. 10.2).

We investigated the prognosis of Caucasian and Japanese patients with hormone therapy in detail. The specific type of hormone therapy each patient received (conventional surgical, medical castration alone, or combined androgen blockade (CAB)) was not available. Details of the patient characteristics of the two ethnic groups are given in Table 10.1. None of the patients received definitive surgical or radiation therapy. Differences in patient characteristics between the two groups were calculated using t-test and the chi-square test. The clinical endpoint was survival. The Kaplan-Meier method was used for overall and cause-specific survival curves, which were compared using log-rank statistics. Age, stage, Gleason score, race, and pretreatment PSA values were assessed as to their interdependence and correlation with the clinical course using Cox's proportional hazard regression model. The hospital's Institutional Research Board approved the study. Median follow-up was 51 months (range 2–126) for Japanese-American men (JAM) and 36 months (range 2–88) for Caucasian men (CM). There were no statistically significant differences in patient characteristics between the two groups (Table 10.1). Forty five JAM and 32 CM died during the follow-up period. At 60 months, the overall survival rate was 65.5% for

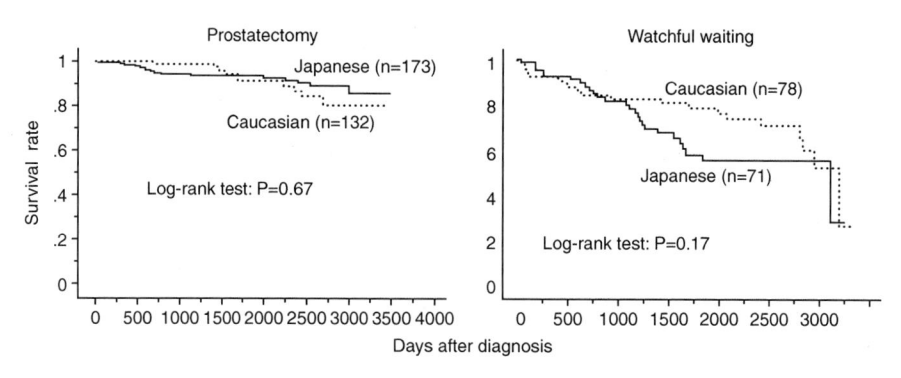

Fig. 10.2 Overall survival rate of the patients with prostatectomy and watchful waiting according to race

Table 10.1 Baseline characteristics of ethnic groups

	Japanese (n = 105)	Caucasian (n = 59)	p value
Age			
Median (range)	77 (53–92)	77 (51–90)	
Mean ± SD	75.8 ± 8.1	76.5 ± 8.2	0.55
PSA			
Median (range)	46.1(3.9–9783)	16.2 (0.6–4000)	
Mean ± SD	351.1 ± 1437.4	152.3 ± 583.9	0.355
Clinical stage[a]			
I	0 (0%)	0 (0%)	
II	53 (50%)	37 (63%)	0.1[b]
III	10 (10%)	1 (2%)	
IV	42 (40%)	21 (36%)	
Gleason score			
2–6	14 (13%)	8 (14%)	
7	33 (31%)	18 (31%)	
8–10	52 (50%)	31 (53%)	
Unknown	6 (6%)	2 (3%)	
Median (range)	8	8	
Mean ± SD	7.7 ± 1.2	7.7 ± 1.4	0.883

[a]Clinical stage followed by 1997 UICC's TNM classification
[b]χ-square test

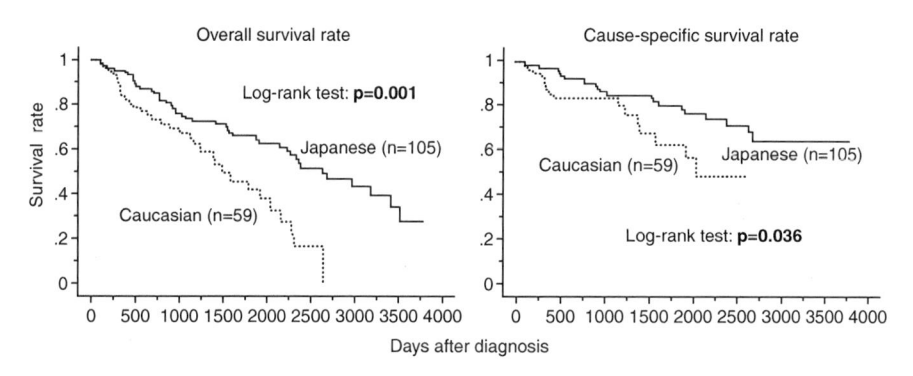

Fig. 10.3 Survival rate after hormone therapy according to race (© 2006, Blackwell Publishing)

JAM and 41.7% for CM ($p = 0.01$). JAM who received hormone therapy had a better overall and cause-specific survival rate compared to CM ($p = 0.001$ and $p = 0.036$, respectively) (Fig. 10.3). For patients with metastasis (CM: 15, JAM: 37) and without metastasis (CM: 44, JAM: 68), the overall survival rate was higher in JAM ($p = 0.032$ and 0.007, respectively). We examined the simultaneous influence of five covariables (age, clinical stage, race, Gleason score, and pretreatment PSA) on time to death. Race was a significant prognostic factor on multivariate analysis ($p = 0.03$) along with pretreatment PSA ($p = 0.03$). The findings suggest a difference in the

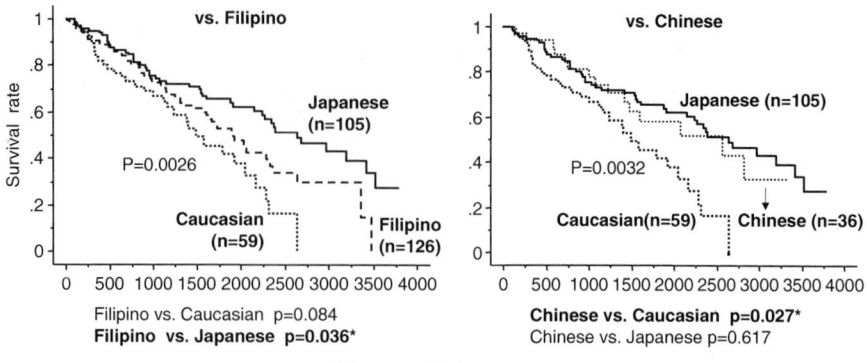

Fig. 10.4 Overall survival rate after hormone therapy according to race: comparison among Japanese, Caucasian, Chinese, and Filipino in Hawaii

effectiveness of hormone therapy of prostate cancer in JAM living in Hawaii compared to CM living in Hawaii. As far as we know, this is the only study comparing the prognosis, particularly after hormone therapy, between Caucasians and Japanese in the United States. Our study consisted of a relatively small number of patients, and the information on progression-free survival rate was not available. All patients were treated by the same group of urologists in a single institution, with follow-up management in cases of relapses. It is also unlikely that only one ethnic group, the Japanese, had a large proportion of CAB treatment because both ethnic groups had almost the same clinical background and were treated by the same urologists. Therefore, we believe that our study findings are significant even though we did not have the information on progression-free survival.

10.3.2 Comparison of Clinical Outcome After Hormone Therapy Among Other Races

After finding that Japanese patients showed better prognosis after hormone therapy, we investigated the clinical outcome after hormone therapy in other races. This research is ongoing. We found 126 Filipino and 36 Chinese who had hormone treatment from same tumor registry in Hawaii. We compared these patients' clinical outcome with that of Caucasians and Japanese. Interestingly, Chinese men show almost the same prognosis as Japanese and better prognosis than CM. Filipinos show worse prognosis after hormonal therapy than Japanese but better than CM (Fig. 10.4).

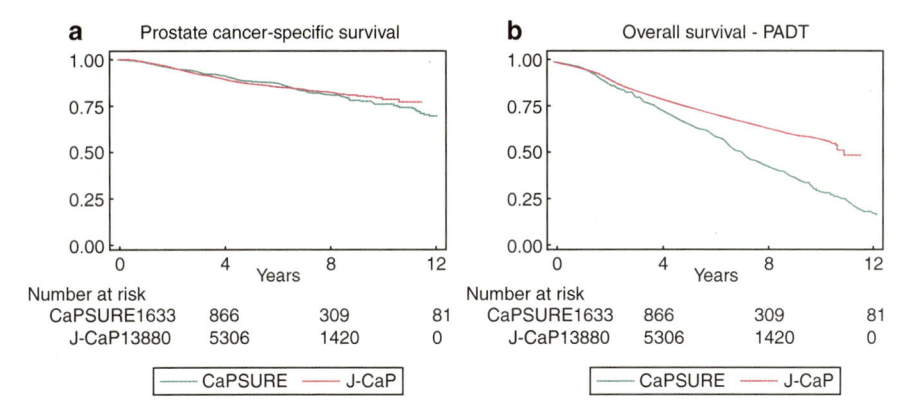

Fig. 10.5 Univariate Kaplan-Meier survival curves showing cancer-specific survival (A, $p = 0.88$, log-rank) and overall survival (B, $p < 0.001$, log-rank) in CaPSURE and J-CaP (© 2016, Blackwell Publishing)

10.4 Comparison of Clinical Outcome After Hormone Therapy Between Japanese in Japan and US Population

Do Japanese prostate cancer patients in Japan have longer survival after hormone therapy than US prostate cancer patients? It is difficult to compare the clinical outcomes between Japanese and US patients because of large differences in prostate cancer screening in each country. The proportion of early-stage prostate cancer at diagnosis has increased in the United States following introduction of the PSA test. Currently, about 50% of men in the United States have a prostate-specific antigen (PSA) test annually, and about 75% of men have had a PSA test [12]. On the other hand, although some Japanese prefectural and city government offices have conducted prostate cancer screening, nationwide the percentage of municipalities conducting prostate cancer screening is still not large. The increase in early-stage cancer, detected in the US medical system, has not yet appeared in the Japanese medical system; thus, Japanese prostate cancer patients have more advanced stage, higher-grade prostate cancer at diagnosis. Consequently, Japanese prostate cancer patients had worse prognosis than US patients.

A recent report by Cooperberg and Akaza successfully compared clinical outcomes after hormone therapy between Japanese and US patients [13]. They compared data directly between men receiving hormone therapy (primary androgen deprivation therapy (PADT)) in the US Cancer of the Prostate Strategic Urologic Research Endeavor (CaPSURE) registry and the Japanese Cancer of the Prostate (J-CaP) registry database. Competing risk regression was used to assess prostate cancer-specific mortality (CSM), adjusting for Japan Cancer of the Prostate Risk Assessment (J-CAPRA) score and other patients' backgrounds. Despite different risk profiles between the cohorts, CSM was similar on univariate analysis (log-rank $p = 0.88$). On multivariable regression, the subhazard ratio for CSM was 0.52 for J-CaP vs. CaPSURE (95% confidence interval 0.40–0.68) (Fig. 10.5). Men on PADT in Japan have less than half the adjusted CSM than those in the United States. This study also showed that at each level of risk according to J-CAPRA score, outcomes were substantially better in J-CaP compared with CaPSURE (log-rank, $p < 0.001$).

10.5 Discussion

We reviewed some studies, including our research, that compared clinical outcomes of Caucasian and Asian prostate cancer patients. These studies indicated that Asian prostate cancer showed longer survival and better response to hormone therapy than Caucasian men in Western countries. Our additional study of other ethnic groups in Hawaii has also shown different prognosis after hormonal therapy. Chinese men show almost the same prognosis as Japanese and better prognosis than CM. Filipinos show worse prognosis after hormonal therapy than Japanese but better than CM. Interestingly, the prognosis after hormonal therapy is inversely correlated with the prostate cancer incidence of the ethnic group. As previously noted, the incidence of prostate cancer within ethnic groups may relate to the exogenous or endogenous hormonal environment, which in turn may also relate to the differences in the effectiveness of hormonal therapy. However, the reasons underlying these differences are poorly understood, as there are many factors that could influence the treatment outcomes of hormone therapy.

We will now explore some factors that influence the ethnic differences of clinical outcomes after hormone therapy for prostate cancer.

10.5.1 The Different Sensitivities for Hormone Therapy with Various Genetic Change

It is well known that prostate cancer shows various genetic changes associated with progression [14, 15]. The findings may indicate different sensitivities for hormonal therapy in Japanese. Several studies have shown racial differences in CAG repeat alleles [16, 17]. Irvine et al. found that the prevalence of short CAG alleles was highest in African-American men with the highest risk for prostate cancer, intermediate in intermediate-risk non-Hispanic whites, and lowest in Asians at very low risk for prostate cancer [16]. Bratt et al. found an association between long CAG repeat length and a good response to hormonal therapy [17]. These findings may explain our results showing better prognosis in Japanese after hormonal therapy, corresponding to the low prevalence of short CAG and the high prevalence of long CAG in Asians. However, other studies report conflicting results. Suzuki et al. found that shorter CAG repeat length was correlated with better response to hormonal therapy and prognosis in Japanese prostate cancer patients [18]. Others also note a higher frequency of short CAG repeat length in African-American men compared with whites and Asians, but no difference in CAG repeat length between whites and Asians [19–21]. Another racial difference in association with androgen levels is 5α-reductase activity. Ross et al. measured serum testosterone, dihydrotestosterone (DHT), and metabolites of DHT among young American blacks and whites and native Japanese [4]. In this study, both black and white men had significantly higher serum levels of DHT metabolites than did native Japanese men. The influence of the different serum levels of DHT metabolites on the effectiveness of hormone treatment is unclear but may potentially have an influence on the different effectiveness of hormone treatment between Japanese and Caucasian men. Fujimoto et al. investigated the association between genetic variations in SLCOs which are polymorphic genes that actively transport testosterone [22]. Their study reported that active androgen transport genotypes of SLCO2B1 (GG allele) occurred more frequently in African and Caucasian populations than in Japanese and Han Chinese populations. Their data suggest that SLCO2B1 rs12422149 variants could provide prognostic value for prostate cancer patients treated with ADT and influence ethnic differences in response to ADT. These molecular differences may be the influence resulting in the different sensitivity to ADT. Further studies are needed to clarify the relation between CAG repeat alleles, 5α-reductase activity, genetic variations in SLCOs, and response to hormonal therapy.

10.5.2 Fewer Side Effects Associated with Hormone Therapy in Asian Patients with Prostate Cancer

It is well known that hormone therapy has side effects. The side effects associated with hormone therapy of sexual dysfunction and hot flashes have been known for decades. More recently, we have become aware of other side effects of hormone therapy: skeletal complications, cardiovascular complications, periodontal disease, and cognition. Whereas these complications are significant and may be associated with increased overall morbidity, skeletal and cardiovascular complications are particularly concerning because of their impact on morbidity as well as mortality. One of the putative reasons for the ethnic morbidity and mortality differences may be fewer side effects, especially bone fracture and cardiovascular disease, associated with hormone therapy in Japanese.

It has been demonstrated that the administration of ADT reduces bone mineral density (BMD), which leads to the increased risk of bone fracture. Also, it is well known that bone fracture was associated with increased mortality risk [23]. Several studies reported hormone treatment produces accelerated bone loss in Japanese patients as well in Western countries [24]. But originally the incidence of hip fracture in Japan is apparently lower than for whites living in north Europe or North America [25]. Hip fractures usually occur after a fall, and differing incidence rates of falls might explain the observed differences in hip fracture rates. To explore this hypothesis, Aoyagi et al.

investigated falls and related conditions among community-dwelling people in Japan and compared the prevalence of falls to Japanese Americans living in Hawaii and to published studies of Caucasians [26]. This study reported that compared with native Japanese, the age-standardized prevalence of falls among Japanese Americans was similar but about twice as high for Caucasians. Considering these results, there is the possibility that the incidence of bone fractures after hormone therapy in Japanese may be lower than in Caucasians. Consequently, this may influence the longer survival seen in Japanese prostate cancer patients treated with hormone therapy.

Another significant side effect that may be associated with increased overall mortality is cardiovascular complications. But this issue is still controversial. Some studies reported a small increased risk of cardiovascular disease in patients undergoing ADT. But some studies did show significantly increased risk. Nanda et al. reported that hormone therapy is significantly associated with an increased risk of all-cause mortality among men with a history of coronary artery disease (CAD)-induced heart failure (CHF) or myocardial infarction (MI) but not among men with no comorbidity or a single CAD risk factor [27]. These studies were all from Western countries, but basic cardiovascular health is better in the Japanese population. The ischemic heart disease mortality of Japanese is much lower than in Western countries [28]. This overall better cardiovascular health in Japanese prostate cancer patients may induce better clinical outcomes after hormone therapy. In fact, Akaza et al. demonstrated that the incidence of cardiovascular death in Japanese patients registered in J-CaP database from 2001 to 2003 and treated with leuprorelin was no greater than that expected in the general Japanese population [29]. Fewer side effects may be contributing to the longer survival of Japanese prostate cancer patients after hormone therapy.

Conclusions

A marked racial difference in clinical outcome after hormonal therapy was observed in our study between Japanese and Caucasians. A prospective study with larger number of patients will be necessary to elucidate the differential effectiveness of hormone therapy of prostate cancer in different races, especially between Japanese and Caucasians. The role of hormone therapy may be different depending on the country or race. These findings support both existing guidelines endorsing hormone treatment in Asia including Japan and those which caution its use in the US and European countries.

References

1. Siegel RL, Miller KD, Jemal A. Cancer statistics, 2017. CA Cancer J Clin. 2017;67:7–30.
2. Wynder EL, Fujita Y, Harris RE, Hirayama T, Hiyama T. Comparative epidemiology of cancer between the United States and Japan. Cancer. 1991;67:746–63.
3. Zaridze DG, Boyle P, Smans M. International trends in prostatic cancer. Int J Cancer. 1984;33:223–30.
4. Ross RK, Bernstein L, Lobo RA, Shimizu H, Stanczyk FZ, Pike MC, Henderson BE. 5-alpha-reductase activity and risk of prostate cancer among Japanese and US white and black males. Lancet. 1992;339:887–9.

5. Platz EA, Rimm EB, Willett WC, Kantoff PW, Giovannucci E. Racial variation in prostate cancer incidence and in hormonal system markers among male health professionals. J Natl Cancer Inst. 2000;92:2009–17.
6. Young JL Jr, Ries LG, Pollack ES. Cancer patient survival among ethnic groups in the United States. J Natl Cancer Inst. 1984;73:341–52.
7. McCracken M, Olsen M, Chen MS Jr, Jemal A, Thun M, Cokkinides V, Deapen D, Ward E. Cancer incidence, mortality, and associated risk factors among Asian Americans of Chinese, Filipino, Vietnamese, Korean, and Japanese ethnicities. CA Cancer J Clin. 2007;57:190–205.
8. Prostate Cancer Trends 1973–1995, SEER Program, National Cancer Institute. https://seer.cancer.gov/archive/publications/prostate/prostate_monograph.pdf. Accessed 30 June 2017.
9. Bernard B, Muralidhar V, Chen YH, Sridhar SS, Mitchell EP, Pettaway CA, Carducci MA, Nguyen PL, Sweeney CJ. Impact of ethnicity on the outcome of men with metastatic, hormone-sensitive prostate cancer. Cancer. 2017;123:1536–44.
10. Holmes L Jr, Chan W, Jiang Z, Ward D, Essien EJ, Du XL. Impact of androgen deprivation therapy on racial/ethnic disparities in the survival of older men treated for locoregional prostate cancer. Cancer Control. 2009;16:176–85.
11. Fukagai T, Namiki ST, Carlile R, Yoshida H, Namiki M. Comparison of the clinical outcome after hormonal therapy for prostate cancer between Japanese and Caucasian men. BJU Int. 2006;97:1190–3.
12. Thompson IM, Canby-Hagino E, Lucia MS. Stage migration and grade inflation in prostate cancer: Will Rogers meets Garrison Keillor. J Natl Cancer Inst. 2005;97:1236–7.
13. Cooperberg MR, Hinotsu S, Namiki M, Carroll PR, Akaza H. Trans-Pacific variation in outcomes for men treated with primary androgen-deprivation therapy (ADT) for prostate cancer. BJU Int. 2016;117:102–9.
14. Wallis CJ, Nam RK. Prostate cancer genetics: a review. EJIFCC. 2015;26:79–91.
15. Bostwick DG, Pacelli A, Lopez-Beltran A. Molecular biology of prostatic intraepithelial neoplasia. Prostate. 1996;29:117–34.
16. Irvine RA, Yu MC, Ross RK, Coetzee GA. The CAG and GGC microsatellites of the androgen receptor gene in linkage disequilibrium in men with prostate cancer. Cancer Res. 1995;55:1937–40.
17. Bratt O, Borg A, Kristoffersson U, Lundgren R, Zhang QX, Olsson H. CAG repeat length in the androgen receptor gene is related to age at diagnosis of prostate cancer and response to endocrine therapy, but not to prostate cancer risk. Br J Cancer. 1999;81:672–6.
18. Suzuki H, Akakura K, Komiya A, Ueda T, Imamoto T, Furuya Y, Ichikawa T, Watanabe M, Shiraishi T, Ito H. CAG polymorphic repeat lengths in androgen9receptor gene among Japanese prostate cancer patients: potential predictor of prognosis after endocrine therapy. Prostate. 2002;51:219–24.
19. Sartor O, Zheng Q, Eastham JA. Androgen receptor gene CAG repeat length varies in a race-specific fashion in men without prostate cancer. Urology. 1999;53:378–80.
20. Jin B, Beilin J, Zajac J, Handelsman DJ. Androgen receptor gene polymorphism and zonal volumes in Australian and Chinese men. J Androl. 2000;21:91–8.
21. Hsing AW, Gao YT, Wu G, Wang X, Deng J, Chen YL, Sesterhenn IA, Mostofi FK, Benichou J, Chang C. Polymorphic CAG and GGN repeat lengths in the androgen receptor gene and prostate cancer risk: a population-based case-control study in China. Cancer Res. 2000;60:5111–6.
22. Fujimoto N, Kubo T, Inatomi H, Bui HT, Shiota M, Sho T, Matsumoto T. Polymorphisms of the androgen transporting gene SLCO2B1 may influence the castration resistance of prostate cancer and the racial differences in response to androgen deprivation. Prostate Cancer Prostatic Dis. 2013;16:336–40.
23. Bliuc D, Nguyen ND, Milch VE, Nguyen TV, Eisman JA, Center JR. Mortality risk associated with low-trauma osteoporotic fracture and subsequent fracture in men and women. JAMA. 2009;301:513–21.
24. Ogawa Y, Fukagai T, Matsui Y, Koshikiya A, Nakasato T, Oshinomi K, Morita J, Aso T, Naoe M, Fuji K, Ogawa Y. The loss of bone mineral density on the long-term androgen-deprivation therapy for the prostate cancer patients. J Showa Univ Soc. 2015;75:445–9.

25. Hagino H, Yamamoto K, Ohshiro H, Nakamura T, Kishimoto H, Nose T. Changing incidence of hip, distal radius, and proximal humerus fractures in Tottori Prefecture, Japan. Bone. 1999;24:265–70.
26. Aoyagi K, Ross PD, Davis JW, Wasnich RD, Hayashi T, Takemoto T. Falls among community-dwelling elderly in Japan. J Bone Miner Res. 1998;13:1468–74.
27. Nanda A, Chen MH, Braccioforte MH, Moran BJ, D'Amico AV. Hormonal therapy use for prostate cancer and mortality in men with coronary artery disease-induced congestive heart failure or myocardial infarction. JAMA. 2009;302:866–73.
28. Health at a Glance 2015 OECD Indicators. http://www.oecd-ilibrary.org/docserver/download/8115071ec008.pdf?expires=1499094285&id=id&accname=guest&checksum=76559C1889D72A784780906659812C5F. Accessed 30 June 2017.
29. Akaza H. Future prospects for luteinizing hormone-releasing hormone analogues in prostate cancer treatment. Pharmacology. 2010;85:110–20.

Androgen Deprivation Therapy in Combination with Radical Prostatectomy

11

Takuya Koie and Chikara Ohyama

Abstract

Radical prostatectomy (RP) is one of the treatment options for patients with localized prostate cancer (PCa). The biochemical recurrence rates in patients with high-risk PCa who underwent RP alone remain high. To date, the clinical benefit, especially with respect to survival, of neoadjuvant therapies, including androgen deprivation therapy (ADT) or chemotherapy, remains unclear. Several prospective, randomized controlled trials showed higher rates of organ-confined disease, reduced rates of extracapsular extension, and reduced rates of positive surgical margins. Although the patients who received neoadjuvant ADT achieved better local tumor control, there were no differences in overall survival (OS) or biochemical recurrence-free survival (BRFS). Patients with locally advanced or seminal vesicle invasion PCa who underwent adjuvant ADT after RP achieved improved 10-year BRFS, local recurrence-free survival, systemic progression-free survival, and cancer-specific survival. However, there was no significant difference in OS. On the contrary, the BRFS rate was higher in high-risk PCa patients treated with neoadjuvant chemohormonal therapy (CHT) than in those treated with RP alone. Neoadjuvant CHT with subsequent RP might reduce the risk of biochemical recurrence.

Keywords

Prostate cancer · Radical prostatectomy · Androgen deprivation therapy Neoadjuvant therapy · Adjuvant therapy

T. Koie (✉) · C. Ohyama
Department of Urology, Hirosaki University Graduate School of Medicine, Hirosaki, Japan
e-mail: goodwin@hirosaki-u.ac.jp

11.1 Introduction

Radical prostatectomy (RP) is one of the treatment options for patients with localized prostate cancer (PCa). Although the goal of RP is complete removal of all cancer cells [1], biochemical recurrence (BCR) rates in patients with high-risk PCa [2] who underwent RP alone remain high, between 55 and 70% [3, 4]. In addition, Loeb et al. reported that 13% of patients with high-risk PCa developed metastatic disease and 6% died of PCa [5]. Treatment options for high-risk PCa include external beam radiation therapy (RT) with androgen deprivation therapy (ADT); trimodal therapy with a combination of brachytherapy, external beam RT, and ADT; and RP with neoadjuvant or adjuvant therapy. In several randomized trials, combination therapy with RT and ADT has been demonstrated to improve oncological outcomes, including overall survival (OS) and biochemical recurrence-free survival (BRFS), compared with RT alone [6, 7]. In contrast, the clinical benefit, especially with respect to survival, of neoadjuvant therapies, including ADT or chemotherapy, remains unclear. This review describes the clinical and oncological outcomes in patients with PCa who received neoadjuvant or adjuvant ADT.

11.2 Neoadjuvant Therapy

Neoadjuvant therapy is established as one of the treatment options for several malignancies, including bladder cancer [8], breast cancer [9], and cervical cancer [10]. Treatment in the neoadjuvant setting has several potential benefits: to eradicate the risk of micrometastases outside the surgical field, to achieve better local tumor control, to reduce the incidence of positive surgical margins after RP, and to assess treatment effect in the surgical specimens.

11.2.1 Neoadjuvant ADT

Several prospective, randomized controlled trials showed that neoadjuvant ADT resulted in higher rates of organ-confined disease, reduced rates of extracapsular extension, and reduced rates of positive surgical margins [11–13]. Although the patients who received neoadjuvant ADT achieved better local tumor control, there were no differences in the OS or BRFS [1, 11, 12].

Shelley et al. reviewed ten randomized clinical trials of neoadjuvant ADT used for localized or locally advanced PCa between 1996 and 2004 (Table 11.1) [13]. The authors showed that neoadjuvant ADT before RP did not improve OS (odds ratio [OR] = 1.11; $p = 0.69$) despite a significant reduction in the positive surgical margin rates (OR = 0.34; $p < 0.001$) and significant improvements in other clinical variables, including lymph node involvement, pathological stage, and organ-confined disease rates [13]. Regarding oncological outcomes, neoadjuvant ADT

Table 11.1 Summary of randomized studies of neoadjuvant androgen deprivation therapy and prostatectomy

Trial	Country	Inclusion criteria	Interventions
Gleave 2001 [1]	Canada	Stage T1b, T1c, T2. Gleason grades <6. No limit on PSA	3 months' ADT followed by RP versus 8 ADT therapy followed by RP
Soloway 2002 [11]	United States	Age <75 years, PSA <50 mg/mL. Normal bone scan. Stage T2b	RP only versus 3 months' ADT followed by RP
Klotz 2003 [12]	Canada	Stages T1–T2. Prostatic acid phosphatase <1.8 u/mL, PSA <50 ng/mL	RP alone versus 3 months' ADT followed by RP
Schulman 2000 [30]	Italy	Stage T2–T3. PSA <100 ng/mL	RP alone versus 3 months' ADT followed by RP
Aus 2002 [5]	Sweden/Denmark	Stage T1b–3a. Aged <75 years	RP alone versus 3 months' ADT followed by RP
Dalkin 1996 [31]	United states	PSA >4.0 ng/mL. Stage T1c, T2a, T2b	RP alone versus 3 months' ADT followed by RP
Prezioso 2004 [32]	Italy	Stage T1a–T2b	RP alone versus 3 months' ADT followed by RP
Labrie 1997 [33]	Canada	Stage B0–2, C1–2	RP alone versus 3 months' ADT followed by RP
Selli 2002 [34]	Italy	Stage T2–T3	RP alone versus 3 months' ADT followed by RP versus 6 months' ADT followed by RP
Van Der Kwast 1999 [35]	The Netherlands/Canada	Stage T1–T3	3 months' ADT followed by RP versus 6 months' ADT followed by RP

PSA prostate-specific antigen, *ADT* androgen deprivation therapy, *RP* radical prostatectomy

resulted in a marginal significant reduction in BRFS (OR = 0.74; $p = 0.05$) [13]. The authors concluded that neoadjuvant ADT is associated with significant clinical benefits for improved local control but does not result in improved OS [13].

O'Shaughnessy et al. reported chronological changes in the rates of neoadjuvant ADT use before RP [14]. The use of neoadjuvant ADT before surgery increased from 6.7% in 1993 to a peak of 17.6% in 1996 [14]. In contrast, the frequency of neoadjuvant ADT use decreased to 13.6% of the patients who underwent RP in 1997 and continued to decline to 12.4% in 2000, 8.6% in 2003, 6.9% in 2005, and 4.6% in 2007 [14]. The downward trend in the use of neoadjuvant ADT after 1996 was due to several reports showing no evidence of benefit in terms of disease recurrence, metastasis, or death [1, 11, 12, 14]. In addition, an increased risk of osteoporotic fractures in patients who received ≥5 doses of ADT has been reported [15], and the risks of cardiovascular and metabolic morbidity were found to be increased as long-term consequences of androgen deprivation [16, 17]. Thus, the evidence of increased harm from ADT may account for the decreased use of neoadjuvant ADT.

11.2.2 Neoadjuvant Chemohormonal Therapy

To improve the oncological outcomes for high-risk PCa, multimodal treatments involving combinations of RP, RT, hormonal therapy, and/or chemotherapy have been investigated. Although the true effect remains controversial because of the lack of results from large randomized trials, neoadjuvant chemohormonal therapy (CHT) may have an important role as one of the treatment options for high-risk PCa.

Narita et al. reported the oncological outcomes in 18 patients with high-risk PCa who received neoadjuvant CHT before RP [17]. Treatment consisted of complete androgen blockade followed by six cycles of docetaxel with estramustine phosphate (EMP) [17]. Two patients (11.1%) had no detectable tumor (pathological complete response [CR]) and surgical margins were negative in all patients [17]. The BRFS was not attained in this study [17].

The patients with high-risk PCa received a gonadotropin-releasing hormone (GnRH) antagonist or luteinizing hormone-releasing hormone (LHRH) agonist with low-dose EMP for at least 6 months before RP at our institution [18–20]. In patients who underwent RP alone, the numbers of patients with lymph node involvement and positive surgical margins were significantly higher than those who received neoadjuvant LHRH and EMP [19]. The 5-year BRFS rates were 90.4% among patients who received neoadjuvant LHRH and EMP and 65.8% among patients who underwent RP alone [19]. The 2-year BRFS rates were 97.8% in patients who received neoadjuvant GnRH and EMP and 87.8% in those with neoadjuvant LHRH and EMP ($p = 0.027$) [20]. Neoadjuvant CHT may potentially achieve long-term BRFS in high-risk PCa patients.

11.2.3 The Rate of Pathological T0 Detected from the Surgical Specimens

In general, PCa patients diagnosed with pathological stage T0 (pT0) based on surgical specimens are assumed to have a good prognosis since BCR does not occur or occurs extremely rarely in these patients. Joung et al. reported that 5.4% of the patients with high-risk PCa who received neoadjuvant ADT before RP achieved pT0 and none of the patients with pT0 showed disease recurrence [21]. However, Kollemann et al. reported that BCR was observed in 18.4% of the patients with pT0 disease who received neoadjuvant ADT before RP during a median follow-up period of 47 months [22]. Of these, three patients had local recurrence or distant metastases [22]. In addition, BRFS was not significantly different between PCa patients with or without pT0 disease [23]. The reasons for the clinical failure of neoadjuvant ADT to improve survival are unclear.

In our previous study, the number of patients who received neoadjuvant LHRH and EMP with lymph node involvement and positive surgical margins was significantly lower than the number of patients who underwent RP alone (Fig. 11.1) [19]. Seventeen patients (8%) who received neoadjuvant LHRH and EMP achieved pT0 (Table 11.2) [19]. On the other hand, pathologic CR was achieved in 11% of the patients who

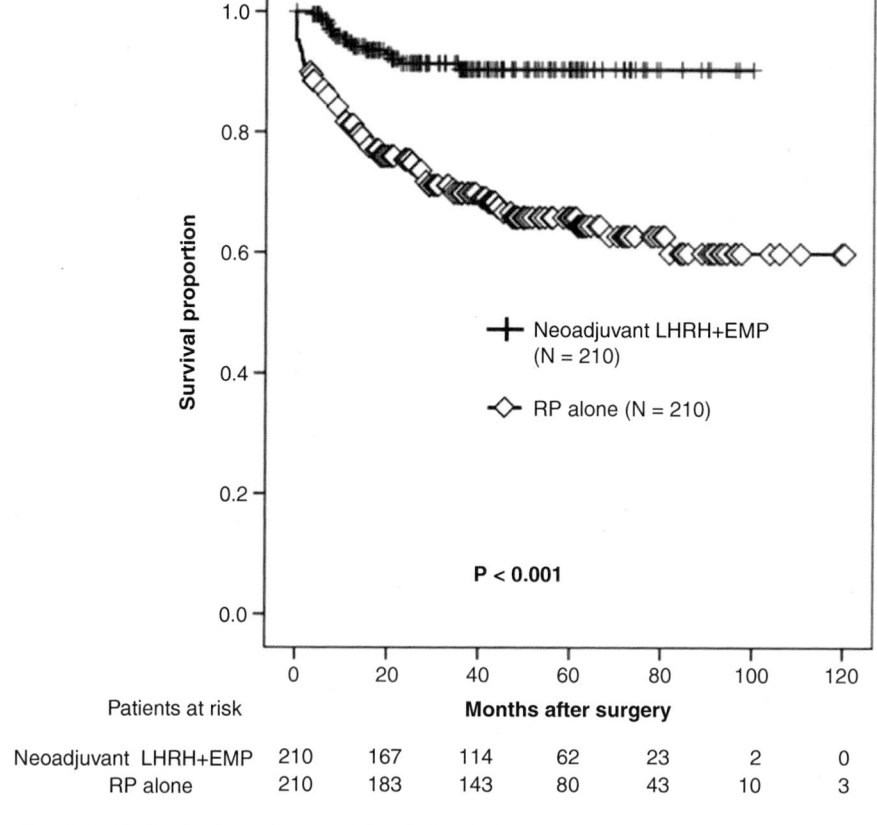

11 Androgen Deprivation Therapy in Combination with Radical Prostatectomy

Patients at risk	0	20	40	60	80	100	120
Neoadjuvant LHRH+EMP	210	167	114	62	23	2	0
RP alone	210	183	143	80	43	10	3

Fig. 11.1 Kaplan–Meier estimates of the biochemical recurrence-free survival (BRFS) in high-risk prostate cancer patients who received radical prostatectomy with or without neoadjuvant therapy. The 5-year BRFS rates were 90.4% among patients who received neoadjuvant luteinizing hormone-releasing hormone plus estramustine and 65.8% among patients who underwent prostatectomy alone ($p < 0.001$)

Table 11.2 Pathological outcomes

	Neoadjuvant LHRH + EMP ($N = 210$)	RP alone ($N = 210$)	p
Pathological stage, number (%)			0.0749
T0	17 (8)	0	
T2a	47 (22)	17 (8)	
T2b	18 (9)	13 (6)	
T2c	50 (24)	84 (40)	
T3a	65 (31)	55 (26)	
T3b	30 (14)	32 (15)	
T4	0	9 (4)	

LHRH luteinizing hormone-releasing hormone, *EMP* estramustine, *RP* radical prostatectomy

received neoadjuvant GnRH and EMP [20]. The pathological T stage was significantly lower in the patients who received neoadjuvant GnRH and EMP than in those who received neoadjuvant LHRH and EMP ($p = 0.007$) [20]. For this reason, the suppression of testosterone levels and follicle-stimulating hormone confers an oncological benefit for PCa, considering its possible role in tumor growth [20].

11.2.4 The Effects of Neoadjuvant Therapy in Patients with PCa Following RP

Although neoadjuvant ADT is associated with significant clinical benefits for improved local control, including positive surgical margin rates, lymph node involvement, pathological stage, and organ-confined disease rates, ADT induces prostatic apoptosis associated with prostatic and periprostatic fibrosis [24]. Therefore, neoadjuvant therapy can alter normal anatomic planes [25], which may lead to greater numbers of patients with positive tumor margins and higher morbidity rates following RP [26].

Williams et al. analyzed the data from 215 consecutive patients with PCa who received neoadjuvant therapy [25]. Of these, 29% experienced a complication of any grade ≤90 days after surgery; 6% experienced grade ≥3, with no significant difference between the cohorts ($p = 0.5$) [25]. Hou et al. reported that neoadjuvant ADT was an independent predictor of prolonged total operating time [26]. In our previous study, we experienced rectal injury in 1 patient (0.4%), leakage from the vesicourethral anastomosis in 35 patients (17%), and surgical site infection in 5 patients (2%); all of these events are considered acceptable complications associated with RP in patients with high-risk PCa [19]. The use of neoadjuvant systemic therapy does not appear likely to increase the risk of perioperative complications [25].

11.3 Adjuvant Therapy

Wirth et al. conducted a randomized clinical trial to assess the efficacy of adjuvant flutamide in patients with locally advanced, lymph node-negative PCa (stage pT3-4N0) after RP [27]. BRFS was better in patients with adjuvant flutamide than in those with RP alone ($p = 0.0041$) [27]. However, there was no significant difference in OS between the groups ($p = 0.92$) [27].

Siddiqui et al. reported the impact of adjuvant ADT on survival in patients with seminal vesicle invasion at the time of RP [28]. A total of 12,115 patients who underwent RP for PCa were identified in this retrospective study. Of these, 191 patients with adjuvant ADT were matched 1:1 to patients with pT3b PCa who received no adjuvant treatment [28]. Patients who underwent adjuvant ADT experienced improved 10-year BRFS, local recurrence-free survival, systemic progression-free survival, and cancer-specific survival (CSS) [28]. However, OS was not significantly different between the groups [28].

Moschini et al. investigated the long-term utility of adjuvant therapy after RP for PCa with seminal vesicle invasion [29]. In this study, 3279 patients with pT3b PCa after RP were included with a median follow-up of 148 months [29]. Overall, adjuvant ADT was associated with improved BCR, cancer-specific mortality (CSM), and overall mortality (OM) [29]. According to an analysis of patients with pT3bN0 PCa, adjuvant ADT was associated with improved BRFS, CSS, and OM [29]. Regarding patients with pT3b and lymph node involvement, adjuvant ADT was associated with an increase in BRFS, but there was no effect on CSM and OM [29].

Adjuvant ADT may improve local and systemic control after RP for pT3b PCa [28]. However, there is no current consensus regarding the optimal adjuvant therapy treatment regimens in patients with high-risk PCa after RP.

Conclusions

Although the patients who received neoadjuvant ADT achieved better local tumor control, there were no differences in OS or BRFS. Likewise, adjuvant ADT may improve local and systemic cancer control after RP for PCa patients with locally advanced disease or seminal vesicle invasion. However, there was no impact on OS. On the other hand, neoadjuvant CHT may potentially achieve long-term BRFS in high-risk PCa patients.

References

1. Gleave ME, Goldenberg SL, Chin JL, et al. Randomized comparative study of 3 versus 8-month neoadjuvant hormonal therapy before radical prostatectomy: biochemical and pathological effects. J Urol. 2001;166:500–6.
2. Lester-Coll NH, Goldhaber SZ, Sher DJ, et al. Death from high-risk prostate cancer versus cardiovascular mortality with hormone therapy. Cancer. 2013;119:1808–15.
3. Yuh B, Artibani W, Heidenreich A, et al. The role of robot-assisted radical prostatectomy and pelvic lymph node dissection in the management of high-risk prostate cancer: a systematic review. Eur Urol. 2013;65:918–27.
4. Yossepowitch O, Eggener SE, Serio AM, et al. Secondary therapy, metastatic progression, and cancer-specific mortality in men with clinically high-risk prostate cancer treated with radical prostatectomy. Eur Urol. 2008;53:950–9.
5. Loeb S, Schaeffer EM, Trock BJ, et al. What are the outcomes of radical prostatectomy for high-risk prostate cancer? Urology. 2010;76:710–4.
6. Mason MD, Parulekar WR, Sydes MR, et al. Final report of the intergroup randomized study of combined androgen-deprivation therapy plus radiotherapy versus androgen-deprivation therapy alone in locally advanced prostate cancer. J Clin Oncol. 2015;33:2143–50.
7. Widmark A, Klepp O, Solberg A, et al. Endocrine treatment, with or without radiotherapy, in locally advanced prostate cancer (SPCG-7/SFUO-3): an open randomized phase III trial. Lancet. 2009;373:301–8.
8. Grossman HB, Natale RB, Tangen CM, et al. Neoadjuvant chemotherapy plus cystectomy compared with cystectomy alone for locally advanced bladder cancer. N Engl J Med. 2003;349:859–66.
9. Bear HD, Anderson S, Brown A, et al. The effect on tumor response of adding sequential preoperative docetaxel to preoperative doxorubicin and cyclophosphamide: preliminary results

from National Surgical Adjuvant Breast and Bowel Project Protocol B-27. J Clin Oncol. 2003;21:4165–674.
10. Benedetti PP, Bellati F, et al. An update in neoadjuvant chemotherapy in cervical cancer. Gynecol Oncol. 2007;107:s20–2.
11. Soloway MS, Pareek K, Sharifi R, et al. Neoadjuvant androgen ablation before radical prostatectomy in cT2bNxMo prostate cancer: 5-year results. J Urol. 2002;167:112–6.
12. Klotz LH, Goldenberg SL, Jewett MA, et al. Long-term followup of a randomized trial of 0 versus 3 months of neoadjuvant androgen ablation before radical prostatectomy. J Urol. 2003;170:791–4.
13. Shelley MD, Kumar S, Wilt T, et al. A systematic review and meta-analysis of randomised trials of neo-adjuvant hormone therapy for localised and locally advanced prostate carcinoma. Cancer Treat Rev. 2009;35:9–17.
14. O'Shaughnessy MJ, Jarosek SL, Virnig BA, et al. Factors associated with reduction in use of neoadjuvant androgen suppression therapy before radical prostatectomy. Urology. 2013;81:745–51.
15. Braga-Basaria M, Dobs AS, Muller DC, et al. Metabolic syndrome in men with prostate cancer undergoing long-term androgen-deprivation therapy. J Clin Oncol. 2006;24:3979–83.
16. Keating NL, O'Malley AJ, Smith MR. Diabetes and cardiovascular disease during androgen deprivation therapy for prostate cancer. J Clin Oncol. 2006;24:4448–56.
17. Narita S, Tsuchiya N, Kumazawa T, et al. Short-term clinicopathological outcome of neoadjuvant chemohormonal therapy comprising complete androgen blockade, followed by treatment with docetaxel and estramustine phosphate before radical prostatectomy in Japanese patients with high-risk localized prostate cancer. World J Surg Oncol. 2012;10:1.
18. Koie T, Ohyama C, Yamamoto H, et al. Safety and effectiveness of neoadjuvant luteinizing hormone-releasing hormone agonist plus low-dose estramustine phosphate in high-risk prostate cancer: a prospective single-arm study. Prostate Cancer Prostatic Dis. 2012;15:397–401.
19. Koie T, Mitsuzuka K, Yoneyama T, et al. Neoadjuvant luteinizing-hormone-releasing hormone agonist plus low-dose estramustine phosphate improves prostate-specific antigen-free survival in high-risk prostate cancer patients: a propensity score-matched analysis. Int J Clin Oncol. 2015;20:1018–25.
20. Hagiwara K, Koie T, Ohyama C. Efficacy of a neoadjuvant gonadotropin-releasing hormone antagonist plus low-dose estramustine phosphate in high-risk prostate cancer: a single-center study. Int Urol Nephrol. 2017;49:811–6.
21. Joung JY, Kim JE, Kim SH, et al. The prevalence and outcomes of pT0 disease after neoadjuvant hormonal therapy and radical prostatectomy in high-risk prostate cancer. BMC Urol. 2015;15:82.
22. Köllermann J, Caprano J, Budde A, et al. Follow-up of nondetectable prostate carcinoma (pT0) after prolonged PSA-monitored neoadjuvant hormonal therapy followed by radical prostatectomy. Urology. 2003;62:476–80.
23. Köllermann J, Hopfenmüller W, Caprano J. Prognosis of stage pT0 after prolonged neoadjuvant endocrine therapy of prostate cancer: a matched-pair analysis. Eur Urol. 2004;45:42–5.
24. Brown JA, Garlitz C, Strup SE, et al. Laparoscopic radical prostatectomy after neoadjuvant hormonal therapy: an apparently safe and effective procedure. J Laparoendosc Adv Surg Tech A. 2004;14:335–8.
25. Williams SB, Davis JW, Wang X, et al. Neoadjuvant systemic therapy before radical prostatectomy in high-risk prostate cancer does not increase surgical morbidity: contemporary results using the Clavien system. Clin Genitourin Cancer. 2016;14:130–8.
26. Hou CP, Lee WC, Lin YH, et al. Neoadjuvant hormone therapy following treatment with robotic-assisted radical prostatectomy achieved favorable in high-risk prostate cancer. Onco Targets Ther. 2015;8:15–9.
27. Wirth MP, Weissbach L, Marx FJ, et al. Prospective randomized trial comparing flutamide as adjuvant treatment versus observation after radical prostatectomy for locally advanced, lymph node-negative prostate cancer. Eur Urol. 2004;45:2672–0.

28. Siddiqui SA, Boorjian SA, Blute ML, et al. Impact of adjuvant androgen deprivation therapy after radical prostatectomy on the survival of patients with pathological T3b prostate cancer. BJU Int. 2011;107:383–8.
29. Moschini M, Sharma V, Gandaglia G, et al. Long-term utility of adjuvant hormonal and radiation therapy for patients with seminal vesicle invasion at radical prostatectomy. BJU Int. 2017;120:69–75.
30. Schulman CC, Debruyne FM, Forster G, et al. 4-year follow-up results of a European prospective randomized study on neoadjuvant hormonal therapy prior to radical prostatectomy in T2-3N0M0 prostate cancer. European Study Group on Neoadjuvant Treatment of Prostate Cancer. Eur Urol. 2000;38:706–13.
31. Dalkin BL, Ahmann FR, Nagle R, et al. Randomized study of neoadjuvant testicular androgen ablation therapy before radical prostatectomy in men with clinically localized prostate cancer. J Urol. 1996;155:1357–60.
32. Prezioso D, Lotti T, Polito M, et al. Neoadjuvant hormone treatment with leuprolide acetate depot 3.75 mg and cyproterone acetate, before radical prostatectomy: a randomized study. Urol Int. 2004;72:189–95.
33. Labrie F, Cusan L, Gomez JL, et al. Neoadjuvant hormonal therapy: the Canadian experience. Urology. 1997;49:56–64.
34. Selli C, Montironi R, Bono A, et al. Effects of complete androgen blockade for 12 and 24 weeks on the pathological stage and resection margin status of prostate cancer. J Clin Pathol. 2002;55:508–13.
35. van der Kwast TH, Têtu B, Candas B, et al. Prolonged neoadjuvant combined androgen blockade leads to a further reduction of prostatic tumor volume: three versus six months of endocrine therapy. Urology. 1999;53:523–9.

ADT in Combination with Radiation Therapy for Clinically Localized Prostate Cancer

12

Takashi Mizowaki

Abstract

External beam radiotherapy (EBRT) is a well-established definitive therapeutic approach for clinically localized prostate cancer (CLPCa). Although CLPCa had been mainly treated with EBRT alone, androgen deprivation therapy (ADT) has been shown to improve not only biochemical control but also survival outcomes when combined with EBRT.

Adding ADT to EBRT using former standard doses (65–70 Gy) significantly improved survival outcomes compared with EBRT alone in patients with intermediate- or high-risk disease. Therefore, ADT is considered to be an essential element in definitive EBRT for most cases of CLPCa.

In terms of intermediate-risk patients, the neoadjuvant combination of ADT for a period of 4–6 months combined with EBRT is recommended. On the other hand, for high- or very-high-risk patients, neoadjuvant ADT for 4–6 months followed by adjuvant ADT for 24–30 months is considered to be the standard treatment for use in combination with EBRT.

However, the optimal duration of ADT in combination with EBRT remains controversial. In addition, the usefulness of ADT is controversial when combined with dose-escalated EBRT. Moreover, ethnic differences in patient sensitivity to ADT have been suggested. Randomized trials are required to clear up these unsolved issues regarding ADT combined with EBRT.

Keywords

Clinically localized prostate cancer · Radiation therapy · Combined androgen deprivation therapy

T. Mizowaki, M.D. Ph.D.
Department of Radiation Oncology and Image-applied Therapy, Kyoto University Graduate School of Medicine, Kyoto, Japan
e-mail: mizo@kuhp.kyoto-u.ac.jp

12.1 Introduction

The impact of the combination of androgen deprivation therapy (ADT) with radiation therapy for clinically localized prostate cancer (CLPCa) has been largely explored with respect to external beam radiation therapy (EBRT) through the use of randomized trials. However, no prospective randomized trial has been conducted to confirm the impact of ADT on brachytherapy for CLPCa, even though ADT is also often clinically combined with brachytherapy. Therefore, this chapter focuses on EBRT as a radiotherapeutic approach for use in combination with ADT.

Thus far, six randomized trials have demonstrated highly significant improvements in survival with combined ADT and EBRT, compared with EBRT alone (Tables 12.1 and 12.2). Combined short-term neoadjuvant ADT (NA-ADT) ± concurrent ADT demonstrated survival advantages over EBRT alone in patients with intermediate- and high-risk CLPCa (Table 12.1). In addition, long-term adjuvant ADT (A-ADT) resulted in significantly better survival outcomes, mainly in high- or very-high-risk cases, compared with those who were treated with EBRT alone (Table 12.2). The radiation doses used in most of these trials were former standard doses (65–70 Gy).

Other randomized studies also confirmed that dose escalations above the former standard doses to the prostate improve prostate-specific antigen (PSA) control rates [1, 2]. However, the impact of dose escalation on survival has not been demonstrated in phase III trials [3, 4]. On the other hand, combined ADT significantly improves survival, as indicated in this chapter. Therefore, ADT is considered to be an essential component of definitive EBRT for CLPCa.

Evidence of definitive EBRT with ADT in East Asian populations, including the Japanese, is rather sparse. In addition, the timing of the start of salvage ADT (S-ADT) in patients who developed a PSA recurrence, which may affect the prognosis [5–7], was not defined in any of the trials conducted in Western countries. Moreover, the impact of combined ADT and dose-escalated EBRT remains controversial [8].

12.2 EBRT Plus ADT Versus EBRT Alone

12.2.1 Overview of the Combination of ADT with EBRT

EBRT alone was previously the main treatment approach in definitive EBRT for prostate cancer [9]. However, not only biochemically recurrence free, but also survival advantages of combined EBRT with AD T over EBRT alone have been proven by randomized trials conducted mainly in the 1980s and 2000s (Tables 12.1 and 12.2). Therefore, combined EBRT with ADT has become a standard approach for patients with intermediate- or high-risk CLPCa. On the other hand, EBRT alone remains as the standard treatment modality for low-risk cases since excellent biochemical control can be achieved by minimizing severe adverse events with dose-escalated EBRT, and, hence, adverse events associated with ADT can be avoided [10, 11].

Table 12.1 Randomized phase III studies comparing NA-ADT plus EBRT versus EBRT alone

Study	n	Clinical stage	RT dose (Gy)	RT field	Arm	PSAF (%)	DM (%)	PCSM (%)	OM (%)	Median FU (years)
RTOG 86-10 [15]	456	Bulky T2-4N0-1M0	65–70	WP	RT alone EBRT + 4M-ADT (NA+C)	80 **65**	47 **35**	36 **23**	66 57	13.2 11.9
RTOG 94-08 [16]	1979	T1b-2bN0M0	66.6	WP	RT alone EBRT + 4M-ADT (NA+C)	41 **26**	8 **6**	8 **4**	43 **38**	9.1
TROG 96-01 [17]	818	T2b-4N0M0	66	PSV	RT alone EBRT + 3M-ADT (NA+C) EBRT + 6M-ADT (NA+C)	74 **60** **53**	14 15 **10**	22 19 **11**	43 37 **29**	10.6
Laverdiere [18]	161	T2-3N0M0	64	PSV	EBRT alone EBRT + 3M-ADT (NA) EBRT + 10M-ADT (NA+C+A)	58 **34** **31**	N/A	N/A	N/A	5
PMH 9907 [19][a]	252	T1b-2N0M0	75.6–79.8	PSV	EBRT alone EBRT + 5M-Anti-A (NA+C)	24 17	N/A	N/A	14 18	9.1
D'Amico [20]	206	T1b-2cN0M0	70	PSV	EBRT alone EBRT + 6M-ADT (NA+C+A)	[b]	N/A	14 **4**	39 **26**	7.6

[a] The study was closed early
[b] ADT use for PSAF was significantly lower in the RT+ADT arm
Bold number: significantly different from the control (EBRT alone)
EBRT external beam radiotherapy, *n* number of patients, *PSAF* prostate-specific antigen failure, *DM* distant metastasis, *PCSM* prostate cancer-specific mortality, *OM* overall mortality, *FU* follow-up period, *M* month, *WP* whole pelvis, *P+SV* prostate plus seminal vesicles, *ADT* androgen deprivation therapy, *NA* neoadjuvant, *C* concurrent, *A* adjuvant, *N/A* not available

Table 12.2 Randomized phase III studies comparing A-ADT plus EBRT versus EBRT alone

Study	n	Clinical stage	RT dose (Gy)	RT field	Arm	PSAF (%)	DM (%)	PCSM (%)	OM (%)	Median FU (years)
RTOG 85-31 [21]	977	T3N0-1M0	65–70	WP	EBRT alone EBRT + permanent ADT (A)	N/A	39 **24**	22 **16**	61 **51**	11
EORTC 22863 [22]	415	T1-4N0M0	70	WP	EBRT alone EBRT + 36M-ADT (C+A)	N/A	70[a] **49**[a]	30 **10**	60 **42**	9.1
EORTC 22991 [23]	819	T1b-2aN0M0	70,74,78	P+SV (WP)	EBRT alone EBRT + 6M-ADT (C+A)	30 **17**	8 4	4 2	12 9	7.2

[a]Distant metastases or all cause of death

Bold number: significantly different from the control (EBRT alone)

EBRT external beam radiotherapy, *n* number of patients, *PSAF* prostate-specific antigen failure, *DM* distant metastasis, *PCSM* prostate cancer-specific mortality, *OM* overall mortality, *FU* follow-up period, *M* month, *WP* whole pelvis, *P+SV* prostate plus seminal vesicles, *ADT* androgen deprivation therapy, *C* concurrent, *A* adjuvant, *N/A* not available

Table 12.3 Randomized phase III studies comparing different durations of NA-ADT in combination with EBRT

Study	n	Clinical stage	RT dose (Gy)	RT field	Arm	PSAF (%)	DM (%)	PCSM (%)	OM (%)	Median FU (years)
TROG 96-01 [17]	818	T2b-4N0M0	66	P+SV	EBRT alone	74	14	22	43	10.6
					EBRT + 3M-ADT (NA+C)	**60**	15	19	37	
					EBRT + 6M-ADT (NA+C)	**53**	**10**	**11**	**29**	
Crook [37]	378	T1c-4N0M0	66–67	P+SV WP	EBRT + 3M-ADT (NA)	42	N/A	6	19	6.6
					EBRT + 8M-ADT (NA)	35		7	21	
ICORG 97-01 [38]	276	T1-4N0M0	70	P+SV	EBRT + 4M-ADT (NA)	34[a]	N/A	4	10	8.5
					EBRT + 8M-ADT (NA)	37[a]		8	17	
RTOG 99-01 [39]	1489	T1b-T4N0M0	70.2	P+SV WP	EBRT + 4M-ADT (NA+C)	27	6	5	34	9.4
					EBRT + 9M-ADT (NA+C)	27	6	4	33	

[a] PSAF or all cause of death

Bold number: significantly different from the control (EBRT alone or EBRT plus short-term ADT)

EBRT external beam radiotherapy, *n* number of patients, *PSAF* prostate-specific antigen failure, *DM* distant metastasis, *PCSM* prostate cancer-specific mortality, *OM* overall mortality, *FU* follow-up period, *M* month, *WP* whole pelvis, *P+SV* prostate plus seminal vesicles, *ADT* androgen deprivation therapy, *NA* neoadjuvant, *C* concurrent, *N/A* not available

There are two major approaches to combining ADT with EBRT: short- and long-term ADT. Short-term ADT is usually combined with EBRT as a neoadjuvant ± concurrent setting with durations of 3–10 months (Tables 12.1, 12.3, and 12.4). On the other hand, long-term ADT is mostly used after EBRT adjuvantly (± concurrently) (Table 12.2). Long-term ADT is also combined with short-term NA-ADT, mainly for patients with locally advanced disease [11] (Table 12.4).

12.2.2 NA-ADT Plus EBRT Versus EBRT Alone

Theoretically, the combination of ADT neoadjuvantly with EBRT has the following benefits. First, improved tumor control can be expected because ADT prior to EBRT enhances tumor eradication compared with EBRT alone, as shown in animal experiments [12]. Second, NA-ADT reduces the volume of the prostate by around 30% on average [13, 14], and this is expected to decrease the risk of adverse effects associated with EBRT by allowing a reduced radiation field size to cover the prostate.

Several randomized phase III studies comparing EBRT plus short-term NA-ADT (± concurrent ADT) with EBRT alone have been conducted [15–20] (Table 12.1). In these studies, intermediate- to moderately high-risk T1-T3N0M0 cases were the main targets. As for the radiation fields, both localized (prostate and seminal vesicles) and whole pelvis followed by a local boost approaches were indicated. The radiation doses were the former standard doses (65–70 Gy) in most studies except for the PMH 9907 study [19], where escalated doses (75.6–79.8 Gy) were used. The duration of NA-ADT in these studies varied from 3 to 10 months. In all but the PMH 9907 study, significantly lower PSA recurrence rates were achieved in combined approaches compared with EBRT alone (Table 12.1). In addition, the combined approach of short-term NA-ADT with EBRT significantly improved both prostate cancer-specific mortality (PCSM) and overall mortality in most studies.

In summary, 4–6 months of NA-ADT significantly improves not only biochemical but also survival outcomes in CLPCa treated with EBRT using the former standard doses. On the other hand, the PMH 9907 study (with a dose-escalated setting) failed to show such benefits. However, the PMH 9970 study only used bicalutamide as hormonal therapy, and the study was closed earlier than planned because subsequent evidence suggested that the relative clinical effectiveness of bicalutamide was inferior to that of standard ADT with luteinizing hormone-releasing hormone agonists [19]. Therefore, the impact of short-term ADT on dose-escalated EBRT remains an open question.

12.2.3 A-ADT Plus EBRT Versus EBRT Alone

There have been three randomized trials comparing A-ADT (± concurrent ADT) plus EBRT versus EBRT alone [21–23] (Table 12.2). Two studies combining long-term (3 years or permanent) A-ADT with EBRT using the former standard doses demonstrated a significant improvement in survival by combining A-ADT

Table 12.4 Randomized phase III studies comparing short-term ADT plus EBRT versus intermediate/long-term ADT plus EBRT

Study	n	Clinical stage	RT dose (Gy)	RT field	Arm	PSAF (%)	DM (%)	PCSM (%)	OM (%)	Median FU (years)
EORTC 22961 [28]	1113	T1c-4N0-1M0	70	WP	EBRT + 6M-ADT (C+A) EBRT + 36M-ADT (C+A)	N/A	N/A	4.7 **3.2**	19 **15**	6.4
RTOG 92-02 [29]	1554	T2c-4N0M0	65–70	WP	EBRT + 4M-ADT (NA+C) EBRT + 28M-ADT (NA+C+A)	61 **45**	26 **17**	22 **16**	73 **70**	19.6
TROG 03-04 [31]	1071	T2b-4N0M0	66–74 46+HDR	P+SV	EBRT + 6M-ADT (NA+C) EBRT + 18M-ADT (NA+C+A)	34 29	15 14	4.1 7.4	17 19	7.4
DART01/05 GICOR [30]	362	T1c-3bN0M0	76–82	P+SV	EBRT + 4M-ADT (NA+C) EBRT + 28M-ADT (NA+C+A)	19[a] **10**[a]	17[b] **6**[b]	3 0	14 **5**	5.3
Ito [32]	280	T3-4N0M0	72	P+SV	EBRT + 14M-ADT (NA+C+A) EBRT + 60M-ADT (NA+C+A)	36[a,c] 42[a,c]	N/A	N/A	20 25	8.2

[a]PSAF or all cause of death
[b]Distant metastases or all cause of death
[c]Non-inferiority unproven
Bold number: significantly different from the control (short-term ADT plus EBRT)
EBRT external beam radiotherapy, *n* number of patients, *PSAF* prostate-specific antigen failure, *DM* distant metastasis, *PCSM* prostate cancer-specific mortality, *OM* overall mortality, *FU* follow-up period, *M* month, *WP* whole pelvis, *P+SV* prostate plus seminal vesicles, *ADT* androgen deprivation therapy, *NA* neoadjuvant, *C* concurrent, *A* adjuvant, *N/A* not available, *HDR* high-dose-rate brachytherapy boost

with EBRT, compared with EBRT alone [21, 22]. The main targets of these studies were patients with locally advanced (T3-4N0M0) CLPCa. Therefore, long-term (2–3 years) ADT is recommended with EBRT for locally advanced CLPCa [10, 11].

The most recent study combined short-term (6 months) A-ADT with EBRT found no significant difference in survival with a median follow-up period of 7.2 years [23]. When compared with the dramatically positive impact of short-term NA-ADT on survival, short-term ADT may need to be administered neoadjuvantly rather than adjuvantly when combined with EBRT using the former standard doses.

12.3 Impact of EBRT on Primary ADT for Locally Advanced Diseases

Locally advanced prostate cancer was formerly treated with primary ADT alone, especially in Japan. In this situation, lifelong ADT is often selected. The significance of adding local EBRT to primary ADT has been debated. However, randomized phase III studies demonstrated the dramatic impact of adding EBRT to primary ADT for locally advanced cases, in terms of not only PSA control, but also survival (Table 12.5). In both the SPCG-7/SFUO-3 and NCIC CTG PR-3/MRC UK PR07 studies, the PCSM rates were reduced by around half when EBRT was added, compared with the rates in those treated by primary ADT alone [24–27]. Because the radiation doses (65–70 Gy) used in these studies can be safely delivered with three-dimensional conformal radiation therapy, EBRT should be combined with long-term ADT for patients with locally advanced prostate cancer, except for patients unfit for EBRT.

12.4 Impact of the Duration of ADT Combined with EBRT

12.4.1 Duration of Short-Term NA-ADT

Table 12.3 summarizes randomized phase III studies comparing different durations of NA-ADT with definitive EBRT for CLPCa. Because ADT is mainly applied to patients with intermediate-risk or moderately high-risk prostate cancer, the duration of ADT is relatively short (6–9 months) even in long-term arms, compared with the duration of long-term arms (28–60 months) in A-ADT studies (Tables 12.3 and 12.4). Although the 3-month ADT arm in the TROG 96-01 study failed to show survival advantages compared to EBRT alone, while the 6-month ADT arm achieved significant improvements in both PSA control and survival outcomes [17], all other studies failed to demonstrate significant differences, not only in survival but also in the PSA failure rate, between shorter (3–4 months) ADT and longer (8–9 months) ADT arms. Therefore, it seems that an ADT duration of 4–6 months will be sufficient for use in combination with EBRT as NA-ADT. Although the role of short-term NA-ADT in a dose escalation setting is unclear, it appears to be reasonable to

Table 12.5 Randomized phase III studies comparing ADT plus EBRT versus primary ADT alone

Study	n	Clinical stage	RT dose (Gy)	RT field	Arm	PSAF (%)	DM (%)	PCSM (%)	OM (%)	Median FU (years)
SPCG-7/SFUO-3 [24, 25]	875	T1b-3N0M0	70 (74–78)	P+SV	Lifelong ADT alone Lifelong ADT plus EBRT	75[a] **26**[a]	N/A	34 **17**	61 **51**	12.2
Mottet [40]	264	T3-4(pT3)N0M0	68–70	WP	36M-ADT alone 36M-ADT + EBRT	85 **35**	11 **3**	14 **7**	28 29	5.6
NCIC CTG PR-3/MRC UK PR07 [26, 27]	1205	T2-4N0M0	65–69	WP	Lifelong ADT alone Lifelong ADT + EBRT	73 **37**	N/A	22 **11**	51 **45**	8

[a] At 7 years
Bold number: significantly different from the control (primary ADT alone)
EBRT external beam radiotherapy, *n* number of patients, *PSAF* prostate-specific antigen failure, *DM* distant metastasis, *PCSM* prostate cancer-specific mortality, *OM* overall mortality, *FU* follow-up period, *M* month, *WP* pelvis, *P+SV* prostate plus seminal vesicles, *ADT* androgen deprivation therapy, *N/A* not available

combine 4–6 months of NA-ADT in view of the striking impact of NA-ADT on survival combined with former standard doses of EBRT because no survival benefit has been proven in any randomized trial using dose-escalated EBRT alone.

12.4.2 Comparison of Short-Term ADT and Intermediate/Long-Term ADT

Randomized trials comparing short-term (4–6 months) ADT with long-term (28–36 months) ADT in combination with EBRT have been mainly conducted in patients with high- or very-high-risk CLPCa (Table 12.4). In those studies, long-term ADT arms demonstrated significant improvement in survival outcomes compared to those with short-term ADT with EBRT [28–30].

In the TROG 03-04 study, intermediate-term (18 months) ADT failed to demonstrate survival advantages over 6 months of ADT, although it was suggested that intermediate-term ADT plus zoledronic acid was more effective than short-term ADT [31]. On the other hand, Ito et al. [32] reported the results of a non-inferiority study comparing long-term (60 months) ADT and intermediate-term ADT (14 months) followed by intermittent ADT (intermittent arm: restart ADT when the PSA value exceeds 5 ng/mL) when combined with EBRT of 72 Gy in patients with locally advanced (T3-4N0M0) disease. Although non-inferiority of the intermittent arm was not proven, there were no statistically significant differences between the arms with regard to not only overall survival but also PSA recurrence-free survival between the arms. Therefore, no consensus has been achieved regarding the usefulness of intermediate-term ADT in EBRT.

Together with the above findings and the impact of short-term NA-ADT over EBRT alone, the current standard treatment for high- or very-high-risk CLPCa is considered to be 4–6 months of NA-ADT followed by EBRT plus an additional 24–30 months of A-ADT [10, 11].

On the other hand, in the subset analyses of both RTOG 92-02 and DART 01/05 GICOR studies, intermediate-risk groups did not show any significant benefits from long-term ADT compared with short-term ADT [30, 33]. Therefore, short-term NA-ADT remains the standard of care with respect to patients with intermediate-risk CLPCa [10, 11].

12.5 Optimal Duration of ADT in Combination with EBRT

There is broad consensus that ADT should not be combined with EBRT in patients with low-risk disease, who can expect to be safely cured by high-dose EBRT alone (in more than 90% of cases) [10, 11]. With respect to the intermediate-risk group, 4–6 months of ADT seems to be optimal, as discussed previously (12.4.2.).

On the other hand, the optimal duration of ADT for high- or very-high-risk groups has yet to be confirmed. As described in Section 12.4.2., the current standard treatment for high- or very-high-risk CLPCa is considered to be 4–6 months of

NA-ADT followed by EBRT plus an additional 24–30 months of A-ADT. However, it has been suggested that the timing of the start of S-ADT could significantly affect survival outcomes in patients who developed PSA recurrence after EBRT [5–7]. In those studies, the survival probabilities were significantly better in patients who were managed by the early initiation (at PSA $\leq$10–20 ng/mL) of S-ADT after the recurrence of PSA. However, none of the studies comparing EBRT alone and EBRT plus ADT, or short-term ADT plus EBRT and long-term ADT plus EBRT, specified the timing of the start of S-ADT.

We treated 120 consecutive cases with T3-4N0M0 disease (about 40% of whom were classified as very high-risk based on the 2017 NCCN classification system) with high-dose (78 Gy in 39 fractions) intensity-modulated radiation therapy combined with an NA-ADT duration of 6 months under an early salvage policy [34]. After completing IMRT, all patients were followed up without the addition of any adjuvant therapy, including A-ADT. S-ADT was started when the PSA values exceeded 4 ng/mL. Although long-term A-ADT was not used, the 8-year prostate cancer-specific and overall survival rates were 96.6% and 89.1%, respectively. Despite the very-high-risk nature of the patients, the PCSM rate was only 3.4% at 8 years. Therefore, future prospective trials should test whether significant survival advantages are still observed in patients treated with long-term ADT plus EBRT compared with those who were treated with short-term NA-ADT plus high-dose EBRT under an early initiation policy of S-ADT after PSA recurrence.

12.6 Ethnic Differences in Sensitivity to ADT

Japanese patients treated with primary ADT have less than half the adjusted PCSM of those in the USA, according to a comparison of registered data between the Japanese Cancer of the Prostate registry database and USA Cancer of the Prostate Strategic Research Endeavor registry [35]. This suggests that Japanese patients, and probably East Asian populations, have better sensitivity to primary ADT than patients in the USA [36]. This finding may also be applicable to sensitivity to S-ADT. Therefore, the outcomes obtained from studies comparing short-term ADT and long-term ADT with EBRT conducted in Western populations should be validated in studies conducted using East Asian populations.

Conclusions

When definitively treating CLPCa with EBRT using former standard doses, ADT should be combined with EBRT, except in low-risk cases. For intermediate-risk cases, the combination of NA-ADT (± concurrent ADT) for a duration of 4–6 months is the current standard treatment approach for definitive EBRT. On the other hand, an NA-ADT (± concurrent ADT) duration of 4–6 months plus A-ADT of 24–30 months is recommended in combination with EBRT for patients with high- or very-high-risk CLPCa. However, these findings should be validated for Japanese and East Asian populations under an early initiation policy of S-ADT, due to the suggestion that there are ethnic differences in sensitivity to

ADT between Japanese and Western populations. In addition, the impact of ADT is controversial when escalated doses are used for EBRT.

References

1. Viani GA, Stefano EJ, Afonso SL. Higher-than-conventional radiation doses in localized prostate cancer treatment: a meta-analysis of randomized, controlled trials. Int J Radiat Oncol Biol Phys. 2009;74(5):1405–18. https://doi.org/10.1016/j.ijrobp.2008.10.091.
2. Zaorsky NG, Palmer JD, Hurwitz MD, Keith SW, Dicker AP, Den RB. What is the ideal radiotherapy dose to treat prostate cancer? A meta-analysis of biologically equivalent dose escalation. Radiother Oncol. 2015;115(3):295–300. https://doi.org/10.1016/j.radonc.2015.05.011.
3. Michalski M, Purd JA, Bosch WR, Bahary J, Lau H, Duclos M, et al. Initial results of a phase 3 randomized study of high dose 3DCRT/IMRT versus standard dose 3D–CRT/IMRT in patients treated for localized prostate cancer (RTOG 0126). Int J Radiat Oncol Biol Phys. 2014;90(5 Suppl 1):1263.
4. Hou Z, Li G, Bai S. High dose versus conventional dose in external beam radiotherapy of prostate cancer: a meta-analysis of long-term follow-up. J Cancer Res Clin Oncol. 2015;141(6):1063–71. https://doi.org/10.1007/s00432-014-1813-1.
5. Shipley WU, Desilvio M, Pilepich MV, Roach M 3rd, Wolkov HB, Sause WT, et al. Early initiation of salvage hormone therapy influences survival in patients who failed initial radiation for locally advanced prostate cancer: a secondary analysis of RTOG protocol 86-10. Int J Radiat Oncol Biol Phys. 2006;64(4):1162–7. https://doi.org/10.1016/j.ijrobp.2005.09.039.
6. Mydin AR, Dunne MT, Finn MA, Armstrong JG. Early salvage hormonal therapy for biochemical failure improved survival in prostate cancer patients after neoadjuvant hormonal therapy plus radiation therapy—a secondary analysis of irish clinical oncology research group 97-01. Int J Radiat Oncol Biol Phys. 2013;85(1):101–8. https://doi.org/10.1016/j.ijrobp.2012.03.001.
7. Souhami L, Bae K, Pilepich M, Sandler H. Timing of salvage hormonal therapy in prostate cancer patients with unfavorable prognosis treated with radiotherapy: a secondary analysis of radiation therapy oncology group 85-31. Int J Radiat Oncol Biol Phys. 2010;78(5):1301–6. https://doi.org/10.1016/j.ijrobp.2009.10.007.
8. Hou WH, Huang CY, Wang CC, Lan KH, Chen CH, Yu HJ, et al. Impact of androgen-deprivation therapy on the outcome of dose-escalation prostate cancer radiotherapy without elective pelvic irradiation. Asian J Androl. 2017;19(5):596–601. https://doi.org/10.4103/1008-682X.183569.
9. Tran E, Paquette M, Pickles T, Jay J, Hamm J, Liu M, et al. Population-based validation of a policy change to use long-term androgen deprivation therapy for cT3-4 prostate cancer: impact of the EORTC22863 and RTOG 85-31 and 92-02 trials. Radiother Oncol. 2013;107(3):366–71. https://doi.org/10.1016/j.radonc.2013.05.003.
10. NCCN.org. NCCN clinical practice guidlines in Oncology: Prostate cancer, version 2.2017. 2017. http://www.nccnorg/professionals/physician_gls/pdf/prostatepdf. Accessed 17 June 2017.
11. Mottet N, Bellmunt J, Bolla M, Briers E, Cumberbatch MG, De Santis M, et al. EAU-ESTRO-SIOG guidelines on prostate cancer. Part 1: screening, diagnosis, and local treatment with curative intent. Eur Urol. 2017;71(4):618–29. https://doi.org/10.1016/j.eururo.2016.08.003.
12. Zietman AL, Nakfoor BM, Prince EA, Gerweck LE. The effect of androgen deprivation and radiation therapy on an androgen-sensitive murine tumor: an in vitro and in vivo study. Cancer J Sci Am. 1997;3(1):31–6.
13. Henderson A, Langley SE, Laing RW. Is bicalutamide equivalent to goserelin for prostate volume reduction before radiation therapy? A prospective, observational study. Clin Oncol. 2003;15(6):318–21.
14. Zelefsky MJ, Leibel SA, Burman CM, Kutcher GJ, Harrison A, Happersett L, et al. Neoadjuvant hormonal therapy improves the therapeutic ratio in patients with bulky prostatic

cancer treated with three-dimensional conformal radiation therapy. Int J Radiat Oncol Biol Phys. 1994;29(4):755–61.
15. Roach M 3rd, Bae K, Speight J, Wolkov HB, Rubin P, Lee RJ, et al. Short-term neoadjuvant androgen deprivation therapy and external-beam radiotherapy for locally advanced prostate cancer: long-term results of RTOG 8610. J Clin Oncol. 2008;26(4):585–91. https://doi.org/10.1200/JCO.2007.13.9881.
16. Jones CU, Hunt D, McGowan DG, Amin MB, Chetner MP, Bruner DW, et al. Radiotherapy and short-term androgen deprivation for localized prostate cancer. N Engl J Med. 2011;365(2):107–18. https://doi.org/10.1056/NEJMoa1012348.
17. Denham JW, Steigler A, Lamb DS, Joseph D, Turner S, Matthews J, et al. Short-term neoadjuvant androgen deprivation and radiotherapy for locally advanced prostate cancer: 10-year data from the TROG 96.01 randomised trial. Lancet Oncol. 2011;12(5):451–9. https://doi.org/10.1016/S1470-2045(11)70063-8.
18. Laverdiere J, Nabid A, De Bedoya LD, Ebacher A, Fortin A, Wang CS, et al. The efficacy and sequencing of a short course of androgen suppression on freedom from biochemical failure when administered with radiation therapy for T2-T3 prostate cancer. J Urol. 2004;171(3):1137–40. https://doi.org/10.1097/01.ju.0000112979.97941.7f.
19. McPartlin AJ, Glicksman R, Pintilie M, Tsuji D, Mok G, Bayley A, et al. PMH 9907: long-term outcomes of a randomized phase 3 study of short-term bicalutamide hormone therapy and dose-escalated external-beam radiation therapy for localized prostate cancer. Cancer. 2016;122(16):2595–603. https://doi.org/10.1002/cncr.30093.
20. D'Amico AV, Chen MH, Renshaw AA, Loffredo M, Kantoff PW. Androgen suppression and radiation vs radiation alone for prostate cancer: a randomized trial. JAMA. 2008;299(3):289–95. https://doi.org/10.1001/jama.299.3.289.
21. Pilepich MV, Winter K, Lawton CA, Krisch RE, Wolkov HB, Movsas B, et al. Androgen suppression adjuvant to definitive radiotherapy in prostate carcinoma—long-term results of phase III RTOG 85-31. Int J Radiat Oncol Biol Phys. 2005;61(5):1285–90. https://doi.org/10.1016/j.ijrobp.2004.08.047.
22. Bolla M, Van Tienhoven G, Warde P, Dubois JB, Mirimanoff R-O, Storme G, et al. External irradiation with or without long-term androgen suppression for prostate cancer with high metastatic risk: 10-year results of an EORTC randomised study. Lancet Oncol. 2010;11(11):1066–73. https://doi.org/10.1016/s1470-2045(10)70223-0.
23. Bolla M, Maingon P, Carrie C, Villa S, Kitsios P, Poortmans PM, et al. Short androgen suppression and radiation dose escalation for intermediate- and high-risk localized prostate cancer: results of EORTC trial 22991. J Clin Oncol. 2016;34(15):1748–56. https://doi.org/10.1200/JCO.2015.64.8055.
24. Widmark A, Klepp O, Solberg A, Damber JE, Angelsen A, Fransson P, et al. Endocrine treatment, with or without radiotherapy, in locally advanced prostate cancer (SPCG-7/SFUO-3): an open randomised phase III trial. Lancet. 2009;373(9660):301–8. https://doi.org/10.1016/S0140-6736(08)61815-2.
25. Fossa SD, Wiklund F, Klepp O, Angelsen A, Solberg A, Damber JE, et al. Ten- and 15-yr prostate cancer-specific mortality in patients with nonmetastatic locally advanced or aggressive intermediate prostate cancer, randomized to lifelong endocrine treatment alone or combined with radiotherapy: final results of the Scandinavian Prostate Cancer Group-7. Eur Urol. 2016;70(4):684–91. https://doi.org/10.1016/j.eururo.2016.03.021.
26. Mason MD, Parulekar WR, Sydes MR, Brundage M, Kirkbride P, Gospodarowicz M, et al. Final report of the intergroup randomized study of combined androgen-deprivation therapy plus radiotherapy versus androgen-deprivation therapy alone in locally advanced prostate cancer. J Clin Oncol. 2015;33(19):2143–50. https://doi.org/10.1200/JCO.2014.57.7510.
27. Warde P, Mason M, Ding K, Kirkbride P, Brundage M, Cowan R, et al. Combined androgen deprivation therapy and radiation therapy for locally advanced prostate cancer: a randomised, phase 3 trial. Lancet. 2011;378(9809):2104–11. https://doi.org/10.1016/S0140-6736(11)61095-7.
28. Bolla M, de Reijke TM, Van Tienhoven G, Van den Bergh AC, Oddens J, Poortmans PM, et al. Duration of androgen suppression in the treatment of prostate cancer. N Engl J Med. 2009;360(24):2516–27. https://doi.org/10.1056/NEJMoa0810095.

29. Lawton CAF, Lin X, Hanks GE, Lepor H, Grignon DJ, Brereton HD, et al. Duration of androgen deprivation in locally advanced prostate cancer: long-term update of NRG oncology RTOG 9202. Int J Radiat Oncol Biol Phys. 2017;98(2):296–303. https://doi.org/10.1016/j.ijrobp.2017.02.004.
30. Zapatero A, Guerrero A, Maldonado X, Alvarez A, Gonzalez San Segundo C, Cabeza Rodriguez MA, et al. High-dose radiotherapy with short-term or long-term androgen deprivation in localised prostate cancer (DART01/05 GICOR): a randomised, controlled, phase 3 trial. Lancet Oncol. 2015;16(3):320–7. https://doi.org/10.1016/S1470-2045(15)70045-8.
31. Denham JW, Joseph D, Lamb DS, Spry NA, Duchesne G, Matthews J, et al. Short-term androgen suppression and radiotherapy versus intermediate-term androgen suppression and radiotherapy, with or without zoledronic acid, in men with locally advanced prostate cancer (TROG 03.04 RADAR): an open-label, randomised, phase 3 factorial trial. Lancet Oncol. 2014;15(10):1076–89. https://doi.org/10.1016/S1470-2045(14)70328-6.
32. Ito K, Suzuki K, Yamanaka H. Oncological outcomes in patients with locally advanced prostate cancer treated with neoadjuvant endocrine and external beam radiation therapy followed by adjuvant continuous/intermittent endocrine therapy in an open-label, randomized, phase III trial. J Urol. 2016;195(4S):e143. https://doi.org/10.1016/j.juro.2016.02.2505.
33. Mirhadi AJ, Zhang Q, Hanks GE, Lepor H, Grignon DJ, Peters CA, et al. Effect of long-term hormonal therapy (vs short-term hormonal therapy): a secondary analysis of intermediate-risk prostate cancer patients treated on NRG oncology RTOG 9202. Int J Radiat Oncol Biol Phys. 2017;97(3):511–5. https://doi.org/10.1016/j.ijrobp.2016.11.002.
34. Mizowaki T, Norihisa Y, Takayama K, Ikeda I, Inokuchi H, Nakamura K, et al. Long-term outcomes of intensity-modulated radiation therapy combined with neoadjuvant androgen deprivation therapy under an early salvage policy for patients with T3-T4N0M0 prostate cancer. Int J Clin Oncol. 2016;21(1):148–55. https://doi.org/10.1007/s10147-015-0867-7.
35. Cooperberg MR, Hinotsu S, Namiki M, Carroll PR, Akaza H. Trans-Pacific variation in outcomes for men treated with primary androgen-deprivation therapy (ADT) for prostate cancer. BJU Int. 2016;117(1):102–9. https://doi.org/10.1111/bju.12937.
36. Fukagai T, Namiki TS, Carlile RG, Yoshida H, Namiki M. Comparison of the clinical outcome after hormonal therapy for prostate cancer between Japanese and Caucasian men. BJU Int. 2006;97(6):1190–3. https://doi.org/10.1111/j.1464-410X.2006.06201.x.
37. Crook J, Ludgate C, Malone S, Perry G, Eapen L, Bowen J, et al. Final report of multicenter Canadian phase III randomized trial of 3 versus 8 months of neoadjuvant androgen deprivation therapy before conventional-dose radiotherapy for clinically localized prostate cancer. Int J Radiat Oncol Biol Phys. 2009;73(2):327–33. https://doi.org/10.1016/j.ijrobp.2008.04.075.
38. Armstrong JG, Gillham CM, Dunne MT, Fitzpatrick DA, Finn MA, Cannon ME, et al. A randomized trial (Irish clinical oncology research group 97-01) comparing short versus protracted neoadjuvant hormonal therapy before radiotherapy for localized prostate cancer. Int J Radiat Oncol Biol Phys. 2011;81(1):35–45. https://doi.org/10.1016/j.ijrobp.2010.04.065.
39. Pisansky TM, Hunt D, Gomella LG, Amin MB, Balogh AG, Chinn DM, et al. Duration of androgen suppression before radiotherapy for localized prostate cancer: radiation therapy oncology group randomized clinical trial 9910. J Clin Oncol. 2015;33(4):332–9. https://doi.org/10.1200/JCO.2014.58.0662.
40. Mottet N, Peneau M, Mazeron JJ, Molinie V, Richaud P. Addition of radiotherapy to long-term androgen deprivation in locally advanced prostate cancer: an open randomised phase 3 trial. Eur Urol. 2012;62(2):213–9. https://doi.org/10.1016/j.eururo.2012.03.053.

13. ADT as Salvage Therapy After Definitive Treatment for Clinically Localized Prostate Cancer

Akira Yokomizo

Abstract

The standard curative treatment is radical prostatectomy (RP) or radiation therapy (RT) in localized prostate cancer (Pca). Unfortunately, at most 30% of the patients develop biochemical recurrent that can be identified by rising prostate-specific antigen (PSA) only but not detectable by CT scan or bone scan. The new technology like chorine PET and ProstaScint could detect the recurrent site, but these modalities are insufficient in low PSA level (less than 1.0 ng/mL) of PSA failure patients after definitive therapy. Many of those patients with biochemical recurrence after RP would initially be treated by salvage RT. But, in patients with biochemical recurrence after RT, salvage RP is performed in only selective patients and most of them are treated by salvage hormone therapy (HT). There are conflicting evidences to support the advantage of salvage ADT; one randomized controlled trial (RCT) showed the benefit of early starting of HT, and another RCT proved the non-inferiority of intermittent ADT to continuous ADT. In this chapter, recent evidences are summarized on salvage ADT after definitive treatment for clinically localized Pca.

Keywords

PSA failure · Salvage hormone therapy · Radical treatment

13.1 Definition of Biochemical Recurrence After RP

RP is one of the curative treatments in localized Pca. Most of the recurrences after RP are detected only by a rise in the PSA level [1]. Recently, robotic surgery has become a standard modality in the world [2], and PSA failure is observed at most of 20% in robotic RP series [1]. The PSA failure is defined by two consecutive PSA values of

A. Yokomizo
Department of Urology, Harasanshin Hospital, Fukuoka, Japan
e-mail: yokoa@harasanshin.or.jp

>0.2 ng/mL and rising in EAU-ESTRO-SIOG guideline [3] and ASCO guideline [4]. On the other hand, NCCN guideline describes "undetectable PSA after RP with a subsequent detectable PSA that increases on 2 or more determinations" [5] and it lacks the PSA value. In general, the former definition seems to be widely accepted in daily practice.

13.2 Definition of Biochemical Recurrence After RT

RT is generally divided into brachytherapy and external beam radiation treatment (EBRT). The EBRT evolves from three-dimensional source to intensity-modulated radiation, and eventually carbon ion radiation therapy can be performed in selective institutes [6]. Basically, the patients' follow-up after RT is performed by PSA measurement, and similarly to RP treatment failure is first discovered by rise of PSA. The definition PSA failure is widely accepted by the American Society for Radiology and Oncology (ASTRO) Phoenix's definition, that is "the lowest value of PSA after treatment (nadir) + 2 ng/mL" [7]. The salvage RP to PSA failure patients after RT is performed only in selective patients and institutes; most of them are treated by salvage HT. Additionally, a high-intensity focused ultrasound therapy and a cryotherapy may be considered in patients that meet very narrow criteria, but it has not been accepted worldwide with lacking of high level of evidences derived from phase 3 studies. If salvage treatment options are not practical or unsuccessful, androgen deprivation therapy (ADT) is a standard option for disease control.

13.3 Identification of Recurrent Sites

13.3.1 A Computed Tomography and Bone Scintigraphy

Most of the recurrences after radical treatments are detected only by a rise in the PSA level [1, 8]. Those who have local recurrence after RP may benefit from RT, whereas those who have metastatic disease may benefit from systemic treatment, the most common of which is ADT [1, 8]. Therefore, identification of recurrent sites is important to select the treatment strategy in PSA failure after definitive therapy. A computed tomography (CT) and bone scintigraphy are most frequently used to detect the metastatic sites. However, these two modalities usually cannot detect the recurrent sites in these cohorts [9]. For example, positive rate of bone scintigraphy was reported to be less than 5% in PSA failure after RP and it can be detectable over PSA 40–45 ng/mL [10].

13.3.2 Choline Positron-Emission Tomography-CT

A recent meta-analysis reported the usefulness of a choline positron-emission tomography (PET)-CT that this modality has a sensitivity of 85% and specificity of 88% [11]. However, the positive predictive value as defined by prolonged PSA-free survival after local salvage is not known. Furthermore, it could detect the recurrence site only in one-third of the patients approximately in PSA values less than 1 ng/mL [12]. Accordingly, in the setting of PSA failure, this modality is considered to be under investigation.

13.3.3 ProstaScint

A monoclonal antibody specifically binds to the intracellular epitope of prostate-specific membrane antigen (PSMA) on prostatic epithelial cells that was developed to detect distant metastasis in both high-risk Pca patients and in patients with increasing PSA levels after RP. When used after RP, ProstaScint had a sensitivity of 75–86% and a specificity of 47–86% in detecting local recurrence in initial studies [13]. However, some conflicting data were reported concerning the effectiveness of ProstaScint in determining the further therapy in the post-RP [13, 14]. Also, there is no difference in PFS in those with a positive scan versus a negative scan [14]. Furthermore, any positive predictive value of ProstaScint is low (27–50%), perhaps due to false-positive scans from postsurgical inflammation and vascular perturbations [13, 15]. Based on the currently published literature, ProstaScint should not be used in recommending salvage radiation therapy after RP [13–15].

13.4 Salvage Hormonal Therapy for PSA Recurrence After Definitive Therapy

13.4.1 Advantage of Salvage ADT

There are conflicting results on the clinical effectiveness of HT after definitive therapy. Some retrospective studies [16, 17] reported a favorable effect of HT, and the only one RCT addressing it [18]. In a subgroup analysis of the RTOG 85–31, 243 patients had PSA recurrence after RT including RP cases. Comparing an early HT group starting with less than 10 ng/mL of PSA and a late HT group starting at 10 ng/mL or more, early HT group had significant longer overall survival with the median observation period of 8.5 years [16]. But there was no significant difference in cancer-specific survival and local recurrence rate [16]. Similarly, in the second analysis of ICORG 97-01 [17], they compared the three subgroups: PSA less than 10 ng/mL with no metastasis, PSA more or 10 ng/mL with no metastasis, and patients with metastasis. As a result, a group of PSA less than 10 ng/mL with no metastasis showed significantly better overall survival rate than the other two groups, and in multivariate analysis on survival timing of salvage therapy, the period from RT to relapse, and PSA nadir value in HT were significant prognostic factors [17]. Finally, there was only one RCT to reveal the advantage of early administration of ADT after curative therapy [18]. They randomized 293 patients to the immediate-therapy arm and to the delayed-therapy arm. They found that 5-year overall survival was 86.4% (95% CI 78.5–91.5) in the delayed-therapy arm versus 91.2% (84.2–95.2) in the immediate-therapy arm (log-rank $p = 0.047$). After Cox regression analysis, the unadjusted HR for overall survival for immediate versus delayed arm assignment was 0.55 (95% CI 0.30–1.00; $p = 0.050$). Other studies did not find any advantage of HT or any differences between early and delayed HT. One retrospective matched cohort study found an unfavorable effect of HT [19]. They separated into five groups for analysis based on the time of hormone therapy initiation of PSA failure after RP. They concluded that the benefit of hormone therapy is lost when ADT is delivered at the time of PSA recurrence or systemic progression. This study may contain the selection bias as clinically unfavorable cases tend to start HT earlier and more intensive follow-up. Boorjian et al. [20] investigated the natural history of the patients with PSA failure after RP. They concluded that older patient age, increased pathologic Gleason score (8–10), advanced tumor stage ('pT3≤), and rapid PSA doubling time (<6 months) predicted systemic progression and death from Pca. Therefore, those young patients who have these risk factors may be beneficial from ADT.

13.4.2 Intermittent Versus Continuous ADT

Once hormone therapy has been started, the next clinical question is whether hormone therapy should be performed intermittently or continuously. The most notable report is a randomized controlled trial study that proved non-inferiority of intermittent therapy to continuous HT [21]. This study [21] consisted of 690 intermittent therapy groups and 696 continuous therapy groups for biochemical recurrence after RT or after RP (approximately 10%). The treatment protocol of the intermittent therapy group was that the patients were off therapy until clinically progressed or increased PSA value (increase of less than 1 ng/mL or less than 4 ng/mL from baseline). One treatment set consisted of a GnRH agonist or a combination of antiandrogen for 8 months. In the median observation period of 6.9 years, the number of death was 268 in the intermittent therapy group whereas 256 cases in the continuous therapy group, and the cumulative mortality rates due to Pca in the 7 years were 18% and 15%, respectively, which were not significantly different ($P = 0.24$). Also, the non-inferiority on median OS was also proved between a continuous (8.8 years) and intermittent therapy group (9.1 years) years, respectively ($p = 0.009$). Regarding QOL, the intermittent therapy group was significantly better in hot flash, sexual desire, and urinary tract symptoms, but not overall QoL outcomes. Furthermore, the proportion of castration resistance was significantly lower in the intermittent group at a hazard ratio of 0.80 ($p = 0.03$). Whereas this report contains a limitation of lacking of any stratifying criteria such as PSA-DT or initial risk factors, it clearly indicates that intermittent HT is useful and beneficial for PSA failure after curative treatment.

13.4.3 Bicalutamide Followed by ADT Versus Radiotherapy

JCOG0401 study was a prospective randomized phase 3 trial to confirm the superiority of radiotherapy ± endocrine therapy over endocrine therapy alone for PSA failure after radical prostatectomy [22] (Fig. 13.1). Two hundred and ten patients were randomly assigned to arm A [endocrine therapy only: bicalutamide (BCL) monotherapy followed

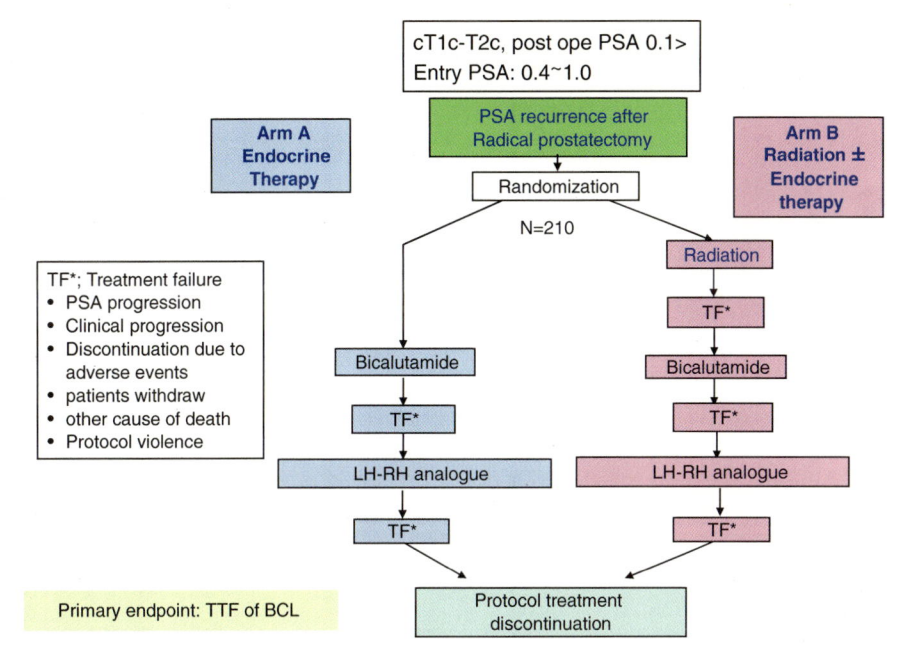

Fig. 13.1 Study design of JCOG0401

by LH-RH agonist in case of BCL failure], or arm B [64.8 Gy of salvage radiotherapy (SRT) followed by same regimen of arm A in case of treatment failure of SRT]. The primary endpoint was time to treatment failure (TTF) of BCL, and secondary endpoints are TTF of protocol treatment, clinical relapse-free survival (RFS), overall survival (OS), and adverse events. As a result, The TTF of BCL was significantly better in arm B (hazard ratio 0.56 90% CI (0.40–0.77); one-sided $p = 0.001$). The 33 patients (32%) of 102 patients with SRT of arm B had no treatment failure of SRT, resulting in being free from hormonal therapy. In addition, TTF of protocol treatment was also significantly better in arm B. However, clinical RFS and OS were similar between the arms. In conclusion, the first SRT had advantage in both TTF of BCL and protocol treatment. Although the clinical outcomes of both arms of salvage therapy were similar with each other in terms of clinical PFS and OS, the SRT was effective in 32% of the patients, which contributed to avoiding the salvage endocrine therapy.

New therapeutic options with improved imaging technology may contribute to change the therapeutic options dramatically in biochemically recurrent Pca patients in the future.

References

1. Carroll P. Rising PSA after a radical treatment. Eur Urol. 2001;40(Suppl 2):9–16. https://doi.org/10.1159/000049879.
2. Ficarra V, Novara G, Ahlering TE, Costello A, Eastham JA, Graefen M, et al. Systematic review and meta-analysis of studies reporting potency rates after robot-assisted radical prostatectomy. Eur Urol. 2012;62(3):418–30. https://doi.org/10.1016/j.eururo.2012.05.046.

3. Mottet N, Bellmunt J, Bolla M, Briers E, Cumberbatch MG, De Santis M, et al. EAU-ESTRO-SIOG Guidelines on prostate cancer. Part 1: Screening, diagnosis, and local treatment with curative intent. Eur Urol. 2017;71(4):618–29. https://doi.org/10.1016/j.eururo.2016.08.003.
4. Freedland SJ, Rumble RB, Finelli A, Chen RC, Slovin S, Stein MN, et al. Adjuvant and salvage radiotherapy after prostatectomy: American Society of Clinical Oncology clinical practice guideline endorsement. J Clin Oncol. 2014;32(34):3892–8. https://doi.org/10.1200/jco.2014.58.8525.
5. NCCN guideline, prostate cancer 2017v2. https://www.nccn.org/professionals/physician_gls/f_guidelines.asp.
6. Shioyama Y, Tsuji H, Suefuji H, Sinoto M, Matsunobu A, Toyama S, et al. Particle radiotherapy for prostate cancer. Int J Urol. 2015;22(1):33–9. https://doi.org/10.1111/iju.12640.
7. Roach M 3rd, Hanks G, Thames H Jr, Schellhammer P, Shipley WU, Sokol GH, et al. Defining biochemical failure following radiotherapy with or without hormonal therapy in men with clinically localized prostate cancer: recommendations of the RTOG-ASTRO Phoenix Consensus Conference. Int J Radiat Oncol Biol Phys. 2006;65(4):965–74. https://doi.org/10.1016/j.ijrobp.2006.04.029.
8. Yokomizo A, Kawamoto H, Nihei K, Ishizuka N, Kakehi Y, Tobisu K, et al. Randomized controlled trial to evaluate radiotherapy +/− endocrine therapy versus endocrine therapy alone for PSA failure after radical prostatectomy: Japan Clinical Oncology Group Study JCOG 0401. Jpn J Clin Oncol. 2005;35(1):34–6. https://doi.org/10.1093/jjco/hyi007.
9. Yokomizo A, Murai M, Baba S, Ogawa O, Tsukamoto T, Niwakawa M, et al. Percentage of positive biopsy cores, preoperative prostate-specific antigen (PSA) level, pT and Gleason score as predictors of PSA recurrence after radical prostatectomy: a multi-institutional outcome study in Japan. BJU Int. 2006;98(3):549–53. https://doi.org/10.1111/j.1464-410X.2006.06379.x.
10. Cher ML, Bianco FJ Jr, Lam JS, Davis LP, Grignon DJ, Sakr WA, et al. Limited role of radionuclide bone scintigraphy in patients with prostate specific antigen elevations after radical prostatectomy. J Urol. 1998;160(4):1387–91.
11. Umbehr MH, Muntener M, Hany T, Sulser T, Bachmann LM. The role of 11C-choline and 18F-fluorocholine positron emission tomography (PET) and PET/CT in prostate cancer: a systematic review and meta-analysis. Eur Urol. 2013;64(1):106–17. https://doi.org/10.1016/j.eururo.2013.04.019.
12. Krause BJ, Souvatzoglou M, Treiber U. Imaging of prostate cancer with PET/CT and radioactively labeled choline derivates. Urol Oncol. 2013;31(4):427–35. https://doi.org/10.1016/j.urolonc.2010.08.008.
13. Zaorsky NG, Yamoah K, Thakur ML, Trabulsi EJ, Showalter TN, Hurwitz MD, et al. A paradigm shift from anatomic to functional and molecular imaging in the detection of recurrent prostate cancer. Future Oncol (London, England). 2014;10(3):457–74. https://doi.org/10.2217/fon.13.196.
14. Koontz BF, Mouraviev V, Johnson JL, Mayes J, Chen SH, Wong TZ, et al. Use of local (111)in-capromab pendetide scan results to predict outcome after salvage radiotherapy for prostate cancer. Int J Radiat Oncol Biol Phys. 2008;71(2):358–61. https://doi.org/10.1016/j.ijrobp.2007.10.020.
15. Petronis JD, Regan F, Lin K. Indium-111 capromab pendetide (ProstaScint) imaging to detect recurrent and metastatic prostate cancer. Clin Nucl Med. 1998;23(10):672–7.
16. Souhami L, Bae K, Pilepich M, Sandler H. Timing of salvage hormonal therapy in prostate cancer patients with unfavorable prognosis treated with radiotherapy: a secondary analysis of Radiation Therapy Oncology Group 85-31. Int J Radiat Oncol Biol Phys. 2010;78(5):1301–6. https://doi.org/10.1016/j.ijrobp.2009.10.007.
17. Mydin AR, Dunne MT, Finn MA, Armstrong JG. Early salvage hormonal therapy for biochemical failure improved survival in prostate cancer patients after neoadjuvant hormonal therapy plus radiation therapy—a secondary analysis of Irish clinical oncology research group 97-01. Int J Radiat Oncol Biol Phys. 2013;85(1):101–8. https://doi.org/10.1016/j.ijrobp.2012.03.001.
18. Duchesne GM, Woo HH, Bassett JK, Bowe SJ, D'Este C, Frydenberg M, et al. Timing of androgen-deprivation therapy in patients with prostate cancer with a rising PSA (TROG 03.06

and VCOG PR 01-03 [TOAD]): a randomised, multicentre, non-blinded, phase 3 trial. Lancet Oncol. 2016;17(6):727–37. https://doi.org/10.1016/s1470-2045(16)00107-8.
19. Siddiqui SA, Boorjian SA, Inman B, Bagniewski S, Bergstralh EJ, Blute ML. Timing of androgen deprivation therapy and its impact on survival after radical prostatectomy: a matched cohort study. J Urol. 2008;179(5):1830–7.; discussion 7. https://doi.org/10.1016/j.juro.2008.01.022.
20. Boorjian SA, Thompson RH, Tollefson MK, Rangel LJ, Bergstralh EJ, Blute ML, et al. Long-term risk of clinical progression after biochemical recurrence following radical prostatectomy: the impact of time from surgery to recurrence. Eur Urol. 2011;59(6):893–9. https://doi.org/10.1016/j.eururo.2011.02.026.
21. Crook JM, O'Callaghan CJ, Duncan G, Dearnaley DP, Higano CS, Horwitz EM, et al. Intermittent androgen suppression for rising PSA level after radiotherapy. N Engl J Med. 2012;367(10):895–903. https://doi.org/10.1056/NEJMoa1201546.
22. Yokomizo A, Satoh T, Hashine K, Inoue T, Fujimoto K, Egawa S, et al. Randomized controlled trial comparing radiotherapy +/− endocrine therapy versus endocrine therapy alone for PSA failure after radical prostatectomy: Japan Clinical Oncology Group Study JCOG0401. Ann Oncol. 2017;28(Suppl 5):v269–94. https://doi.org/10.1093/annonc/mdx370.

Androgen Deprivation Therapy for Clinically Localized Prostate Cancer

Yoichi Arai and Koji Mitsuzuka

Abstract

Androgen deprivation therapy (ADT) has been widely used as primary monotherapy in men with localized prostate cancer (PCa). Since most new cases of PCa are diagnosed in the early stages in the prostate-specific antigen (PSA) era, the situation has gradually changed toward earlier and longer use of hormone therapy. Emerging evidence suggests the potential harm associated with long-term use of ADT, such as increased risks of osteoporosis, cardiovascular disease, and metabolic change. It is important to understand the impact of primary ADT (PADT) on survival among men who do not undergo definitive treatment.

Large, population-based studies suggest that PADT does not improve survival in men with localized PCa, and there are data suggesting reduced overall survival with ADT. Many of the randomized, controlled trials (RCTs) of immediate versus deferred ADT failed to show a survival benefit of immediate use of ADT for localized PCa. In the most recent RCT, immediate ADT resulted in a modest but statistically significant increase in overall survival, but no significant difference in PCa mortality or symptom-free survival. A subset of men with localized PCa may benefit from immediate PADT, but this must be weighed against the adverse effects of long-term ADT.

Keywords

Androgen deprivation therapy · Primary · Prostate cancer · Localized

Y. Arai, M.D., Ph.D. · K. Mitsuzuka
Department of Urology, Tohoku University Graduate School of Medicine, Sendai, Japan
e-mail: yarai@uro.med.tohoku.ac.jp

14.1 Introduction

The incidence of prostate cancer (PCa) in Japan had been considered to be relatively low, but it has been increasing dramatically in recent years. According to the Cancer Information Service of the National Cancer Center, there were 98,400 estimated new cases of PCa in 2015, making this the leading cancer in Japanese men [1]. There is significant controversy about the role of treatment for patients with clinically localized disease. Radical prostatectomy, radiation therapy, or active surveillance can usually be offered to these patients, based on their prostate-specific antigen (PSA) level, clinical stage, Gleason score, age, comorbidities, and preferences. Another potential treatment option is androgen deprivation therapy (ADT) as monotherapy for localized prostate cancer. ADT is the first-line treatment for patients with metastatic disease and is commonly used in combination with radiotherapy for patients with high-risk localized disease [2]. Since its role as monotherapy (i.e., primary ADT [PADT]) in patients with localized PCa has not been established in clinical trials, PADT is not recommended by the European Association of Urology (EAU) guideline or the National Comprehensive Cancer Network for nonmetastatic disease [3, 4]. In daily practice, however, use of ADT has increased as a treatment of choice for these men [5–7].

Since most of the new cases are diagnosed in the early stages in the PSA era, the situation has gradually changed toward earlier and longer use of hormone therapy. On the other hand, emerging evidence suggests the potential harm associated with long-term ADT, such as increased risks of osteoporosis, cardiovascular disease, and metabolic change [8, 9]. It is important to understand the impact of PADT on survival among men who do not undergo definitive treatment. The aim of this chapter is to review the existing literature concerning PADT for localized PCa and to understand whether there is objective evidence showing that PADT is beneficial in terms of quantity and quality of life.

14.2 Trends in PADT for Clinically Localized PCa in Japan

Historically, PADT continued to be used for numerous localized PCa cases in Japan. The concept that cardiovascular adverse reactions to administration of estrogen were relatively uncommon in Japan has long been believed to play a part in this situation. Another concept, that there is a difference in response to PADT between Japanese and Western men, may have contributed to wide use of PADT even for localized PCa in Japan [5]. A recent study on trans-Pacific variations in outcomes showed that men on PADT in Japan have less than half the adjusted PCa-specific mortality (PCSM) than men in the USA [10].

Trends in PADT for clinically localized PCa in Japan were first reported in 2005 [11]. The Japanese Urological Association (JUA) initiated computer-based registration of PCa patients in Japan from 2001. The aim of the registration system was to examine etiology, diagnosis, initial planned treatment, pathological findings, and final outcome. A total of 4529 patients newly diagnosed with prostate cancer were registered in 2000. Since it was estimated that there were approximately 14,000 new prostate cancer patients in Japan that year [12], this registry covered about 30% of the new cases. For cases of T1c to T3N0M0, 44.5% underwent PADT without any other additional treatment. PADT was used in 35.7% of T1c patients and in 41.6% of T2 patients.

The Japan Prostate Cancer Study Group (J-CaP) conducted a study named "J-CaP 2010 surveillance" and reported recent trends in the initial therapy for newly diagnosed PCa [13]. PADT was used in 25% of T1 patients and in 36% of T2 patients, showing a decreasing trend in the use of PADT for early-stage disease compared with the 2001 JUA registration data. Although combined androgen blockade (CAB) was much more frequently chosen in patients with poorer risk factors or in higher risk categories, it was frequently used even for stage I (T1, T2a) disease (63.5%) and in D'Amico's low-risk category (56.7%) [14]. There are considerable differences in the treatment patterns for localized disease among countries. Analysis of the Cancer of the Prostate Strategic Urologic Research Endeavor (CaPSURE) data 2010 showed that 49.9% of patients underwent prostatectomy, 24.5% radiation, and 14.4% ADT [6]. Although a trend in the treatment patterns toward more curative treatments was observed in Japan, there are still large differences between Japan and the USA [13].

14.3 The Role of PADT for Localized PCa: Population-Based Study

ADT has been widely used as primary monotherapy in men with localized PCa. During the last decade, however, potential long-term toxicities associated with ADT have been well recognized [8, 9]. Furthermore, the body of literature on the long-term survival impact of PADT in men with localized PCa has been growing rapidly (Table 14.1).

Using the Surveillance, Epidemiology, and End Results (SEER) Medicare data, Wong et al. measured the impact of PADT compared to observation on overall survival in men with localized PCa [15]. The cohort consisted of 16,535 men with organ-confined well-differentiated or moderately differentiated PCa at diagnosis who survived >1 year past diagnosis and did not undergo definitive treatment within 6 months of diagnosis. After propensity score adjustment, PADT did not improve overall survival, but instead resulted in worse outcomes compared with observation (hazard ratio [HR]: 1.20; 95% confidence interval [CI]: 1.13–1.27). Interestingly, patients who received PADT had a higher risk of PCSM (subdistribution hazard ratio [sHR]: 2.22; 95% CI: 1.87–2.65) compared to those who were observed. Non-PCSM appeared similar in both groups (sHR: 1.06; 95% CI: 1.00–1.13; $p = 0.057$). Patients who receive PADT may be at higher risk of developing androgen-independent disease earlier than those who do not receive PADT.

Regarding this issue, Lu-Yao et al. reported that early treatment of low-risk, localized PCa with PADT does not delay the receipt of subsequent palliative therapies and is associated with increased use of chemotherapy [16]. Men with low-risk

Table 14.1 Population-based cohort studies of the role of PADT for patients with localized PCa

Authors	Population — Clinical stage	n	Data source	Follow-up, median	Key findings
Wong et al. [15]	Men aged 65–80 years at diagnosis with organ-confined, well-differentiated or moderately differentiated PCa who survived >1 year past diagnosis. They were diagnosed between 1991 and 1999	16,535	Surveillance, Epidemiology, and End Results (SEER) Medicare data	NA	PADT did not improve overall survival, but instead resulted in worse outcomes compared with observation (hazard ratio [HR]: 1.20; 95% confidence interval [CI]: 1.13–1.27) Patients who received PADT had a higher risk of PCSM (subdistribution hazard ratio [sHR]: 2.22; 95% CI: 1.87–2.65) compared to those who were observed. Non-PCSM appeared similar in both groups (sHR:1.06; 95% CI: 1.00–1.13; $p = 0.057$)
Lu-Yao et al. [17]	Men aged 66 years or older diagnosed as having stage T1-T2 PCa between 1992 and 2009	66,717	Surveillance, Epidemiology, and End Results (SEER) Medicare data	110 months	PADT was not associated with improved 15-year overall or PCa-specific survival following the diagnosis of localized PCa
Potosky et al. [18]	Men diagnosed with clinically localized PCa between 1995 and 2008	15,170	Three integrated healthcare delivery systems within the HMO Cancer Research Network	PADT: 54 months Non-PADT: 64 months	PADT was associated with neither a risk of all-cause mortality (HR: 1.04; 95% CI: 0.97–1.11) nor PCSM (HR: 1.03; 95% CI: 0.89–1.19) PADT was associated with a decreased risk of all-cause mortality only among the subgroup of men with a high risk of cancer progression (HR: 0.88; 95% CI: 0.78–0.97)

PADT primary androgen deprivation therapy, *OS* overall survival, *PCS* prostate cancer-specific survival, *PCSM* prostate cancer-specific mortality, *NA* not available

PCa who were started on PADT shortly after diagnosis received subsequent palliative cancer therapy, especially chemotherapy, more frequently than men who delayed the use of PADT. They expanded their study to include more Surveillance, Epidemiology and End Results (SEER) regions and extended the follow-up for an additional 6 years, from 2003 to 2009 [17]. The study cohort consisted of 66,717 Medicare patients from the SEER database. The patients were 66 years or older who received no definitive local therapy within 180 days of PCa diagnosis. The instrumental variable comprised combined health services areas with various usage rates of primary ADT. With a median follow-up of 110 months, PADT was not associated with improved 15-year overall or PCa-specific survival following the diagnosis of localized PCa. They underlined that PADT should be used only to palliate symptoms of disease or prevent imminent symptoms associated with disease progression. The study was limited to men 66 years or older; the results could differ for younger men.

Potosky et al. conducted a retrospective cohort study using comprehensive utilization and cancer registry data from three integrated health plans [18]. The study cohort included 15,170 men with newly diagnosed localized PCa who did not receive curative intent therapy; 23% of the men had PADT initiated within the first year after diagnosis. After adjusting for all sociodemographic and clinical characteristics, PADT was associated with neither a risk of all-cause mortality (HR: 1.04; 95% CI: 0.97–1.11) nor PCSM (HR: 1.03; 95% CI: 0.89–1.19). PADT was associated with a decreased risk of all-cause mortality only among the subgroup of men with a high risk of cancer progression (HR: 0.88; 95% CI: 0.78–0.97). Interestingly, there was an increased risk of cardiovascular deaths in the PADT group (13% vs. 8%; unadjusted HR: 1.81; 95% CI: 1.61–2.02), although, after adjustment, this difference was not significant (HR: 1.11; 95% CI: 0.95–1.27).

14.4 Immediate Versus Deferred ADT for Patients with Localized PCa: Randomized Trial

14.4.1 Veterans Administration Cooperative Urological Research Group (VACURG) Study 1

The earliest controlled trial was VACURG Study 1 reported in 1973 [19]. This was a placebo-controlled, blinded trial that compared patients treated with placebo to treatment with orchiectomy plus placebo, diethylstilbestrol 5 mg daily, or orchiectomy plus diethylstilbestrol. Patients treated with diethylstilbestrol alone or orchiectomy plus diethylstilbestrol were excluded, since these men had significantly increased cardiovascular mortality, and diethylstilbestrol is rarely used as PADT. Thus, the discussion is limited only to patients who were in the placebo and orchiectomy treatment groups. Of men with locally advanced (T3-T4M0, stage III disease), 262 were assigned to placebo and 266 to orchiectomy. At 9 years, there was no difference in PCa-specific survival or overall survival between the two treatment groups. Interestingly, similar findings were observed in men with metastatic disease (M1, stage IV). In this study, at the time of symptomatic progression, patients were eligible for treatment with other regimens, and in the placebo group 65% of the patients with locally advanced disease received active treatment. Therefore, the study is actually considered to be an examination of the survival benefit of immediate versus deferred ADT. Although the study was conducted in the pre-PSA era, the results suggest that there is little advantage to immediate ADT in men with locally advanced or metastatic disease.

14.4.2 The Medical Research Council Trial

The Medical Research Council Prostate Cancer Working Party Investigator Group conducted a randomized trial of immediate versus deferred ADT in 676 M0 and 261 M1 patients [20]. Early results suggested a survival benefit in favor of immediate ADT for M0 patients. In contrast to the interim analysis, however, the final analysis showed that the difference in overall survival was no longer significant in M0 patients [21]. The immediate patients died more from non-prostatic cancer. The study also suggested a possible survival benefit with immediate ADT in M1 patients (Table 14.2).

14.4.3 The Swiss Group for Clinical Cancer Research (SAKK) Trial

The SAKK conducted a prospective randomized trial involving 197 patients: 67% with T3-T4 tumors, 20% with lymph node metastases, and 22% with distant metastases at randomization [22]. The study showed a trend toward improved PCa-specific survival with immediate orchiectomy ($p = 0.09$), but overall survival was not significantly different between the two treatment groups ($p = 0.96$) (Table 14.2).

14.4.4 The European Organization for Research and Treatment of Cancer (EORTC) Trial 30891

Most recently, the EORTC Trial 30891 attempted to demonstrate equivalent overall survival in patients with localized prostate cancer not suitable for local curative treatment treated with immediate or deferred ADT [23] (Table 14.2). A total of 985 patients with newly diagnosed PCa T0-4N0-2M0 were randomly assigned to receive ADT either immediately ($n = 493$) or on symptomatic disease progression or occurrence of serious complications ($n = 492$). Their median age was 73 years (range, 52–81 years). At a median follow-up of 7.8 years, immediate ADT resulted in a modest but significant increase in overall survival, but no significant difference in prostate cancer mortality or symptom-free survival. Interestingly, the differences in survival were observed predominantly in patients who died within 3–5 years after random assignment, and the overall survival difference was apparently due to increased non-PCa-related mortality. Moreover, many patients in the deferred ADT

Table 14.2 Randomized, controlled trials of immediate versus deferred ADT for patients with localized PCa conducted in the post-PSA era

Data source	Population - Clinical stage	n	Intervention	Follow-up, y, median	Key findings
The Medical Research Council Trial [20, 21]	M0	667	Immediate orchiectomy or LH-RH analogue compared to deferred ADT	NA	Better OS with immediate ADT for M0 patients in the initial results. Difference in OS was no longer significant after longer follow-up
	M1	261			Possible survival benefit with immediate ADT in M1 patients
The Swiss Group for Clinical Cancer Research (SAKK) Trail [22]	T0-4N0-2M0-1	197	Immediate orchiectomy compared to deferred ADT	NA	Trend toward improved PCS with immediate orchiectomy ($p = 0.09$), but OS was not significantly different between the two treatment groups ($p = 0.96$)
The European Organization for Research and Treatment of Cancer (EORTC) Trial 30891 [23–25]	T0-4N0-2M0	985	Immediate orchiectomy or LH-RH analogue compared to deferred ADT	12.8	Deferred ADT was inferior to immediate ADT in terms of overall survival (HR: 1.21; 95% CI: 1.05–1.39; $p = 0.0085$). Deferred ADT was significantly worse than immediate ADT for time to first objective disease progression, but time to objective castration-resistant disease after deferred ADT did not differ significantly ($p = 0.42$) from that after immediate ADT. Consequently, PCSM did not differ significantly, except in patients with aggressive PCa resulting in death within 3–5 years after diagnosis
					Sub-analysis revealed that patients with a baseline PSA >50 ng/mL and/or a PSA doubling time (PSADT) <12 months were at increased risk to die from PCa and might have benefited from immediate ADT

ADT androgen deprivation therapy, *OS* overall survival, *PCS* prostate cancer-specific survival, *PCSM* prostate cancer-specific mortality, *NA* not available

arm did not require ADT because they died before becoming symptomatic. Thus, despite the overall survival benefit, immediate ADT may not be needed in all patients with M0 PCa who are not candidates for local therapy. Then, sub-analyses showed that patients with a baseline PSA >50 ng/mL and/or a PSA doubling time (PSADT) <12 months were at increased risk to die from PCa and might have benefited from immediate ADT [24].

The long-term (median follow-up: 12.9 years) results of EORTC trial 30891 were reported in 2014 [25]. Again, deferred ADT was inferior to immediate ADT in terms of overall survival (HR: 1.21; 95% CI: 1.05–1.39; $p = 0.0085$). Deferred ADT was significantly worse than immediate ADT for time to first objective disease progression, but time to objective castration-resistant disease after deferred ADT did not differ significantly ($p = 0.42$) from that after immediate ADT. Consequently, PCa mortality did not differ significantly, except in patients with aggressive PCa resulting in death within 3–5 years after diagnosis. The reasons why the significant survival benefit with immediate ADT was apparently due to less non-PCa-related mortality and not due to prostate cancer-related deaths are not clear. Interestingly, the number of cardiovascular related deaths was unexpectedly, although slightly, greater in the deferred ADT arm than in the immediate ADT arm (133 vs. 121 deaths).

Importantly, there was a big difference in ADT modality (orchiectomy or LHRH agonist) chosen by the patient: 52% of patients on immediate ADT were effectively orchiectomized compared with only 34% of the 275 patients who started deferred ADT (chi-squared $p < 0.0001$), because LHRH treatment became more popular over time. The most recent study using a population-based cohort of 3295 men with metastatic PCa showed that LHRH agonist therapy is associated with higher risks of cardiac related complications, peripheral arterial disease, and fracture compared with orchiectomy [26]. In EORTC trial 30891, therefore, ADT modalities were not well balanced between the two treatment arms in terms of possible risks of clinically relevant adverse effects.

14.5 Efficacy of PADT for Japanese Men with Localized or Locally Advanced PCa

Although PADT has been widely used even for localized PCa in Japan, there have been sparse data supporting its efficacy in terms of survival advantage. Unfortunately, there have been no well-controlled trials of immediate versus deferred ADT for localized PCa in Japan. Akaza et al. reported 10-year survival rates for men with localized or locally advanced PCa treated with PADT or prostatectomy [27]. Between February 1993 and March 1995, men with T1b, T1c, or T2-3N0M0 prostate cancer were enrolled. In all, 176 men who underwent prostatectomy were assigned to Study 1 and were given adjuvant LHRH agonist therapy; 151 men who did not undergo prostatectomy were assigned to Study 2 and had LHRH agonist monotherapy or CAB. With a median of 10.4 years of follow-up, in Study 1, the 10-year overall survival rate was 73%, and the 10-year cause-specific survival rate was 86%, vs. 41% and 78%, respectively, in Study 2. Overall survival curves were similar to expected survival curves in both studies. There was no significant difference between studies in cause-specific survival. They concluded that, with PADT or prostatectomy, the men had a life expectancy similar to that of the normal population.

However, it is hard to clearly draw conclusions that the life expectancy of men with localized or locally advanced PCa can be improved by PADT, since no deferred therapy group was included in the study, and natural history data are not available for Japanese patients with PCa. Furthermore, when evaluating the life expectancy of PCa patients, a healthy screener effect should be taken into account in the PSA era [28]. Generally, people who undergo screening have better overall health behaviors than those who do not. Patients choosing PSA screening may have better diets and healthier lifestyles and may more often choose definitive treatment when diagnosed with PCa [29]. Actually, comparison of other-cause survival to US life tables showed a survival benefit for patients with locoregional PCa over the baseline population [28]. Therefore, their findings that men had a life expectancy similar to that of the normal population do not guarantee that PADT has a survival advantage.

Conclusions

PADT has been widely used in men with localized PCa in Japan, despite a lack of clinical trials supporting its use. Large, population-based studies suggest that PADT does not improve survival in men with localized PCa, and there are data suggesting reduced overall survival with ADT. Many of the RCTs of immediate versus deferred ADT failed to show a survival benefit of immediate use of ADT for localized PCa. In the most recent RCT, immediate ADT resulted in a modest but significant increase in overall survival, but no significant difference in PCa mortality or symptom-free survival. A subset of men with localized PCa may benefit from immediate PADT, but this must be weighed against the adverse effects of long-term ADT.

References

1. http://ganjoho.jp/reg_stat/statistics/stat/short_pred.html
2. Pagliarulo V, Bracarda S, Eisenberger MA, Mottet N, Schröder FH, Sternberg CN, Studer UE. Contemporary role of androgen deprivation therapy for prostate cancer. Eur Urol. 2012;61(1):11–25. https://doi.org/10.1016/j.eururo.2011.08.026.
3. http://uroweb.org/guidelines/
4. https://www.nccn.org/about/
5. Akaza H. Trends in primary androgen depletion therapy for patients with localized and locally advanced prostate cancer: Japanese perspective. Cancer Sci. 2006;97(4):243–7.
6. Cooperberg MR, Broering JM, Carroll PR. Time trends and local variation in primary treatment of localized prostate cancer. J Clin Oncol. 2010;28:1117–23. https://doi.org/10.1200/JCO.2009.26.0133.
7. Hinotsu S, Akaza H, Usami M, Ogawa O, Kagawa S, Kitamura T, Tsukamoto T, Naito S, Namiki M, Hirao Y, Murai M, Yamanaka H. Japan Study Group of Prostate Cancer (J-CaP). Current status of endocrine therapy for prostate cancer in Japan analysis of primary androgen

deprivation therapy on the basis of data collected by J-CaP. Jpn J Clin Oncol. 2007;37:775–81. https://doi.org/10.1093/jjco/hym098.
8. Isbarn H, Boccon-Gibod L, Carroll PR, Montorsi F, Schulman C, Smith MR, Sternberg CN, Studer UE. Androgen deprivation therapy for the treatment of prostate cancer: consider both benefits and risks. Eur Urol. 2009;55(1):62–75. https://doi.org/10.1016/j.eururo.2008.10.008.
9. Mitsuzuka K, Kyan A, Sato T, Orikasa K, Miyazato M, Aoki H, Kakoi N, Narita S, Koie T, Namima T, Toyoda S, Fukushi Y, Habuchi T, Ohyama C, Arai Y. Tohoku Evidence-Based Medicine Study Group; Michinoku Urological Cancer Study Group. Influence of 1 year of androgen deprivation therapy on lipid and glucose metabolism and fat accumulation in Japanese patients with prostate cancer. Prostate Cancer Prostatic Dis. 2016;19(1):57–62. https://doi.org/10.1038/pcan.2015.50.
10. Cooperberg MR, Hinotsu S, Namiki M, Carroll PR, Akaza H. Trans-Pacific variation in outcomes for men treated with primary androgen-deprivation therapy (ADT) for prostate cancer. BJU Int. 2016;117(1):102–9. https://doi.org/10.1111/bju.12937.
11. Cancer Registration Committee of Japanese Urological Association. Clinicopathological statistics on registered prostate cancer patients in Japan: 2000 report from the Japanese Urological Association. Int J Urol. 2005;12:46–61.
12. The Research Group for Population-based Cancer Registration in Japan. Cancer incidence and incidence rates in Japan in 1997: estimates based on data from 12 population-based cancer registries. Jpn J Clin Oncol. 2002;32:318–22.
13. Onozawa M, Hinotsu S, Tsukamoto T, Oya M, Ogawa O, Kitamura T, Suzuki K, Naito S, Namiki M, Nishimura K, Hirao Y, Akaza H. Recent trends in the initial therapy for newly diagnosed prostate cancer in Japan. Jpn J Clin Oncol. 2014;44(10):969–81. https://doi.org/10.1093/jjco/hyu104.
14. D'Amico AV, Whittington R, Malkowicz SB, Schultz D, Blank K, Broderick GA, Tomaszewski JE, Renshaw AA, Kaplan I, Beard CJ, Wein A. Biochemical outcome after radical prostatectomy, external beam radiation therapy, or interstitial radiation therapy for clinically localized prostate cancer. JAMA. 1998;280:969–74.
15. Wong YN, Freedland SJ, Egleston B, Vapiwala N, Uzzo R, Armstrong K. The role of primary androgen deprivation therapy in localized prostate cancer. Eur Urol. 2009;56(4):609–16. https://doi.org/10.1016/j.eururo.2009.03.066.
16. Lu-Yao GL, Albertsen PC, Li H, Moore DF, Shih W, Lin Y, DiPaola RS, Yao SL. Does primary androgen-deprivation therapy delay the receipt of secondary cancer therapy for localized prostate cancer? Eur Urol. 2012;62(6):966–72. https://doi.org/10.1016/j.eururo.2012.05.003.
17. Lu-Yao GL, Albertsen PC, Moore DF, Shih W, Lin Y, DiPaola RS, Yao SL. Fifteen-year survival outcomes following primary androgen-deprivation therapy for localized prostate cancer. JAMA Intern Med. 2014;174(9):1460–7. https://doi.org/10.1001/jamainternmed.2014.3028.
18. Potosky AL, Haque R, Cassidy-Bushrow AE, Ulcickas Yood M, Jiang M, Tsai HT, Luta G, Keating NL, Smith MR, Van Den Eeden SK. Effectiveness of primary androgen-deprivation therapy for clinically localized prostate cancer. J Clin Oncol. 2014;32(13):1324–30. https://doi.org/10.1200/JCO.2013.52.5782.
19. Byar DP. The Veterans Administration Cooperative Urological Research Group's studies of cancer of the prostate. Cancer. 1973;32:1126–30.
20. The Medical Research Council Prostate Cancer Working Party Investigator Group. Immediate versus deferred treatment for advanced prostatic cancer: initial results of the Medical Research Council trial. Br J Urol. 1997;79:235–46.
21. D. Kirk on behalf of the Medical Research Council Prostate Cancer Working Party Investigators Group. Immediate vs. deferred hormone treatment for prostate cancer: how safe is androgen deprivation? Br J Urol. 2000:S220.
22. Studer UE, Hauri D, Hanselmann S, Chollet D, Leisinger HJ, Gasser T, Senn E, Trinkler FB, Tscholl RM, Thalmann GN, Dietrich D. Immediate versus deferred hormonal treatment for patients with prostate cancer who are not suitable for curative local treatment: results of the randomized trial SAKK 08/88. J Clin Oncol. 2004;22(20):4109–18.

23. Studer UE, Whelan P, Albrecht W, Casselman J, de Reijke T, Hauri D, Loidl W, Isorna S, Sundaram SK, Debois M, Collette L. Immediate or deferred androgen deprivation for patients with prostate cancer not suitable for local treatment with curative intent: European Organisation for Research and Treatment of Cancer (EORTC) trial 30891. J Clin Oncol. 2006;24(12):1868–76.
24. Studer UE, Collette L, Whelan P, Albrecht W, Casselman J, de Reijke T, Knönagel H, Loidl W, Isorna S, Sundaram SK, Debois M, EORTC Genitourinary Group. Using PSA to guide timing of androgen deprivation in patients with T0-4 N0-2 M0 prostate cancer not suitable for local curative treatment (EORTC 30891). Eur Urol. 2008;53(5):941–9. https://doi.org/10.1016/j.eururo.2007.12.032.
25. Studer UE, Whelan P, Wimpissinger F, Casselman J, de Reijke TM, Knönagel H, Loidl W, Isorna S, Sundaram SK, Collette L, EORTC Genitourinary Cancer Group. Differences in time to disease progression do not predict for cancer-specific survival in patients receiving immediate or deferred androgen-deprivation therapy for prostate cancer: final results of EORTC randomized trial 30891 with 12 years of follow-up. Eur Urol. 2014;66(5):829–38. https://doi.org/10.1016/j.eururo.2013.07.024.
26. Sun M, Choueiri TK, Hamnvik OP, Preston MA, De Velasco G, Jiang W, Loeb S, Nguyen PL, Trinh QD. Comparison of gonadotropin-releasing hormone agonists and orchiectomy: effects of androgen-deprivation therapy. JAMA Oncol. 2016;2(4):500–7. https://doi.org/10.1001/jamaoncol.2015.4917.
27. Akaza H, Homma Y, Usami M, Hirao Y, Tsushima T, Okada K, Yokoyama M, Ohashi Y, Aso Y. Prostate Cancer Study Group. Efficacy of primary hormone therapy for localized or locally advanced prostate cancer: results of a 10-year follow-up. BJU Int. 2006;97(5):997–1001.
28. Sammon JD, Abdollah F, D'Amico A, Gettman M, Haese A, Suardi N, Vickers A, Trinh QD. Predicting life expectancy in men diagnosed with prostate cancer. Eur Urol. 2015;68(5):756–65. https://doi.org/10.1016/j.eururo.2015.03.020.
29. Kramer BS. The science of early detection. Urol Oncol. 2004;22:344–7.

Complications of ADT for Prostate Cancer: Hot Flashes

15

Hideki Sakai and Tomoaki Hakariya

Abstract

Hot flashes are often a lasting and distressing side effect of androgen deprivation therapy (ADT) for men with prostate cancer. Hot flashes have been reported in as many as 80% of men with prostate cancer treated with ADT. In men treated with ADT, endorphins may be reduced because of suppression of testosterone levels. This reduction in endorphins may mediate the process of lowering the thermoregulatory set point and ultimately the activation of heat loss mechanisms, resulting in a hot flash. A variety of treatments have been assessed for managing hot flashes, including hormonal therapies, complementary treatments, and nonhormonal drug treatments, such as clonidine, gabapentin, and selective serotonin reuptake inhibitors. However, for hot flashes, there are presently no highly effective mitigating interventions without adverse events.

Keywords

Prostate cancer · Androgen deprivation therapy · Hot flash · Steroidal antiandrogen · Gabapentin · Venlafaxine · Acupuncture · Cognitive-behavioral therapy

15.1 Introduction

Hot flashes are often a lasting and distressing side effect of androgen deprivation therapy (ADT) for men with prostate cancer. Hot flashes have been reported in as many as 80% of men with prostate cancer treated with ADT [1]. Hot flashes, flushing or hot flushes, are synonymous words for episodes of heat sensation that are

H. Sakai (✉) · T. Hakariya
Department of Urology, Nagasaki University Graduate School of Biomedical Sciences, Nagasaki, Japan
e-mail: hsakai@nagasaki-u.ac.jp

associated with objective signs of cutaneous vasodilation and a subsequent drop in core temperature [2]. The vasomotor symptoms that characterize hot flashes (e.g., feelings of intense heat, profuse sweating, and flushing) have a negative effect on sleep, energy, sexuality, and overall quality of life [3]. This relatively common side effect of ADT may persist for several years. In a study of 63 men treated with orchiectomy or luteinizing hormone-releasing hormone agonists, 68% of patients reported hot flashes and 48% still had hot flashes 5 years after treatment [4].

Moreover, hot flashes may be one of the reasons that patients treated with ADT discontinue treatment prematurely and lose the potential survival benefit conferred by these therapies. The persistence of hot flashes in men has been associated with their decision to discontinue ADT [5]. Thus, it is important to manage hot flashes in men receiving ADT for prostate cancer.

15.2 Mechanisms of Hot Flashes

It is presumed that the physiological mechanism of hot flashes in men treated with ADT is similar to that in menopausal women and women treated with antiestrogens. A hot flash may be described as a subjective feeling of heat, accompanied by profuse sweating and shivering that may last a few minutes. In addition, patients may experience reddening of the skin of the face, head, and neck secondary to increased skin blood flow during these episodes. These phenomena occur as a result of a decreased set point of the hypothalamic thermoregulatory center and the resultant heat loss mechanisms. This change in set point is likely due to aberrations in endorphin and serotonin levels in the central nervous system [6, 7]. Several authors have reported that estrogen and testosterone stimulate endorphin production and that decreased estrogen levels are associated with decreased serotonin levels in the blood [7]. In the hypothalamus, it is thought that the thermoregulatory set point is lowered by norepinephrine. Endorphins are known to tonically inhibit norepinephrine production and release in the thermoregulatory centers of the hypothalamus. In men treated with ADT, endorphins may be reduced because of suppression of testosterone levels. This reduction in endorphins may mediate the process of lowering the thermoregulatory set point and ultimately the activation of heat loss mechanisms, resulting in a hot flash [7]. While the role of serotonin in the thermoregulatory pathway is not completely understood, it is known that activation of certain serotonin receptors in the hypothalamus mediates heat loss. Thus, a relationship between androgens and vasomotor tone regulation may exist. However, the exact physiologic mechanisms of hot flashes are still uncertain.

15.3 Signs and Symptoms of Hot Flashes

Hot flashes occur with a reddening of the skin and often sweating. The episodes may last anywhere from a few seconds to several minutes; however, most episodes usually last 2–3 min. Symptoms associated with hot flashes can be graded

Table 15.1 Hot flash scoring scale

Severity	Score	Duration (min)	Observations
Mild	1	<1	– Warm, slightly uncomfortable
			– No sweating
Moderate	2	<5	– Warmer, perspiration
			– Removal of some clothing
Severe	3	>5	– Burning, warmth
			– Disruption of normal life
			– Difficulty sleeping
			– Excessive perspiration

from mild to severe, as shown in Table 15.1 [8]. Subjective measures of hot flashes include assessing the frequency, severity, intensity, distress, and interference with daily activities. A study of 138 medically or surgically castrated men showed that hot flashes occurred an average of four times per day [9]. Younger men were more likely to report hot flashes than older men. In addition to flushing and sweating, most men reported warmth, dry mouth, and clammy skin. Fatigue and weakness were experienced in 45% of men, whereas emotional symptoms, such as distress, anxiety, and irritability, were reported by less than 40% [9].

15.4 Treatments for Hot Flashes

A variety of treatments have been assessed for managing hot flashes, including hormonal therapies, complementary treatments, and nonhormonal drug treatments, such as clonidine, gabapentin, and selective serotonin reuptake inhibitors. Most of these treatments have been evaluated predominantly in postmenopausal women and those receiving therapy for breast cancer.

15.4.1 Gabapentin

Several randomized, controlled clinical trials have demonstrated the efficacy of gabapentin in reducing hot flashes in women with breast cancer [10, 11]. In addition, a randomized crossover study of gabapentin and venlafaxine in women with breast cancer revealed that both agents decreased hot flashes. However, gabapentin was associated with more dizziness ($p = 0.005$) and increased appetite ($p < 0.001$) [12]. Moraska et al. described the efficacy of low-dose gabapentin in treating hot flashes in men treated with ADT [13]. This self-report of 117 men with prostate cancer who received gabapentin 600 mg per day showed moderately decreased hot flash scores without substantial toxicities.

15.4.2 Venlafaxine

Several randomized, controlled trials have demonstrated the efficacy of venlafaxine, a selective serotonin reuptake inhibitor antidepressant, in reducing hot flashes. A 12-week, double-blind trial comparing clonidine, venlafaxine, and a placebo in 80 women with breast cancer found that venlafaxine and clonidine were slightly more effective than the placebo in reducing hot flash symptoms [14]. However, all study groups showed significant reductions in symptoms at 12 weeks, including the placebo group, which reported a 29% decrease in hot flashes. In men treated with ADT for prostate cancer, venlafaxine was not found to be superior to cyproterone acetate or medroxyprogesterone acetate in a double-blind randomized study ($n = 109$). However, no placebo control group was included in this study [15].

15.4.3 Steroidal Antiandrogens

The preventive and therapeutic effects of steroidal antiandrogens against hot flashes have been investigated in a combined androgen blockade (CAB) setting [16, 17]. Recently, Sakai et al. reported that CAB using the steroidal antiandrogen chlormadinone acetate might reduce distressing hot flashes to a greater extent than CAB with bicalutamide in a prospective, randomized controlled study ($n = 124$) [18]. Bicalutamide is a pure antiandrogen, and chlormadinone is a progestin with progestational, as well as antiandrogenic, properties, which could partly explain the clinical differences between the two antiandrogens. Irani et al. conducted a 12-week double-blind study of three drugs to manage hot flashes in men receiving ADT for prostate cancer: venlafaxine 75 mg per day ($n = 102$), medroxyprogesterone acetate 20 mg per day ($n = 108$), or cyproterone acetate 100 mg per day ($n = 101$). No comparator placebo control arm was included. All three drugs were found to reduce hot flashes in men, but cyproterone acetate and medroxyprogesterone were most effective [15].

15.4.4 Clonidine

In a systematic review, Rada et al. reported that clonidine reduced hot flashes in women with breast cancer [11]. However, a similar placebo-controlled trial in men treated with orchiectomy for prostate cancer found no significant benefit of clonidine treatment [17].

15.4.5 Acupuncture

Acupuncture has also been evaluated. A systematic review identified six studies using acupuncture to treat hot flashes, of which none were randomized and placebo controlled [19]. One prospective study of 60 men receiving auricular acupuncture weekly for 10 weeks found that 95% of men experienced a decrease in symptoms

[20]. A more recent study of 14 men found that acupuncture decreased hot flash scores by 89.2% from 37.41 to 4.05 ($p = 0.0078$) after 6 weeks [21]. The clinical improvement is likely related to acupuncture's ability to stimulate the release of endorphins, norepinephrine, and serotonin in the hypothalamic thermoregulatory nucleus and modulate the peripheral autonomic nervous system, leading to peripheral vascular dilatation. These results must be considered preliminary, and randomized placebo-controlled trials are needed to further evaluate the role of acupuncture in the treatment of ADT-related hot flashes.

15.4.6 Cognitive Behavioral Therapy

There is evidence that cognitive behavioral therapy (CBT) is a safe and effective intervention for reducing the impact of hot flashes and night sweats (HFNS) and improving psychosocial functioning for menopausal women [22] and breast cancer survivors [23, 24]. Another author reported that 96 symptomatic women seen in a breast cancer clinic were enrolled in a randomized trial in which individualized "usual care" by breast care nurses was compared to usual care plus group CBT intervention [23]. Group CBT incorporated group discussions, handouts, and weekly homework with audio instructions for daily relaxation and paced breathing exercises at home. Little difference in hot flash frequency and night sweats was found between the two groups at weeks 9 and 26. Recently, Stefanopoulou et al. reported a randomized controlled trial of guided self-help CBT ($n = 33$) on HFNS problem rating compared with treatment as usual ($n = 35$) in patients undergoing ADT [25]. They revealed that CBT significantly reduced HFNS problem rating ($p = 0.001$) and HFNS frequency ($p = 0.02$) at 6 weeks compared with treatment as usual. They concluded that further research should test this intervention in a multicenter trial and include a range of ethnicities.

15.4.7 Other Treatments

Alternative remedies have also been tested to try to reduce hot flashes. Soy protein was tested in a randomized trial of 33 men undergoing ADT but showed no improvement in vasomotor symptoms [26]. A 2 × 2 randomized trial of soy protein, venlafaxine, and a combination of the two found no reduction in hot flashes for either soy protein or venlafaxine compared with placebo [27].

> **Conclusions**
>
> Although ADT can improve survival for men in certain settings, it also has a variety of potential disadvantages. For hot flashes, there are presently no highly effective mitigating interventions without adverse events. At this point, the only way to prevent hot flashes is to avoid unnecessary use of ADT. ADT is not recommended as therapy for low-risk cancer or neoadjuvant therapy before radical prostatectomy. For situations in which ADT is necessary, clinicians should intervene to reduce the negative outcomes following ADT.

References

1. Frisk J. Managing hot flushes in men after prostate cancer. A systematic review. Maturitas. 2010;65:15–22.
2. Boekhout AH, Beijnen JH, Schellens JH. Symptoms and treatment in cancer therapy-induced early menopause. Oncologist. 2006;11:641–54.
3. Kadakia KC, Loprinzi CL, Barton DL. Hot flashes: the ongoing search for effective interventions. Menopause. 2012;19:719–21.
4. Karling P, Hammar M, Varenhorst E. Prevalence and duration of hot flushes after surgical or medical castration in men with prostatic carcinoma. J Urol. 1994;152:1170–3.
5. Engstrom CA. Hot flashes in prostate cancer: state of the science. Am J Mens Health. 2008;2:122–32.
6. Spetz AC, Zetterlund EL, Varenhorst E, Hammer M. Incidence and management of hot flashes in prostate cancer. J Upport. Oncologia. 2003;1:263–73.
7. Shanafelt TD, Barton DL, Adjei AA, Loprinzi CL. Pathophisiology and treatment of hot flashes. Mayo Clin Proc. 2002;77:1207–18.
8. Baum N, Torti D. Management of hot flashes in men with prostate cancer. Geriatri. Aging. 2003;6(2):43–6.
9. Kagee A, Kruus LK, Malkowicz S, Vaughn DJ, Coyne JC. The experience of hot flashes among prostate cancer patients receiving hormone treatment. Proceedings of the. Proc Am Soc Clin Oncol. 2001;20(2):2999.
10. Kaplan M, Mahon S, Cope D, Keating E, Hill S, Jacobson M. Putting evidence into practice: evidence-based interventions for hot flashes resulting from cancer therapies. Clin J Oncol Nurs. 2011;15:149–57.
11. Rada G, Capurro D, Pantoja T, Corbalán J, Moreno G, Letelier LM, et al. Non-hormonal interventions for hot f lushes in women with a history of breast cancer. Cochrane Database Syst Rev. 2010;9:CD004923.
12. Bordeleau L, Pritchard KI, Loprinzi CL, Ennis M, Jugovic O, Warr D, et al. Multicenter, randomized, cross-over clinical trial of venlafaxine versus gabapentin for the management of hot flashes in breast cancer survivors. J Clin Oncol. 2010;28:5147–52.
13. Moraska AR, Atherton PJ, Szydlo DW, Barton DL, Stella PJ, Rowland KM, et al. Gabapentin for the management of hot flashes in prostate cancer survivors: a longitudinal continuation study-NCCTG trial N00CB. J Support Oncol. 2010;8:128–32.
14. Boekhout AH, Vincent AD, Dalesio OB, van den Bosch J, Foekema-Töns JH, Adriaansz S, et al. Management of hot flashes in patients who have breast cancer with venlafaxine and clonidine: a randomized, double-blind, placebocontrolled trial. J Clin Oncol. 2011;29:3862–8.
15. Irani J, Salomon L, Oba R, Bouchard P, Mottet N. Efficacy of venlafaxine, medroxyprogesterone acetate, and cyproterone acetate for the treatment of vasomotor hot flushes in men taking gonadotropin-releasing hormone analogues for prostate cancer: a double-blind, randomised trial. Lancet Oncol. 2010;11:147–54.
16. Thorpe SC, Azmatullah S, Fellows GJ, Gingell JC, O'Boyle PJ. A prospective, randomized study to compare goserelin acetate (Zoladex) versus cyproterone acetate (Cyprostat) versus a combination of the two in the treatment of metastatic prostatic carcinoma. Eur Urol. 1996;29:47–54.
17. Loprinzi CL, Michalak JC, Quella SK, O'Fallon JR, Hatfield AK, Nelimark RA, et al. Megestrol acetate for the prevention of hot flashes. N Engl J Med. 1994;331:347–52.
18. Sakai H, Igawa T, Tsurusaki T, Yura M, Kusaba Y, Hayashi M, et al. Hot flashes during androgen deprivation therapy with luteinizing hormone-releasing hormone agonist combined with steroidal or nonsteroidal antiandrogen for prostate cancer. Urology. 2009;73:635–40.
19. Lee MS, Kim KH, Shin BC, Choi SM, Ernst E. Acupuncture for treating hot flushes in men with prostate cancer: a systematic review. Support Care Cancer. 2009;17:763–70.

20. Harding C, Harris A, Chadwick D. Auricular acupuncture: a novel treatment for vasomotor symptoms associated with luteinizing hormone releasing hormone agonist treatment for prostate cancer. BJU Int. 2009;103:186–90.
21. Ashamalla H, Jiang ML, Guirguis A, Peluso F, Ashamalla M. Acupuncture for the alleviation of hot flashes in men treated with androgen ablation therapy. Int J Radiat Oncol Biol Phys. 2011;79:1358–63.
22. Ayers B, Smith M, Hellier J, Mann E, Hunter MS. Effectiveness of group and self-help cognitive behavior therapy in reducing problematic menopausal hot flushes and night sweats (MENOS 2): a randomized controlled trial. Menopause. 2012;19(7):749–59.
23. Mann E, Smith MJ, Hellier J, Balabanovic JA, Hamed H, Grunfeld EA, et al. Cognitive behavioural treatment for women who have menopausal symptoms after breast cancer treatment (MENOS 1): a randomised controlled trial. Lancet Oncol. 2012;13(3):309–18.
24. Duijts SF, van Beurden M, Oldenburg HS, Hunter MS, Kieffer JM, Stuiver MM, et al. Efficacy of cognitive behavioral therapy and physical exercise in alleviating treatmentinduced menopausal symptoms in patients with breast cancer: results of a randomized, controlled, multicenter trial. J Clin Oncol. 2012;30(33):4124–33.
25. Stefanopoulou E, Yousaf O, Grunfeld EA, Hunter MSA. Randomised controlled trial of a brief cognitive behavioural intervention for men who have hot flushes following prostate cancer treatment (MANCAN). Psycho-Oncology. 2015;24:1159–66.
26. Sharma P, Wisniewski A, Braga-Basaria M, Xu X, Yep M, Denmeade S, et al. Lack of an effect of high dose isoflavones in men with prostate cancer undergoing androgen deprivation therapy. J Urol. 2009;182:2265–72.
27. Vitolins MZ, Griffin L, Tomlinson WV, Vuky J, Adams PT, Moose D, et al. Randomized trial to assess the impact of venlafaxine and soy protein on hot flashes and quality of life in men with prostate cancer. J Clin Oncol. 2013;31:4092–8.

Complications of ADT for Prostate Cancer: Osteoporosis and the Risk of Fracture

Hiroji Uemura

Abstract

Patients with advanced disease usually receive hormonal therapy, such as androgen deprivation therapy (ADT). Although ADT is initially very effective for prostate cancer, long-term ADT is known to be associated with various side effects. Among them ADT is associated with the deterioration of bone health, including an increased risk of fracture from osteoporosis and the development of bone metastasis. For patients with conditions associated with fragility, such as osteoporosis in patients treated with ADT, it is important to estimate the risk of fracture. In order to identify the patients who require bone-supportive treatment for osteoporosis, the bone mineral density is assessed by dual-energy X-ray absorptiometry. The Fracture Risk Assessment Tool (FRAX) has been developed to evaluate the risk of fracture, and likely improves the assessment of the risk of fracture through the inclusion of patient characteristics. The maintenance of bone health is very important for achieving long survival because skeletal fractures are associated with shortened survival. Clinicians must pay attention to bone health and provide specific management for osteoporosis in prostate cancer patients.

Keywords

ADT · Osteoporosis · Bone fracture · FRAX score

H. Uemura, M.D., Ph.D
Department of Urology and Renal Transplantation,
Yokohama City University Medical Center,
Yokohama, Japan
e-mail: hu0428@yokohama-cu.ac.jp

16.1 Introduction

In Japan, the number of prostate cancer patients has dramatically increased because of widespread PSA screening and aging of the population. After the Caucasian countries and the countries in the Asia Pacific (such as Australia and New Zealand), Japan has the highest prevalence of prostate cancer. The proportion of patients with advanced-stage prostate cancer is higher in comparison to the United States. Patients with advanced disease usually receive hormonal therapy, such as androgen deprivation therapy (ADT) including GnRH analogue or surgical castration.

Although ADT is initially very effective for prostate cancer, long-term ADT is known to be associated with various side effects, including vasomotor flushing, cardiovascular complications, metabolic syndrome, a decreased sexual function, increased fat mass, and decreased muscle strength [1]. Furthermore, it is well known that ADT is associated with the deterioration of bone health, including an increased risk of fracture from osteoporosis and the development of bone metastasis. Most prostate cancer patients are >70 years of age. Osteoporosis and osteopenia become advanced in association with aging. A prospective cohort study in a semi-urban city in Australia revealed that all major fractures (i.e., proximal femur or vertebral fractures) were associated with increased mortality, even in elderly men [2]. Thus, the maintenance of bone health is very important for achieving long survival because skeletal fractures are associated with shortened survival [3].

16.2 The Risk of Osteoporosis and Bone Fractures in Patients Undergoing ADT

In healthy adults, an appropriate bone mass is maintained by the balance between bone formation by osteoblasts and bone resorption by osteoclasts. For instance, in vertebral bones, micro-fractures constantly occur due to gravity; through this, bone formation and resorption are equally maintained. Osteoblasts secrete receptor activator of nuclear factor-κB ligand (RANKL), which binds to RANK on the surfaces of osteoclast precursors, leading to the triggering of maturation, activation, and prolonged survival of osteoclasts [4]. Osteoprotegerin (OPG) plays a role as a decoy receptor, by binding and neutralizing RANKL, and essentially inhibits bone resorption [5]. In patients receiving vitamin D3, parathyroid hormone, tumor necrosis factor-a, activated T-cells, and glucocorticoid therapies increase the ratio of RANKL to OPG, promoting bone resorption [5, 6]. Testosterone stimulates the osteoblasts and inhibits the apoptosis of osteoblasts and osteoclasts. In contrast, in male patients with hypogonadism (e.g., patients who have undergone orchiectomy or who are receiving ADT), the decreased testosterone and estrogen levels induce bone resorption [7, 8]. A previous study showed that the rates of other femur, hip/femoral neck, upper and lower arm, spine, and pelvic bone fractures were significantly increased in patients undergoing ADT treatment in comparison to ADT nonusers [9]. Furthermore, independent predictors of fragility and fracture were revealed, including aging, prior bone thinning medications, chronic kidney disease, prior dementia, prior fragility fracture, and a prior diagnosis of osteoporosis ($P < 0.05$).

Morote et al. investigated the prevalence of osteoporosis in hormone-naïve patients with prostate cancer. The results showed that the prevalence of osteoporosis increased in accordance with the duration of ADT, finally reaching >80% after 10 years of ADT [10]. The other patients showed osteopenia, which means no patient on long-term ADT had a normal bone mass. Osteoporosis can be detected based on the bone mineral density (BMD), which can be measured by dual-energy X-ray absorptiometry (DEXA). Numerous reports have discussed the relationship between the BMD and bone fractures. Patients with prostate cancer who received ADT showed a significantly decreased hip BMD in comparison to patients who had not started ADT ($P = 0.02$) [11]. Similar findings were reported in Japanese patients, in that the BMD/young adult mean ratio was inversely correlated with the duration of ADT. The ratio was found to decrease by approximately 3% every 12 months [12]. A large study of Medicare records indicated that the overall fracture rate after 5 years was 19.4% among patients treated with ADT within 6 months of their diagnosis, while that in patients who did not receive ADT was 12.6% ($P < 0.001$) [13]. Cox proportional hazards analyses revealed a statistically significant relationship between the number of doses of gonadotropin-releasing hormone (GnRH) that were received in the year after diagnosis and the subsequent risk of fracture [13].

16.3 The FRAX Tool

In patients with conditions associated with fragility, such as osteoporosis in patients treated with ADT, it is important to estimate the risk of fracture. In order to identify the patients who require bone-supportive treatment for osteoporosis, the bone mineral density (BMD) is assessed by dual-energy X-ray absorptiometry (DEXA). A patient's standardized scale T-score is determined by comparing their femoral neck BMD with that of the young adult population of the same sex. Osteoporosis is diagnosed in patients with a T-score of <−2.5 standard deviations (SD). Osteopenia (low bone mass) is diagnosed in patients with a score of −1 to −2.5 SDs, while a score of −1 SD is considered normal. However, the T-score does not reflect the need for preventive treatment to reduce the risk of fracture in patients with osteoporosis [14].

The Fracture Risk Assessment Tool (FRAX) has been developed to evaluate the risk of fracture, and likely improves the assessment of the risk of fracture through the inclusion of patient characteristics, with or without BMD [15]. The patient characteristics include age, sex, weight, height, previous fracture, parental fracture, smoking, glucocorticoids, rheumatoid arthritis, secondary osteoporosis, alcohol, and BMD (https://www.sheffield.ac.uk/FRAX/tool.jsp?locationValue=). The FRAX was used to calculate the 10-year probability of hip and major osteoporotic fractures with or without BMD. The probability of fracture is adjusted for patients from different countries, including Japanese patients.

An early retrospective study reported that the ADT for prostate cancer was associated with the increase in >2 risk factors for osteoporosis. These risk factors include >70 years of age, Caucasian ancestry, BMI <25, smoking/alcohol intake, steroid exposure, and secondary risk factors for osteoporosis (excluding ADT). For instance, the risk of sustaining a major fracture increased from 4 to 5.6% after the initiation of ADT ($P \leq 0.001$), while the risk of hip fracture increased from 1.3 to 2.2% ($P \leq 0.001$) [16]. However, compliance with the national osteoporosis guideline recommendations was found to be very low; DEXA was only performed in 9% of cases and calcium supplementation and vitamin D supplementation were only administered to 5% and 3% of patients, respectively [16]. Another report indicated the importance of using FRAX to identify patients who require treatment to improve bone health. Based on the results of DEXA alone, 33% of men would need treatment, while the number of men who met the criteria for treatment was decreased when the femoral neck T-score was included in the FRAX calculation [17]. Without the T-score in the FRAX calculation, the number of patients who met the criteria for treatment increased in comparison to when DEXA was used alone [17]. James et al. reported the comparison of the FRAX tool score to the BMD in patients with advanced prostate cancer on ADT [18]. When the FRAX was used with the BMD, the number of patients who were identified as requiring therapy was higher in comparison to when patients were identified based on the T-score alone. Furthermore, they emphasized that the T-score may be suboptimal in patients who truly require bone tropic therapy. Although age was identified as a profound risk factor for bone fracture, elderly patients, specifically patients >80 years of age, do not always require treatment because all such patients are found to be at risk of fracture without the evaluation of the BMD.

Kawahara et al. assessed the FRAX score in Japanese prostate cancer patients who had undergone several types of therapy, including brachytherapy, radical prostatectomy, external beam radiation therapy (EBRT), and hormonal therapy, at a single institution [19]. The FRAX score data indicated that the median 10-year probability of a major osteoporotic fracture was 7.9%, while the 10-year probability of hip fracture was 2.7%. As shown in Fig. 16.1, the EBRT and ADT monotherapy groups showed significantly higher FRAX scores in comparison to the brachytherapy group ($p < 0.001$, $p < 0.001$, respectively). The EBRT and ADT monotherapy groups showed higher FRAX scores than both the brachytherapy group ($p < 0.001$, $p < 0.001$, respectively) and the prostatectomy group ($p < 0.05$, $p < 0.001$, respectively). The duration of ADT in the ADT cohort was correlated with the risk of both types of fracture ($p < 0.001$ [$R^2 = 0.141$] and $P < 0.001$ [$R^2 = 0.166$]), respectively (Fig. 16.2a, b). When the risk of fracture was compared between ADT and non-ADT cohorts, the risks of both types of fracture were increased in the ADT cohort in comparison to the non-ADT cohort ($p < 0.001$ [$R^2 = 0.141$] and $P < 0.001$ [$R^2 = 0.166$]), respectively. As expected, the duration of ADT was found to influence the FRAX score and patients undergoing ADT required additional treatment because of bone loss.

16 Complications of ADT for Prostate Cancer: Osteoporosis and the Risk of Fracture

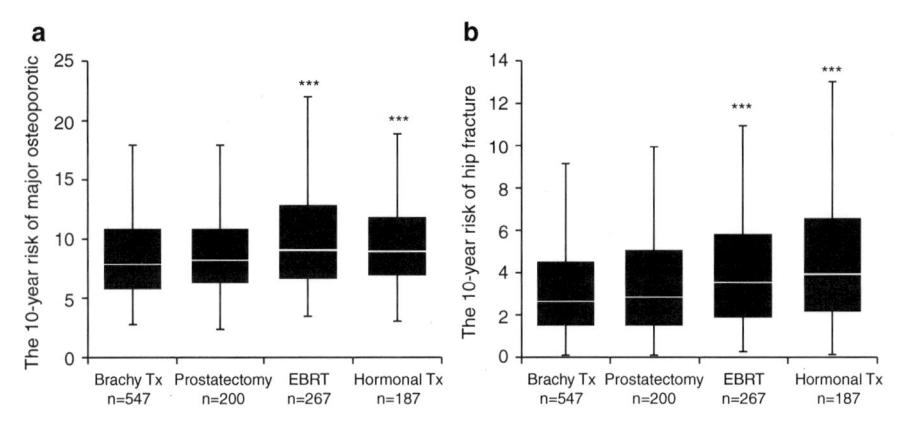

Fig. 16.1 The FRAX score among various prostate cancer therapies. (**a**) The 10-year risk of major osteoporotic. (**b**) The 10-year risk of hip fracture

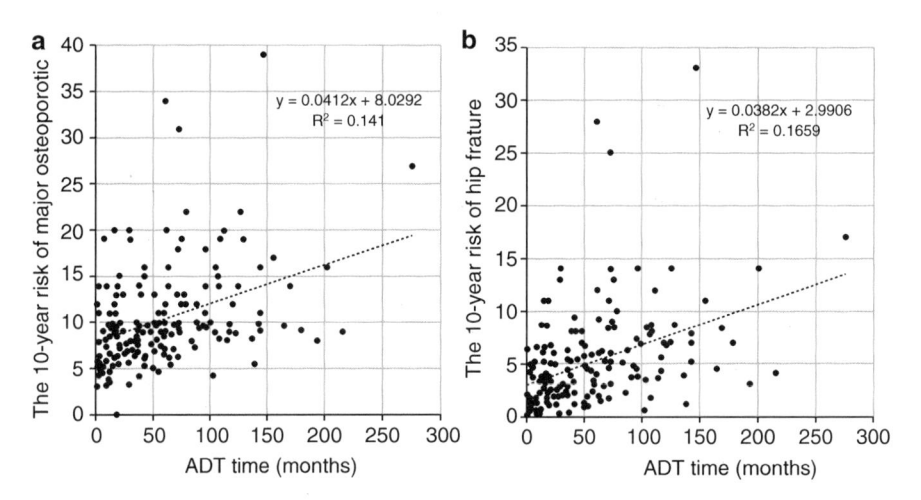

Fig. 16.2 The correlation between FRAX score and duration of ADT. (**a**) The 10-year risk of major osteoporosis. (**b**) The 10-year risk of hip fracture

16.4 The Prevention of Bone Fracture in Patients Undergoing ADT

Denosumab is a human monoclonal antibody that binds to RANKL and which is usually used to treat bone metastasis. Denosumab has been known to have the potential to increase the BMD, and was shown to increase the BMD of women receiving hormonal therapy for breast cancer at multiple skeletal sites [20]. Furthermore, the use of denosumab by postmenopausal women increased their BMD and reduced their bone turnover marker levels [21, 22]. Smith et al. investigated the effects of denosumab on BMD and fractures in men treated with ADT for prostate cancer [23]. In their randomized phase 3 trial, patients were assigned to receive denosumab (60 mg every 6 months) or a placebo. The study showed that the BMD of the lumbar spine increased by 5.6% in the denosumab group but decreased by 1.0% in the placebo group ($P < 0.001$), and significant differences between the two groups were consistently recognized from 1 month to 36 months. Similarly, the significant differences were shown in the BMD of the total hip, femoral neck, and distal third of the radius. In association with the increasing BMD of the vertebral body, patients treated with denosumab showed a decreased incidence of new vertebral fractures at 36 months in comparison to patients treated with placebo (1.5% vs. 3.9%, $P = 0.006$).

With regard to bisphosphonates, an oral agent—risedronate—was shown to lead to the recovery from bone loss in Japanese patients treated with ADT in a small clinical study. The mean percentage of change in the BMD/young adult mean ratio in patients treated with risedronate was higher than that of the control group after 1 year of treatment (2.6 ± 4.5% and −2.8 ± 2.6%, respectively; $P = 0.0001$) [12]. Zoledronic acid therapy was also reported to prevent fracture in men with osteoporosis [24]. In a multicenter, double-blind, placebo-controlled trial, Boonen et al. randomly assigned men with primary or hypogonadism-associated osteoporosis to receive zoledronic acid or a placebo at baseline and at 12 months. Concurrently, participants received daily calcium and vitamin D supplementation. As a primary endpoint, their data revealed that the zoledronic acid group showed a significant decrease in new morphometric vertebral fractures in comparison to the placebo group at 24 months (1.6% and 4.9%, respectively; relative risk, 0.33; $P = 0.002$). In addition, men who received zoledronic acid showed significantly higher BMD values and lower bone turnover marker levels than men who received the placebo ($P < 0.05$). Another clinical trial demonstrated the usefulness of zoledronic acid in the treatment of glucocorticoid-induced osteoporosis. The 1-year randomized, double-blind, non-inferiority study tested the effectiveness of zoledronic acid versus oral bisphosphonate in the prevention and treatment of glucocorticoid-induced osteoporosis [25]. The results indicated that zoledronic acid was non-inferior and superior with regard to promoting an increase in the BMD of the lumbar vertebrae—in both the treatment and prevention of glucocorticoid-induced bone loss. Because the long-term use of glucocorticoid has become common, especially in patients receiving treatment for castration-resistant prostate cancer (such as abiraterone or docetaxel therapy), prevention and treatment using bone-modifying agents are very important.

The Japanese Society for Bone Mineral Research investigated the predictors for glucocorticoid induced bone fracture in 903 Japanese patients using a Cox hazards model. Four risk factors for fracture were identified: aging, dose of glucocorticoid, %YAM (Young Adult Mean) level, and prior fracture [26]. The fracture risk was proven to increase by 2.4% for each year of age, by 3.8% with a glucocorticoid dose of 1 mg/day, and by 3.4 times in patients with a history of fracture, while a BMD increase of 1% reduced the FR by 2.1%. Bisphosphonate treatment reduced the FR by 52.8% (Table 16.1).

Table 16.1 Predictors of the risk of bone fracture: 2014 guidelines of the Japanese Society for Bone Mineral Research

Risk factors		Hazard ratio	95% CI	P-value
Age	1-year increase	1.024	1.008–1.040	0.025
Dose of GC[a]	1 mg/day increase	1.038	1.024–1.051	<0.0001
Lumbar BMD (%YAM)	1% increase	0.979	0.968–0.991	0.006
Prior fragility fracture	yes	3.412	2.409–4.832	<0.0001
BP therapy	yes	0.472	0.302–0.738	0.001

GC glucocorticoid, *BMD* bone mineral density, *BP* bisphosphonate, *CI* confidence interval
[a]Conversion of prednisolone (mg/day)

16.5 The Prevention of Bone Metastasis by Bone-Modifying Agents

Bone metastasis is a critical issue for the survival of prostate cancer patients; thus, the development of bone metastasis in a nonmetastatic situation represents an important turning point for the initiation of systematic treatment in patients with metastatic disease. Smith et al. reported the natural history of patients with nonmetastatic prostate cancer whose PSA levels increased despite ADT in a study that evaluated the effects of zoledronic acid [27]. One-third of the placebo patients developed bone metastasis at 2 years and the median bone metastasis-free survival (BMFS) was 30 months. The baseline PSA level (>10 ng/mL) and PSA velocity independently predicted a shorter time to first bone metastasis as well as OS and metastasis-free survival. Furthermore, in a randomized, placebo-controlled, phase trial of men with nonmetastatic CRPC and a high risk of progression, denosumab significantly improved the BMFS, the time to first bone metastasis, and the time to symptomatic bone metastasis [28]. However, denosumab improved neither the OS nor the progression-free survival, while denosumab increased the time to bone metastasis through the PSA doubling time (PSADT) [29]. A study of patients with nonmetastatic CRPC revealed that, in the placebo group, the cohort with shorter BMFS showed a decreased PSADT (<8 months) [29]. Neither denosumab nor zoledronic acid increased the OS of patients with nonmetastatic CRPC in comparison to patients who received a placebo.

16.6 Bone Management for Prostate Cancer Patients

In prostate cancer, bone management has been focused on aspects such as maintaining the quality of life (QOL) and the prognosis. Even if patients newly diagnosed with prostate cancer have healthy bone situation, their bones will become fragile in association with the decrease in BMD during long-term hormonal therapy. Thus, the BMD and FRAX score should be measured at the start of prostate cancer treatment, as shown in Fig. 16.3. The bone should be evaluated, through methods such as the measurement of the BMD or FRAX score, at the start of hormonal therapy. Patients with osteopenia should receive the treatments with bone-modifying agents such as denosumab or bisphosphonate to prevent osteoporosis. Furthermore, monitoring to detect bone metastasis is very important during hormonal therapy because of the considerable association between the progression to castration-resistant prostate cancer (CRPC) and bone metastasis. Once bone metastasis occurs, the physician must take account of the skeletal related events (SREs), including pathological fracture, radiotherapy for bone metastasis, and surgery for bone and spinal cord compression, which may lead to a reduced QOL and an increased risk of death. Under these conditions, bone-modifying agents have been used to prevent SRE regardless of their lack of benefit in terms of prolonged survival. Radium-223, alpha emitter, selectively targets bone metastases and has been proven to improve overall survival (OS) in CRPC patients with bone metastasis [30]. In addition, the combination of radium-223 and denosumab may prolong OS in CRPC patients [31]. Such combined multimodality therapies that specifically target bone metastasis can improve OS as well as the QOL.

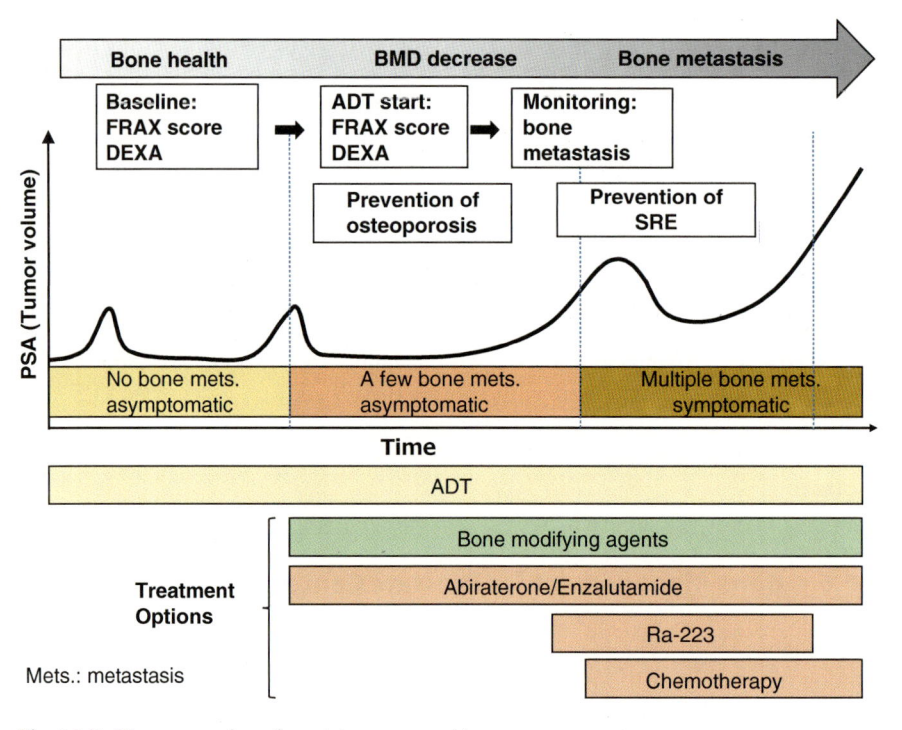

Fig. 16.3 The progression of prostate cancer and bone management

Conclusion

Long-term ADT for prostate cancer induces osteoporosis, leading to fragility fracture and other types of fracture, particularly in older patients. Clinicians must pay attention to bone health and provide specific management for osteoporosis in prostate cancer patients. Simultaneously, clinicians must discuss bone management with their patients. The evaluation of the conditions of the bone and the administration of appropriate supportive and adjuvant therapies are important matters in clinical practice.

References

1. Bolam KA, Galvao DA, Spry N, Newton RU, Taaffe DR. AST-induced bone loss in men with prostate cancer: exercise as a potential countermeasure. Prostate Cancer Prostatic Dis. 2012;15(4):329–38.
2. Center JR, Nguyen TV, Schneider D, Sambrook PN, Eisman JA. Mortality after all major types of osteoporotic fracture in men and women: an observational study. Lancet. 1999;353(9156):878–82.
3. Oefelein MG, Ricchiuti VS, Conrad PW, Goldman H, Bodner D, Resnick MI, Seftel A. Clinical predictors of androgen-independent prostate cancer and survival in the prostate-specific antigen era. Urology. 2002;60(1):120–4.
4. Egerdie B, Saad F. Bone health in the prostate cancer patient receiving androgen deprivation therapy: a review of present and future management options. Can Urol Assoc J. 2010;4(2):129–35.
5. Boyle WJ, Simonet WS, Lacey DL. Osteoclast differentiation and activation. Nature. 2003;423(6937):337–42.
6. Hofbauer LC, Schoppet M. Clinical implications of the osteoprotegerin/RANKL/RANK system for bone and vascular diseases. JAMA. 2004;292(4):490–5.
7. Higano CS. Androgen-deprivation-therapy-induced fractures in men with nonmetastatic prostate cancer: what do we really know? Nat Clin Pract Urol. 2008;5(1):24–34.
8. Perez EA, Weilbaecher K. Aromatase inhibitors and bone loss. Oncology (Williston Park). 2006;20(9):1029–39; discussion 1039–40, 1042, 1048
9. Alibhai SM, Duong-Hua M, Cheung AM, Sutradhar R, Warde P, Fleshner NE, Paszat L. Fracture types and risk factors in men with prostate cancer on androgen deprivation therapy: a matched cohort study of 19,079 men. J Urol. 2010;184(3):918–23.
10. Morote J, Morin JP, Orsola A, Abascal JM, Salvador C, Trilla E, Raventos CX, Cecchini L, Encabo G, Reventos J. Prevalence of osteoporosis during long-term androgen deprivation therapy in patients with prostate cancer. Urology. 2007;69(3):500–4.
11. Kiratli BJ, Srinivas S, Perkash I, Terris MK. Progressive decrease in bone density over 10 years of androgen deprivation therapy in patients with prostate cancer. Urology. 2001;57(1):127–32.
12. Izumi K, Mizokami A, Sugimoto K, Narimoto K, Miwa S, Maeda Y, Kadono Y, Takashima M, Koh E, Namiki M. Risedronate recovers bone loss in patients with prostate cancer undergoing androgen-deprivation therapy. Urology. 2009;73(6):1342–6.
13. Shahinian VB, Kuo YF, Freeman JL, Goodwin JS. Risk of fracture after androgen deprivation for prostate cancer. N Engl J Med. 2005;352(2):154–64.
14. Seeman E, Bianchi G, Khosla S, Kanis JA, Orwoll E. Bone fragility in men—where are we? Osteoporos Int. 2006;17(11):1577–83.
15. Kanis JA, Johnell O, Oden A, Johansson H, McCloskey E. FRAX and the assessment of fracture probability in men and women from the UK. Osteoporos Int. 2008;19(4):385–97.

16. Dhanapal V, Reeves DJ. Bone health management in prostate cancer patients receiving androgen deprivation therapy. J Oncol Pharm Pract. 2012;18(1):84–90.
17. Adler RA, Hastings FW, Petkov VI. Treatment thresholds for osteoporosis in men on androgen deprivation therapy: T-score versus FRAX. Osteoporos Int. 2010;21(4):647–53.
18. James H 3rd, Aleksic I, Bienz MN, Pieczonka C, Iannotta P, Albala D, Mariados N, Mouraviev V, Saad F. Comparison of fracture risk assessment tool score to bone mineral density for estimating fracture risk in patients with advanced prostate cancer on androgen deprivation therapy. Urology. 2014;84(1):164–8.
19. Kawahara T, Fusayasu S, Izumi K, Yokomizo Y, Ito H, Ito Y, Kurita K, Furuya K, Hasumi H, Hayashi N, et al. Bone management in Japanese patients with prostate cancer: hormonal therapy leads to an increase in the FRAX score. BMC Urol. 2016;16(1):32.
20. Ellis GK, Bone HG, Chlebowski R, Paul D, Spadafora S, Smith J, Fan M, Jun S. Randomized trial of denosumab in patients receiving adjuvant aromatase inhibitors for nonmetastatic breast cancer. J Clin Oncol. 2008;26(30):4875–82.
21. McClung MR, Lewiecki EM, Cohen SB, Bolognese MA, Woodson GC, Moffett AH, Peacock M, Miller PD, Lederman SN, Chesnut CH, et al. Denosumab in postmenopausal women with low bone mineral density. N Engl J Med. 2006;354(8):821–31.
22. Miller PD, Bolognese MA, Lewiecki EM, McClung MR, Ding B, Austin M, Liu Y, San Martin J, AMG Bone Loss Study Group. Effect of denosumab on bone density and turnover in postmenopausal women with low bone mass after long-term continued, discontinued, and restarting of therapy: a randomized blinded phase 2 clinical trial. Bone. 2008;43(2):222–9.
23. Smith MR, Egerdie B, Hernandez Toriz N, Feldman R, Tammela TL, Saad F, Heracek J, Szwedowski M, Ke C, Kupic A, et al. Denosumab in men receiving androgen-deprivation therapy for prostate cancer. N Engl J Med. 2009;361(8):745–55.
24. Boonen S, Reginster JY, Kaufman JM, Lippuner K, Zanchetta J, Langdahl B, Rizzoli R, Lipschitz S, Dimai HP, Witvrouw R, et al. Fracture risk and zoledronic acid therapy in men with osteoporosis. N Engl J Med. 2012;367(18):1714–23.
25. Reid DM, Devogelaer JP, Saag K, Roux C, Lau CS, Reginster JY, Papanastasiou P, Ferreira A, Hartl F, Fashola T, et al. Zoledronic acid and risedronate in the prevention and treatment of glucocorticoid-induced osteoporosis (HORIZON): a multicentre, double-blind, double-dummy, randomised controlled trial. Lancet. 2009;373(9671):1253–63.
26. Suzuki Y, Nawata H, Soen S, Fujiwara S, Nakayama H, Tanaka I, Ozono K, Sagawa A, Takayanagi R, Tanaka H, et al. Guidelines on the management and treatment of glucocorticoid-induced osteoporosis of the Japanese Society for Bone and Mineral Research: 2014 update. J Bone Miner Metab. 2014;32(4):337–50.
27. Smith MR, Kabbinavar F, Saad F, Hussain A, Gittelman MC, Bilhartz DL, Wynne C, Murray R, Zinner NR, Schulman C, et al. Natural history of rising serum prostate-specific antigen in men with castrate nonmetastatic prostate cancer. J Clin Oncol. 2005;23(13):2918–25.
28. Smith MR, Saad F, Coleman R, Shore N, Fizazi K, Tombal B, Miller K, Sieber P, Karsh L, Damiao R, et al. Denosumab and bone-metastasis-free survival in men with castration-resistant prostate cancer: results of a phase 3, randomised, placebo-controlled trial. Lancet. 2012;379(9810):39–46.
29. Smith MR, Saad F, Oudard S, Shore N, Fizazi K, Sieber P, Tombal B, Damiao R, Marx G, Miller K, et al. Denosumab and bone metastasis-free survival in men with nonmetastatic castration-resistant prostate cancer: exploratory analyses by baseline prostate-specific antigen doubling time. J Clin Oncol. 2013;31(30):3800–6.
30. Parker C, Nilsson S, Heinrich D, Helle SI, O'Sullivan JM, Fossa SD, Chodacki A, Wiechno P, Logue J, Seke M, et al. Alpha emitter radium-223 and survival in metastatic prostate cancer. N Engl J Med. 2013;369(3):213–23.
31. Saad F, Carles J, Gillessen S, Heidenreich A, Heinrich D, Gratt J, Levy J, Miller K, Nilsson S, Petrenciuc O, et al. Radium-223 and concomitant therapies in patients with metastatic castration-resistant prostate cancer: an international, early access, open-label, single-arm phase 3b trial. Lancet Oncol. 2016;17(9):1306–16.

Metabolic Health for Patients with Prostate Cancer During Androgen Deprivation Therapy

17

Koji Mitsuzuka and Yoichi Arai

Abstract

Androgen deprivation therapy (ADT) continues to be widely used for the treatment of prostate cancer despite the appearance of new-generation androgen receptor-targeting drugs after 2000. ADT can alleviate symptoms in patients with metastatic prostate cancer and may have a survival benefit in some patients, but it causes undesirable changes in lipid and sugar metabolism. Moreover, these metabolic changes could be related to new onset or worsening of diseases such as diabetes mellitus or cardiovascular disease. Several studies examining the influence of ADT in Japanese patients with prostate cancer also showed that metabolic changes such as weight gain, dyslipidemia, or fat accumulation can occur as in patients in Western countries. Efforts to decrease these unfavorable changes and events are important. First, overuse of ADT for localized or elderly prostate cancer patients should be reconsidered. Second, intermittent ADT may be beneficial for selected patients who suffer from impaired quality of life (QOL) due to continuous ADT. Third, education and instruction, such as diet or exercise, to decrease metabolic changes before initiating ADT are important, because metabolic changes can occur in the early ADT period.

Keywords

Prostate cancer · Androgen deprivation therapy · Metabolic change · Obesity · Sarcopenia

K. Mitsuzuka (✉) · Y. Arai
Department of Urology, Tohoku University School of Medicine, Sendai, Japan
e-mail: mitsuzuka@uro.med.tohoku.ac.jp

Abbreviations

ADT   Androgen deprivation therapy
CT   Computed tomography
CVD   Cardiovascular disease
GnRH   Gonadotropin-releasing hormone
HDL   High-density lipoprotein
LDL   Low-density lipoprotein
QOL   Quality of life

17.1 Metabolic Changes During ADT

17.1.1 Lipid and Glucose Metabolism

Influence of ADT on lipid and glucose metabolisms has been widely well known. Previous studies showed a mean increase of 3.2–10.6% in total cholesterol and 3.8–46.6% in triglycerides [1–10], with the duration of ADT ranging from 24 weeks to 12 months (Table 17.1). These changes in lipid and glucose levels were noticeable in the first 3 or 6 months of ADT (Figs. 17.1 and 17.2) [2, 5–7, 10]. Only one study compared the differences in lipid profile according to treatment modality [10]. The study showed that there were no significant differences between GnRH agonist alone and maximal androgen blockade with bicalutamide, while changes in total cholesterol and triglyceride were greater in GnRH agonist alone than in maximal androgen blockade. ADT also affects sugar metabolism, and it is associated with worsening blood sugar control and incidence of diabetes mellitus [1, 3, 4, 6, 7, 11]. Smith et al. reported that ADT decreased insulin sensitivity and increased serum insulin levels in patients who received 12 weeks of ADT [4]. These changes in lipid and glucose metabolism are related to the risk of type 2 diabetes mellitus. Keating et al. conducted an observational study of 37,443 population-based men who were diagnosed with local or regional prostate cancer. Of these, 14,597 (39%) were treated with ADT. The incidence of diabetes mellitus was 159.4 events per 1000 person-years for the ADT group and 87.5 events for the no-ADT group (adjusted hazard ratio = 1.28) [12].

17.1.2 Metabolic Syndrome

Metabolic changes caused by ADT are associated with the incidence of metabolic syndrome. Braga-Basaria et al. found that more than half of the men receiving long-term (at least 12 months) ADT had metabolic syndrome compared with one-fifth of the men in the control groups [13]. Recently, Bosco et al. performed a meta-analysis of metabolic syndrome caused by ADT and showed that ADT significantly increased the risk of metabolic syndrome (relative risk = 1.75) [14].

Table 17.1 Changes in lipid and sugar metabolic profiles by androgen deprivation therapy

	Region	Year	Study design	No. of pts	Indications	Methods of ADT	ADT duration	Age (mean or median)	Weight	Abdominal circumference	Triglyceride	Total cholesterol	LDL cholesterol	HDL cholesterol	Fasting blood sugar	HbA1c
Nowicki et al. [15]	Poland	2001	Prospective	18	Stage D	GnRH agonists with flutamide	12 weeks	67	+2.7 kg (3.8%)							
Smith et al. [1]	United Kingdom	2001	Prospective	22	Nonmetastatic	GnRH agonists [21] orchiectomy [1]	3 months	67	Unchanged		+13.3%	+3.2%	−2.3%	+8.3%	+3.5%	
Smith et al. [2]	United States	2002	Prospective	32	No bone metastasis	GnRH agonists with bicalutamide	48 weeks	66	+2.3 kg (2.4%)		+26.5%	+9.0%	+7.3%	+11.3%		
Smith [16]	United States	2004	Prospective	79	Nonmetastatic	GnRH agonists or orchiectomy with or without antiandrogen	48 weeks	71	+1.4 kg (1.8%)							
Nishiyama et al. [3]	Japan	2005	Prospective	49	Nonmetastatic	GnRH agonists or orchiectomy with flutamide	6 months	69	+0.5 kg (8.3%)		+8.2%	+6.1%	+5.0%		+3.5%	
Smith et al. [4]	United States	2006	Prospective	25	Nonmetastatic	GnRH agonists with bicalutamide	12 weeks	68	+0.6 kg (0.4%)		+23.0%	+9.4%	+8.7%	+9.9%	+2.0%	
Torimoto et al. [5]	Japan	2011	Prospective	39	Any stage	GnRH agonists with or without bicalutamide	12 months	74	+1.37 kg	+2.0 cm	+14.1%	+4.1%	+14.8%	−3.2%		+2.9%

(continued)

at 36 months. Weight gain was significantly higher in patients younger than 65 years. Seible et al. examined factors associated with weight gain after 1 year of ADT [18]. They found that age <65 years, body mass index <30 kg/m [2], and nondiabetic status were risk factors for weight gain on univariate analyses, and that age <65 years and body mass index <30 kg/m [2] were independent predictors of weight gain on multivariate analysis.

ADT induces not only fat accumulation but also decrease of lean mass. These changes in body composition are called "sarcopenic obesity." Previous studies examined decrease of lean mass, while methods of measuring of fat or lean mass were different among the studies (Table 17.2) [1, 2, 4–7, 11, 16, 19, 20]. In several studies, accumulation of adipose tissue was more noticeable in subcutaneous fat than in visceral fat in patients treated with ADT, whereas visceral fat increases predominantly compared to subcutaneous fat in usual metabolic syndrome. Smith et al. measured the cross-sectional area of subcutaneous and visceral fat by CT and showed that subcutaneous fat increased by 11.1%, but intra-abdominal fat did not change significantly in patients treated with ADT for 48 weeks [2]. We also confirmed this phenomenon in an observational study that measured areas of subcutaneous and visceral fat using CT in 88 patients who underwent 1-year treatment with ADT. In that study, the median increases in visceral and subcutaneous fat were 21.2% and 29.8%, respectively ($P = 0.028$) [7]. Cheung et al. reported that ADT increased fat mass, but visceral fat was unchanged after 12 months of ADT using dual-energy X-ray absorptiometry [11]. Although a predominant increase in subcutaneous fat compared to visceral fat was not seen in all studies and methods of measuring fat or lean mass were not consistent among the studies, the mechanisms of ADT-related obesity might be different from those of usual obesity.

Sarcopenia caused by ADT has not been as well studied as weight gain, but several studies reported the effect of ADT on lean mass. In 2004, Smith et al. reported that the percent lean mass decreased by 3.8% after 1 year of ADT using dual-energy X-ray absorptiometry [16]. In another study, they compared changes in thigh muscle area using CT between patients treated with leuprolide and patients treated with bicalutamide monotherapy, and they showed that thigh muscle area decreased 2.7% in the leuprolide group and 2.2% in the bicalutamide group [19]. Recently, Chang et al. studied muscle attenuation in 39 men using CT measurement of the rectus femoris, sartorius, and quadriceps muscles. There was a significant decrease in the muscle cross-sectional area of the sartorius, quadriceps, and rectus femoris muscles, with decreases of 21.8%, 15.4%, and 16.6%, respectively [21]. The skeletal changes caused by ADT lead to impairments in physical function or quality of life (QOL). Alibhai et al. showed that endurance, upper extremity strength, and physical components of QOL were affected within 3 months of starting ADT [22]. Moreover, these changes in body compositions due to ADT may be related to increase of risk of falls or fractures. Wu et al. reported that the incidence rates of falls were significantly higher in patients treated with ADT (13.37 per 1000 person-years) than those without ADT (6.44 per 1000 person-years) [23].

Table 17.2 Changes in body composition by androgen deprivation therapy

	Region	Year	Study design	No. of pts.	Indications	Methods of ADT	ADT duration	Age (mean or median)	Methods	Visceral fat	Subcutaneous fat	Lean mass
Smith et al. [1]	United Kingdom	2001	Prospective	22	Nonmetastatic	GnRH agonist (21) orchiectomy (1)	3 months	67	Bioelectrical impedance analysis	+8.4% (fat mass)		−2.7% (lean mass)
Smith et al. [2]	United States	2002	Prospective	32	No bone metastasis	GnRH agonists with bicalutamide	48 weeks	66	CT (L4 level)	−0.3%	+11.1%	−3.2% (paraspinal muscle)
Smith et al. [19]	United States	2004	Prospective	52	Nonmetastatic	Leuprolide (50%) Bicalutamide (50%)	12 months	52	Dual-energy X-ray absorptiometry	Leuprolide +11.2% (fat mass) Bicalutamide +6.4% (fat mass)		Leuprolide −3.6% (lean mass) Bicalutamide −2.4% (lean mass)
Lee et al. [20]	United States	2005	Prospective	65	Including previous ADT (35%)	GnRH agonist	12 months	66	Dual-energy X-ray absorptiometry	+6.6% (fat mass)		−2.0% (lean mass)
Smith [16]	United States	2004	Prospective	79	Nonmetastatic	GnRH agonists or orchiectomy with or without antiandrogen	48 weeks	71	Dual-energy X-ray absorptiometry	+11.0% (fat mass)		−3.8% (lean mass)
Smith et al. [4]	United States	2006	Prospective	25	Nonmetastatic	GnRH agonists with bicalutamide	12 weeks	68	Dual-energy X-ray absorptiometry	+4.3% (fat mass)		−1.4% (lean mass)

(continued)

Table 17.2 (continued)

	Region	Year	Study design	No. of pts.	Indications	Methods of ADT	ADT duration	Age (mean or median)	Methods	Visceral fat	Subcutaneous fat	Lean mass
Torimoto et al. [5]	Japan	2011	Prospective	39	Any stage	GnRH agonists with or without bicalutamide	12 months	74	Bioelectrical impedance analysis	+2.08 kg (fat mass) +17.24 cm^2 (visceral fat)		−0.57 kg (lean mass)
Hamilton et al. [6]	Australia	2011	Prospective	26	Nonmetastatic	N.A.	12 months	71	Dual-energy X-ray absorptiometry	+22% +14% (fat mass)	+13%	−3–6% (lean mass)
Mitsuzuka et al. [7]	Japan	2016	Prospective	177	Any stage	GnRH agonists with or without bicalutamide	12 months	75	CT (umbilical level)	+21.2%	+29.8%	−8.0%[a] (psoas muscle)
Cheung et al. [11]	Australia	2016	Prospective	34	Nonmetastatic	N.A.	12 months	68	Dual-energy X-ray absorptiometry	+3.5 kg (fat mass) unchanged (visceral fat)		−1.49 kg (lean mass)

N.A. not available
[a]Data not published

17.1.4 Incidence of Cardiovascular Disease

These metabolic changes may lead to cardiovascular events, but the association between ADT and cardiovascular disease is controversial. In 2006, Keating et al. reported that ADT increased the risks of coronary heart disease, myocardial infarction, and sudden death in patients >65 years and prostate cancer in 2006 [24]. In 2010, they again showed that ADT was associated with an increased risk of diabetes and cardiovascular disease in men of all ages with prostate cancer in an observational study of 37,443 population-based men who were diagnosed with local or regional prostate cancer in the Veterans Healthcare Administration [12]. In 2013, they examined the influence of comorbidities on cardiovascular disease (CVD) risk in a population-based observational study of 185,106 US men ≥66 years diagnosed with local/regional prostate cancer from 1992 to 2007, including 49.9% of patients who were treated with ADT and 50.1% of patients who were treated without ADT [25]. Among men with no comorbidities, ADT was associated with an increase in the adjusted hazard ratio of myocardial infarction (adjusted hazard ratio = 1.09), whereas among patients with comorbidities such as previous myocardial infarction, congestive heart failure, peripheral arterial disease, stroke, hypertension, chronic obstructive pulmonary disease, and renal disease, CVD risks increased similarly regardless of ADT use. Several recent studies also showed relationships between CVD risks and comorbidities in patients treated with ADT. In a trial of 206 men with localized but unfavorable-risk prostate cancer randomized to radiation therapy or to radiation therapy plus 6 months of ADT, cardiac death occurred in 13 patients in each treatment group. In those who received ADT, most cardiac deaths occurred among those with moderate-to-severe comorbidities [26]. On the other hand, other groups did not find an association between ADT and CVD risks. Alibhai et al. performed a matched-cohort study comparing patients aged 66 years or older with prostate cancer given continuous ADT for at least 6 months or who underwent bilateral orchiectomy ($n = 19,079$) with patients with prostate cancer who had never received ADT. They showed that, although ADT treatment was associated with an increased risk of diabetes mellitus (hazard ratio, 1.16), neither use of ADT nor duration of ADT treatment was associated with an increased risk of myocardial infarction or sudden cardiac death [27]. Thus, metabolic changes by ADT were confirmed in many previous studies, but whether these changes lead to CVD events has not yet been determined, probably due to differences in patient populations, study design, or selection bias in men offered ADT among the studies [28]. Interestingly, Jespersen et al. reported that ADT increased the risk of myocardial infarction and stroke, but orchiectomy did not increase these risks [29]. Gonadotropin-releasing hormone (GnRH) agonists might have a direct role on the cardiac receptors regulating cardiac contractile function and lead to a dysfunction of this system [30]. Several studies reported differences in disease control or adverse effects between agonists and antagonists. Albertsen et al. analyzed the six phase III prospective randomized trials and concluded that the risk of cardiac events within 1 year of initiating therapy was significantly lower for treatments with GnRH antagonists than for treatments with GnRH agonists in patients with preexisting CVD [31].

17.2 Effects of ADT in Japanese Patients

Onozawa et al. investigated the initial therapy of 8291 newly diagnosed prostate cancer patients in 2010 who were registered in a Japanese multi-institutional observation study [32]. ADT was most frequently used as the initial therapy (40.2%) for newly diagnosed prostate cancer patients, but information related to ADT-related adverse effects is sparse in Japanese patients. Metabolic changes caused by ADT were considered to be lower in Japanese patients than in Caucasian patients, possibly because the prevalence of severe obesity or metabolic syndrome is lower in Asian countries than in Western countries [33]. However, some Japanese studies demonstrated that significant changes in metabolism can occur in Japanese patients. Nishiyama et al. described metabolic changes among 49 Japanese patients who received 6 months of ADT in 2005 [3]. In that study, the mean increase in weight was 0.8%, and the mean increases in total cholesterol, high-density lipoprotein (HDL) cholesterol, triglycerides, and fasting blood sugar were 6.1%, 5.0%, 8.2%, and 3.5%, respectively. Torimoto et al. described the effects of ADT on lipid metabolism and body composition as measured by bioelectrical impedance analysis among 32 Japanese patients who received 1 year of ADT [5]. In that study, the weight increase was 1.37 kg, and increases in total cholesterol, low-density lipoprotein (LDL), HDL cholesterol, and triglycerides were 4.1%, 14.8%, −3.2%, and 14.1%, respectively. We recently conducted a prospective observational study that examined changes in lipid and glucose metabolism and body composition in Japanese patients with prostate cancer [7]. In that study, patients with prostate cancer who were hormone naive and scheduled to receive long-term ADT were recruited between 2011 and 2013. Of 177 patients who completed 1 year of ADT, mean increases in body weight and abdominal circumference were 2.9% and 3.0%, respectively. Mean increases in total, LDL, and HDL cholesterol and triglycerides were 10.6%, 14.3%, 7.8%, and 16.2%, respectively. Mean increases in fasting blood sugar and hemoglobin A1c were 3.9% and 2.7%, respectively. Lipid alterations were noted in patients without comorbidities, whereas changes in hemoglobin A1c were noted in patients with diabetes mellitus at baseline. These lipid and glucose alterations were prominent in the early ADT period. Both visceral and subcutaneous fat, as measured by CT, increased by >20%. The increase was significantly greater in subcutaneous fat than in visceral fat ($P = 0.028$). These studies showed that metabolic changes caused by ADT could be similar in Japanese patients and Caucasian patients, but the incidence of diabetes mellitus or cardiovascular events in Japanese patients may not always be similar to that in Caucasian patients, because the possible risks of diabetes mellitus or cardiovascular events including insulin sensitivity, prevalence of obesity, metabolic syndrome, and diabetes mellitus among the general population or genetic status may differ between Japanese and Caucasian populations [34]. Future studies are expected to clarify whether the incidence of diabetes mellitus or CVD risks in Japanese patients treated with ADT are similar to those of Caucasian patients.

17.3 Management of Metabolic Changes During ADT (Metabolic Health)

17.3.1 Overuse of ADT

Adverse effects of ADT have been widely recognized by physicians, and now interest regarding the adverse effects of ADT is moving to how we can decrease them. The most important issue is to select appropriate patients who really need ADT. As previously described, about 40% of Japanese patients with newly diagnosed localized prostate cancer underwent primary ADT [32]. Moreover, the percentage of primary ADT in patients >80 years old and with low-risk prostate cancer was 59%. Such overuse of ADT for patients who may not need ADT should be reconsidered when considering ADT-related adverse effects.

17.3.2 Instruction or Education Before Initiating ADT

Instruction or education for patients treated with ADT is also very important to avoid unfavorable metabolic changes or events during ADT. Metabolic changes by ADT are noticeable in the early period of ADT, and the Swedish group recently showed that the risk of cardiovascular events was highest in the first 6 months [35]. Therefore, such instruction or education should be performed before initiating ADT, especially in patients who have risk factors like diabetes mellitus or previous CVD.

17.3.3 Intermittent ADT

Intermittent ADT may have some merits compared to continuous ADT. Calais et al. showed that intermittent ADT did not decrease overall survival and caused no clinical impairment of QOL, and patients had better sexual activity and considerable economic benefit [36]. Crook et al. assessed overall survival and QOL in patients who had PSA recurrence after radiotherapy and received intermittent or continuous ADT. Although median overall survival was not significantly different between patients treated with intermittent and continuous ADT, QOL factors including physical function, fatigue, urinary symptoms, hot flashes, sexual activity, and erections improved with intermittent therapy [37]. Recently, Rezaei et al. reported that the incidence of metabolic syndrome in patients treated with 12 months of intermittent ADT was 14.7%, which was lower than the incidence in previous studies of continuous ADT [38]. Although no studies have directly compared the effects of intermittent ADT on metabolic changes with those of continuous ADT, intermittent ADT could be an option for patients with undesirable metabolic changes or QOL impairment with continuous ADT.

17.3.4 Monitoring or Intervention During ADT

Monitoring or intervention for metabolic changes during ADT is of course essential. Routine measurements of weight, laboratory data including lipid or sugar levels, blood pressure, and bone density are necessary to avoid unfavorable events. If the metabolic changes are significant, instructions including diet or exercise and intervention using medications should be considered. Several studies demonstrated the utility of exercise to decrease or prevent the metabolic changes due to ADT. In 2003, Segal et al. performed a randomized trial which studied the effects of 12 weeks of resistance exercise on ADT-related adverse effects. They showed that resistance exercise reduced fatigue, QOL, and muscular fitness in patients treated with ADT compared to no-exercise intervention [39]. Recently, Cormie et al. also performed a randomized trial to determine if supervised exercise minimizes treatment toxicity due to ADT. They showed that a 3-month exercise program prevented gains in fat mass, and maintained cardiovascular fitness, muscular strength, lower body function, or serum cholesterol level compared to usual care [40]. Thus, exercise intervention seems to be effective to reduce adverse effects derived from ADT, but exercise type, intensity, frequency, and duration differed among the studies and need to be further examined in future studies [41].

> **Conclusions**
>
> The use of ADT may be expected to continue in the future despite the appearance of new-generation androgen receptor-targeting drugs or chemotherapy agents. Many existing studies have shown that ADT has non-negligible changes through suppressing testosterone almost completely. Prostate cancer has a relatively better prognosis than other malignancies, and it also has aspects of chronic disease even when metastatic. We physicians need to be conscious with "*metabolic health*," which means avoiding unfavorable results due to ADT, as well as maintaining cancer control. Metabolic changes can occur in Japanese patients with prostate cancer treated with ADT, but subsequent events such as diabetes mellitus or cardiovascular events need to be further investigated. Future studies should be planned to elucidate the associations between ADT and such events in Japanese patients with prostate cancer.

References

1. Smith JC, Bennett S, Evans LM. The effects of induced hypogonadism on arterial stiffness, body composition, and metabolic parameters in males with prostate cancer. J Clin Endocrinol Metab. 2001;86:4261–7.
2. Smith MR, Finkelstein JS, McGovern FJ, et al. Changes in body composition during androgen deprivation therapy for prostate cancer. J Clin Endocrinol Metab. 2002;87:599–603.
3. Nishiyama T, Ishizaki F, Anraku T, Shimura H, Takahashi K. The influence of androgen deprivation therapy on metabolism in patients with prostate cancer. J Clin Endocrinol Metab. 2005;90:657–60.
4. Smith MR, Lee H, Nathan DM. Insulin sensitivity during combined androgen blockade for prostate cancer. J Clin Endocrinol Metab. 2006;91:1305–8.

5. Torimoto K, Samma S, Kagebayashi Y, et al. The effects of androgen deprivation therapy on lipid metabolism and body composition in Japanese patients with prostate cancer. Jpn J Clin Oncol. 2011;41:577–81.
6. Hamilton EJ, Gianatti E, Strauss BJ, et al. Increase in visceral and subcutaneous abdominal fat in men with prostate cancer treated with androgen deprivation therapy. Clin Endocrinol. 2011;74:377–83.
7. Mitsuzuka K, Kyan A, Sato T, et al. Influence of 1 year of androgen deprivation therapy on lipid and glucose metabolism and fat accumulation in Japanese patients with prostate cancer. Prostate Cancer Prostatic Dis. 2016;19:57–62.
8. Eri LM, Urdal P, Bechensteen AG. Effects of the luteinizing hormone-releasing hormone agonist leuprolide on lipoproteins, fibrinogen and plasminogen activator inhibitor in patients with benign prostatic hyperplasia. J Urol. 1995;154:100–4.
9. Dockery F, Bulpitt CJ, Agarwal S, Donaldson M, Rajkumar C. Testosterone suppression in men with prostate cancer leads to an increase in arterial stiffness and hyperinsulinaemia. Clin Sci (Lond). 2003;104:195–201.
10. Salvador C, Planas J, Agreda F, et al. Analysis of the lipid profile and atherogenic risk during androgen deprivation therapy in prostate cancer patients. Urol Int. 2013;90:41–4.
11. Cheung AS, Hoermann R, Dupuis P, Joon DL, Zajac JD, Grossmann M. Relationships between insulin resistance and frailty with body composition and testosterone in men undergoing androgen deprivation therapy for prostate cancer. Eur J Endocrinol. 2016;175:229–37.
12. Keating NL, O'Malley AJ, Freedland SJ, Smith MR. Diabetes and cardiovascular disease during androgen deprivation therapy: observational study of veterans with prostate cancer. J Natl Cancer Inst. 2010;102:39–46.
13. Braga-Basaria M, Dobs AS, Muller DC, et al. Metabolic syndrome in men with prostate cancer undergoing long-term androgen-deprivation therapy. Clin Oncol. 2006;24:3979–83.
14. Bosco C, Crawley D, Adolfsson J, Rudman S, Van Hemelrijck M. Quantifying the evidence for the risk of metabolic syndrome and its components following androgen deprivation therapy for prostate cancer: a meta-analysis. PLoS One. 2015;10:e0117344.
15. Nowicki M, Bryc W, Kokot F. Hormonal regulation of appetite and body mass in patients with advanced prostate cancer treated with combined androgen blockade. J Endocrinol Investig. 2001;24:31–6.
16. Smith MR. Changes in fat and lean body mass during androgen-deprivation therapy for prostate cancer. Urology. 2004;63:742–5.
17. Timilshina N, Breunis H, Alibhai SM. Impact of androgen deprivation therapy on weight gain differs by age in men with nonmetastatic prostate cancer. J Urol. 2012;188:2183–8.
18. Seible DM, Gu X, Hyatt AS, et al. Weight gain on androgen deprivation therapy: which patients are at highest risk? Urology. 2014;83:1316–21.
19. Smith MR, Goode M, Zietman AL, McGovern FJ, Lee H, Finkelstein JS. Bicalutamide monotherapy versus leuprolide monotherapy for prostate cancer: effects on bone mineral density and body composition. J Clin Oncol. 2004;22:2546–53.
20. Lee H, McGovern K, Finkelstein JS, Smith MR. Changes in bone mineral density and body composition during initial and long-term gonadotropin-releasing hormone agonist treatment for prostate carcinoma. Cancer. 2005;104:1633–7.
21. Chang D, Joseph DJ, Ebert MA, et al. Effect of androgen deprivation therapy on muscle attenuation in men with prostate cancer. J Med Imaging Radiat Oncol. 2014;58:223–8.
22. Alibhai SM, Breunis H, Timilshina N, et al. Impact of androgen-deprivation therapy on physical function and quality of life in men with nonmetastatic prostate cancer. J Clin Oncol. 2010;28:5038–45.
23. FJ W, Sheu SY, Lin HC, Chung SD. Increased fall risk in patients receiving androgen deprivation therapy for prostate cancer. Urology. 2016;95:145–50.
24. Keating NL, O'Malley AJ, Smith MR. Diabetes and cardiovascular disease during androgen deprivation therapy for prostate cancer. J Clin Oncol. 2006;24:4448–56.
25. Keating NL, O'Malley AJ, Freedland SJ, Smith MR. Does comorbidity influence the risk of myocardial infarction or diabetes during androgen-deprivation therapy for prostate cancer? Eur Urol. 2013;64:159–66.

26. D'Amico AV, Chen MH, Renshaw AA, Loffredo M, Kantoff PW. Androgen suppression and radiation vs radiation alone for prostate cancer: a randomized trial. JAMA. 2008;299:289–95.
27. Alibhai SM, Duong-Hua M, Sutradhar R, et al. Impact of androgen deprivation therapy on cardiovascular disease and diabetes. J Clin Oncol. 2009;27:3452–8.
28. Levine GN, D'Amico AV, Berger P, et al. Androgen-deprivation therapy in prostate cancer and cardiovascular risk: a science advisory from the American Heart Association, American Cancer Society, and American Urological Association: endorsed by the American Society for Radiation Oncology. Circulation. 2010;121:833–40.
29. Jespersen CG, Nørgaard M, Borre M. Androgen-deprivation therapy in treatment of prostate cancer and risk of myocardial infarction and stroke: a nationwide Danish population-based cohort study. Eur Urol. 2014;65:704–9.
30. Dong F, Skinner DC, Wu TJ, Ren J. The heart: a novel gonadotrophin-releasing hormone target. J Neuroendocrinol. 2011;23:456–63.
31. Albertsen PC, Klotz L, Tombal B, Grady J, Olesen TK, Nilsson J. Cardiovascular morbidity associated with gonadotropin releasing hormone agonists and an antagonist. Eur Urol. 2014;65:565–73.
32. Onozawa M, Hinotsu S, Tsukamoto T, et al. Recent trends in the initial therapy for newly diagnosed prostate cancer in Japan. Jpn J Clin Oncol. 2014;44:969–81.
33. Hoang KC, Le TV, Wong ND. The metabolic syndrome in east Asians. J Cardiometab Syndr. 2007;2:276–82.
34. Wei FY, Tomizawa K. Functional loss of Cdkal1, a novel tRNA modification enzyme, causes the development of type 2 diabetes. Endocr J. 2011;58(10):819–25.
35. O'Farrell S, Garmo H, Holmberg L, Adolfsson J, Stattin P, Van Hemelrijck M. Risk and timing of cardiovascular disease after androgen-deprivation therapy in men with prostate cancer. J Clin Oncol. 2015;33:1243–51.
36. Calais da Silva FE, Bono AV, Whelan P, et al. Intermittent androgen deprivation for locally advanced and metastatic prostate cancer: results from a randomised phase 3 study of the South European Uroncological Group. Eur Urol. 2009;55:1269–77.
37. Crook JM, O'Callaghan CJ, Duncan G, et al. Intermittent androgen suppression for rising PSA level after radiotherapy. N Engl J Med. 2012;367:895–903.
38. Rezaei MM, Rezaei MM, Ghoreifi A, Kerigh BF. Metabolic syndrome in patients with prostate cancer undergoing intermittent androgen-deprivation therapy. Can Urol Assoc J. 2016;10:e300–5.
39. Segal RJ, Reid RD, Courneya KS, et al. Resistance exercise in men receiving androgen deprivation therapy for prostate cancer. J Clin Oncol. 2003;21(9):1653.
40. Cormie P, Galvão DA, Spry N, et al. Can supervised exercise prevent treatment toxicity in patients with prostate cancer initiating androgen-deprivation therapy: a randomised controlled trial. BJU Int. 2015;115:256–66.
41. Gardner JR, Livingston PM, Fraser SF. Effects of exercise on treatment-related adverse effects for patients with prostate cancer receiving androgen-deprivation therapy: a systematic review. J Clin Oncol. 2014;32:335–46.

Bone Scan Index as a Biomarker of Bone Metastasis

18

Kenichi Nakajima and Lars Edenbrandt

Abstract

Bone metastasis in patients with prostate cancer can be screened and followed up using bone scintigraphy, and the role of quantitative bone imaging has recently become important. The bone scan index (BSI) is defined as the amount (%) of bone metastasis to the whole-body bones determined using an artificial neural network (ANN). It is currently recognized as a reproducible and practical means of quantifying bone metastasis and as an *imaging biomarker* of bone metastasis. This chapter summarizes the principles and application of BSI determined using dedicated software (EXINI bone in Europe and North America; BONENAVI in Japan), and its advantages and disadvantages. The BSI could serve as a reliable marker of disease progression and treatment effects as well as a prognostic indicator. The index can also reflect the effects of new drugs and internal radiation therapy on bone metastasis and help in its management.

Keywords

Nuclear imaging · Scintigraphy · Artificial neural network · Quantitation

K. Nakajima (✉)
Department of Nuclear Medicine, Kanazawa University, Kanazawa, Japan
e-mail: nakajima@med.kanazawa-u.ac.jp

L. Edenbrandt
Department of Clinical Physiology and Nuclear Medicine, University of Gothenburg, Gothenburg, Sweden

Abbreviations

ANN	Artificial neural network
BSI	Bone scan index
mCRPC	Metastatic castration-resistant prostate cancer
MDP	Methylenediphosphonate
OS	Overall survival
PSA	Prostate-specific antigen
ROC	Receiver operating characteristics

A biomarker is an objective metric of disease condition and severity and it is derived from pathophysiological responses. Biomarkers are therefore convenient to monitor therapeutic responses and support decisions regarding subsequent treatment strategies. Although chemical and tumor markers have become quite commonplace, medical imaging modalities have not been applied for these purposes partly due to insufficient methods of quantitation. The bone scan index (BSI) is a new imaging biomarker for integrating the total amount of bone metastasis in patients with metastatic castration-resistant prostate cancer (mCRPC) [1].

Bones are the most common sites of metastatic prostate cancer involvement, which significantly worsens the quality of life due to skeletal related events such as bone pain, pathological fractures, and finally shortening overall survival (OS). Early diagnosis of bone metastasis is therefore essential to start appropriate therapy, and surrogate markers linked to relevant outcomes are particularly important for a correct diagnosis and subsequent treatment [2].

18.1 Bone Scintigraphy as First-Line Imaging

The bone scan index (BSI) was developed as a marker of the total amount of bone metastasis on whole-body scintigraphic images generated using ^{99m}Tc-methylenediphosphonate (MDP) [3, 4]. The BSI is now considered as an imaging biomarker of the extent of bone metastasis in the whole body.

Since then, planar images and whole-body scintigraphic images continued to be the first-line approach to surveying bone metastasis. Single-photon emission computed tomography (SPECT) imaging has also become popular for additional nuclear imaging. Whereas X-ray CT and magnetic resonance imaging (MRI) have also become prevalent for detecting bone and bone marrow metastasis in clinical practice, whole-body imaging using bone scintigraphy remains a convenient choice for patients with suspected metastasis [5]. Osteoblastic metastasis is dominant in patients with bone metastasis of prostate cancer, and therefore bone scintigraphy can visualize abnormalities as hot spots or as localized accumulation. Based on scintigraphic images, the criteria for the exacerbation of metastasis published by the Prostate Cancer Clinical Trials Working Group 2 include counting the number of bone metastases, and ≥2 metastatic lesions compared with a previous imaging assessment are judged as signs of exacerbation [6]. One idea for expressing the extent of disease (EOD) is to count the numbers of hot spots on images [7–9]. Despite the simplicity of this method, a more objective quantitative approach is needed for clinical and investigative purposes and this is recommended in the EANM practice guidelines for bone scintigraphy [5].

18.2 Bone Scan Index

The idea of a BSI was first introduced by investigators at Memorial Sloan-Kettering Cancer Center (New York, NY, USA) during 1977 [3]. A Swedish group subsequently developed a method of quantitation using an artificial neural network (ANN), which resulted in a completely automated method of analyzing whole-body bone images. The ANN is an artificial intelligence that is learned from the expert assessment of bone images collected from large databases accumulated from around 1000 studies [10]. The software is now available as EXINI bone (EXINI Diagnostics, Lund, Sweden) in Europe and North America and BONENAVI software in Japan (FUJIFILM RI Pharma Co. Ltd., Tokyo, Japan) [1, 11]. The ability to diagnose bone metastasis has been enhanced and adjusted to the Japanese practice of bone scintigraphy, with sensitivity and specificity of nearly 90% for prostate cancer [12].

Understanding the calculation steps is important to appropriately interpret changes in the BSI.

Segmentation of whole-body images: Whole-body bone scintigraphic images are fit to a whole-body gender-specific bone template consisting of 12 regions including the skull, ribs, vertebrae, pelvis, and extremities.

Detection of hot spots: Potentially abnormal regions are identified based on a specific algorithm for detecting hot spots, which incorporates a count threshold as well as surrounding structures and physiological distribution.

Standardization of display: Normal bone counts are standardized so that bone images are displayed in the same count density format.

Hot-spot quantitation and classification: Hot spots are quantified in all possible abnormal regions and segments. Features of hot spots include variations in their size, shape, intensity, and distribution, and ANN analysis classifies all hot areas into high (≥0.5, shown as red) and low (<0.5, shown as blue) probabilities of metastasis.

Calculation of BSI: The BSI is an indicator of the total amount of bone metastasis expressed as a ratio (%) of high probability (>0.5) fractions within the sum of all bone fractions.

Display format: In the final output page (Fig. 18.1), the three major indices are the probability of abnormalities (ANN values; range 0–1), the total ratio (%) of bone metastasis to the whole bones (BSI), and the number of hot spots (HS). Serial changes in the BSI and the HS number can be displayed as graphs to understand the clinical course of bone metastasis in patients.

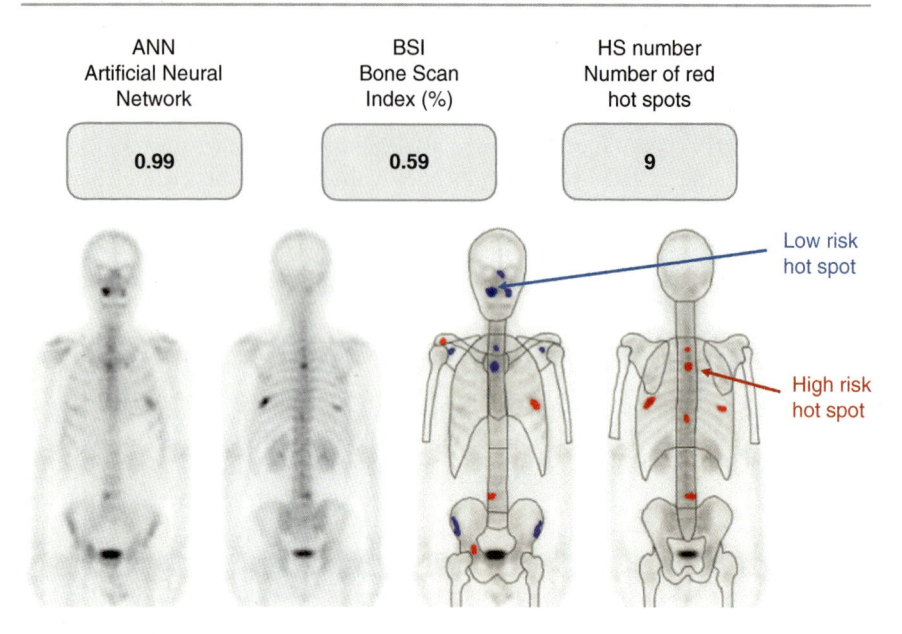

Fig. 18.1 Major indices of bone metastasis in artificial neural network analysis

18.3 Tips for Using Bone Scan Index

Manual adjustments can be made when a judgment of metastasis by the ANN is false. The BSI can be automatically calculated [13], but an operator can change it manually if a judgment of metastasis is inappropriate. Although automatic processing usually works well, atypical urinary contamination, active degenerative changes in the vertebrae, and traumatic regions for example could be misinterpreted as metastasis. Considering that BSI is a marker of the total amount of bone metastasis, modifications of all interpretations in a series of studies are impractical, and we recommend modification only when artifactual mistakes in judgment are apparent.

Understanding the general relationship between a visual impression of metastasis and BSI values is clinically useful (Fig. 18.2). A BSI of 0% means that bone metastasis is unlikely. A BSI of $\geq 1\%$ usually corresponds to multiple-bone metastases, whereas a BSI of $\geq 5\%$ indicates multiple hot spots.

18.4 Clinical Applications of Bone Scan Index

18.4.1 Diagnostic Application of BSI

The ability to diagnose bone metastasis is essential for calculating the BSI, although the purpose of the BSI is not to decide whether or not a specific hot spot represents metastasis. After the initial development of BSI with EXINI bone [10, 14] its

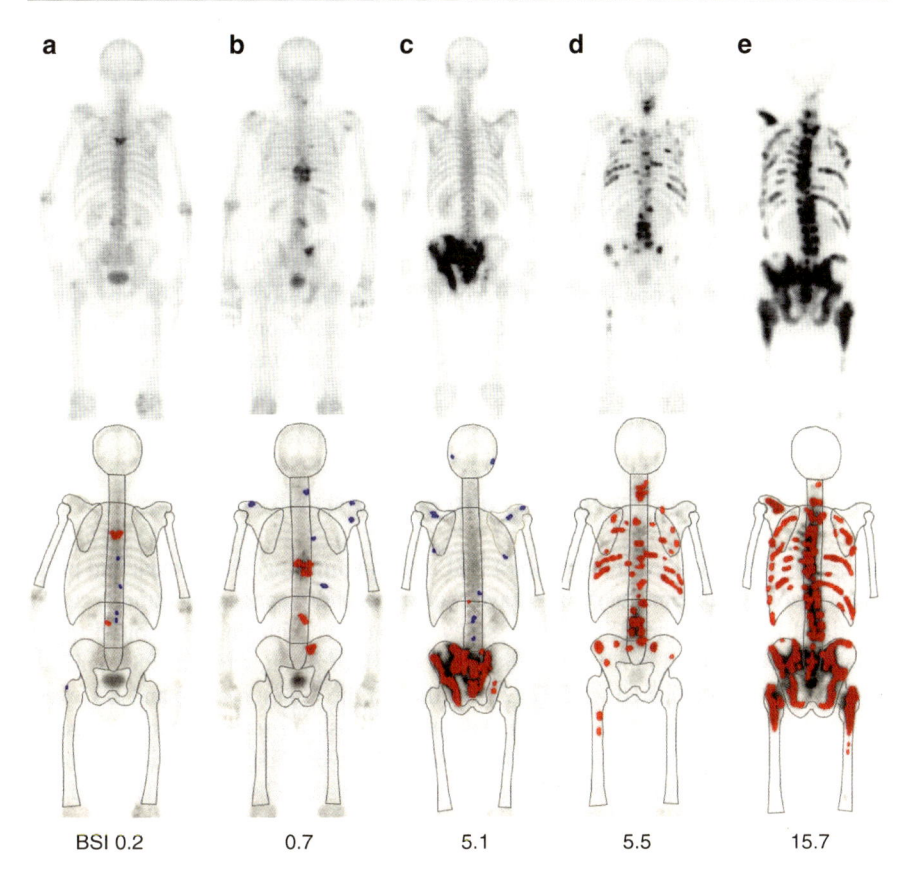

18 Bone Scan Index as a Biomarker of Bone Metastasis

Fig. 18.2 Relationship between extent of bone metastasis and bone scan index (%). Although panels (**c**) and (**d**) show similar BSI of ~5, panel (**c**) shows large pelvic metastasis, and (**d**) shows multiple hot spots in vertebrae, rib, pelvis, and extremities. Total amount of metastasis can be expressed more appropriately than simple counting of the number of hot spots in these patients

diagnostic utility was further validated for BONENAVI software in Japan. Retraining based on a database from a single institution resulted in diagnostic sensitivity of 90% and specificity of 81% [15], and the comparison with EOD as described above closely agreed with semiautomated BSI partly modified by radiologists [11]. Subsequently, a new ANN database was created based on 1532 patients, among whom 451 had prostate cancer. When the finally retrained ANN system was validated, a diagnostic accuracy with an area under the receiver operating characteristics (ROC) curve (AUC) of 0.93 was achieved for both men and women. The AUC in patients with prostate cancer was 0.96, with 94% sensitivity and 89% specificity [12]. Regional segmentation was further improved in the current version without the loss of diagnostic accuracy [16]. The correlation between the BSI and several metabolic markers is optimal for bone alkaline phosphatase, whereas the correlation with prostate-specific antigen (PSA) is only fair [17].

Table 18.1 (continued)

Author	BSI calculation	Patients or study setting (number of patients)	BSI and prognosis	Reference no.
Miyoshi Y	BONENAVI	Hormone-naive prostate cancer patients with bone metastases ($n = 60$)	Median OS: not reached in patients with a BSI $\leq$ 1.9; 34.8 months in patients with a BSI > 1.9	BMC Cancer 2016 [33]
Poulsen MH	EXINI bone	Patients with prostate cancer awaiting initiation of androgen deprivation therapy ($n = 88$)	Patients with a BSI $\geq$ 1, significantly shorter OS than patients with a BSI < 1	BJU Int 2016 [34]
Anand	EXINI bone	Prediction of OS in mCRPC treated with enzalutamide ($n = 80$)	Combined predictive model of percent PSA change and change in automated BSI was significantly higher than PSA change alone	EJNMMI Res 2016 [25]
Reza	EXINI bone	Outcome evaluation in mCRPC patients on treatment with abiraterone ($n = 104$)	BSI change $\leq$0.30 had significantly longer median survival	European Urology Focus 2016 [26]
Alva	EXINI bone	Consecutive non-trial mCRPC patients who received $\geq$1 dose of radium-223 ($n = 145$)	Baseline BSI <5, significantly associated with OS	Prostate 2017 [27]

Abbreviations: *BSI* bone scan index, *mCRPC* metastatic castration-resistant prostate cancer, *OS* overall survival

Conclusion

The new imaging biomarker BSI is a quantitative measure of the total amount of bone metastasis determined using an artificial intelligence of neural network. The BSI could be a surrogate marker of bone metastasis and will be effective for the development of new drugs and internal radiation therapy. Because the BSI is becoming increasingly popular in clinical applications, appropriate understanding and effective use of a computer-assisted diagnostic and management system will be required.

References

1. Nakajima K, Edenbrandt L, Mizokami A. Bone scan index: a new biomarker for bone metastasis in patients with prostate cancer. Int J Urol. 2017;24(9):668–73. https://doi.org/10.1111/iju.13386.
2. Scher HI, Morris MJ, Larson S, Heller G. Validation and clinical utility of prostate cancer biomarkers. Nat Rev Clin Oncol. 2013;10:225–34.
3. Erdi YE, Humm JL, Imbriaco M, Yeung H, Larson SM. Quantitative bone metastases analysis based on image segmentation. J Nucl Med. 1997;38:1401–6.

4. Imbriaco M, Larson SM, Yeung HW, et al. A new parameter for measuring metastatic bone involvement by prostate cancer: the Bone Scan Index. Clin Cancer Res. 1998;4:1765–72.
5. Van den Wyngaert T, Strobel K, Kampen WU, et al. The EANM practice guidelines for bone scintigraphy. Eur J Nucl Med Mol Imaging. 2016;43:1723–38.
6. Scher HI, Halabi S, Tannock I, et al. Design and end points of clinical trials for patients with progressive prostate cancer and castrate levels of testosterone: recommendations of the Prostate Cancer Clinical Trials Working Group. J Clin Oncol. 2008;26:1148–59.
7. Jorgensen T, Muller C, Kaalhus O, Danielsen HE, Tveter KJ. Extent of disease based on initial bone scan: important prognostic predictor for patients with metastatic prostatic cancer. Experience from the Scandinavian Prostatic Cancer Group Study No. 2 (SPCG-2). Eur Urol. 1995;28:40–6.
8. Noguchi M, Kikuchi H, Ishibashi M, Noda S. Percentage of the positive area of bone metastasis is an independent predictor of disease death in advanced prostate cancer. Br J Cancer. 2003;88:195–201.
9. Soloway MS, Hardeman SW, Hickey D, et al. Stratification of patients with metastatic prostate cancer based on extent of disease on initial bone scan. Cancer. 1988;61:195–202.
10. Sadik M, Jakobsson D, Olofsson F, Ohlsson M, Suurkula M, Edenbrandt L. A new computer-based decision-support system for the interpretation of bone scans. Nucl Med Commun. 2006;27:417–23.
11. Takahashi Y, Yoshimura M, Suzuki K, et al. Assessment of bone scans in advanced prostate carcinoma using fully automated and semi-automated bone scan index methods. Ann Nucl Med. 2012;26:586–93.
12. Nakajima K, Nakajima Y, Horikoshi H, et al. Enhanced diagnostic accuracy for quantitative bone scan using an artificial neural network system: a Japanese multi-center database project. EJNMMI Res. 2013;3:83.
13. Ulmert D, Kaboteh R, Fox JJ, et al. A novel automated platform for quantifying the extent of skeletal tumour involvement in prostate cancer patients using the Bone Scan Index. Eur Urol. 2012;62:78–84.
14. Sadik M, Hamadeh I, Nordblom P, et al. Computer-assisted interpretation of planar whole-body bone scans. J Nucl Med. 2008;49:1958–65.
15. Horikoshi H, Kikuchi A, Onoguchi M, Sjostrand K, Edenbrandt L. Computer-aided diagnosis system for bone scintigrams from Japanese patients: importance of training database. Ann Nucl Med. 2012;26:622–6.
16. Koizumi M, Miyaji N, Murata T, et al. Evaluation of a revised version of computer-assisted diagnosis system, BONENAVI version 2.1.7, for bone scintigraphy in cancer patients. Ann Nucl Med. 2015;29(8):659–65.
17. Wakabayashi H, Nakajima K, Mizokami A, et al. Bone scintigraphy as a new imaging biomarker: the relationship between bone scan index and bone metabolic markers in prostate cancer patients with bone metastases. Ann Nucl Med. 2013;27:802–7.
18. Watanabe S, Nakajima K, Mizokami A, et al. Bone scan index of the jaw: a new approach for evaluating early-stage anti-resorptive agents-related osteonecrosis. Ann Nucl Med. 2017;31: 201–10.
19. Anand A, Morris MJ, Kaboteh R, et al. A preanalytic validation study of automated Bone Scan Index: effect on accuracy and reproducibility due to the procedural Variabilities in bone scan image acquisition. J Nucl Med. 2016;57:1865–71.
20. Anand A, Morris MJ, Kaboteh R, et al. Analytic validation of the automated Bone Scan Index as an imaging biomarker to standardize quantitative changes in bone scans of patients with metastatic prostate cancer. J Nucl Med. 2016;57:41–5.
21. Sabbatini P, Larson SM, Kremer A, et al. Prognostic significance of extent of disease in bone in patients with androgen-independent prostate cancer. J Clin Oncol. 1999;17:948–57.
22. Dennis ER, Jia X, Mezheritskiy IS, et al. Bone scan index: a quantitative treatment response biomarker for castration-resistant metastatic prostate cancer. J Clin Oncol. 2012;30:519–24.
23. Kaboteh R, Damber JE, Gjertsson P, et al. Bone Scan Index: a prognostic imaging biomarker for high-risk prostate cancer patients receiving primary hormonal therapy. EJNMMI Res. 2013;3:9.

24. Mitsui Y, Shiina H, Yamamoto Y, et al. Prediction of survival benefit using an automated bone scan index in patients with castration-resistant prostate cancer. BJU Int. 2012;110:E628–34.
25. Anand A, Morris MJ, Larson SM, et al. Automated Bone Scan Index as a quantitative imaging biomarker in metastatic castration-resistant prostate cancer patients being treated with enzalutamide. EJNMMI Res. 2016;6:23.
26. Reza M, Ohlsson M, Kaboteh R, et al. Bone scan index as an imaging biomarker in metastatic castration-resistant prostate cancer: a multicentre study based on patients treated with abiraterone acetate (Zytiga) in clinical practice. Eur Urol Focus. 2016;2:540–6.
27. Alva A, Nordquist L, Daignault S, et al. Clinical correlates of benefit from Radium-223 therapy in metastatic castration resistant prostate cancer. Prostate. 2017;77:479–88.
28. Armstrong AJ, Kaboteh R, Carducci MA, et al. Assessment of the bone scan index in a randomized placebo-controlled trial of tasquinimod in men with metastatic castration-resistant prostate cancer (mCRPC). Urol Oncol. 2014;32:1308–16.
29. Meirelles GS, Schoder H, Ravizzini GC, et al. Prognostic value of baseline [18F] fluorodeoxyglucose positron emission tomography and 99mTc-MDP bone scan in progressing metastatic prostate cancer. Clin Cancer Res. 2010;16:6093–9.
30. Kaboteh R, Gjertsson P, Leek H, et al. Progression of bone metastases in patients with prostate cancer—automated detection of new lesions and calculation of bone scan index. EJNMMI Res. 2013;3:64.
31. Reza M, Bjartell A, Ohlsson M, et al. Bone Scan Index as a prognostic imaging biomarker during androgen deprivation therapy. EJNMMI Res. 2014;4:58.
32. Uemura K, Miyoshi Y, Kawahara T, et al. Prognostic value of a computer-aided diagnosis system involving bone scans among men treated with docetaxel for metastatic castration-resistant prostate cancer. BMC Cancer. 2016;16:109.
33. Miyoshi Y, Yoneyama S, Kawahara T, et al. Prognostic value of the bone scan index using a computer-aided diagnosis system for bone scans in hormone-naive prostate cancer patients with bone metastases. BMC Cancer. 2016;16:128.
34. Poulsen MH, Rasmussen J, Edenbrandt L, et al. Bone Scan Index predicts outcome in patients with metastatic hormone-sensitive prostate cancer. BJU Int. 2016;117:748–53.

Genetic Polymorphism Analysis in Predicting Prognosis of Advanced Prostate Cancer

19

Norihiko Tsuchiya

Abstract

The human genome project has revealed significant interindividual genomic variation, including over ten million single-nucleotide polymorphisms (SNP). The finding accelerated a large number of studies exploring genes involved in the predisposition of various types of cancer. Previous case-control studies or genome-wide association studies discovered hundreds of prostate cancer (PC)-associated genes. Meanwhile, clinical applications of the genetic polymorphisms have been investigated. Polymorphisms associated with early-onset aggressive phenotypes, prognosis of hormone-sensitive metastatic or castration-resistant prostate cancer, and outcomes after specific treatments are expected as useful markers, which are of great help in the therapeutic decision making of PC.

Keywords

Advanced prostate cancer · Metastatic prostate cancer · Castration-resistant prostate cancer · Genetic polymorphism · Single-nucleotide polymorphism · Prostate cancer-associated gene polymorphism · Hormone therapy · Androgen receptor-targeting agent · Docetaxel

19.1 Introduction

The development of PC is known to be associated with aging, ethnicity, and family history, which are explained by inheritable disposition, the so-called genetic polymorphisms, as well as environmental factors. After a quarter

N. Tsuchiya
Department of Urology, Yamagata University Faculty of Medicine, Yamagata, Japan
e-mail: ntsuchiya@med.id.yamagata-u.ac.jp

© Springer Nature Singapore Pte Ltd. 2018
Y. Arai, O. Ogawa (eds.), *Hormone Therapy and Castration Resistance of Prostate Cancer*, https://doi.org/10.1007/978-981-10-7013-6_19

century into the exploration of PC-related genetic polymorphisms, its extreme complexity beyond the initial estimate has become apparent, and the exploratory studies continue till date.

Approximately 30% of males aged over 50 years harbor latent prostate cancers, only a part of which progresses to clinically significant PC [1]. Most studies dealing with PC-related genetic polymorphisms target clinical cancers, so that genetic polymorphisms for the risk of progression to clinical PC could be assessed. Considering that many latent PCs do not progress to clinical cancers, additional environmental and/or genetic factors could affect the development of the clinically significant cancer. The clinical stage of PCs could be affected by the initiation and frequency of screening. Even in recent years when prostate-specific antigen (PSA) tests are widely being conducted, a small, but not negligible, number of men are diagnosed with locally advanced or metastatic PC (mPC). The 5-year survival rate of PC patients with metastasis at diagnosis is still as low as 30–50% [2–4]. Therefore, to explore the genetic polymorphisms specific to mPC, it is important to discriminate fatal PCs from others. To accomplish this genetic screening for an aggressive/fatal cancer is highly expected.

Prognosis of an advanced or mPC is thought to be influenced by cancer host-dependent factors, as well as clinical and biological characteristics of the cancer. As per the meta-analytic studies involving several types of cancer, genetic polymorphisms, either specific or nonspecific to the treatment targets, have been associated with either the treatment outcome or the survival of the patients, although most of the results have not been validated [5, 6]. However, polymorphisms identified as risk factors for cancer development do not always predict treatment outcome or survival. The standard treatment for patients with mPC is a sequential or combined therapy with hormonal and chemotherapeutic agents, and the response to each agent differs among individuals. The differences in the response to treatment are not explained only by the diversity in the characteristics of cancer cells and their surrounding micromilieus but also by drug-related polymorphisms that are associated with drug disposition and polymorphisms common between the germ cells and cancer cells. Thus, genetic polymorphisms that are associated with prognosis in advanced or mPC patients may be important genetic markers in devising an effective personalized treatment strategy.

19.2 Genetic Polymorphisms Associated with Early Onset of PC

The prevalence of diagnosed PC in European-American men under 56 years is less than 1%. Because the age at diagnosis may depend on the initial time of PSA screening, early-onset PC does not necessarily exhibit poor prognosis. In multiple studies, however, the effect of risk polymorphisms for early PC was in the same direction as for aggressive PC. According to a large cohort study, PC diagnosed under 55 years increased from 2.3% in around 1990 to 9.0% in early 2000s, and younger patients had a shorter overall survival (OS) and cancer-specific survival (CSS) compared with older patients, especially in patients with high-grade and locally advanced cancer [7].

Table 19.1 Genetic polymorphisms associated with early-onset (≤60 years old) prostate cancer

Author	Year	Country, subjects	Genetic polymorphisms	Risk allele/ genotype	Odds ratio
Kote-Jarai, Z	2001	UK, <56 years old	GSTP1 105 Ile > Val	Ile/Val, Val/Val	1.3, 1.80
Edwards, SM	2003	UK, <56 years old	BRCA2	Various mutations	N/R
Camp, N	2005	USA, <60 years old	ELAC2	Combination of three haplotypes	2.23
Forrest MS	2005	UK, <56 years old	AR (CAG)n, SRD5A2 V > L	≤22 rpts, L/L	1.47
Agalliu, I	2007	USA, <55 years old	BRCA2	Protein-truncating mutations	7.8
Levin, AM	2007	USA, FH or <56ears old	AMACAR rs3195676	TT/TC	1.72
Levin, AM	2008	USA, FH or <56 years old	TCF2 rs4430796	A allele	1.40
Camp, N	2009	USA, ≤60 years old	PRCA rs10993994	N/R	2.20
Hughes, L	2012	USA, ≤60 years old AA	8q24, rs6983561	CC	3.34
Lange EM	2012	USA, ≤55 years old	rs6983267, rs10993994, rs7931342, rs2735839, rs5945619	N/R	1.60, 1.49, 1.37, 1.45, 1.50
Ewing, CM	2012	USA, ≤50 years old	HOXB13 rs138213197 (G84E)	E allele	9.5
Al Olama, AA	2014	USA, ≤55 years old	PEX14 rs636291	N/R	1.18
Gomez, R	2016	Mexico, <60 years old	AR (CAG)n	<19 rpts	2.31

N/R not reported, *rpts* repeats, *FH* family history, *AA* African-American

Several studies assessed the significance of candidate SNPs, for PCs identified by genome-wide association study (GWAS), as risk SNPs for overall or early-onset PC. Representative studies that investigated genetic polymorphisms associated with early-onset (≤60 years) PC are shown in Table 19.1. One study validated five SNPs previously reported to be a risk for early-onset PC in a different cohort, and found that the association of rs6983561 with earlier time to PC diagnosis was significant [8]. Two studies validated whether risk-SNP for overall PC is identical to that in early-onset PC. The first study demonstrated that 13 of the 14 SNPs were significantly associated with early-onset PC and that a cumulative effect of those SNPs was observed, suggesting that those risk-SNPs for PC also have an important role in the early-onset PC [9]. The second study demonstrated that rs10993994 at 10q11 has a significant association both with the aggressive and early-onset PC [10]. Interestingly, rs10993994 is a common risk-SNP validated in both studies for early-onset PC.

Meanwhile, some genetic polymorphisms may be involved specifically in the early-onset PC. Recent meta-analyses of GWAS identified a SNP rs636291 at 1q35. The SNP, located in intron 2 of the PEX14 gene, is in linkage equilibrium to rs616488, which was identified as the risk-SNP for breast cancer [11, 12].

19.3 Genetic Polymorphisms Associated with Aggressiveness of PC

To find genetic polymorphisms associated with the aggressiveness of PC, two approaches are considered. The first approach is to compare germline genome data between pathologically aggressive, clinically advanced, PC (or mPC) with indolent cancers, and the second approach is to explore genetic polymorphisms associated with the recurrence, progression, or survival of PC. In this chapter, GWAS and GWAS replication studies are considered (Table 19.2). An overview of studies conducted to find candidate SNPs, predicting aggressive or fatal PC in men treated with definitive treatments or androgen deprivation therapy (ADT), will be dealt later.

Recently, several studies investigated the effect of SNPs, previously reported to be associated with a predisposition of PC, on aggressive clinicopathological features, disease progression, and survival. Those SNPs are summarized in Table 19.2. With regard to the first approach, Gudmundsson et al. demonstrated that A allele of rs721048 at 2p15 was significantly associated with aggressive PC (defined variously as Gleason ≥7; T3 or higher; node positive; and/or metastatic disease) [13]. The 8q24 is a well-known region harboring multiple SNPs identified as risk of PC. Cheng I et al. reported a meta-analysis in which SNPs in 8a24 region were compared between

Table 19.2 Genetic polymorphisms associated with aggressive PCa (GWAS or GWAS replication study)

Author	Year	Genetic polymorphisms	Risk allele/ genotype	Outcome	Odds ratio
Cheng, I	2008	rs10090154, rs16901979, rs6983267	T, A, G allele	Aggressiveness	1.42, 1.52, 1.25
Kaeder, AK	2009	rs2735839, rs10993994	G, T	Aggressiveness	1.38, 1.10
Cheng, I	2010	rs12621278, rs629242, rs9364554, rs4430796, rs5945572	G, T, T, A, A	Biochemical recurrence	2.43, 1.23, 1.27, 1.14, 1.45
FitzGerald, LM	2010	rs6497287	C	Aggressiveness	1.46
Pomerantz, MM	2011	rs2735839, rs7679673	AA, CC	CSS	1.92, 1.56
Liu, X	2011	rs17160911	N/R	Gleason score	N/R
McGuire, BB	2012	rs1447295, rs1571801	AA, AA	Aggressive pathology	2.3, 3.9

CSS cancer-specific survival, *N/R* not reported

patients with aggressive PC and controls. In that study, three SNPs, rs10090154, rs16901979, and rs6983267, were associated with advanced PC with Gleason score ≥7, TNM stage >T2c, or PSA >10 ng/mL [14]. Another GWAS study by FitzGerald et al. discovered nine SNPs by comparing aggressive PC with controls and validated that rs6497287at 15q13 was associated only with aggressive PC—defined as PSA level ≥20 ng/mL, regional/distant stage, Gleason score ≥7 (3 + 4), recurrence/progression event, and/or PC-specific death—but not with less aggressive PC [15]. More aggressive PC (Gleason scores ≥4 + 3, or stage ≥T3b, or N+) was also assessed in comparison with less aggressive PC. The G allele of rs2735839 in KLK3 gene and T allele of rs10993994 in MSMB gene were reported to be risk alleles for more aggressive clinicopathological feature [16]. Liu X et al. performed a fine mapping analysis to explore PC aggressiveness loci. They narrowed the 7q22-35 locus down to a 370 kb region and found nonsynonymous SNP rs17160911 (Gly339Ala) in KLRG2, which had a significant association with Gleason score. In patients with less aggressive PC, who are candidates for active surveillance, rs1447295 at 8q24 and rs1571801 at 9q33 were shown to be a risk for unfavorable pathology with Gleason score ≥7 and/or ≥pT2b in the prostatectomy specimen [17].

As the second approach, several studies reported risk SNPs related with progression after definitive treatments for localized PC. Cheng I et al. demonstrated that rs12621278, rs629242, rs9364554, rs4430796, and rs5945572 were associated with biochemical recurrence after radical prostatectomy or radiotherapy in patients with aggressive PC defined as Gleason score of >7, tumor-node-metastasis stage >T2c, or as a diagnostic PSA level of >10 ng/mL [15]. PC harboring BRCA1 and BRCA2 germline mutations are known to be more aggressive. Edwards SM et al. reported that BRCA2 germline mutation was an independent prognostic factor of poor overall survival and the status of BRCA2 mutation may be useful in identifying the patients who need more intense treatment [18].

We should be aware of an ascertainment bias when the risk-SNP possibly exerts influence on cancer screening. Pomerantz et al. reported that two SNPs, rs2735839 at19q13 and rs7679673 at 4q24, were associated with CSS [19]. The rs2735839 is located in the intergenic region of KLK2 and KLK3, which codes PSA, and interestingly the risk allele of rs2735839 for CSS was inversely reported as a protective allele for PC diagnosis in a previous GWAS study [20]. This SNP may not directly lead to the aggressiveness of PC, and an ascertainment bias due to the lower PSA in men with a risk allele of rs2735839 is believed to cause a delayed diagnosis which could lead to a poor survival.

19.4 Genetic Polymorphisms Associated with Prognosis of Metastatic PC at Diagnosis

The median overall survival of patients with newly diagnosed metastatic PC treated with conventional hormone therapy ranges from 44 to 54 months. The survival time varies among patients and 20–50% of those patients achieve long-term survival beyond 5 years [2, 3]. It has been known that the survival is affected by the extent of bone metastasis, visceral metastasis, and other clinicopathological factors. The standard treatment for hormone-sensitive mPC has been hormone therapy. Recent clinical studies demonstrated the efficacy of early chemotherapy with docetaxel, and the treatment strategy for those patients is changing from stereotypic treatment to a more personalized treatment. In accordance with this change, more accurate prognostic evaluation and prediction of treatment effect in each individual patient are required. Efforts have been made to explore genetic polymorphisms, involved in the prognosis of mPC, in order to utilize them for better decision making in the selection of treatment options and intensity.

Shimbo et al. focused on the CAG repeat polymorphism, which reportedly had an association in response to hormone therapy, and demonstrated that D2 patients with shorter CAG repeat (<23 repeats) had a shorter CSS than those with longer CAG repeat (≥23 repeats) [21]. Furthermore, CCS was compared between the patients with lower and higher serum testosterone levels (cutoff of 4.33 ng/mL) at diagnosis. They found that the combination of serum testosterone level and CAG repeat length was an independent prognostic factor of stage D2 patients. In another study targeting D2 disease, reported by Tsuchiya et al., the association between 13 polymorphisms, previously reported to be a risk for PC and CSS, was analyzed [22]. Both the long alleles of the two polymorphisms, insulin growth factor-I (IGF-I) and cytochrome P450 19 (CYP19), were related to worse CSS.

Several studies have demonstrated the association between genetic polymorphisms and CSS or OS of D2 disease in subgroup analyses. These studies are listed in Table 19.3 [23–28]. Huang et al. genotyped 29 PC-associated SNPs and picked up four SNPs most relevant to CSS after ADT, and showed that the number of unfavorable genotypes among those SNPs implicated CSS in patients with or without distant metastasis [27]. Similarly, Tsuchiya et al. retrospectively conducted an exploratory study using SNP panel to identify SNPs as prognosticator of mPC [29]. They found 14 candidate SNPs in six genes, and the three patients groups stratified according to the number of risk genotypes demonstrated significantly separate CSS curves.

Recently, Shiota et al. reported the significance of a SRD5A2 polymorphism with a possible role as regulator of serum testosterone during ADT in hormone-naive mPC [30, 31]. SRD5A2 encodes 5α-reductase type 2, which converts testosterone into DHT and the GG allele of functional SNP rs523349 is related to higher enzymatic activity. The GG allele indicated worst survival in patients with mPC, and demonstrated a higher serum testosterone level during ADT than the other genotypes. These findings are consistent with the function of the SNP and the clinical observation that men with lower testosterone during ADT had a better prognosis.

Table 19.3 Genetic polymorphisms associated with prognosis of newly diagnosed metastatic PCa

Author	Year	Analysis	Genetic polymorphisms	Risk allele/genotype	Outcome	Hazard ratio
Shimbo, M	2004	M	AR (CAG)n	<23 rpts	CSS	3.635 (combined with TS)
Tsuchiya, N	2005	M	CYP17 (TTTA)n, IGF-1 (CA)n	>3 rpts, >7 rpts	CSS	2.012, 1.976
Fukuda, H	2007	S	VEGF T-460C	C allele	CSS	2.463
Narita, N	2008	S	OPG T950C	T allele	CSS	2.157
Wang, W	2009	S	Mel-18 A1805G	G allele	CSS	4.658
Suzuki, M	2011	S	rs6983561 (8q24)	AA	CSS, OS	3.353, 3.361
Huang, SP	2012	S	rs3734444 (BMP5), rs3118536 (RXRA), rs7986346 (IRS2), rs2836370 (ERG)	GG, CA or AA, TG or GG, TT or TC	OS	No. of UF genotypes 1: 1.94, 2: 3.90 (vs. 0)
Tsuchiya, N	2013	M	rs2891980 (XRCC4), rs256550 (PMS1), rs570730 (GATA3), rs1295686 (IL-13), rs2293554 (CASP8), rs2162679 (IGF-1)	GG, AG or GG, AG or GG, AA or AG, AA, AG or GG	CSS	No. of UF genotypes 4–6: 3.06 (vs. 0–1)
Kanda, S	2013	S	rs4775936 (CYP19)	GA or AA	CSS	1.737
Shiota, M	2015	M	rs523349 (SRD5A2)	GG	PFS, OS	1.72, 1.85

M main analysis, *rpts* repeats, *CSS* cancer-specific survival, *TS* testosterone, *S* subanalysis, *OS* overall survival, *UF* unfavorable, *PFS* progression-free survival

19.5 Genetic Polymorphisms Associated with Outcome After Specific Drug Therapy in Castration-Resistant PC (CRPC)

In an era of precision medicine, it is essential to predict the effect and adverse events of a specific treatment. Several specific drugs are used for the treatment of PC. Table 19.4 indicates previously reported genetic polymorphisms associated with their outcomes after specific drug therapy in CRPC patients.

Abiraterone acetate (AA) is one of the novel androgen receptor (AR)-targeted agents that inhibit cytochrome P450 17 (CYP17), a key enzyme in androgen synthesis. AA blocks the synthetic pathway of DHT from the adrenal gland-derived androgens, the so-called backdoor pathway, and exhibits growth inhibition of androgen-dependent PC cells. Phase III studies of AA have demonstrated a significant extension of progression-free survival (PFS) and OS in castration-resistant PC (CRPC) before and after chemotherapy [32, 33]. A retrospective study demonstrated

Table 19.4 Genetic polymorphisms associated with outcome after specific drug therapy in CRPC patients

Author	Year	Drug	Genetic polymorphisms	Risk allele/ genotype	Outcome	Hazard ratio
Suzuki, M	2005	Estramustine phosphate	COMT Val158Met	Val/Met or Met/Met	PFS	4.784
Hahn, NM	2006	Docetaxel-based regimens	ABCG2 C421CA	A allele	OS >15 m	N/A
Sissung, TM	2008	Docetaxel	ABCB1	1236C-2677G-3435C	OS	N/A
Pastina, I	2010	Docetaxel	CYP1B1 C4326G	GG	PFS, OS	N/A
Sissung, TM	2011	Docetaxel-based regimens	rs2234693, rs9340799 (ERα)	TC or CC, GG	PFS	N/A
			rs700519 (CYP19)	CT or TT	OS	
Orlandi, P	2015	Cyclophosphamide	VEGF-A A-2578C, C-634G	CC, CC	RR, PFS	N/A
Joerger, M	2015	Metformin	rs622342 (OCT1)	C allele	RR	N/A
Binder, M	2016	Abiraterone acetate	rs2486758 (CYP17A1)	CT or CC	PFS	2.22

PFS progression-free survival, *OS* overall survival, *N/A* not assessed, *RR* response rate

that rs2486758, which is located in the promoter region of CYP17A1, and shown to be a risk-SNP by a meta-analysis [34], was associated with the response to AA and biochemical PFS [35]. Meanwhile, other SNPs reported to be associated with a PC risk had no association with the outcome of AA treatment [35, 36].

Docetaxel (DTX) is a substrate for cytochrome P450 3A (CYP3A) and DTX metabolized in the liver by hepatic CYP3A is excreted into the bile duct system through membrane transporters of the ABC family, especially the ATP-binding cassette subfamily B member 1 (ABCB1) and ATP-binding cassette subfamily G member 2 (ABCG2). ABCB1 harbors well-known genetic variants such as 1236C > T, 2677G > T/A, and 3435C > T. Sissung et al. reported that in CRPC patients treated with DTX, patients with C-G-C (with reference to 1236-2677-3435) haplotype had a significantly longer OS than those with T-T-T haplotype [37]. Hahn et al. assessed the survival after treatments with docetaxel-based regimens, docetaxel plus vinorelbine, and docetaxel plus estramustine phosphate, in pharmacogenetic analysis [38]. Among eight polymorphisms in six taxane-associated genes, A allele of the ABCG2 C421A polymorphism was predictive for a chance of being alive beyond 15 months after the docetaxel-based therapies. Although many studies demonstrated the association of ABCB1 polymorphisms with drug disposition, clinical response, or drug toxicity, the clinical significance is limited due to conflicting results and their biological implications are yet to be determined.

Meanwhile, cytochrome P4501B1 (CYP1B1) is responsible for the interaction of docetaxel with microtubules. The G (Val) allele of the functional SNP 4326C > G (Leu432Val) is thought to increase the expression and catalytic activity of CYP1B1 [39]. Pastina I et al. reported that CRPC patients with 432ValVal genotype experienced a lower response rate, shorter PFS, and shorter OS. A strong inhibition of the polymerization of microtubules by CYP1B1 estrogen metabolites, and estradiol-3,4-quinine originated from 4-OHE2, reduces the anticancer effect of docetaxel, which stabilizes tubulin polymerization. Docetaxel also forms the 4-OHE2-docetaxel adduct by reacting with estradiol-3,4-quinine [40]. Thus, CYC1B1 polymorphism is suggested to influence the clinical response to docetaxel through the structural alteration of docetaxel and its interaction with 4-OHE2 [41].

Estramustine phosphate (EMP) is a conjugate of 17β-estradiol and nitrogen mustard and is one of the mostly used drugs for CRPC that was used before the novel AR-targeted drugs. 17β-Estradiol is hydroxylated by CYP1A1 and sequentially methylated by catechol-O-methyltransferase (COMT) to yield 2-methoxyestradiol, which possesses antiproliferative effect on PC. Suzuki et al. investigated the association of COMT polymorphism Val158Met, of which Met allele leads to a reduction in the enzymatic activity and biochemical PFS [42]. They found that EPM-treated patients with the Met allele had a significantly shorter PFS compared with those with Val/Val.

With regard to other chemotherapeutic agents that lack convincing evidence, some studies demonstrated the association of SNPs with survival in CRPC patients. Orlandi et al. genotyped three SNPs in the VEGF-A gene to assess the genetic effect on the response to metronomic cyclophosphamide (CTX), celecoxib, and dexamethasone, on PFS, and OS after treatment [43]. Among the SNPs, -2578CC genotype was associated with a poor response and -634CC genotype was associated with both a poor response and shorter PFS. Metformin is used to treat type 2 diabetes mellitus and recently came to be known as a possible anticancer drug for PC. A mechanism of direct anticancer effect is the activation of adenosine monophosphate-activated protein kinase (AMPK) through the inhibition of the mitochondrial electron transport chain (ETC) [44]. Another mechanism is leading to a downregulation of the phosphoinositide-3-kinase (PI3K) axis by lowering systemic insulin levels [44]. Joerger et al. investigated the genetic effect of transporter of metformin, organic cation transporter 1 (OCT1), and multidrug and toxin extrusion transporter 1 (MATE1), and demonstrated that the C allele of rs622342 in the OCT1 gene was associated with the response to metformin [45].

19.6 Genetic Polymorphisms Associated with Prognosis of CRPC

Continuous hormone therapy is the standard treatment for mPC at diagnosis, but the hormone therapy fails in such patients with an average of 2 years. Although recent advances in drug therapy prolonged the survival after the failure in the first-line treatment, the survival rate remains as short as 22–38 months [46, 47]. Even in the localized PC patients who underwent radical prostatectomy, more than 30% of those exhibit a progression to advanced disease [48], following which they were subjected to hormone therapy or chemotherapy. Since most of the advanced PC patients eventually acquired CRPC, studies have assessed the genetic polymorphisms, as well as clinical and pathological factors, for predicting the survival after CRPC.

There are few studies investigating the genetic effect on the prognosis of CRPC. Zhang et al. examined the effect of 84 SNPs in 14 genes—that are implicated in the risk, OS, or response to ADT—on the survival of CRPC patients [49]. Among those SNPs, 11 of 18 SNPs in the JAK2 gene were independently associated with OS. JAK2 has been known to be involved in the growth and progression of PC through both androgen receptor-dependent and -independent mechanisms, leading to an activation of STAT signaling pathway. A multivariate prognostic model for predicting survival using two SNPs, rs2149556 and rs4372063, concurrent with age and Gleason score, could accurately discriminate good and poor survival of CRPC patients [49].

AA was recently shown to induce a somatic mutation in HSD3B1, which encodes 3β-hydroxysteroid dehydrogenase (3βHSD). 3βHSD is one of the key enzymes capable of synthesizing DHT from precursors that are secreted from the adrenal gland, which is involved both in the classical and backdoor pathways [50]. Meanwhile, HSD3B1 harbors a conspicuous germline SNP 1245 A > C (367 N > T), which is the same somatic mutation caused by AA. Both somatic and germline mutations of 1245C stabilize the enzyme by an inhibition of ubiquitination and increase metabolic cascade from DHEA to DHT. This SNP or somatic mutation is thought to be associated with resistance to drug therapies in CRPC patients [50]. One recent study demonstrated that HSD3B1 1245C is associated with shorter PFS, as well as metastatic-free survival and OS, in hormone-sensitive PC patients in an allele dose-dependent manner [51]. However, the effect of this SNP on CRPC needs further evaluation.

19.7 Summary

Numerous studies that explored PC-associated genes, through the GWAS, have contributed to understanding its ethiology. However, issues with respect to the genetic predisposition related to the prognosis and therapeutic outcome remain poorly explored. The available evidence has several limitations, and therefore validation of the results obtained thus far is mandatory for clinical application. A genetic polymorphism is a unique marker that is not altered by intrinsic and extrinsic environments. Genetic markers, along with somatic gene alterations and conventional clinicopathological factors, will be of much significance in that management of PC—a disease that continues to evolve. In the coming era of precision medicine, this approach will be of great help for therapeutic decision making of advanced PC.

References

1. Stemmermann GN, Nomura AM, Chyou PH, et al. A prospective comparison of prostate cancer at autopsy and as a clinical event: the Hawaii Japanese experience. Cancer Epidemiol Biomarkers Prev. 1992;1(3):189–93.
2. Sweeney CJ, Chen YH, Carducci M, et al. Chemohormonal therapy in metastatic hormone-sensitive prostate cancer. N Engl J Med. 2015;373(8):737–46.
3. Gravis G, Fizazi K, Joly F, et al. Androgen-deprivation therapy alone or with docetaxel in non-castrate metastatic prostate cancer (GETUG-AFU 15): a randomised, open-label, phase 3 trial. Lancet Oncol. 2013;14(2):149–58.
4. Gandaglia G, Karakiewicz PI, Briganti A, et al. Impact of the site of metastases on survival in patients with metastatic prostate cancer. Eur Urol. 2015;68(2):325–34.
5. Smith CG, Fisher D, Harris R, et al. Analyses of 7,635 patients with colorectal cancer using independent training and validation cohorts show that rs9929218 in CDH1 is a prognostic marker of survival. Clin Cancer Res. 2015;21(15):3453–61.
6. Megias-Vericat JE, Herrero MJ, Rojas L, et al. A systematic review and meta-analysis of the impact of WT1 polymorphism rs16754 in the effectiveness of standard chemotherapy in patients with acute myeloid leukemia. Pharmacogenomics J. 2016;16(1):30–40.
7. Lin DW, Porter M, Montgomery B. Treatment and survival outcomes in young men diagnosed with prostate cancer: a Population-based Cohort Study. Cancer. 2009;115(13):2863–71.
8. Hughes L, Zhu F, Ross E, et al. Assessing the clinical role of genetic markers of early-onset prostate cancer among high-risk men enrolled in prostate cancer early detection. Cancer Epidemiol Biomarkers Prev. 2012;21(1):53–60.
9. Lange EM, Salinas CA, Zuhlke KA, et al. Early onset prostate cancer has a significant genetic component. Prostate. 2012;72(2):147–56.
10. Camp NJ, Farnham JM, Wong J, et al. Replication of the 10q11 and Xp11 prostate cancer risk variants: results from a Utah pedigree-based study. Cancer Epidemiol Biomarkers Prev. 2009;18(4):1290–4.
11. Al Olama AA, Kote-Jarai Z, Berndt SI, et al. A meta-analysis of 87,040 individuals identifies 23 new susceptibility loci for prostate cancer. Nat Genet. 2014;46(10):1103–9.
12. Shui IM, Mucci LA, Kraft P, et al. Vitamin D-related genetic variation, plasma vitamin D, and risk of lethal prostate cancer: a prospective nested case-control study. J Natl Cancer Inst. 2012;104(9):690–9.
13. Gudmundsson J, Sulem P, Rafnar T, et al. Common sequence variants on 2p15 and Xp11.22 confer susceptibility to prostate cancer. Nat Genet. 2008;40(3):281–3.
14. Cheng I, Plummer SJ, Jorgenson E, et al. 8q24 and prostate cancer: association with advanced disease and meta-analysis. Eur J Hum Genet. 2008;16(4):496–505.
15. Cheng I, Plummer SJ, Neslund-Dudas C, et al. Prostate cancer susceptibility variants confer increased risk of disease progression. Cancer Epidemiol Biomarkers Prev. 2010;19(9):2124–32.
16. Kader AK, Sun J, Isaacs SD, et al. Individual and cumulative effect of prostate cancer risk-associated variants on clinicopathologic variables in 5,895 prostate cancer patients. Prostate. 2009;69(11):1195–205.
17. McGuire BB, Helfand BT, Kundu S, et al. Association of prostate cancer risk alleles with unfavourable pathological characteristics in potential candidates for active surveillance. BJU Int. 2012;110(3):338–43.
18. Narod SA, Neuhausen S, Vichodez G, et al. Rapid progression of prostate cancer in men with a BRCA2 mutation. Br J Cancer. 2008;99(2):371–4.
19. Pomerantz MM, Werner L, Xie W, et al. Association of prostate cancer risk Loci with disease aggressiveness and prostate cancer-specific mortality. Cancer Prev Res. 2011;4(5):719–28.
20. Gudmundsson J, Besenbacher S, Sulem P, et al. Genetic correction of PSA values using sequence variants associated with PSA levels. Sci Transl Med. 2010;2(62):62ra92.

Local Therapy in Combination with Androgen Deprivation Therapy for Metastatic Prostate Cancer

20

Hideyasu Tsumura, Ken-Ichi Tabata, and Masatsugu Iwamura

Abstract

There is growing interest in the role of local therapy for the prostate in patients with metastatic disease. Several retrospective studies indicated that cytoreductive therapy for the prostate in addition to androgen deprivation therapy (ADT) had better oncological outcomes than ADT alone in patients with newly diagnosed metastatic prostate cancer. Others reported the benefit of prior local therapy with curative intention for patients who eventually developed treatment failure and subsequently progressed to metastatic disease. When local therapy, including radical prostatectomy and prostate radiotherapy, could improve the survival and palliate the obstructive symptoms/conditions in patients with newly diagnosed metastatic prostate cancer, this treatment option should be offered. The concept of local therapy for the prostate in those patients remains controversial, however, and lacks level 1 evidence. Several prospective studies are now under way to investigate whether a combination of local therapy and ADT has survival benefit when compared to ADT alone. The results from these prospective studies may propose a new concept in the treatment of newly diagnosed metastatic prostate cancer.

Keywords

Local therapy · Cytoreductive therapy · Metastatic prostate cancer · Androgen deprivation therapy

H. Tsumura, M.D. (✉) · K.-I. Tabata · M. Iwamura
Department of Urology, Kitasato University School of Medicine, Sagamihara, Kanagawa, Japan
e-mail: tsumura@med.kitasato-u.ac.jp

Abbreviations

ADT	Androgen deprivation therapy
BT	Brachytherapy
CSS	Cancer-specific survival
EBRT	External beam radiation therapy
mCRPC	Metastatic castration-resistant prostate cancer
mCSPC	Metastatic castration-sensitive prostate cancer
mPCa	Metastatic prostate cancer
NSR	No surgery or radiation therapy
OS	Overall survival
RP	Radical prostatectomy
RT	Radiotherapy
SEER	Surveillance Epidemiology and End Results
TURP	Transurethral resection of prostate

20.1 Introduction

Since Huggins found that metastatic prostate cancer (mPCa) responded to androgen deprivation therapy (ADT) in the 1940s, surgical or pharmacological castration with/without an antiandrogen agent was the standard of care for metastatic castration-sensitive prostate cancer (mCSPC) [1]. Once the disease developed into metastatic castration-resistant prostate cancer (mCRPC), there were only a few drugs that could be expected to prolong the prognosis. The use of these drugs was not based on high-level evidence. In the early twenty-first century, the treatment for mCRPC began to change as novel agents, including docetaxel [2], abiraterone acetate [3, 4], enzalutamide [5, 6], cabazitaxel [7], radium-223 [8], and sipuleucel-T [9], have been shown to prolong overall survival (OS). Although these agents have offered new treatment options for patients with mCRPC, their efficacy is limited.

While therapeutic options are increasing for mCRPC, there has been a paradigm shift in the treatment of newly diagnosed mPCa. First, the standard of care for those patients may change from ADT alone to combined use of ADT and up-front docetaxel. Early chemotherapy with docetaxel has been shown to improve the prognosis of patients with newly diagnosed mPCa [10–12]. Second, a role of local therapy for the prostate is being increasingly explored in the setting of newly diagnosed mPCa. Although it is controversial whether local therapy in combination with ADT for mPCa delays time to CRPC and consequently improves survival, several retrospective studies have demonstrated the benefit of local treatment in this setting [13–15]. When cytoreductive therapy for the prostate could improve the survival in patients with newly diagnosed mPCa, this option should be offered. In addition, there are reports that indicated the benefit of prior local therapy with curative intention for patients who eventually developed treatment failure and subsequently progressed to mPCa [16].

In this chapter, we review the relevant literature on the role of local therapy in combination with ADT for mPCa. We also describe the therapeutic implications of local therapy for the prostate in this setting.

20.2 Rationale for Primary Local Treatment in mPCa

Although curative treatment is almost impossible for various metastatic cancers, some studies proved the survival benefit of a combined therapy with primary excision and systemic therapy for metastatic diseases including ovarian, colorectal, and renal cell cancers [17–19]. For example, Mickisch et al. conducted a randomized study of metastatic renal carcinoma in which patients received either combined treatment of radical nephrectomy and immunotherapy or immunotherapy alone; the combined therapy delayed time to progression and improved OS [19].

The mechanisms underlying a survival benefit of cytoreductive therapy for various metastatic diseases are not well understood, although there are some possible explanations for the benefit of primary therapy [13]. First, cytoreductive therapy for a primary lesion could decrease the total tumor burden and allow for an improved response to systemic therapy. Second, a primary tumor could be a source of disseminated tumor cells and thus cytoreductive therapy could eliminate the source of metastasis [20]. Third, a primary tumor may help to not only disseminate the cancer cells but also to prepare the metastatic soil. Thus, therapy directed at the primary tumor could delay the formation and the growth of distant metastases [21, 22].

In the setting of newly diagnosed mPCa, there exists no level 1 evidence supporting the survival benefit of local therapy in addition to systemic therapy when compared with systemic therapy alone. However, some experimental findings suggested the benefit of combined therapy. Kadmon et al. demonstrated the principle of surgical adjuvant chemotherapy in metastatic rat prostatic tumor [23]. They compared treatment efficacy among single-dose chemotherapy, surgical excision of the primary tumor, or a combination of surgical excision and single-dose chemotherapy. Only the combined therapy substantially prolonged survival and produced cures at an early metastatic stage.

In the field of radiotherapy (RT), the abscopal effect is observed in some metastatic cancers, including hepatocellular carcinoma and melanoma [24–26]. The abscopal effect is a phenomenon in which local RT at a particular tumor site causes a response in a site distant to the irradiated volume. It results in a non-irradiated tumor being spontaneously reduced. Lock et al. reported the abscopal effect with focal liver RT alone causing regression of distant lung metastasis in a systemic treatment-naïve patient with hepatocellular carcinoma [26]. Others demonstrated that immune checkpoint inhibition alone or RT alone did not result in an abscopal effect. However, a combined fractionated RT with immune checkpoint inhibition resulted in an abscopal effect [24, 25].

The mechanism underlying the abscopal effect is not clearly understood. Some experimental reports suggested that local RT results in the release of circulating tumor antigens and subsequently recruits tumor-specific T lymphocytes and dendritic cells, which seem to play an important role in remission of tumors, and then the induced immune response delivers an attack to non-irradiated malignant sites that express the same tumor antigens [26, 27]. If these kinds of immune responses actually occur in clinical practice, it may be one possible explanation for the benefit of local RT in mPCa patients. Nesslinger et al. reported on autoantibody responses to tumor proteins in patients with nonmetastatic prostate cancer [28]. They revealed the development of treatment-associated autoantibody responses in patients undergoing neoadjuvant hormone therapy (29.2%), external beam radiation therapy (EBRT) (13.8%), brachytherapy (BT) (25%), and radical prostatectomy (RP) (0%). They showed that ADT and prostate RT strongly induce antigen-specific immune responses when compared with surgery in clinically nonmetastatic diseases. These results support previous reports that the use of neoadjuvant ADT with prostate RT contributes to better OS or cancer-specific survival (CSS) in men with locally advanced or localized unfavorable-risk prostate cancer compared to RT alone [29–31], whereas the combined therapy of prostatectomy and neoadjuvant ADT does not contribute to the prognosis [32, 33]. While the combination of prostate RT and ADT has shown survival benefit for patients with nonmetastatic diseases, it is not clear whether this combined therapy contributes to better prognosis in those with mPCa. Further research is needed to clarify whether prostate RT induces the immune response for an attack on non-irradiated metastatic sites and subsequently contributes to better prognosis.

20.3 Cytoreductive Therapy for the Prostate in mCSPC

20.3.1 The Role of Transurethral Resection of Prostate (TURP)

Historically, TURP was generally performed to relieve bladder outlet obstruction caused by locally advanced prostate cancer. Palliative TURP may be effective to relieve the bladder outlet symptoms even if patients have metastatic disease [34]. However, the survival benefit of palliative TURP is not clear because long-term follow-up studies that assess the oncological outcomes are lacking.

Qin et al. retrospectively investigated the oncological impact of TURP as a cytoreductive surgery in patients with newly diagnosed mPCa [35]. All patients ($n = 146$) received complete androgen blockade as the initial systematic therapy. Thirty-nine patients underwent TURP for a relief of bladder outlet obstruction, and the others ($n = 107$) were treated with androgen blockade alone. Age, biopsy Gleason Score, and prostate-specific antigen at diagnosis were comparable among the two groups. Patients in the non-TURP group had a greater risk for CRPC than those in the TURP group (52% vs. 33%, $P = 0.007$). While no statistical significance was found for OS, there was a trend towards longer OS in the TURP group ($P = 0.071$). In addition, all patients in the TURP group improved voiding function without serious complications. Although this study is limited by its retrospective nature, it seems to support the concept that cytoreductive surgery results in a better response to systemic therapy and prolongs time to CRPC even in mCSPC patients.

The potential disadvantage of TURP for mPCa may be a risk of disseminating cancer cells due to extravasation of the irrigating medium into the circulation system [36]. However, it is still controversial whether the procedure can provoke hematogenous spillage of prostate cancer cells and subsequently increase metastatic foci in this setting. In addition, TURP is not always safe because it requires anesthesia and has a risk of bleeding and total/stress urinary incontinence.

20.3.2 The Role of Prostate RT and Radical Prostatectomy

Tabata et al. retrospectively analyzed the efficacy of prostate RT for patients diagnosed with mPCa (M1a-c) using propensity score matching analysis [37]. Among the patients, 146 received hormonal therapy without prostate RT (no-RT group) and 103 received hormonal therapy and prostate RT (RT group). Either EBRT or a combined high-dose-rate BT with EBRT was used for RT for the prostate. Propensity score matching identified 104 matched pairs of patients. There were no significant differences in baseline characteristics including age, prostate-specific antigen at diagnosis, Gleason scores, level of hemoglobin, alkaline phosphatase, and lactase dehydrogenase between the two groups. The 3-year OS rates were 50.3% and 91.3% in the no-RT and RT group, respectively ($P = 0.0062$), and the 3-year CSS rates were 59.6% and 93.3% ($P = 0.0082$). These findings suggest that RT for prostate prolongs survival even in mPCa patients.

Using the National Cancer Database, Rusthoven et al. retrospectively evaluated survival benefit of patients with mPCa treated with ADT with or without prostate RT [14]. Patients receiving prostate RT and ADT had significantly longer OS than those treated with ADT alone. In addition, survival analyses demonstrated that patients with higher dose RT ($\geq$65 Gy; median, 75.6 Gy) had significantly longer OS than those with lower dose RT (<65 Gy; median, 40 Gy).

Culp et al. evaluated the survival of patients diagnosed with mPCa (M1a-c) based on definitive therapy for the prostate by using the Surveillance Epidemiology and End Results (SEER) database (2004–2010) [13]. Patients were divided based on definitive treatment for the prostate: RP ($n = 245$), BT ($n = 129$), and no surgery or RT (NSR, $n = 7811$). The 5-year OS and predicted CSS were each significantly higher in patients undergoing RP (67.4% and 75.8%, respectively) or BT (52.6% and 61.3%) compared with NSR patients (22.5% and 48.7%; $P < 0.001$). RP and BT were each independently associated with decreased prostate cancer-specific mortality ($P < 0.01$). Gratzke et al. evaluated the role of RP in patients diagnosed with mPCa using data from the Munich Cancer Registry (1998–2010) [15]. In this series, 1464 patients (95%) did not undergo RP and 74 patients (5%) underwent RP. Patients undergoing RP showed a 55% 5-year OS rate compared with 21% in those who did not ($P < 0.01$). The data from the Munich Cancer Registry reproduced the results from the SEER database. However, these two studies have some limitations because there was no information about performance status, comorbidity, use of chemotherapy, and extent of bone or visceral metastasis. Although the extent of metastasis does not always reflect the prognosis in mPCa, patients with polymetastatic disease usually have poorer prognosis than those with oligometastatic disease [10]. In addition, 3–5% of selected patients who received definitive treatment for the prostate were compared with 95% those who did not [15].

In summary, some retrospective studies showed a survival benefit of cytoreductive treatment for the prostate in mPCa patients. This definitive therapy for the prostate may have a role in treatment in this setting. However, further prospective studies are needed to identify those patients likely to receive a benefit for definitive therapy in this setting.

20.4 The Role of Primary Local Therapy for Obstructive Uropathy

Local extension of prostate cancer and lymph node metastases causes obstructive uropathy and local symptomatic progression. Treatment interventions such as urethral catheterization, indwelling ureteral stent placement, and TURP are needed to resolve the urinary retention or hydronephrosis [34]. Obstructive uropathy secondary to local progression of prostate cancer is generally considered to be associated with reduced OS [38] and apparently decreases the quality of life. If a local therapy can effectively prevent mPCa patients from developing an obstructive condition and local symptomatic progression, it may have both therapeutic and palliative value.

Several reports evaluated the efficacy of prior local therapy including RP and definitive RT for reducing the risk of obstructive uropathy in the setting of subsequent development of mPCa. Won et al. evaluated whether local prostate therapy gave palliative benefit to patients who eventually developed CRPC [16]. Patients were divided into three groups: RP, definitive EBRT, and no local treatment. RP and definitive EBRT were conducted with curative intention at the time of clinically nonmetastatic condition, and all eligible patients were treated with ADT. The endpoint of the study was the development of local complications including ureteric obstruction, bladder outlet obstruction, hematuria, pelvic pain, or prostatitis. Patients who received local treatment for the prostate by either RP or definitive EBRT had significantly fewer local complications when compared to those who did not receive treatment for the prostate. RP showed the most effective palliation effect compared to the EBRT and no local treatment groups.

Oefelein retrospectively evaluated the impact of prior local therapy on the development of obstructive uropathy [38]. He compared the probability of obstructive uropathy between 80 patients undergoing local therapy with salvage ADT and 180 patients who received primary ADT. Either RP or EBRT (60–72 Gy) was used for local therapy at the time of clinically nonmetastatic disease. Of those, skeletal metastasis was identified in 110 and lymph node metastasis in 55. The author concluded that patients treated with salvage ADT followed by local therapy had no statistically significant risk reduction for the development of obstructive uropathy compared with those who received primary ADT alone. However, this study examined the risk of developing obstructive uropathy only in patients with progression who required ADT followed by local therapy. In addition, most bladder neck obstruction was observed in those who received EBRT. A dose of 60–72 Gy might not be adequate for local control.

In the setting of stage D1 (TxN+M0), Grimm et al. conducted a retrospective study in 82 patients undergoing pelvic lymph node dissection for prostate cancer. Thirty-two patients were treated with ADT alone, 50 patients underwent RP, and 42 of them received ADT as well. They concluded that patients undergoing RP may have a possible benefit with regard to the necessity for secondary interventions when compared to ADT alone [39]. Schmeller and Lubos conducted a retrospective study in a series of 76 consecutive patients who underwent pelvic lymphadenectomy and had pathological stage D1 (T1-3, pN1-2, M0) prostate cancer; 37 patients underwent early ADT and 39 underwent combined therapy of RP with immediate ADT. They concluded that the combined therapy offered no advantage over ADT alone either for curative or palliative intent [40].

Although there exists no clear evidence to support the use of local therapy for the prostate to prevent mPCa patients from developing obstructive uropathy, several retrospective studies suggest that primary local prostatic treatment reduces the risk of obstructive uropathy. The reduced risk is more likely to be observed in patients undergoing RP than in those without RP. However, it seems that the dose of RT was much lower than that of contemporary doses. In addition, these retrospective observations may be biased by more advanced diseases assigned to ADT alone [39]. Further prospective research is warranted.

20.5 Future Perspectives for Primary Local Therapy in mCSPC

Several prospective studies are now under way to determine whether patients presenting mPCa should have primary local therapy in combination with ADT (Table 20.1). In addition, we have to identify the best timing and candidates for the local therapy in this setting. Should we offer the local therapy for the prostate only in patients with obstructive symptoms or in patients who eventually failed to respond to primary ADT? Which patients are the best candidates for the local therapy, patients with limited metastatic lesions or those with widely metastatic disease? Does the local therapy prevent mCSPC patients from developing obstructive uropathy or delay the time to CRPC? Because mPCa is an extremely heterogeneous disease, well-designed and large clinical trials are needed to answer these questions.

The Systemic Therapy in Advancing or Metastatic Prostate Cancer: Evaluation of Drug Efficacy (STAMPEDE) trial was launched to investigate multimodal therapy in the treatment of mPCa. Arm H was newly proposed to investigate whether RT for the primary tumor delays metastatic progression and subsequently prolongs survival in patients presenting with mPCa (NCT00268476) [41]. Arm H is ADT plus RT for the prostate. Nonmetastatic patients and patients who have failed to respond to prior local therapy cannot be allocated to Arm H. Only patients with newly diagnosed mPCa and no contraindication to RT can be enrolled. As with all the existing arms, Arm H will be compared only to the same subset of patients who

Table 20.1 Prospective randomized clinical trials for the treatment of newly diagnosed mPCa with local therapy for the prostate

Identifier	Acronym	Purpose	Primary endpoint	Secondary endpoint	Arms (intervention)
NCT 00268476	STAMPEDE	Learn if RT for the primary tumor delays metastatic progression and subsequently prolongs survival	OS	1. Toxicity 2. Complications	1. RT + ADT 2. ADT alone
ISRCTN 06890529	HORRAD	A randomized study about the effect on survival of ADT versus ADT plus RT for the prostate	Survival	1. bF 2. Quality of life	1. RT + ADT 2. ADT alone
NCT 01751438		Learn if ADT in combination with RP or RT is more effective than ADT alone	PFS	1. Quality of life 2. Time to CRPC	1. BST + RP or RT 2. BST alone
ISRCTN 15704862	TRoMbone	Testing RP in men with prostate cancer and oligometastases to the bone	Feasibility to randomization	1. Quality of life 2. Time to CRPC	1. RP + SoC 2. SoC alone

Abbreviations: *mPCa* metastatic prostate cancer, *RT* radiotherapy, *OS* overall survival, *ADT* androgen deprivation therapy, *bF* biochemical failure, *RP* radical prostatectomy, *PFS* progression-free survival, *BST* best systemic therapy, *CRPC* castration-resistant prostate cancer, *SoC* standard of care (defined as ADT with or without chemotherapy)

are allocated to the control arm, hormone therapy alone (Arm A). A relative improvement of 25% in OS is the target. Secondary outcome measures will be toxicity and the complications of uncontrolled pelvic disease such as the need for ureteric stents, TURP, or colostomy.

A prospective randomized phase 3 study is under way to learn if treatment with standard systemic therapy (ADT or bilateral orchiectomy) in combination with RP or RT is more effective at controlling prostate cancer than standard systemic therapy alone (NCT01751438). Group 1 will continue to receive best systemic therapy. Group 2 will receive best systemic therapy in addition to RP or prostate RT. The primary endpoint is progression-free survival, defined as the time interval from the start of initial best systemic therapy treatment to the date of disease progression or death, whichever occurs first.

A UK-based trial, TRoMbone, was launched to investigate the role for treatment of the primary tumor in patients with oligometastatic prostate cancer (ISRCTN15704862). Participants will be randomly allocated to standard-of-care treatment (ADT with or without chemotherapy) versus standard-of-care treatment plus surgery. Eligible patients are <75 years old with newly diagnosed prostate cancer and one to three skeletal lesions. TRoMbone trials will assess technical feasibility, safety, and complications of surgery in oligometastatic prostate cancer, and examine ways to improve recruitment in this pilot study. Secondary outcome measures will be time to CRPC.

Conclusion

Although some retrospective studies suggested a survival benefit of cytoreductive treatment for the prostate in mCSPC, the concept of local therapy for the prostate in these patients remains controversial and lacks level 1 evidence. Neither the European Association of Urology nor the American Urological Association guidelines recommend local therapy for the prostate in newly diagnosed mPCa for the purpose of prolonged survival. Although there is growing interest in the role of local therapy for newly diagnosed mPCa, so far, only upfront docetaxel with ADT have been prospectively shown to improve the prognosis when compared with ADT alone in this setting [11]. Several prospective studies are now under way to investigate whether combination of local therapy for the prostate and ADT has survival benefit when compared to ADT alone. The results from these prospective studies may provide a new avenue for the treatment of newly diagnosed mPCa patients.

References

1. Huggins C, Stephens R, Hodges C. Studies on prostatic cancer. 2. The effects of castration on advanced carcinoma of the prostate gland. Arch Surg. 1941;43:209–23.
2. Tannock IF, de Wit R, Berry WR, Horti J, Pluzanska A, Chi KN, et al. Docetaxel plus prednisone or mitoxantrone plus prednisone for advanced prostate cancer. N Engl J Med. 2004;351(15):1502–12. https://doi.org/10.1056/NEJMoa040720.
3. de Bono JS, Logothetis CJ, Molina A, Fizazi K, North S, Chu L, et al. Abiraterone and increased survival in metastatic prostate cancer. N Engl J Med. 2011;364(21):1995–2005. https://doi.org/10.1056/NEJMoa1014618.
4. Ryan CJ, Smith MR, de Bono JS, Molina A, Logothetis CJ, de Souza P, et al. Abiraterone in metastatic prostate cancer without previous chemotherapy. N Engl J Med. 2013;368(2):138–48. https://doi.org/10.1056/NEJMoa1209096.
5. Scher HI, Fizazi K, Saad F, Taplin ME, Sternberg CN, Miller K, et al. Increased survival with enzalutamide in prostate cancer after chemotherapy. N Engl J Med. 2012;367(13):1187–97. https://doi.org/10.1056/NEJMoa1207506.
6. Beer TM, Armstrong AJ, Rathkopf DE, Loriot Y, Sternberg CN, Higano CS, et al. Enzalutamide in metastatic prostate cancer before chemotherapy. N Engl J Med. 2014;371(5):424–33. https://doi.org/10.1056/NEJMoa1405095.
7. de Bono JS, Oudard S, Ozguroglu M, Hansen S, Machiels JP, Kocak I, et al. Prednisone plus cabazitaxel or mitoxantrone for metastatic castration-resistant prostate cancer progressing after docetaxel treatment: a randomised open-label trial. Lancet. 2010;376(9747):1147–54. https://doi.org/10.1016/S0140-6736(10)61389-X.
8. Parker C, Nilsson S, Heinrich D, Helle SI, O'Sullivan JM, Fossa SD, et al. Alpha emitter radium-223 and survival in metastatic prostate cancer. N Engl J Med. 2013;369(3):213–23. https://doi.org/10.1056/NEJMoa1213755.

9. Cheever MA, Higano CS. PROVENGE (Sipuleucel-T) in prostate cancer: the first FDA-approved therapeutic cancer vaccine. Clin Cancer Res. 2011;17(11):3520–6. https://doi.org/10.1158/1078-0432.CCR-10-3126.
10. Sweeney CJ, Chen YH, Carducci M, Liu G, Jarrard DF, Eisenberger M, et al. Chemohormonal therapy in metastatic hormone-sensitive prostate cancer. N Engl J Med. 2015;373(8):737–46. https://doi.org/10.1056/NEJMoa1503747.
11. James ND, Sydes MR, Clarke NW, Mason MD, Dearnaley DP, Spears MR, et al. Addition of docetaxel, zoledronic acid, or both to first-line long-term hormone therapy in prostate cancer (STAMPEDE): survival results from an adaptive, multiarm, multistage, platform randomised controlled trial. Lancet. 2016;387(10,024):1163–77. https://doi.org/10.1016/S0140-6736(15)01037-5.
12. Tucci M, Bertaglia V, Vignani F, Buttigliero C, Fiori C, Porpiglia F, et al. Addition of docetaxel to androgen deprivation therapy for patients with hormone-sensitive metastatic prostate cancer: a systematic review and meta-analysis. Eur Urol. 2016;69(4):563–73. https://doi.org/10.1016/j.eururo.2015.09.013.
13. Culp SH, Schellhammer PF, Williams MB. Might men diagnosed with metastatic prostate cancer benefit from definitive treatment of the primary tumor? A SEER-based study. Eur Urol. 2014;65(6):1058–66. https://doi.org/10.1016/j.eururo.2013.11.012.
14. Rusthoven CG, Jones BL, Flaig TW, Crawford ED, Koshy M, Sher DJ, et al. Improved survival with prostate radiation in addition to androgen deprivation therapy for men with newly diagnosed metastatic prostate cancer. J Clin Oncol. 2016;34(24):2835–42. https://doi.org/10.1200/JCO.2016.67.4788.
15. Gratzke C, Engel J, Stief CG. Role of radical prostatectomy in metastatic prostate cancer: data from the Munich Cancer Registry. Eur Urol. 2014;66(3):602–3. https://doi.org/10.1016/j.eururo.2014.04.009.
16. Won AC, Gurney H, Marx G, De Souza P, Patel MI. Primary treatment of the prostate improves local palliation in men who ultimately develop castrate-resistant prostate cancer. BJU Int. 2013;112(4):E250–5. https://doi.org/10.1111/bju.12169.
17. Bristow RE, Tomacruz RS, Armstrong DK, Trimble EL, Montz FJ. Survival effect of maximal cytoreductive surgery for advanced ovarian carcinoma during the platinum era: a meta-analysis. J Clin Oncol. 2002;20(5):1248–59. https://doi.org/10.1200/JCO.2002.20.5.1248.
18. Temple LK, Hsieh L, Wong WD, Saltz L, Schrag D. Use of surgery among elderly patients with stage IV colorectal cancer. J Clin Oncol. 2004;22(17):3475–84. https://doi.org/10.1200/JCO.2004.10.218.
19. Mickisch GH, Garin A, van Poppel H, de Prijck L, Sylvester R, European Organisation for Research and Treatment of Cancer (EORTC) Genitourinary Group, et al. Radical nephrectomy plus interferon-alfa-based immunotherapy compared with interferon alfa alone in metastatic renal-cell carcinoma: a randomised trial. Lancet. 2001;358(9286):966–70.
20. Comen E, Norton L, Massague J. Clinical implications of cancer self-seeding. Nat Rev Clin Oncol. 2011;8(6):369–77. https://doi.org/10.1038/nrclinonc.2011.64.
21. Kaplan RN, Riba RD, Zacharoulis S, Bramley AH, Vincent L, Costa C, et al. VEGFR1-positive haematopoietic bone marrow progenitors initiate the pre-metastatic niche. Nature. 2005;438(7069):820–7. https://doi.org/10.1038/nature04186.
22. Psaila B, Lyden D. The metastatic niche: adapting the foreign soil. Nat Rev Cancer. 2009;9(4):285–93. https://doi.org/10.1038/nrc2621.
23. Kadmon D, Heston WD, Fair WR. Treatment of a metastatic prostate derived tumor with surgery and chemotherapy. J Urol. 1982;127(6):1238–42.
24. Dewan MZ, Galloway AE, Kawashima N, Dewyngaert JK, Babb JS, Formenti SC, et al. Fractionated but not single-dose radiotherapy induces an immune-mediated abscopal effect when combined with anti-CTLA-4 antibody. Clin Cancer Res. 2009;15(17):5379–88. https://doi.org/10.1158/1078-0432.CCR-09-0265.
25. Postow MA, Callahan MK, Barker CA, Yamada Y, Yuan J, Kitano S, et al. Immunologic correlates of the abscopal effect in a patient with melanoma. N Engl J Med. 2012;366(10):925–31. https://doi.org/10.1056/NEJMoa1112824.

26. Lock M, Muinuddin A, Kocha WI, Dinniwell R, Rodrigues G, D'Souza D. Abscopal effects: case report and emerging opportunities. Cureus. 2015;7(10):e344. https://doi.org/10.7759/cureus.344.
27. Shiraishi K, Ishiwata Y, Nakagawa K, Yokochi S, Taruki C, Akuta T, et al. Enhancement of antitumor radiation efficacy and consistent induction of the abscopal effect in mice by ECI301, an active variant of macrophage inflammatory protein-1alpha. Clin Cancer Res. 2008;14(4):1159–66. https://doi.org/10.1158/1078-0432.CCR-07-4485.
28. Nesslinger NJ, Sahota RA, Stone B, Johnson K, Chima N, King C, et al. Standard treatments induce antigen-specific immune responses in prostate cancer. Clin Cancer Res. 2007;13(5):1493–502. https://doi.org/10.1158/1078-0432.CCR-06-1772.
29. D'Amico AV, Manola J, Loffredo M, Renshaw AA, DellaCroce A, Kantoff PW. 6-month androgen suppression plus radiation therapy vs radiation therapy alone for patients with clinically localized prostate cancer: a randomized controlled trial. JAMA. 2004;292(7):821–7. https://doi.org/10.1001/jama.292.7.821.
30. Roach M 3rd, Bae K, Speight J, Wolkov HB, Rubin P, Lee RJ, et al. Short-term neoadjuvant androgen deprivation therapy and external-beam radiotherapy for locally advanced prostate cancer: long-term results of RTOG 8610. J Clin Oncol. 2008;26(4):585–91. https://doi.org/10.1200/JCO.2007.13.9881.
31. Denham JW, Steigler A, Lamb DS, Joseph D, Turner S, Matthews J, et al. Short-term neoadjuvant androgen deprivation and radiotherapy for locally advanced prostate cancer: 10-year data from the TROG 96.01 randomised trial. Lancet Oncol. 2011;12(5):451–9. https://doi.org/10.1016/S1470-2045(11)70063-8.
32. Aus G, Abrahamsson PA, Ahlgren G, Hugosson J, Lundberg S, Schain M, et al. Three-month neoadjuvant hormonal therapy before radical prostatectomy: a 7-year follow-up of a randomized controlled trial. BJU Int. 2002;90(6):561–6.
33. Soloway MS, Pareek K, Sharifi R, Wajsman Z, McLeod D, Wood DP Jr, et al. Neoadjuvant androgen ablation before radical prostatectomy in cT2bNxMo prostate cancer: 5-year results. J Urol. 2002;167(1):112–6.
34. Friedlander JI, Duty BD, Okeke Z, Smith AD. Obstructive uropathy from locally advanced and metastatic prostate cancer: an old problem with new therapies. J Endourol. 2012;26(2):102–9. https://doi.org/10.1089/end.2011.0227.
35. Qin XJ, Ma CG, Ye DW, Yao XD, Zhang SL, Dai B, et al. Tumor cytoreduction results in better response to androgen ablation: a preliminary report of palliative transurethral resection of the prostate in metastatic hormone sensitive prostate cancer. Urol Oncol. 2012;30(2):145–9. https://doi.org/10.1016/j.urolonc.2010.02.010.
36. Levine ES, Cisek VJ, Mulvihill MN, Cohen EL. Role of transurethral resection in dissemination of cancer of prostate. Urology. 1986;28(3):179–83.
37. Tabata K, Satoh T, Tsumura H, Ishii D, Fujita T, Matsumoto K, et al. Radiotherapy for prostate in men with metastatic prostate cancer: a propensity-score matching analysis. Paper presented at the 111th Annual Meeting of the American Urological Association; 2016.
38. Oefelein MG. Prognostic significance of obstructive uropathy in advanced prostate cancer. Urology. 2004;63(6):1117–21. https://doi.org/10.1016/j.urology.2004.01.026.
39. Grimm MO, Kamphausen S, Hugenschmidt H, Stephan-Odenthal M, Ackermann R, Vogeli TA. Clinical outcome of patients with lymph node positive prostate cancer after radical prostatectomy versus androgen deprivation. Eur Urol. 2002;41(6):628–34; discussion 34
40. Schmeller N, Lubos W. Early endocrine therapy versus radical prostatectomy combined with early endocrine therapy for stage D1 prostate cancer. Br J Urol. 1997;79(2):226–34.
41. Parker CC, Sydes MR, Mason MD, Clarke NW, Aebersold D, de Bono JS, et al. Prostate radiotherapy for men with metastatic disease: a new comparison in the Systemic Therapy in Advancing or Metastatic Prostate Cancer: Evaluation of Drug Efficacy (STAMPEDE) trial. BJU Int. 2013;111(5):697–9. https://doi.org/10.1111/bju.12087.

Oxidative Stress and Castration-Resistant Prostate Cancer

21

Masaki Shiota

Abstract

Androgen deprivation therapy can induce oxidative stress by increasing reactive oxygen species levels and/or decreasing cellular antioxidant capacity, which in turn cause genetic and epigenetic effects in prostate cancer. Oxidative stress increases androgen receptor (AR) activation through several possible mechanisms, including AR overexpression, AR activation by co-regulators and intracellular signal transduction pathways, mutation of AR and AR-related proteins, expression of AR splice variants, de novo androgen synthesis, and changes in non-AR signaling. Alterations in AR and non-AR signaling appear to have pro-survival and anti-apoptotic effects on prostate cancer cells, resulting in the development of castration-resistant prostate cancer. Thus, antioxidant therapy could be a promising strategy for the treatment of prostate cancer. Oxidative stress also influences the activity of several prostate cancer therapies, such as taxanes, radiotherapy, and AR-targeting agents. Taken together, these observations suggest that oxidative stress-induced AR signaling is a critical resistance factor and a crucial target for prostate cancer treatment.

Keywords

Androgen deprivation therapy · Androgen receptor · Castration-resistant prostate cancer · Oxidative stress · Reactive oxygen species

M. Shiota, M.D., Ph.D.
Department of Urology, Graduate School of Medical Sciences, Kyushu University, Fukuoka, Japan
e-mail: shiota@uro.med.kyushu-u.ac.jp

21.1 Introduction

Reactive oxygen species (ROS), which include superoxide (O_2^-), hydrogen peroxide (H_2O_2), and hydroxyl radicals (HO·), are produced by the partial reduction of oxygen and are generated endogenously mainly during mitochondrial oxidative phosphorylation and exogenously predominantly from xenobiotic compounds. ROS levels are controlled through the activity of endogenous antioxidant defense systems such as superoxide dismutase (SOD), catalase, and peroxiredoxin, as well as through exogenous antioxidants such as isoflavones, catechins, carotenes, vitamins, and selenium [1]. Oxidative stress occurs when the cellular antioxidant defense systems are overwhelmed by an increase in ROS levels or a decrease in the antioxidant capacity. Excessive ROS levels lead to damage of macromolecules such as DNA, RNA, proteins, and lipids, which is in part rescued by the DNA repair system and the thioredoxin and glutathione detoxification systems [2]. Damage to DNA can cause genetic aberrations, such as mutations and chromosomal rearrangements, while damage to other molecules can affect epigenetic processes, largely through dysregulation of proteins containing redox-reactive cysteine residues. Oxidation of cysteine produces reactive sulfenic acid (–SOH), which forms disulfide bonds with nearby cysteine residues (–S–S–) or undergoes further oxidation to sulfinic (–SO_2H) or sulfonic (–SO_3H) acids. With the exception of –SO_3H formation, each of these redox modifications can be reversed by reducing systems [3]. These oxidative modifications of cysteines alter the protein structure and function, thereby directly or indirectly affecting a range of events, including intracellular signal transduction and gene expression pathways that modulate various cellular processes (Fig. 21.1) [4].

Oxidative stress not only plays an important role in prostate carcinogenesis and progression of prostate cancer [5–7] but also is involved in the resistance of prostate cancer to therapy, especially androgen deprivation therapy (ADT) [1, 7, 8]. ADT, which consists of surgical or pharmacological castration or anti-androgen therapy, has been commonly used for the treatment of advanced or recurrent prostate cancer

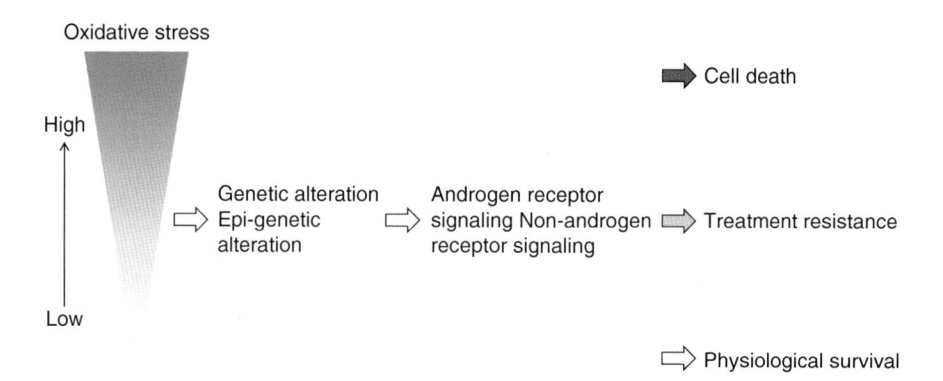

Fig. 21.1 Relationship between treatment resistance and oxidative stress

since 1941 [9]. Although ADT is initially effective for most prostate cancer patients, therapy resistance invariably develops and the disease becomes lethal castration-resistant prostate cancer (CRPC). Increasing evidence suggests the existence of functional cross talk between oxidative stress and CRPC. Here, we summarize our current knowledge in this area.

21.2 Oxidative Stress Induced by ADT in Prostate Cancer

Several experiments in vitro and in vivo have indicated that castration leads to oxidative stress by promoting increased ROS production and decreased ROS-detoxifying enzyme activity [10–13]. However, there are also several conflicting studies showing that androgens can induce oxidative stress [14, 15]. This discrepancy may be due to differences in the physiological and nonphysiological conditions in the various studies (Fig. 21.2). For example, Ripple et al. demonstrated that oxidative stress was decreased or increased by physiological or excessive androgen levels, respectively, suggesting that stress can be induced nonspecifically under nonphysiological conditions [16]. Several molecular mechanisms may be responsible for castration-induced oxidative stress, as shown by a reduction in the antioxidant molecules thioredoxin 1, peroxiredoxin 5, and SOD2 in rats after castration [11], a reduction in SOD2 in human prostate cancer tissue after ADT [10], and upregulation of pro-oxidant nicotinamide adenine dinucleotide phosphate oxidases (Noxs) in rat prostate after castration [13]. Collectively, these studies suggest that epigenetic alterations in gene expression and protein function lead to a redox imbalance and induction of oxidative stress in prostate cancer; this is supported by the finding of elevated oxidative stress levels in prostate cancer cells and surgically resected prostate cancer tissues [8, 17]. Thus, ADT-induced oxidative stress can lead to wide-ranging genetic and epigenetic alterations in prostate cancer, as described in more depth in the following sections.

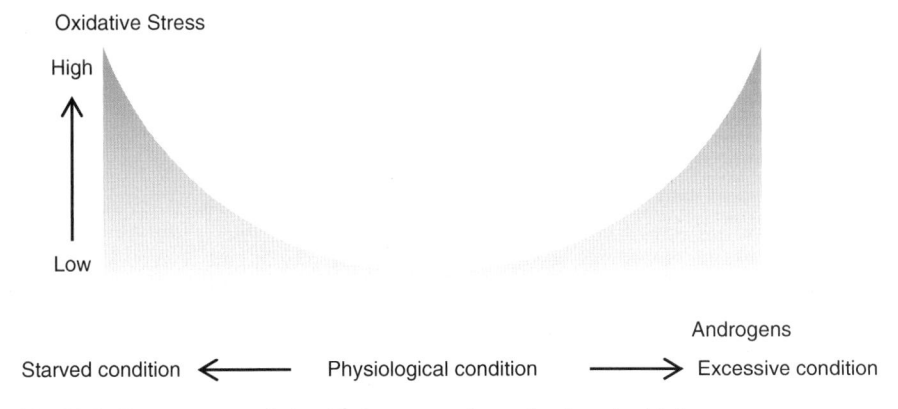

Fig. 21.2 Dose-response relationship between androgen levels and oxidative stress

21.3 Effects of Oxidative Stress on AR and Non-AR Signaling

21.3.1 Effects of Oxidative Stress on AR Signaling

In CRPC, AR signaling is aberrantly augmented by the low androgen milieu via a number of mechanisms, including AR overexpression, AR activation by co-regulators and intracellular signal transduction pathways, mutation of AR and AR-related proteins, expression of AR splice variants, and de novo androgen synthesis. Over the last decade, ADT-induced oxidative stress has been shown to influence AR signaling in prostate cancer. Sharifi et al. showed that suppression of the antioxidant enzyme SOD2 and increased ROS production activated AR signaling through changes in the expression of genes related to steroid metabolism, nuclear receptor co-regulators, and interleukin-6 receptor [7]. We also independently found that ROS play a crucial role in AR signaling and the development of CRPC [1, 8]. Thus, oxidative stress could contribute to castration resistance through AR reactivation by several mechanisms.

21.3.1.1 AR Overexpression

AR overexpression is thought to be a major cause of CRPC [18]. Indeed, many studies have shown that CRPC progression is associated with increased AR expression [19–22], which may be attributed to gene amplification, increased transcription and translation, and decreased degradation. Among these, transcriptional upregulation is a particularly important mechanism of increased AR expression. As we summarized previously [1, 18], several transcription factors activated by oxidative stress, including Twist1 [8], YB-1 [23], NF-κB [24], Sp1 [25, 26], Myc [27, 28], CREB [29], and Foxo3a [30], are also known to regulate AR expression, suggesting that ADT-induced oxidative stress may act through these factors to upregulate AR transcription [8].

Many other molecules have also been reported to be involved in regulating AR expression. For example, a pathway linked to 12-hydroxyeicosatetraenoic acid and leukotriene B4 receptor 2 was shown to increase ROS production and upregulate AR expression via the Nox4 pathway [31]. Conversely, treatment with diphenyleneiodonium chloride, an antioxidant that inhibits Nox-mediated ROS production, reduced AR expression via SREBP-1 [32]. The oxidative stress inducers cadmium and zinc chloride increase AR expression in dysplastic prostate glands of rats [33], while the synthetic antimicrobial chemical mequindox induces oxidative stress and AR overexpression in rat testes [34]. Paradoxically, other inducers of oxidative stress, such as a curcumin analog [35] and thymoquinone [36], were reported to suppress AR expression. However, these agents may act through non-redox signaling since the effects were poorly suppressed by the antioxidant N-acetyl cysteine (NAC), an electrophile that supports the production of a major intracellular antioxidant, glutathione.

Collectively, these data suggest that oxidative stress induced by internal and external stimuli induces AR overexpression through stress-induced transcription factors and other pathways.

21.3.1.2 AR Activation by Co-regulators and Intracellular Signal Transduction Pathways

The transcriptional activity of AR is modulated by co-regulators [37], several of which, including peroxiredoxin, Hsp27, and EGR-1, are activated by oxidative stress [1]. We previously showed that cysteine residues in peroxiredoxin are critical for its AR co-regulatory function [1], supporting the possibility that ROS-mediated modification of AR co-regulators affects AR signaling.

In addition, several intracellular signaling pathways play a role in AR transactivation. AR function can be augmented by growth factors and cytokines such as insulin-like growth factor, fibroblast growth factor, epidermal growth factor, and IL-6, as well as key components of their downstream signaling pathways, such as mitogen-activated protein kinase (MAPK), JAK/STAT, protein kinase A, phosphatidylinositol-3-kinase (PI3K)/Akt, and protein kinase C, which may itself be activated by oxidative stress [1]. In fact, we have shown that the ε isoform of protein kinase C increases AR expression through NF-κB signaling and contributes to cellular resistance to castration [38, 39]. Thus, oxidative stress also influences intracellular signaling pathways that interact with transcription factors and co-regulators to modulate AR activity.

21.3.1.3 Mutation of AR-Related Proteins and Generation of AR Splice Variants

Mutations in the *AR* gene have been shown to change the protein's ligand-binding affinity, permitting activation by non-cognate steroids and even by anti-androgen agents [6, 40, 41]. Although oxidative stress induces mutations in DNA, it is not yet known whether the *AR* gene is affected [6]. However, mutations in genes related to AR signaling, including FASN, CYP11B1, HSD17B4 (androgen metabolism), NCOR1, and FOXOA1 (AR cofactors), have been detected in CRPC tissues [42, 43]. Such mutations, probably induced by oxidative stress, may contribute to the development of CRPC through aberrant activation of AR signaling.

Several splice variants of AR exhibit transcriptional activity in the absence of androgen and play a key role in promoting CRPC [44–48]. Although possible, a relationship between expression of the AR splice variants and oxidative stress has not yet been documented. However, we recently reported that the redox-sensitive nuclear factor YB-1 [49] and its upstream kinase RSK [50] regulate the expression of an AR variant [51], supporting a direct link. Based on these intriguing observations, further studies of the effects of oxidative stress on mutation of the *AR* gene and expression of AR splice variants are warranted.

21.3.1.4 De Novo Androgen Synthesis

De novo synthesis of androgens in the adrenal glands and prostate tumors has been recognized as a potential cause of CRPC [52–54], and this was confirmed by clinical trials of abiraterone acetate, an inhibitor of a critical enzyme in androgen biosynthesis, cytochrome P17 (CYP17) [55, 56]. H_2O_2 regulates androgen synthesis in rat Leydig cells in a biphasic manner, indicating that physiological levels of oxidative stress promote steroidogenesis [57]. Nevertheless, there is no direct evidence at present for the existence of a relationship between oxidative stress and de novo androgen synthesis.

21.3.2 Effects of Oxidative Stress on Non-AR Signaling

In addition to AR signaling, numerous non-AR signaling pathways are activated by oxidative stress and many have been reported to be involved in the development to CRPC through genetic and epigenetic mechanisms. The genotoxic effects of oxidative stress include aberrations such as DNA point mutations and chromosomal rearrangements. In fact, genetic alterations in non-AR signaling molecules, such as PIK3CA, SPOP, RET, RICTOR, and CTNNB1, have been identified in tissues from patients with CRPC [42, 43, 58, 59].

Oxidative stress also causes epigenetic alterations that activate signaling independently of the AR [60]. For example, in prostate cancer, oxidative stress activates PI3K/Akt [61] and MAPK [62] and elevates the transcriptional activity of NF-κB [63], which promotes survival and inhibits apoptosis. However, many components of these pathways are also involved in AR signaling and show elevated activity in CRPC cells and tissues, as is the case for PI3K/Akt [64], MAPK [65], and NF-κB [66]. Additional non-AR-related mechanisms that contribute to the development of CRPC include inflammation, epithelial–mesenchymal transition, and cancer stem-like characteristics of prostate cancer cells [67]. Intriguingly, these phenomena are also affected by oxidative stress, further supporting the multiple mechanisms through which oxidative stress is involved in CRPC development.

21.4 Oxidative Stress and the Development of CRPC

As described above, the mutual link between oxidative stress and AR signaling supports a role for oxidative stress in CRPC development; indeed, there is direct evidence of such a relationship. We chronically exposed LNCaP, an androgen-dependent prostate cancer cell line, to oxidative stress to generate H_2O_2-resistant sublines, and found that they expressed increased levels of AR mRNA and protein and exhibited a castration-resistant phenotype [8]. Whereas castration-resistant cells normally exhibit elevated antioxidant protein levels [70, 71] and ROS-scavenging activity [72], overexpression of AR in such cells increases oxidative stress, as indicated by higher intracellular ROS levels [68, 69].

A connection between oxidative stress and CRPC is also supported by clinical findings. Compared with prostate specimens from patients who had undergone radical prostatectomy without ADT, prostate cancer tissues obtained from patients post-ADT show increased 4-hydroxy-2-nonenal levels, indicative of elevated oxidative stress [17]. In addition, a genetic polymorphism in the *GSTM3* gene, which encodes an antioxidant enzyme glutathione S-transferase, was recently reported to be associated with increased risk of progression of metastatic prostate cancer to CRPC, which was validated in nonmetastatic prostate cancer [69].

Collectively, these experimental and clinical data are consistent with a close link between oxidative stress and progression to CRPC.

21.5 Clinical Implications of Antioxidant Therapy in CRPC

Given the accumulating evidence that oxidative stress contributes to CRPC, it has been speculated that antioxidant therapy could have therapeutic effects in prostate cancer patients receiving ADT.

Various naturally occurring antioxidative compounds, including isoflavones, catechins, carotenes, vitamins, and selenium, have been investigated as possible prophylactic agents for prostate carcinogenesis and as therapeutic agents for prostate cancer [73, 74]. Among these compounds, the carotenoid lycopene was shown to prevent oxidative damage to proteins, lipids, and DNA. In a preclinical study, lycopene suppressed AR activity and had antitumor effects [75]. In clinical studies, lycopene augmented the therapeutic effects of orchiectomy in advanced prostate cancer patients [76]. A phase II study showed that administration of lycopene at 10 mg per day suppressed elevation of prostate-specific antigen (PSA) in 41 men with prostate cancer [75]. In addition, a case report of a CRPC patient described a reduction in serum PSA levels and disease-associated symptoms after intake of saw palmetto and lycopene supplements [77]. Although the number of patients in these clinical studies was small, the findings support the potential use of lycopene combined with castration in the treatment of prostate cancer, including CRPC. The antioxidants vitamin E and α-tocopherol have also been reported to decrease the risk of prostate cancer mortality, suggesting that they may prevent disease progression [78].

In addition to naturally occurring compounds, synthetic antioxidants might also be useful for the treatment of prostate cancer. In the TRAMP mouse model of prostate cancer, NAC administration reduced 8-hydroxy-2'-deoxyguanosine, nitrotyrosine, and 4-hydroxy-2-nonenal levels in the prostate [79]. In addition, we previously showed that NAC reduced AR expression and that NAC plus ADT successfully suppressed tumor growth in a mouse xenograft model of prostate cancer [17]. SOD mimetics have been shown to reduce oxidative stress, reduce the expression of AR and AR splice variants, and have a therapeutic effect in prostate cancer cells [80]. Finally, the anti-angiogenic agent endostatin inhibits CRPC growth by augmenting antioxidant enzyme activity and suppressing ROS levels [81].

An alternative therapeutic strategy to counter oxidative stress in CRPC is inhibition of ROS production. In support of this, the Nox inhibitor diphenyleneiodonium decreases the viability of prostate cancer cells, including LNCaP cells [82] and another Nox inhibitor, apocynin, suppresses prostate cancer cell invasion [83].

These observations highlight several options for antioxidant therapy, including natural and synthetic antioxidants and ROS inhibitors. However, a critical obstacle for the clinical use of antioxidants is their rapid oxidative degradation under physiological conditions, resulting in poor stability and bioavailability. One potential solution to this problem might be to encapsulate the antioxidant compounds in nanoparticles that also act as oxygen radical scavengers. For example, it was recently reported that curcumin-loaded pH-sensitive redox nanoparticles exert excellent antitumor activity in prostate cancer [84].

21.6 Novel Agents for CRPC and Oxidative Stress

Taxanes such as docetaxel and cabazitaxel, AR-targeting agents such as abiraterone acetate and enzalutamide, and the radiopharmaceutical radium-223 all show benefit in prolonging progression-free and overall survival and have been approved globally for use in CRPC [37, 85].

Similar to other cytotoxic anticancer agents, taxanes have been shown to cause oxidative stress in cancer cells [86]. Moreover, many molecules implicated in oxidative stress signaling, including PI3K/Akt [87], MAPK [88], and NF-κB [89], and their downstream effectors such as Twist1 [90] and YB-1 [91, 92], are all involved in the resistance of prostate cancer to taxanes. In addition, the status of TMPRSS2-ERG fusion gene caused by inflammation-induced oxidative stress through DNA breaks [93] was reported to be associated with the therapeutic effect of taxanes [94, 95]. Thus, oxidative stress appears to contribute to taxane resistance in prostate cancer through various mechanisms.

Radiation is known to induce oxidative stress in prostate cancer [96]; however, this is not necessarily beneficial because irradiation-induced oxidative stress can activate pro-survival and anti-apoptotic signaling through molecules such as PI3K/Akt [97], MAPK [98], and NF-κB [99], resulting in resistance to irradiation. Radium-223 is an α particle-emitting isotope [100] and appears to induce oxidative stress in prostate cancer cells. Although the therapeutic effect of this isotope may be affected by oxidative stress-induced signaling, there is currently no direct evidence for this.

Little is known about the interaction between oxidative stress and AR-targeting agents, including abiraterone acetate and enzalutamide. However, oxidative stress levels are increased in enzalutamide-resistant prostate cancer cells established in vitro [69], warranting further investigation. Clinical trials have been initiated for several additional promising agents, including immune checkpoint inhibitors and the poly (ADP-ribose) polymerase inhibitor olaparib. To those agents, biomarkers such as the presence of somatic mutations in DNA repair genes and the number of missense somatic mutations which may be caused by oxidative stress are postulated, and then oxidative stress may commit to the sensitivity to those emerging agents.

21.7 Conclusions and Future Directions

Oxidative stress induced by ADT can activate both AR and non-AR signaling, resulting in the acquisition of castration resistance. Treatment-induced oxidative stress also appears to be involved in the resistance of prostate cancer to therapy. Thus, oxidative stress is a critical resistance factor and a crucial target for prostate cancer treatment. Suppression of oxidative stress signaling by antioxidants or inhibitors of ROS production may thus be a promising strategy to overcome treatment resistance in prostate cancer. However, the relationship between oxidative stress and CRPC is a vast and underexplored area of research, and further investigation is warranted. Such studies will undoubtedly lead to some remarkable discoveries.

References

1. Shiota M, Yokomizo A, Naito S. Oxidative stress and androgen receptor signaling in the development and progression of castration-resistant prostate cancer. Free Radic Biol Med. 2011;51:1320–8. https://doi.org/10.1016/j.freeradbiomed.2011.07.011.
2. Trachootham D, Alexandre J, Huang P. Targeting cancer cells by ROS-mediated mechanisms: a radical therapeutic approach? Nat Rev. Drug Discov. 2009;8:579–91. https://doi.org/10.1038/nrd2803.
3. Roos G, Messens J. Protein sulfenic acid formation: from cellular damage to redox regulation. Free Radic Biol Med. 2011;51:314–26. https://doi.org/10.1016/j.freeradbiomed.2011.04.031.
4. Ray PD, Huang BW, Tsuji Y. Reactive oxygen species (ROS) homeostasis and redox regulation in cellular signaling. Cell Signal. 2012;24:981–90. https://doi.org/10.1016/j.cellsig.2012.01.008.
5. Bostwick DG, Alexander EE, Singh R, Shan A, Qian J, Santella RM, et al. Antioxidant enzyme expression and reactive oxygen species damage in prostatic intraepithelial neoplasia and cancer. Cancer. 2000;89:123–34.
6. Khandrika L, Kumar B, Koul S, Maroni P, Koul HK. Oxidative stress in prostate cancer. Cancer Lett. 2009;282:125–36. https://doi.org/10.1016/j.canlet.2008.12.011.
7. Sharifi N, Hurt EM, Thomas SB, Farrar WL. Effects of manganese superoxide dismutase silencing on androgen receptor function and gene regulation: implications for castration-resistant prostate cancer. Clin Cancer Res. 2008;14:6073–80. https://doi.org/10.1158/1078-0432.CCR-08-0591.
8. Shiota M, Yokomizo A, Tada Y, Inokuchi J, Kashiwagi E, Masubuchi D, et al. Castration resistance of prostate cancer cells caused by castration-induced oxidative stress through Twist1 and androgen receptor overexpression. Oncogene. 2010;29:237–50. https://doi.org/10.1038/onc.2009.322.
9. Miyamoto H, Messing EM, Chang C. Androgen deprivation therapy for prostate cancer: current status and future prospects. Prostate. 2004;61:332–53. https://doi.org/10.1002/pros.20115.
10. Best CJ, Gillespie JW, Yi Y, Chandramouli GV, Perlmutter MA, Gathright Y, et al. Molecular alterations in primary prostate cancer after androgen ablation therapy. Clin Cancer Res. 2005;11:6823–34. https://doi.org/10.1158/1078-0432.CCR-05-0585.
11. Pang ST, Dillner K, Wu X, Pousette A, Norstedt G, Flores-Morales A. Gene expression profiling of androgen deficiency predicts a pathway of prostate apoptosis that involves genes related to oxidative stress. Endocrinology. 2002;143:4897–906. https://doi.org/10.1210/en.2002-220327.
12. Shan W, Zhong W, Zhao R, Oberley TD. Thioredoxin 1 as a subcellular biomarker of redox imbalance in human prostate cancer progression. Free Radic Biol Med. 2010;49:2078–87. https://doi.org/10.1016/j.freeradbiomed.2010.10.691.
13. Tam NN, Gao Y, Leung YK, Ho SM. Androgenic regulation of oxidative stress in the rat prostate: involvement of NAD(P)H oxidases and antioxidant defense machinery during prostatic involution and regrowth. Am J Pathol. 2003;163:2513–22. https://doi.org/10.1016/S0002-9440(10)63606-1.
14. Pathak S, Singh R, Verschoyle RD, Greaves P, Farmer PB, Steward WP, et al. Androgen manipulation alters oxidative DNA adduct levels in androgen-sensitive prostate cancer cells grown in vitro and in vivo. Cancer Lett. 2008;261:74–83. https://doi.org/10.1016/j.canlet.2007.11.015.
15. Pinthus JH, Bryskin I, Trachtenberg J, Lu JP, Singh G, Fridman E, et al. Androgen induces adaptation to oxidative stress in prostate cancer: implications for treatment with radiation therapy. Neoplasia. 2007;9:68–80.
16. Ripple MO, Henry WF, Rago RP, Wilding G. Prooxidant-antioxidant shift induced by androgen treatment of human prostate carcinoma cells. J Natl Cancer Inst. 1997;89:40–8.
17. Shiota M, Song Y, Takeuchi A, Yokomizo A, Kashiwagi E, Kuroiwa K, et al. Antioxidant therapy alleviates oxidative stress by androgen deprivation and prevents conversion from

androgen dependent to castration resistant prostate cancer. J Urol. 2012;187:707–14. https://doi.org/10.1016/j.juro.2011.09.147.
18. Shiota M, Yokomizo A, Naito S. Increased androgen receptor transcription: a cause of castration-resistant prostate cancer and a possible therapeutic target. J Mol Endocrinol. 2011;47:R25–41. https://doi.org/10.1530/JME-11-0018.
19. Chen CD, Welsbie DS, Tran C, Baek SH, Chen R, Vessella R, et al. Molecular determinants of resistance to antiandrogen therapy. Nat Med. 2004;10:33–9. https://doi.org/10.1038/nm972.
20. Gregory CW, Hamil KG, Kim D, Hall SH, Pretlow TG, Mohler JL, et al. Androgen receptor expression in androgen-independent prostate cancer is associated with increased expression of androgen-regulated genes. Cancer Res. 1998;58:5718–24.
21. Scher HI, Sawyers CL. Biology of progressive, castration-resistant prostate cancer: directed therapies targeting the androgen-receptor signaling axis. J Clin Oncol. 2005;23:8253–61. https://doi.org/10.1200/JCO.2005.03.4777.
22. Zegarra-Moro OL, Schmidt LJ, Huang H, Tindall DJ. Disruption of androgen receptor function inhibits proliferation of androgen-refractory prostate cancer cells. Cancer Res. 2002;62:1008–13.
23. Shiota M, Takeuchi A, Song Y, Yokomizo A, Kashiwagi E, Uchiumi T, et al. Y-box binding protein-1 promotes castration-resistant prostate cancer growth via androgen receptor expression. Endocr Relat Cancer. 2011;18:505–17. https://doi.org/10.1530/ERC-11-0017.
24. Zhang L, Altuwaijri S, Deng F, Chen L, Lal P, Bhanot UK, et al. NF-kappaB regulates androgen receptor expression and prostate cancer growth. Am J Pathol. 2009;175:489–99. https://doi.org/10.2353/ajpath.2009.080727.
25. Faber PW, van Rooij HC, Schipper HJ, Brinkmann AO, Trapman J. Two different, overlapping pathways of transcription initiation are active on the TATA-less human androgen receptor promoter. The role of Sp1. J Biol Chem. 1993;268:9296–301.
26. Yuan H, Gong A, Young CY. Involvement of transcription factor Sp1 in quercetin-mediated inhibitory effect on the androgen receptor in human prostate cancer cells. Carcinogenesis. 2005;26:793–801. https://doi.org/10.1093/carcin/bgi021.
27. Grad JM, Dai JL, Wu S, Burnstein KL. Multiple androgen response elements and a Myc consensus site in the androgen receptor (AR) coding region are involved in androgen-mediated up-regulation of AR messenger RNA. Mol Endocrinol. 1999;13:1896–911.
28. Lee JG, Zheng R, McCafferty-Cepero JM, Burnstein KL, Nanus DM, Shen R. Endothelin-1 enhances the expression of the androgen receptor via activation of the c-myc pathway in prostate cancer cells. Mol Carcinog. 2009;48:141–9. https://doi.org/10.1002/mc.20462.
29. Mizokami A, Yeh SY, Chang C. Identification of 3′,5′-cyclic adenosine monophosphate response element and other cis-acting elements in the human androgen receptor gene promoter. Mol Endocrinol. 1994;8:77–88.
30. Yang L, Xie S, Jamaluddin MS, Altuwaijri S, Ni J, Kim E, et al. Induction of androgen receptor expression by phosphatidylinositol 3-kinase/Akt downstream substrate, FOXO3a, and their roles in apoptosis of LNCaP prostate cancer cells. J Biol Chem. 2005;280:33558–65. https://doi.org/10.1074/jbc.M504461200.
31. Lee JW, Kim GY, Kim JH. Androgen receptor is up-regulated by a BLT2-linked pathway to contribute to prostate cancer progression. Biochem Biophys Res Commun. 2012;420:428–33. https://doi.org/10.1016/j.bbrc.2012.03.012.
32. Huang WC, Li X, Liu J, Lin J, Chung LW. Activation of androgen receptor, lipogenesis, and oxidative stress converged by SREBP-1 is responsible for regulating growth and progression of prostate cancer cells. Mol Cancer Res. 2012;10:133–42. https://doi.org/10.1158/1541-7786.MCR-11-0206.
33. Arriazu R, Pozuelo JM, Martín R, Rodríguez R, Santamaría L. Quantitative and immunohistochemical evaluation of PCNA, androgen receptors, apoptosis, and Glutathione-S-Transferase P1 on preneoplastic changes induced by cadmium and zinc chloride in the rat ventral prostate. Prostate. 2005;63:347–57. https://doi.org/10.1002/pros.20192.

34. Ihsan A, Wang X, Liu Z, Wang Y, Huang X, Liu Y, et al. Long-term mequindox treatment induced endocrine and reproductive toxicity via oxidative stress in male Wistar rats. Toxicol Appl Pharmacol. 2011;252:281–8. https://doi.org/10.1016/j.taap.2011.02.020.
35. Fajardo AM, MacKenzie DA, Ji M, Deck LM, Vander Jagt DL, Thompson TA, et al. The curcumin analog ca27 down-regulates androgen receptor through an oxidative stress mediated mechanism in human prostate cancer cells. Prostate. 2012;72:612–25. https://doi.org/10.1002/pros.21464.
36. Koka PS, Mondal D, Schultz M, Abdel-Mageed AB, Agrawal KC. Studies on molecular mechanisms of growth inhibitory effects of thymoquinone against prostate cancer cells: role of reactive oxygen species. Exp Biol Med. 2010;235:751–60. https://doi.org/10.1258/ebm.2010.009369.
37. Shiota M, Yokomizo A, Fujimoto N, Naito S. Androgen receptor cofactors in prostate cancer: potential therapeutic targets of castration-resistant prostate cancer. Curr Cancer Drug Targets. 2011;11:870–81. https://doi.org/10.2174/156800911796798904.
38. Shiota M, Yokomizo A, Takeuchi A, Imada K, Kashiwagi E, Song Y, et al. Inhibition of protein kinase C/Twist1 signaling augments anticancer effects of androgen deprivation and enzalutamide in prostate cancer. Clin Cancer Res. 2014;20:951–61. https://doi.org/10.1158/1078-0432.CCR-13-1809.
39. Shiota M, Yokomizo A, Takeuchi A, Kashiwagi E, Dejima T, Inokuchi J, et al. Protein kinase C regulates Twist1 expression via NF-κB in prostate cancer. Endocr Relat Cancer. 2017. https://doi.org/10.1530/ERC-16-0384.
40. Brooke GN, Bevan CL. The role of androgen receptor mutations in prostate cancer progression. Curr Genomics. 2009;10:18–25. https://doi.org/10.2174/138920209787581307.
41. Azad AA, Volik SV, Wyatt AW, Haegert A, Le Bihan S, Bell RH, et al. Androgen receptor gene aberrations in circulating cell-free DNA: biomarkers of therapeutic resistance in castration-resistant prostate cancer. Clin Cancer Res. 2015;21:2315–24. https://doi.org/10.1158/1078-0432.CCR-14-2666.
42. Grasso CS, Wu YM, Robinson DR, Cao X, Dhanasekaran SM, Khan AP, et al. The mutational landscape of lethal castration-resistant prostate cancer. Nature. 2012;487:239–43. https://doi.org/10.1038/nature11125.
43. Robinson D, Van Allen EM, Wu YM, Schultz N, Lonigro RJ, Mosquera JM, et al. Integrative clinical genomics of advanced prostate cancer. Cell. 2015;161:1215–28. https://doi.org/10.1016/j.cell.2015.05.001.
44. Dehm SM, Schmidt LJ, Heemers HV, Vessella RL, Tindall DJ. Splicing of a novel androgen receptor exon generates a constitutively active androgen receptor that mediates prostate cancer therapy resistance. Cancer Res. 2008;68:5469–77. https://doi.org/10.1158/0008-5472.CAN-08-0594.
45. Hu R, Dunn TA, Wei S, Isharwal S, Veltri RW, Humphreys E, et al. Ligand-independent androgen receptor variants derived from splicing of cryptic exons signify hormone-refractory prostate cancer. Cancer Res. 2009;69:16–22. https://doi.org/10.1158/0008-5472.CAN-08-2764.
46. Guo Z, Yang X, Sun F, Jiang R, Linn DE, Chen H, et al. A novel androgen receptor splice variant is up-regulated during prostate cancer progression and promotes androgen depletion-resistant growth. Cancer Res. 2009;69:2305–13. https://doi.org/10.1158/0008-5472.CAN-08-3795.
47. Sun S, Sprenger CC, Vessella RL, Haugk K, Soriano K, Mostaghel EA, et al. Castration resistance in human prostate cancer is conferred by a frequently occurring androgen receptor splice variant. J Clin Invest. 2010;120:2715–30. https://doi.org/10.1172/JCI41824.
48. Watson PA, Chen YF, Balbas MD, Wongvipat J, Socci ND, Viale A, et al. Constitutively active androgen receptor splice variants expressed in castration-resistant prostate cancer require full-length androgen receptor. Proc Natl Acad Sci U S A. 2010;107:16759–65. https://doi.org/10.1073/pnas.1012443107.
49. Hayakawa H, Uchiumi T, Fukuda T, Ashizuka M, Kohno K, Kuwano M, et al. Binding capacity of human YB-1 protein for RNA containing 8-oxoguanine. Biochemistry. 2002;41:12739–44.

50. Siebel A, Cubillos-Rojas M, Santos RC, Schneider T, Bonan CD, Bartrons R, et al. Contribution of S6 K1/MAPK signaling pathways in the response to oxidative stress: activation of RSK and MSK by hydrogen peroxide. PLoS One. 2013;8:e75523. https://doi.org/10.1371/journal.pone.0075523.
51. Shiota M, Fujimoto N, Imada K, Yokomizo A, Itsumi M, Takeuchi A, et al. Potential role for YB-1 in castration-resistant prostate cancer and resistance to enzalutamide through the androgen receptor V7. J Natl Cancer Inst. 2016;108:djw005. https://doi.org/10.1093/jnci/djw005.
52. Locke JA, Guns ES, Lubik AA, Adomat HH, Hendy SC, Wood CA, et al. Androgen levels increase by intratumoral de novo steroidogenesis during progression of castration-resistant prostate cancer. Cancer Res. 2008;68(15):6407. https://doi.org/10.1158/0008-5472.CAN-07-5997.
53. Montgomery RB, Mostaghel EA, Vessella R, Hess DL, Kalhorn TF, Higano CS, et al. Maintenance of intratumoral androgens in metastatic prostate cancer: a mechanism for castration-resistant tumor growth. Cancer Res. 2008;68:4447–54. https://doi.org/10.1158/0008-5472.CAN-08-0249.
54. Stanbrough M, Bubley GJ, Ross K, Golub TR, Rubin MA, Penning TM, et al. Increased expression of genes converting adrenal androgens to testosterone in androgen-independent prostate cancer. Cancer Res. 2006;66:2815–25. https://doi.org/10.1158/0008-5472.CAN-05-4000.
55. de Bono JS, Logothetis CJ, Molina A, Fizazi K, North S, Chu L, et al. Abiraterone and increased survival in metastatic prostate cancer. N Engl J Med. 2011;364:1995–2005. https://doi.org/10.1056/NEJMoa1014618.
56. Ryan CJ, Smith MR, de Bono JS, Molina A, Logothetis CJ, de Souza P, et al. Abiraterone in metastatic prostate cancer without previous chemotherapy. N Engl J Med. 2013;368:138–48. https://doi.org/10.1056/NEJMoa1209096.
57. Zhao Y, Ao H, Chen L, Sottas CM, Ge RS, Li L, Zhang Y. Mono-(2-ethylhexyl) phthalate affects the steroidogenesis in rat Leydig cells through provoking ROS perturbation. Toxicol In Vitro. 2012;26:950–5. https://doi.org/10.1016/j.tiv.2012.04.003.
58. Beltran H, Yelensky R, Frampton GM, Park K, Downing SR, MacDonald TY, et al. Targeted next-generation sequencing of advanced prostate cancer identifies potential therapeutic targets and disease heterogeneity. Eur Urol. 2013;63:920–6. https://doi.org/10.1016/j.eururo.2012.08.053.
59. Beltran H, Prandi D, Mosquera JM, Benelli M, Puca L, Cyrta J, et al. Divergent clonal evolution of castration-resistant neuroendocrine prostate cancer. Nat Med. 2016;22:298–305. https://doi.org/10.1038/nm.4045.
60. Zhang Z, Hou X, Shao C, Li J, Cheng JX, Kuang S, et al. Plk1 inhibition enhances the efficacy of androgen signaling blockade in castration-resistant prostate cancer. Cancer Res. 2014;74:6635–47. https://doi.org/10.1158/0008-5472.CAN-14-1916.
61. Ning P, Zhong JG, Jiang F, Zhang Y, Zhao J, Tian F, et al. Role of protein S in castration-resistant prostate cancer-like cells. Endocr Relat Cancer. 2016;23:595–607. https://doi.org/10.1530/ERC-16-0126.
62. Kumar B, Koul S, Khandrika L, Meacham RB, Koul HK. Oxidative stress is inherent in prostate cancer cells and is required for aggressive phenotype. Cancer Res. 2008;68:1777–85. https://doi.org/10.1158/0008-5472.CAN-07-5259.
63. Zhang J, Johnston G, Stebler B, Keller ET. Hydrogen peroxide activates NFkappaB and the interleukin-6 promoter through NFκB-inducing kinase. Antioxid Redox Signal. 2001;3:493–504.
64. Chung S, Furihata M, Tamura K, Uemura M, Daigo Y, Nasu Y, et al. Overexpressing PKIB in prostate cancer promotes its aggressiveness by linking between PKA and Akt pathways. Oncogene. 2009;28:2849–59. https://doi.org/10.1038/onc.2009.144.
65. Mukherjee R, McGuinness DH, McCall P, Underwood MA, Seywright M, Orange C, et al. Upregulation of MAPK pathway is associated with survival in castrate-resistant prostate cancer. Br J Cancer. 2011;104:1920–8. https://doi.org/10.1038/bjc.2011.163.

66. McCall P, Bennett L, Ahmad I, Mackenzie LM, Forbes IW, Leung HY, et al. NFκB signalling is upregulated in a subset of castrate-resistant prostate cancer patients and correlates with disease progression. Br J Cancer. 2012;107:1554–63. https://doi.org/10.1038/bjc.2012.372.
67. Zong Y, Goldstein AS. Adaptation or selection--mechanisms of castration-resistant prostate cancer. Nat Rev. Urol. 2013;10:90–8. https://doi.org/10.1038/nrurol.2012.237.
68. Shigemura K, Sung SY, Kubo H, Arnold RS, Fujisawa M, Gotoh A, et al. Reactive oxygen species mediate androgen receptor- and serum starvation-elicited downstream signaling of ADAM9 expression in human prostate cancer cells. Prostate. 2007;67:722–31. https://doi.org/10.1002/pros.20565.
69. Shiota M, Fujimoto N, Itsumi M, Takeuchi A, Inokuchi J, Tatsugami K, et al. Gene polymorphisms in antioxidant enzymes correlate with the efficacy of androgen-deprivation therapy for prostate cancer with implications of oxidative stress. Ann Oncol. 2016. https://doi.org/10.1093/annonc/mdw646.
70. Kuruma H, Egawa S, Oh-Ishi M, Kodera Y, Satoh M, Chen W, et al. High molecular mass proteome of androgen-independent prostate cancer. Proteomics. 2005;5:1097–112. https://doi.org/10.1002/pmic.200401115.
71. Shiota M, Yokomizo A, Kashiwagi E, Takeuchi A, Fujimoto N, Uchiumi T, et al. Peroxiredoxin 2 in the nucleus and cytoplasm distinctly regulates androgen receptor activity in prostate cancer cells. Free Radic Biol Med. 2011;51:78–87. https://doi.org/10.1016/j.freeradbiomed.2011.04.001.
72. Wu CT, Chen WC, Liao SK, Hsu CL, Lee KD, Chen MF. The radiation response of hormone-resistant prostate cancer induced by long-term hormone therapy. Endocr Relat Cancer. 2007;14:633–43. https://doi.org/10.1677/ERC-07-0073.
73. Hori S, Butler E, McLoughlin J. Prostate cancer and diet: food for thought? BJU Int. 2011;107:1348–59. https://doi.org/10.1111/j.1464-410X.2010.09897.x.
74. Itsumi M, Shiota M, Takeuchi A, Kashiwagi E, Inokuchi J, Tatsugami K, et al. Equol inhibits prostate cancer growth through degradation of androgen receptor by S-phase kinase-associated protein 2. Cancer Sci. 2016;107:1022–8. https://doi.org/10.1111/cas.12948.
75. Zhang X, Wang Q, Neil B, Chen X. Effect of lycopene on androgen receptor and prostate-specific antigen velocity. Chin Med J. 2010;123:2231–6.
76. Ansari MS, Gupta NP. A comparison of lycopene and orchidectomy vs orchidectomy alone in the management of advanced prostate cancer. BJU Int. 2003;92:375–8.
77. Matlaga BR, Hall MC, Stindt D, Torti FM. Response of hormone refractory prostate cancer to lycopene. J Urol. 2001;166:613.
78. Watters JL, Gail MH, Weinstein SJ, Virtamo J, Albanes D. Associations between alpha-tocopherol, beta-carotene, and retinol and prostate cancer survival. Cancer Res. 2009;69:3833–41. https://doi.org/10.1158/0008-5472.CAN-08-4640.
79. Tam NN, Nyska A, Maronpot RR, Kissling G, Lomnitski L, Suttie A, et al. Differential attenuation of oxidative/nitrosative injuries in early prostatic neoplastic lesions in TRAMP mice by dietary antioxidants. Prostate. 2006;66:57–69. https://doi.org/10.1002/pros.20313.
80. Thomas R, Sharifi N. SOD mimetics: a novel class of androgen receptor inhibitors that suppresses castration-resistant growth of prostate cancer. Mol Cancer Ther. 2012;11:87–97. https://doi.org/10.1158/1535-7163.MCT-11-0540.
81. Lee JH, Kang M, Wang H, Naik G, Mobley JA, Sonpavde G, et al. Endostatin inhibits androgen-independent prostate cancer growth by suppressing nuclear receptor-mediated oxidative stress. FASEB J. 2017. https://doi.org/10.1096/fj.201601178R.
82. Chaiswing L, Bourdeau-Heller JM, Zhong W, Oberley TD. Characterization of redox state of two human prostate carcinoma cell lines with different degrees of aggressiveness. Free Radic Biol Med. 2007;43:202–15. https://doi.org/10.1016/j.freeradbiomed.2007.03.031.
83. Chaiswing L, Zhong W, Cullen JJ, Oberley LW, Oberley TD. Extracellular redox state regulates features associated with prostate cancer cell invasion. Cancer Res. 2008;68:5820–6. https://doi.org/10.1158/0008-5472.CAN-08-0162.

84. Thangavel S, Yoshitomi T, Sakharkar MK, Nagasaki Y. Redox nanoparticles inhibit curcumin oxidative degradation and enhance its therapeutic effect on prostate cancer. J Control Release. 2015;209:110–9. https://doi.org/10.1016/j.jconrel.2015.04.025.
85. Fujimoto N. Novel agents for castration-resistant prostate cancer: early experience and beyond. Int J Urol. 2016;23:114–21. https://doi.org/10.1111/iju.12907.
86. Bellezza I, Grottelli S, Gatticchi L, Mierla AL, Minelli A. α-Tocopheryl succinate pretreatment attenuates quinone toxicity in prostate cancer PC3 cells. Gene. 2014;539:1–7. https://doi.org/10.1016/j.gene.2014.02.009.
87. Kosaka T, Miyajima A, Shirotake S, Suzuki E, Kikuchi E, Oya M. Long-term androgen ablation and docetaxel up-regulate phosphorylated Akt in castration resistant prostate cancer. J Urol. 2011;185:2376–81. https://doi.org/10.1016/j.juro.2011.02.016.
88. Shiota M, Itsumi M, Yokomizo A, Takeuchi A, Imada K, Kashiwagi E, et al. Targeting ribosomal S6 kinases/Y-box binding protein-1 signaling improves cellular sensitivity to taxane in prostate cancer. Prostate. 2014;74:829–38. https://doi.org/10.1002/pros.22799.
89. Tantivejkul K, Loberg RD, Mawocha SC, Day LL, John LS, Pienta BA, et al. PAR1-mediated NFkappaB activation promotes survival of prostate cancer cells through a Bcl-xL-dependent mechanism. J Cell Biochem. 2005;96:641–52. https://doi.org/10.1002/jcb.20533.
90. Shiota M, Izumi H, Tanimoto A, Takahashi M, Miyamoto N, Kashiwagi E, et al. Programmed cell death protein 4 down-regulates Y-box binding protein-1 expression via a direct interaction with Twist1 to suppress cancer cell growth. Cancer Res. 2009;69:3148–56. https://doi.org/10.1158/0008-5472.CAN-08-2334.
91. Shiota M, Zoubeidi A, Kumano M, Beraldi E, Naito S, Nelson CC, et al. Clusterin is a critical downstream mediator of stress-induced YB-1 transactivation in prostate cancer. Mol Cancer Res. 2011;9:1755–66. https://doi.org/10.1158/1541-7786.MCR-11-0379.
92. Shiota M, Kashiwagi E, Yokomizo A, Takeuchi A, Dejima T, Song Y, et al. Interaction between docetaxel resistance and castration resistance in prostate cancer: implications of Twist1, YB-1, and androgen receptor. Prostate. 2013;73:1336–44. https://doi.org/10.1002/pros.22681.
93. Mani RS, Amin MA, Li X, Kalyana-Sundaram S, Veeneman BA, Wang L, et al. Inflammation-induced oxidative stress mediates gene fusion formation in prostate cancer. Cell Rep. 2016;17:2620–31. https://doi.org/10.1016/j.celrep.2016.11.019.
94. Galletti G, Matov A, Beltran H, Fontugne J, Miguel Mosquera J, Cheung C, et al. ERG induces taxane resistance in castration-resistant prostate cancer. Nat Commun. 2014;5:5548. https://doi.org/10.1038/ncomms6548.
95. Reig Ò, Marín-Aguilera M, Carrera G, Jiménez N, Paré L, García-Recio S, et al. TMPRSS2-ERG in blood and docetaxel resistance in metastatic castration-resistant prostate cancer. Eur Urol. 2016;70:709–13. https://doi.org/10.1016/j.eururo.2016.02.034.
96. Josson S, Xu Y, Fang F, Dhar SK, St Clair DK, St Clair WH. RelB regulates manganese superoxide dismutase gene and resistance to ionizing radiation of prostate cancer cells. Oncogene. 2006;25:1554–9. https://doi.org/10.1038/sj.onc.1209186.
97. Goldberg Z, Rocke DM, Schwietert C, Berglund SR, Santana A, Jones A, et al. Human in vivo dose-response to controlled, low-dose low linear energy transfer ionizing radiation exposure. Clin Cancer Res. 2006;12:3723–9. https://doi.org/10.1158/1078-0432.CCR-05-2625.
98. Yacoub A, McKinstry R, Hinman D, Chung T, Dent P, Hagan MP. Epidermal growth factor and ionizing radiation up-regulate the DNA repair genes XRCC1 and ERCC1 in DU145 and LNCaP prostate carcinoma through MAPK signaling. Radiat Res. 2003;159:439–52.
99. Kim BY, Kim KA, Kwon O, Kim SO, Kim MS, Kim BS, et al. NF-κB inhibition radiosensitizes Ki-Ras-transformed cells to ionizing radiation. Carcinogenesis. 2005;26:1395–403. https://doi.org/10.1093/carcin/bgi081.
100. Shore ND. Radium-223 dichloride for metastatic castration-resistant prostate cancer: the urologist's perspective. Urology. 2015;85:717–24. https://doi.org/10.1016/j.urology.2014.11.031.

Alternative Antiandrogen Therapy for CRPC

22

Takanobu Utsumi, Naoto Kamiya, Masashi Yano, Takumi Endo, and Hiroyoshi Suzuki

Abstract

Androgen deprivation therapy continues to be a mainstream treatment for prostate cancer. Failure after initial hormonal treatment including combined androgen blockade (CAB)/maximum androgen blockade (MAB) does not necessarily imply treatment-refractory disease progression. Antiandrogen withdrawal syndrome (AWS) is a manifestation of a prostate-specific antigen (PSA) decrease with or without subjective or objective symptomatic improvement on discontinuation of the antiandrogen. In general, the incidence of this effect has been reported to be 10–30%, and it lasts for 3–5 months. Some patients with progressive disease who have undergone initial CAB/MAB therapy respond to second- and third-line hormonal therapy after AWS is recognized. Mutations in the androgen receptor (AR) gene are thought to account for this phenomenon by enabling the previous antiandrogens to act as receptor agonists. Alternative antiandrogens probably have different functional interactions with the AR. Alternative antiandrogen therapy has been shown to improve symptoms and decrease pain in patients with prior antiandrogen therapy. A 50% PSA decrease has been reported after second-line treatment with nonsteroidal antiandrogens in 35–50% of cases. Responders to second-line hormonal treatment are expected to survive significantly longer than nonresponders. Responsiveness to second-line regimens is the most important prognostic factor for increased cause-specific and overall survival.

Keywords

Androgen receptor · Alternative antiandrogen therapy · Antiandrogen withdrawal syndrome · Castration-resistant prostate cancer · Combined androgen blockade

---

T. Utsumi · N. Kamiya · M. Yano · T. Endo · H. Suzuki, M.D., Ph.D. (✉)
Department of Urology, Toho University Sakura Medical Center, Chiba, Japan
e-mail: hiroyoshi.suzuki@med.toho-u.ac.jp

22.1 General

Androgen deprivation therapy (ADT) continues to be a mainstream treatment for prostate cancer. Although most patients with prostate cancer respond to ADT initially, its efficacy is temporary for almost all patients, and they finally develop castration-resistant prostate cancer (CRPC) despite castration levels of testosterone [1, 2]. CRPC is thought to be mediated through two main overlapping mechanisms, androgen-receptor (AR)-independent and AR-dependent [1, 2]. Prostate cancer deaths are typically the result of metastatic CRPC, and historically the median survival for patients with metastatic CRPC has been less than 2 years [2, 3]. The treatment of patients with metastatic CRPC has changed dramatically over the past decade.

The addition of oral antiandrogens to luteinizing hormone-releasing hormone agonists or surgical castration, an approach termed "combined androgen blockade" (CAB) or "maximum androgen blockade" (MAB), has been developed to synergistically target AR signaling [1–3]. Oral steroidal antiandrogens, such as cyproterone acetate and chlormadinone acetate, or nonsteroidal antiandrogens, such as flutamide, bicalutamide, and nilutamide, competitively block testosterone and/or dihydrotestosterone binding to the AR [1]. CAB/MAB can slightly but significantly improve survivals in patients with advanced prostate cancer [4]. CAB/MAB using a nonsteroidal antiandrogen tends to be superior to that using cyproterone acetate in delaying progression [1–4]. However, the therapeutic benefit from CAB/MAB is also at best transient, and inevitably almost all patients ultimately develop CRPC.

In the past, once patients failed primary ADT including CAB/MAB, palliative treatments were mainly administered. However, failure after initial hormonal treatment does not necessarily mean treatment-refractory disease progression. Antiandrogen withdrawal syndrome (AWS) is a manifestation of a prostate-specific antigen (PSA) decrease with or without subjective or objective symptomatic improvement on discontinuation of the antiandrogen flutamide [5]. A PSA decrease has also been observed after discontinuing nonsteroidal antiandrogens, such as bicalutamide and nilutamide, and after discontinuing steroidal antiandrogens [6–8]. This effect has been reported to occur in 10–30% of cases, and it lasts for approximately 3–5 months [9]. The precise molecular mechanisms underlying AWS have not been identified, but AR mutations or gene amplification of the AR might result in an altered response to antiandrogens [10–13]. However, androgen independence does not necessarily mean that the tumor is resistant to further hormonal manipulation [6, 10, 11].

Some patients with progressive disease who have undergone initial CAB/MAB therapy respond to second- and third-line hormonal therapy after AWS is recognized [6, 14–19]. Mutations in the AR gene are thought to account for this phenomenon by enabling the previous antiandrogens to act as receptor agonists [20]. Alternative antiandrogens probably have different functional interactions with the AR. It has been reported that antiandrogen therapy alters responses to subsequent hormonal agents [14, 16]. Alternative antiandrogen therapy has been shown to improve symptoms and decrease pain in patients who are resistant to prior antiandrogen therapy [1, 6, 14–17]. A 50% PSA decrease has been described after second-line treatment with nonsteroidal antiandrogens in 35–50% of cases [1, 6, 14–19]. Responders to second-line hormonal treatment are expected to survive significantly longer than nonresponders. Responsiveness to second-line regimens is one of the most important prognostic factors for increased cause-specific survival (CSS), as measured from the time of initiation of first-line therapy to the time of relapse after first-line therapy [18].

The more recently developed highly active hormonal agents abiraterone and enzalutamide have been proven to provide survival benefits to CRPC patients [21–23]. As a result of the availability of these newer and highly active agents, the clinical utility of the vintage drugs, such as flutamide, bicalutamide, and nilutamide, might need to be reconsidered. In this chapter, alternative antiandrogen therapy for CRPC is described in this new era of treatment for CRPC.

22.2 Antiandrogen Withdrawal Syndrome

AWS, which was first described by Kelly and Scher in 1993, is a phenomenon characterized by tumor regression and a PSA decrease due to interruption of antiandrogen or other hormonal treatment [3, 5, 14, 24–26]. The mechanism of AWS suggests one possibility for treating patients after androgen-independent progression: mutations of the AR gene and/or its amplification might cause an altered response to antiandrogens and the acquisition of agonist properties [12, 13, 27, 28]. Withdrawal of antiandrogen stimulation can result in tumor regression and decreased serum PSA levels [11, 29]. Androgen independence after first-line antiandrogen therapy does not always mean that such tumors are resistant to further hormonal therapy [30]. Although AWS was first reported in association with flutamide (previously called flutamide withdrawal syndrome), it can occur with other antiandrogens and hormonal agents, including bicalutamide, nilutamide, and chlormadinone acetate [5, 23–26].

The largest prospective study of patients with AWS enrolled 210 patients whose disease progressed on CAB/MAB with bicalutamide, flutamide, or nilutamide (SWOG 9426) [31]. PSA level decreases of ≥50% were confirmed in 21% of the patients in the SWOG 9426 study, although no radiological responses were reported. Moreover, progression-free survival (PFS) of at least 1 year after interruption of antiandrogen therapy was confirmed in 19% of patients.

Table 22.1 shows the clinical studies of AWS. These data demonstrate that around 10–30% of patients with AWS had ≥50% PSA decreases from baseline, and the median duration of response was 3–5 months. In general, radiological response was rare. Inconsistency among radiological and clinical progression and PSA decrease was reported, although symptomatic patients can experience relief of their symptoms under PSA suppression associated with AWS [32, 33]. The timeframe between antiandrogen interruption and PSA response varies, depending on the different half-life of each agent (5.2 h for flutamide and 1 week for bicalutamide). Responses can be clarified within the first day after flutamide withdrawal, while time periods up to 8 weeks are needed in the patients treated with bicalutamide [34].

Table 22.2 Clinical studies of alternative antiandrogen therapy

Study group	Number of enrolled patients	First-line antiandrogen	Second-line antiandrogen	Total response rate (%)	Duration of response (months)
Joyce et al. [16]	14	FLT	BCA	42.9	No data
Kojima et al. [17]	40	CMA (n = 22)	FLT (n = 6)	37.9	8.8
			BCL (n = 16)		
		FLT (n = 8)	CMA (n = 5)		
			BCL (n = 17)		
		BCL (n = 10)	FLT (n = 10)		
Okihara et al. [43]	59	CMA (n = 6)	FLT (n = 3)	44.1	No data
			BCL (n = 3)		
		FLT (n = 22)	CMA (n = 5)		
			BCL (n = 17)		
		BCL (n = 31)	FLT (n = 29)		
			CMA (n = 2)		
Suzuki et al. [18]	232	BCL (n = 193)	FLT (n = 193)	35.8	6.6
		FLT (n = 39)	BCL (n = 39)		
Okegawa et al. [44]	112	BCL (n = 82)	FLT (n = 79)	35.7	No data
			CMA (n = 2)		
		FLT (n = 22)	BCL (n = 20)		
			CMA (n = 2)		
		CMA (n = 8)	BCL (n = 6)		
			FLT (n = 2)		
Choi et al. [45]	47	BCL or CA	CA or BCL	48.9	13.4
Momozono et al. [30]	231	BCA	FLT	37.9	No data

BCL bicalutamide, *CA* cyproterone acetate, *CMA* chlormadinone acetate, *FLT* flutamide
Total response rate is defined as ≥50% or greater decrease of PSA after alternative antiandrogen therapy

In the NASA-PC study group, we reported that, consistent with the PSA response to second-line therapy, not only the patients with PSA decreases of ≥50%, but also patients with PSA decreases from 0 to 50% showed significantly better cause-specific survival (CSS) than nonresponders [18]. Moreover, a recent study reported that a PSA decrease following alternative antiandrogen therapy was an independent predictor of CSS and overall survival. This suggests that the PSA response to alternative antiandrogens is one of the most important prognostic factors for increased survival in patients with CRPC. The response to second-line therapy was the most important factor, followed by response to first-line therapy, AWS, and Gleason score (≤7 vs. ≥8), indicating the potential predictive value of responsiveness to second-line therapies in the NASA-PC study [18].

Recently, we developed a novel nomogram to predict a PSA decrease of ≥50% in response to alternative nonsteroidal antiandrogen therapy [19]. We incorporated five independent risk factors (initial serum PSA level, hemoglobin, C-reactive protein, PSA nadir to second hormone therapy, and Gleason sum) into this nomogram. Clinicians can use the nomogram to select the further therapies followed by first-line CAB/MAB and/or early treatment with new generation hormonal therapy or chemotherapy, because patients who do not respond to second-line therapy showed the worst survival. In general, a further antiandrogen switch (third-line antiandrogen) is much less effective than an early switch, with a response rate of 13–29% in our and other studies [17, 18, 43]. However, third-line CAB/MAB was effective in 80% of second-line responders [17].

Unfortunately, resistance to new generation hormonal agents inevitably occurs. Some researchers reported a novel mutation of AR codon 876 that specifically confers resistance to enzalutamide by rendering it agonist [47, 48]. Interestingly, enzalutamide-resistant models that have the mutation of AR codon 876 maintain sensitivity to bicalutamide [47, 48].

EAU-ESTRO-SIOG guidelines recommend that clinicians should interrupt antiandrogen therapy once PSA progression occurs and observe AWS for 4–6 weeks after discontinuation of flutamide or bicalutamide as evidence level 2a and recommendation grade A [49]. However, according to recent guidelines on CRPC, alternative antiandrogen therapy was excluded as a treatment option for patients with CRPC [2, 49, 50]. On the other hand, the consensus of opinion from panel member experts in the St Gallen Advanced Prostate Cancer Consensus Conference shows that vintage hormonal agents, such as flutamide and bicalutamide, can be used for patients with CRPC who cannot undergo treatment with new generation hormonal agents for economic reasons [51].

In conclusion, treatment decisions need to be individualized based on clinical and social characteristics and to maximize the efficacy of ADT with the use of even more effective agents. AWS and alternative antiandrogen therapy for CRPC can still be a treatment option for some patients with CRPC who may benefit. Clinicians should take the benefits into account and treat patients with CRPC in clinical practice.

References

1. Suzuki H, Kamiya N, Imamoto T, Kawamura K, Yano M, Takano M, et al. Current topics and perspectives relating to hormone therapy for prostate cancer. Int J Clin Oncol. 2008;13:401–10.
2. Lowrance WT, Roth BJ, Kirkby E, Murad MH, Cookson MS. Castration-resistant prostate cancer: AUA guideline amendment 2015. J Urol. 2016;195:1444–52.
3. Lorente D, Mateo J, Zafeiriou Z, Smith AD, Sandhu S, Ferraldeschi R, et al. Switching and withdrawing hormonal agents for castration-resistant prostate cancer. Nat Rev Urol. 2015; 12:37–47.
4. Maximum androgen blockade in advanced prostate cancer: an overview of the randomised trials. Prostate Cancer Trialsts' Collaborative Group. Lancet. 2000;355:1491–8.
5. Kelly WK, Scher HI. Prostate specific antigen decline after antiandrogen withdrawal: the flutamide withdrawal syndrome. J Urol. 1933;149:607–9.
6. Scher HI, Zhang ZF, Nanus D, Kelly WK. Hormone and antihormone withdrawal: implications for the management of androgen-independent prostate cancer. Urology. 1996;47:61–9.
7. Small EJ, Carroll PR. Prostate-specific antigen decline after casodex withdrawal: evidence for an antiandrogen withdrawal syndrome. Urology. 1994;43:408–10.
8. Akakura K, Akimoto S, Ohki T, Shimazaki J. Antiandrogen withdrawal syndrome in prostate cancer after treatment with steroidal antiandrogen chlormadinone acetate. Urology. 1995; 45(4):700.

9. Lam JS, Leppert JT, Vemulapalli SN, Shvarts O, Belldegrun AS. Secondary hormonal therapy for advanced prostate cancer. J Urol. 2006;175:27–34.
10. Suzuki H, Ueda T, Ichikawa T, Ito H. Androgen receptor involvement in the progression of prostate cancer. Endocr Relat Cancer. 2003;10:209–16.
11. Taplin ME, Bubley GJ, Shuster TD, Frantz ME, Spooner AE, Ogata GK, et al. Mutation of the androgen-receptor gene in metastatic androgen-independent prostate cancer. N Engl J Med. 1995;332:1393–8.
12. Buchanan G, Greenberg NM, Scher HI, Harris JM, Marshall VR, Tilley WD. Collocation of androgen receptor gene mutations in prostate cancer. Clin Cancer Res. 2001;7:1273–81.
13. Palmberg C, Koivisto P, Kakkola L, Tammela TL, Kallioniemi OP, Visakorpi T. Androgen receptor gene amplification at primary progression predicts response to combined androgen blockade as second line therapy for advanced prostate cancer. J Urol. 2000;164:1992–5.
14. Scher HI, Kelly WK. Flutamide withdrawal syndrome: its impact on clinical trials in hormone-refractory prostate cancer. J Clin Oncol. 1993;11:1566–72.
15. Desai A, Stadler WM, Vogelzang NJ. Nilutamide: possible utility as a second-line hormonal agent. Urology. 2001;58:1016–20.
16. Joyce R, Fenton MA, Rode P, Constantine M, Gaynes L, Kolvenbag G, et al. High dose bicalutamide for androgen independent prostate cancer: effect of prior hormonal therapy. J Urol. 1998;159:149–53.
17. Kojima S, Suzuki H, Akakura K, Shimbo M, Ichikawa T, Ito H. Alternative antiandrogens to treat prostate cancer relapse after initial hormone therapy. J Urol. 2004;171:679–83.
18. Suzuki H, Okihara K, Miyake H, Fujisawa M, Miyoshi S, Matsumoto T, et al. Alternative nonsteroidal antiandrogen therapy for advanced prostate cancer that relapsed after initial maximum androgen blockade. J Urol. 2008;180:921–7.
19. Kamiya N, Suzuki H, Nishimura K, Fujii M, Okegawa T, Matsuda T, et al. Development of nomogram to non-steroidal antiandrogen sequential alternation in prostate cancer for predictive model. Jpn J Clin Oncol. 2014;44:263–9.
20. Yoshida T, Kinoshita H, Segawa T, Nakamura E, Inoue T, Shimizu Y, et al. Antiandrogen bicalutamide promotes tumor growth in a novel androgen-dependent prostate cancer xenograft model derived from a bicalutamide-treated patient. Cancer Res. 2005;65:9611–6.
21. Ryan CJ, Smith MR, de Bono JS, Molina A, Logothetis CJ, de Souza P, et al. Abiraterone in metastatic prostate cancer without previous chemotherapy. N Engl J Med. 2013;368:138–48.
22. de Bono JS, Logothetis CJ, Molina A, Fizazi K, North S, Chu L, et al. Abiraterone and increased survival in metastatic prostate cancer. N Engl J Med. 2011;364:1995–2005.
23. Scher HI, Fizazi K, Saad F, Taplin ME, Sternberg CN, Miller K, et al. Increased survival with enzalutamide in prostate cancer after chemotherapy. N Engl J Med. 2012;367:1187–97.
24. Akakura K, Akimoto S, Furuya Y, Ito H. Incidence and characteristics of antiandrogen withdrawal syndrome in prostate cancer after treatment with chlormadinone acetate. Eur Urol. 1998;33:567–71.
25. Huan SD, Gerridzen RG, Yau JC, Stewart DJ. Antiandrogen withdrawal syndrome with nilutamide. Urology. 1997;49(4):632.
26. Dupont A, Gomez JL, Cusan L, Koutsilieris M, Labrie F. Response to flutamide withdrawal in advanced prostate cancer in progression under combination therapy. J Urol. 1993;150:908–13.
27. Suzuki H, Akakura K, Komiya A, Aida S, Akimoto S, Shimazaki J. Codon 877 mutation in the androgen receptor gene in advanced prostate cancer: relation to antiandrogen withdrawal syndrome. Prostate. 1996;29:153–8.
28. Suzuki H, Sato N, Watabe Y, Masai M, Seino S, Shimazaki J. Androgen receptor gene mutations in human prostate cancer. J Steroid Biochem Mol Biol. 1993;46:759–65.
29. Gaddipati JP, McLeod DG, Heidenberg HB, Sesterhenn IA, Finger MJ, Moul JW, et al. Frequent detection of codon 877 mutation in the androgen receptor gene in advanced prostate cancers. Cancer Res. 1994;54:2861–4.
30. Momozono H, Miyake H, Tei H, Harada KI, Fujisawa M. Clinical outcomes of anti-androgen withdrawal and subsequent alternative anti-androgen therapy for advanced prostate cancer following failure of initial maximum androgen blockade. Mol Clin Oncol. 2016;4:839–44.

31. Sartor AO, Tangen CM, Hussain MH, Eisenberger MA, Parab M, Fontana JA, et al. Antiandrogen withdrawal in castrate-refractory prostate cancer: a Southwest Oncology Group trial (SWOG 9426). Cancer. 2008;112:2393–400.
32. Herrada J, Dieringer P, Logothetis CJ. Characterization of patients with androgen-independent prostatic carcinoma whose serum prostate specific antigen decreased following flutamide withdrawal. J Urol. 1996;155:620–3.
33. Small EJ, Halabi S, Dawson NA, Stadler WM, Rini BI, Picus J, et al. Antiandrogen withdrawal alone or in combination with ketoconazole in androgen-independent prostate cancer patients: a phase III trial (CALGB 9583). J Clin Oncol. 2004;22:1025–33.
34. Schellhammer PF, Venner P, Haas GP, Small EJ, Nieh PT, Seabaugh DR, et al. Prostate specific antigen decreases after withdrawal of antiandrogen therapy with bicalutamide or flutamide in patients receiving combined androgen blockade. J Urol. 1997;157(5):1731.
35. Tran C, Ouk S, Clegg NJ, Chen Y, Watson PA, Arora V, et al. Development of a second-generation antiandrogen for treatment of advanced prostate cancer. Science. 2009;324:787–90.
36. Mosca A. Enzalutamide withdrawal syndrome: is there a rationale? BJU Int. 2015;115:348–9.
37. von Klot CA, Kuczyk MA, Merseburger AS. No androgen withdrawal syndrome for enzalutamide: a report of disease dynamics in the postchemotherapy setting. Eur Urol. 2014;65:258–9.
38. Phillips R. Prostate cancer: an enzalutamide antiandrogen withdrawal syndrome. Nat Rev Urol. 2014;11:366.
39. Rodriguez-Vida A, Bianchini D, Van Hemelrijck M, Hughes S, Malik Z, Powles T, et al. Is there an antiandrogen withdrawal syndrome with enzalutamide? BJU Int. 2015;115:373–80.
40. Hara T, Miyazaki J, Araki H, Yamaoka M, Kanzaki N, Kusaka M, et al. Novel mutations of androgen receptor: a possible mechanism of bicalutamide withdrawal syndrome. Cancer Res. 2003;63:149–53.
41. Nishiyama T, Hashimoto Y, Takahashi K. The influence of androgen deprivation therapy on dihydrotestosterone levels in the prostatic tissue of patients with prostate cancer. Clin Cancer Res. 2004;10:7121–6.
42. Nazareth LV, Weigel NL. Activation of the human androgen receptor through a protein kinase a signaling pathway. J Biol Chem. 1996;271:19900–7.
43. Okihara K, Ukimura O, Kanemitsu N, Mizutani Y, Kawauchi A, Miki T, Kyoto Prefectural University of Medicine Prostate Cancer Research Group. Clinical efficacy of alternative antiandrogen therapy in Japanese men with relapsed prostate cancer after first-line hormonal therapy. Int J Urol. 2007;14:128–32.
44. Okegawa T, Nutahara K, Higashihara E. Alternative antiandrogen therapy in patients with castration-resistant prostate cancer: a single-center experience. Int J Urol. 2010;17:950–5.
45. Choi JI, Kim YB, Yang SO, Lee JK, Jung TY. Efficacy of alternative antiandrogen therapy for prostate cancer that relapsed after initial maximum androgen blockade. Korean J Urol. 2011;52:461–5.
46. Yasui M, Uemura K, Yoneyama S, Kawahara T, Hattori Y, Teranishi JI, et al. Predictors of poor response to secondary alternative antiandrogen therapy with flutamide in metastatic castration-resistant prostate cancer. Jpn J Clin Oncol. 2016 [Epub ahead of print].
47. Joseph JD, Lu N, Qian J, Sensintaffar J, Shao G, Brigham D, et al. A clinically relevant androgen receptor mutation confers resistance to second-generation antiandrogens enzalutamide and ARN-509. Cancer Discov. 2013;3(9):1020.
48. Korpal M, Korn JM, Gao X, Rakiec DP, Ruddy DA, Doshi S, et al. An F876 L mutation in androgen receptor confers genetic and phenotypic resistance to MDV3100 (enzalutamide). Cancer Discov. 2013;3:1030–43.
49. Cornford P, Bellmunt J, Bolla M, Briers E, De Santis M, Gross T, et al. EAU-ESTRO-SIOG Guidelines on Prostate Cancer. Part II: Treatment of relapsing, metastatic, and castration-resistant prostate cancer. Eur Urol. 2017;71:630–42.
50. Cookson MS, Lowrance WT, Murad MH, Kibel AS, American Urological Association. Castration-resistant prostate cancer: AUA guideline amendment. J Urol. 2015;193:491–9.
51. Gillessen S, Omlin A, Attard G, de Bono JS, Efstathiou E, Fizazi K, et al. Management of patients with advanced prostate cancer: Recommendations of the St.Gallen Advanced Prostate Cancer Consensus Conference (APCCC) 2015. Ann Oncol. 2015;26:1589–604.

Optimization of Sequential AR Targeted Therapy for CRPC

23

Naoki Terada

Abstract

Abiraterone and enzalutamide are novel hormonal treatments for castration-resistant prostate cancer that have been demonstrated to improve overall survival. Although their mechanisms are different, the clinical efficacy of these drugs appears very similar. Elucidating an appropriate treatment sequence of these therapies is important for maximizing the clinical benefit of castration-resistant prostate cancer patients. Currently, there is a trend to use these novel hormonal therapies before chemotherapy because of better tolerability, especially for the patients with long duration to resistance to first-line androgen deprivation therapy. Recent reports have shown that the abiraterone-to-enzalutamide sequence might have more favorable efficacy in terms of combined prostate-specific antigen progression-free survival than the enzalutamide-to-abiraterone sequence. However, there was no significant difference in overall survival. Based on these studies, the optimal sequence of these novel hormonal therapies is discussed.

Keywords

Abiraterone · Enzalutamide · Sequence

23.1 Introduction

Recently, there has recently been a rapid increase in the number of effective systemic agents for castration-resistant prostate cancer (CRPC), including novel hormonal therapies. Abiraterone (ABI) and enzalutamide (ENZ) are novel hormonal

N. Terada, M.D., Ph.D.
Department of Urology, Miyazaki University, Miyazaki, Japan
e-mail: naoki_terada@med.miyazaki-u.ac.jp

Y. Arai, O. Ogawa (eds.), *Hormone Therapy and Castration Resistance of Prostate Cancer*, https://doi.org/10.1007/978-981-10-7013-6_23

treatments for CRPC that have been reported to improve overall survival [1, 2]. ABI is a CYP17 inhibitor, and ENZ is a novel antiandrogen that targets multiple steps in the AR signaling pathway. Although their mechanisms are different, the clinical efficacies of these drugs are similar. Elucidating an appropriate treatment sequence of these therapies is important for maximizing clinical benefit of CRPC patients.

23.2 Abiraterone and Enzalutamide

The discovery that prostate cancers remain dependent upon AR-mediated signaling for their growth and survival has opened the door to the development of several targeted agents [3]. ABI is a potential inhibitor of CYP17, an enzyme essential for androgen synthesis. Improved OS has been demonstrated with the use of ABI in both the pre- and post-docetaxel setting. ABI was first evaluated by the COU-AA-301 study in the post-docetaxel setting [1] and then later in the pre-docetaxel setting by the COU-AA-302 study [4]. ENZ is a next-generation hormonal therapy that acts by fourfold inhibition of AR signaling. ENZ blocks AR interaction, inhibits translocation of the AR to the nucleus, impairs AR binding to DNA, and inhibits coactivator recruitment and receptor-mediated DNA transcription. Thus compared with ABI, ENZ targets androgen-AR signaling through binding of the AR itself, rather than through CYP17 inhibition, and so ENZ has the added benefit of no requirement for corticosteroids. Like ABI, ENZ has shown increased OS when used pre- and post-docetaxel. The AFFIRM study evaluated ENZ in the post-docetaxel setting [2], and the PREVEIL study examined ENZ in the pre-docetaxel setting [5].

There are no reports yet that have directly compared the efficacy of these two agents. Table 23.1 shows the 50% PSA reduction rate and median PSA progression free-survival (PSA-PFS) time in each study of ABI and ENZ. In the pre-docetaxel setting, the 50% PSA reduction rate appeared higher with ENZ (78%) than ABI (62%); however, the PSA-PFS time was similar between ABI (11.1 months) and ENZ (11.2 months). In the post-docetaxel setting, the 50% PSA reduction rate and PSA-PFS time showed differences between groups, which were probably caused by the difference in the patients' background. Based on these results, the efficacy of ABI and ENZ as first-line treatment was considered to be almost similar.

Table 23.1 PSA reduction and PSA-PFS time of ABI and ENZ

Study	References	N	>50% PSA reduction (%)	Median PSA-PFS time (months)
COU-AA-302(ABI/pre-DTX)	Ryan et al. NEJM 2013	546	62	11.1
PREVAIL(ENZA/pre-DTX)	Beer et al. NEJM 2014	872	78	11.2
COU-AA-301(ABI/post-DTX)	De bono et al. NEJM 2011	797	29	10.2
AFFIRM(ENZA/post-DTX)	Scher et al. NEJM 2012	800	54	8.3

23.3 Should AR Target Therapies Be Used Before Chemotherapy?

There is currently a trend to use these novel hormonal therapies before chemotherapy, because of better tolerability [6]. However, whether they should be used before chemotherapy for all CRPC patients has not been determined. Antonarakis et al. reported that the detection of AR-V7 in circulating tumor cells (CTCs) of CRPC patients was associated with resistance to ABI and ENZ [7]. The PSA response rate was 0% for AR-V7-positive patients in the context of both therapies. These results have now been expanded to a larger sample of 202 patients, in whom the negative prognostic impact of CTC-specific AR-V7 detection has been confirmed [8]. These results suggest that the presence of AR-V7 might explain the mechanism of primary resistance to ABI and ENZ in many cases. In contrast, the presence of AR-V7 does not appear to correlate with poor treatment responses in patients receiving docetaxel or cabazitaxel [9–11]. These results indicated that chemotherapy should be used before AR target therapies for patients with positive AR-V7 in CTCs. However, in clinical practice, it is difficult to extract CTCs and measure AR-V7. Therefore, we need to use clinically available predictive markers. Loriot et al. reported that the duration of response to first-line androgen deprivation therapy (ADT) was a predictor of sensitivity to novel AR axis-targeted drugs in CRPC patients [12]. However, the efficacy of docetaxel was not correlated with the duration of first-line ADT [13]. We evaluated the parameters predicting efficacy of ABI or ENZ treatment in the 465 patients in our retrospective study [14, 15]. The only parameter significantly associated with PSA-PFS of both ABI and ENZ in multivariate Cox proportional hazard analyses was time to resistance to first-line ADT of less than 1 year. These results indicated that for CRPC patients with short duration to resistance to first-line ADT, chemotherapy should be used before AR target therapies.

23.4 What Is the Optimal Sequence of AR Target Therapies for Prostate Cancer?

Guidelines for the treatment of CRPC have not outlined the optimal sequence of these therapies. The question, thus, remains as to which approach should be first for the treatment of CRPC, ABI, or ENZ? This question is one of the major concerns in considering a treatment strategy for CRPC. Several retrospective studies have demonstrated the decreased efficacy of the second-line AR-targeting therapy after progression on the first-line therapy, and ENZ was superior to ABI in their efficacy as the second-line setting [16]. Maughan et al. performed a retrospective analysis of 81 consecutive CRPC patients, which included 65 patients treated with ABI-to-ENZ and 16 patients treated with ENZ-to-ABI. The ABI-to-ENZ group tended to have a better PSA-PFS compared with the ENZ-to-ABI group. The difference was significant only in the multivariate analysis not in the univariate analysis [17]. We collaborated with these authors (Kyoto-Baltimore collaboration) and evaluated the efficacy of ABI and ENZ in each sequence, including 113 patients treated with ABI-to-ENZ and 85 patients treated with ENZ-to-ABI in the pre-docetaxel setting. Our results showed that PSA-PFS was not significantly different between the two groups in the first-line setting. However, in the second-line setting, PSA-PFS was significantly longer in ENZ than in ABI; the combined PSA-PFS was significantly longer in the ABI-to-ENZ group (median 15 months) compared with the ENZ-to-ABI group (median 10 months). The difference was significant both in univariate and multivariate analyses. However, there was no statistical difference in OS between the two sequences [15]. Miyake et al. also performed a retrospective analysis in 108 consecutive patients with CRPC who sequentially received ABI and ENZ, including 49 patients with ABI-to-ENZ treatment and 59 patients with ENZ-to-ABI treatment. The combined PSA-PFS in the ABI-to-ENZ group (median 18 months) was significantly superior to that of the ENZ-to-ABI group (median 13 months) [18]. Although these studies were all retrospective and showed no significant difference in OS, these results might affect our treatment strategy in CRPC patients. Although the ABI-to-ENZ sequence might have more favorable efficacy in terms of combined PSA-PFS than the ENZ-to-ABI sequence, the results did not conclusively demonstrate that ABI should be used before ENZ for all the CRPC patients. Without useful predictive biomarkers, we need to select first-line or second-line therapies by discussing not only the efficacy but also the prevalence of the adverse effects with the patients.

23.5 Future Prospectives

There have been rapid advancements in the treatment of CRPC, with a resulting improvement in the prognosis of patients. Further research is needed with respect to selection and sequencing of therapy [16, 19] to determine the optimal series of treatments for an individual patient.

Acknowledgments We thank Edanz Group (www.edanzediting.com) for editing a draft of this manuscript.

References

1. de Bono JS, Logothetis CJ, Molina A, et al. Abiraterone and increased survival in metastatic prostate cancer. N Engl J Med. 2011;364:1995–2005.
2. Scher HI, Fizazi K, Saad F, et al. Increased survival with enzalutamide in prostate cancer after chemotherapy. N Engl J Med. 2012;367:1187–97.
3. Mohler JL. Castration-recurrent prostate cancer is not androgen-independent. Adv Exp Med Biol. 2008;617:223–34.
4. Ryan CJ, Smith MR, de Bono JS, et al. Abiraterone in metastatic prostate cancer without previous chemotherapy. N Engl J Med. 2013;368:138–48.
5. Beer TM, Armstrong AJ, Rathkopf DE, et al. Enzalutamide in metastatic prostate cancer before chemotherapy. N Engl J Med. 2014;371:424–33.

6. Flaig TW, Potluri RC, Ng Y, Todd MB, Mehra M. Treatment evolution for metastatic castration-resistant prostate cancer with recent introduction of novel agents: retrospective analysis of real-world data. Cancer Med. 2016;5:182–91.
7. Antonarakis ES, Lu C, Wang H, et al. AR-V7 and resistance to enzalutamide and abiraterone in prostate cancer. N Engl J Med. 2014;371:1028–38.
8. Antonarakis ESLC, Luber B. Clinical significance of AR-V7 mRNA detection in circulating tumor cells of men with metastatic castration-resistant prostate cancer treated with first- and second-line abiraterone and enzalutamide. J Clin Oncol. 2017;35(19):2149–56.
9. Antonarakis ES, Lu C, Luber B, et al. Androgen receptor splice variant 7 and efficacy of taxane chemotherapy in patients with metastatic castration-resistant prostate cancer. JAMA Oncol. 2015;1:582–91.
10. Onstenk W, Sieuwerts AM, Kraan J, et al. Efficacy of Cabazitaxel in castration-resistant prostate cancer is independent of the presence of AR-V7 in circulating tumor cells. Eur Urol. 2015;68:939–45.
11. Scher HI, Lu D, Schreiber NA, et al. Association of AR-V7 on circulating tumor cells as a treatment-specific biomarker with outcomes and survival in castration-resistant prostate cancer. JAMA Oncol. 2016;2:1441–9.
12. Loriot Y, Eymard JC, Patrikidou A, et al. Prior long response to androgen deprivation predicts response to next-generation androgen receptor axis targeted drugs in castration resistant prostate cancer. Eur J Cancer. 2015;51:1946–52.
13. van Soest RJ, Templeton AJ, Vera-Badillo FE, et al. Neutrophil-to-lymphocyte ratio as a prognostic biomarker for men with metastatic castration-resistant prostate cancer receiving first-line chemotherapy: data from two randomized phase III trials. Ann Oncol. 2015;26:743–9.
14. Terada N, Akamatsu S, Okada Y, et al. Factors predicting efficacy and adverse effects of enzalutamide in Japanese patients with castration-resistant prostate cancer: results of retrospective multi-institutional study. Int J Clin Oncol. 2016;21:1155–61.
15. Terada N, Maughan BL, Akamatsu S, et al. Exploring the optimal sequence of abiraterone and enzalutamide in patients with chemotherapy-naive castration-resistant prostate cancer: the Kyoto-Baltimore collaboration. Int J Urol. 2017;24:441–8.
16. Lorente D, Mateo J, Perez-Lopez R, de Bono JS, Attard G. Sequencing of agents in castration-resistant prostate cancer. Lancet Oncol. 2015;16:e279–92.
17. Maughan BL, Luber B, Nadal R, Antonarakis ES. Comparing sequencing of abiraterone and enzalutamide in men with metastatic castration-resistant prostate cancer: a retrospective study. Prostate. 2017;77:33–40.
18. Miyake H, Hara T, Terakawa T, Ozono S, Fujisawa M. Comparative assessment of clinical outcomes between abiraterone acetate and enzalutamide in patients with docetaxel-naive metastatic castration-resistant prostate cancer: experience in real-world clinical practice in Japan. Clin Genitourin Cancer. 2017;15:313–9.
19. Handy CE, Antonarakis ES. Sequencing treatment for castration-resistant prostate cancer. Curr Treat Options in Oncol. 2016;17:64.

Enzalutamide Therapy for mCRPC in Japanese Men

24

Go Kimura

Abstract

Enzalutamide, which inhibits androgen receptor signaling at multiple steps, was approved for metastatic castration-resistant prostate cancer (mCRPC) in Japan in 2014. Since then, we have treated mCRPC patients with enzalutamide; however, limited information is available as to clinical outcomes of enzalutamide in Japanese patients. In this chapter, I will review the efficacy, safety, and pharmacokinetics of enzalutamide in Japanese patients first from clinical trials, including the PREVAIL and phase I/II study in Japanese patients and then from retrospective studies of real-world data in Japan. Treatment effects and safety of enzalutamide in Japanese patients were generally consistent with the overall results from non-Japanese populations. However, in daily clinical practice, the patients often complain of such difficulties as swallowing due to the big size of capsule, fatigue, and appetite loss. In order to continue this effective enzalutamide therapy without discontinuation due to these subjective symptoms, dose reduction seems to be the best way.

Keywords

Enzalutamide · Castration-resistant prostate cancer · Japanese patients

24.1 Introduction

Since Huggins's report [1], androgen deprivation therapy (ADT) has been used as the gold standard of systemic therapy for metastatic prostate cancer. Although initially ADT is effective in most patients, it becomes refractory [2] and progresses to

G. Kimura
Department of Urology, Nippon Medical School, Tokyo, Japan
e-mail: gokimura@nms.ac.jp

Y. Arai, O. Ogawa (eds.), *Hormone Therapy and Castration Resistance of Prostate Cancer*, https://doi.org/10.1007/978-981-10-7013-6_24

fatal castration-resistant prostate cancer (CRPC) in nearly all patients [3]. Despite castration levels of testosterone, CRPC can continue to grow through activation of an androgen-androgen receptor (AR) signal pathway by mechanisms of testosterone synthesis from adrenal-derived weak androgens and/or from cholesterol by de novo synthesis [4, 5] and the amplification of their androgen receptors [6, 7]. Enzalutamide targets AR signaling at multiple steps, AR binding, nuclear translocation of the ARs, DNA binding, and coactivator recruitment. Enzalutamide has been shown to have favorable clinical outcomes, including prolonged overall survival (OS) and safety in pivotal phase III trials in mCRPC patients before and after docetaxel treatment [8, 9].

In Japan, enzalutamide for mCRPC received insurance coverage in 2014. Since then, we have treated mCRPC patients with enzalutamide in daily clinical practice; however, limited information is available as to efficacy and safety of enzalutamide in Japanese patients with mCRPC. In this chapter, I will review the efficacy, safety, and pharmacokinetics (PK) of enzalutamide in Japanese patients first from the clinical trial data, including a post hoc analysis of the PREVAIL trial and phase I/II study in Japanese CRPC patients and then from retrospective studies of real-world clinical practice data in Japan.

24.1.1 Enzalutamide

Enzalutamide is an AR-signaling inhibitor distinct from the vintage antiandrogen agents in that it inhibits nuclear translocation of the AR, DNA binding, and coactivator recruitment. Enzalutamide also has an eightfold greater affinity for AR compared to bicalutamide, induces tumor shrinkage in xenograft models, in which vintage antiandrogen agents only retard growth [10, 11].

One XTANDI™ (brand name of enzalutamide) soft capsule contains 40 mg enzalutamide. The recommended dose is 160 mg enzalutamide (four 40 mg capsules) as a single oral daily dose. It is absorbed promptly by oral administration and is not affected by diet, so it can be administered either before or after a meal. Unlike abiraterone acetate, there is no need to take additional steroids while taking enzalutamide. XTANDI™ was approved in Japan in May 2014 for the treatment of men with mCRPC refractory to docetaxel. Since October 2014, XTANDI™ is also available for docetaxel-naive settings. By the drug price revision made in April 2016, the price of XTANDI™ was lowered by 25%, with one capsule costing 2354.1 yen and 30 days costing 282,492 yen.

One of the most important side effects of enzalutamide is the occurrence of seizures, which are a known dose-dependent toxicity. In the phase I/II study, there were three cases of seizures (2%), and all of these three cases took equal to or more than 360 mg/day dosages [12]. Although incidence of seizures in the two pivotal phase III trials was low, extreme caution is required for administration in patients with a risk of seizures, such as those with a history of seizures, brain injury, stroke, brain metastases, alcoholism, and concomitant medications known to lower the seizure threshold.

24.1.2 Phase III Trials of Enzalutamide

24.1.2.1 AFFIRM Trial [12]

The AFFIRM trial was a double-blind, phase III study comparing the efficacy and safety between enzalutamide and placebo in men with mCRPC after chemotherapy. 1199 men were stratified according to the Eastern Cooperative Oncology Group (ECOG) performance status (PS) score and pain intensity and were randomly assigned in a 2:1 ratio to receive oral enzalutamide at a dose of 160 mg per day (800 patients) or placebo (399 patients). The primary endpoint was OS, and secondary endpoints were measures of response in the prostate-specific antigen (PSA) level, in soft tissue, and in the quality of life (QOL) score and measures of progression including time to PSA progression, radiographic progression-free survival (rPFS), and time to the first skeletal-related event (SRE).

The median OS was 18.4 months in the enzalutamide group versus 13.6 months in the placebo group (hazard ratio (HR) for death in the enzalutamide group, 0.63; 95% confidence interval (CI), 0.53–0.75; $P < 0.001$). The superiority of enzalutamide over placebo was shown with respect to all secondary endpoints. The rates of adverse events (AEs) were similar in the two groups. Incidence of all grades of fatigue, diarrhea, hot flashes, musculoskeletal pain, and headache was higher in the enzalutamide group. Hypertension or increased blood pressure was observed in 6.6% of patients in the enzalutamide group and 3.3% of those in the placebo group. The enzalutamide group had a lower incidence of AEs of grade 3 or above (45.3%, vs. 53.1% in the placebo group). Seizures were reported in five patients (0.6%) receiving enzalutamide.

It was concluded that enzalutamide significantly prolonged OS in men with mCRPC after chemotherapy.

24.1.2.2 PREVAIL Trial [9, 13]

The PREVAIL trial was a double-blind, phase III study comparing the efficacy and safety between enzalutamide and placebo in men with mCRPC before chemotherapy. The 1717 patients were randomly assigned to receive either enzalutamide (at a dose of 160 mg) or placebo once daily. The coprimary endpoints were rPFS and OS. The secondary endpoints included the time until the initiation of cytotoxic chemotherapy, the time until the first SRE, the best overall soft-tissue response, the time until PSA progression, and a decline in the PSA level of 50% or more from baseline. Prespecified exploratory endpoints included QOL and a decline in the PSA level of 90% or more from baseline.

The rate of rPFS at 12 months was 65% in the enzalutamide group, compared to 14% in the placebo group (HR in the enzalutamide group, 0.19; 95% CI, 0.15 to 0.23; $P < 0.001$). Treatment with enzalutamide resulted in a 29% decrease in the risk of death compared to placebo (HR, 0.71; 95% CI, 0.60–0.84; $P < 0.001$). The benefit of enzalutamide was shown with respect to all secondary and prespecified exploratory endpoints. AEs that occurred in $\geq 20\%$ of patients receiving enzalutamide at a rate at least 2% higher than that in the placebo group were fatigue, back pain, constipation, and arthralgia. After adjustment for the length of exposure, events with a higher rate in the enzalutamide group than in the placebo group were hot flash, hypertension, and falls. The most common event of ≥grade 3 in the enzalutamide group was hypertension (7%). One patient in each study group had a seizure.

It was concluded that enzalutamide significantly decreased the risk of rPFS and OS and delayed the initiation of chemotherapy in men with mCRPC before chemotherapy.

24.1.3 The Outcome of the PREVAIL Trial in Japanese Patients [14]

A post hoc analysis of the PREVAIL trial was done to evaluate the treatment effects, safety, and PK of enzalutamide in Japanese patients. Of 1717 patients, 61 were enrolled in Japan (enzalutamide, $n = 28$; placebo, $n = 33$). Among Japanese patients, baseline demographic and disease characteristics were well balanced between the enzalutamide and placebo treatment arms, except that more enzalutamide-treated patients had at least ten bone metastases (50.0 vs. 36.4%) and soft-tissue metastases (46.4 vs. 36.4%). Some differences in baseline disease characteristics were observed between Japanese patients and the overall study population. Japanese patients had lower bodyweight and body mass index, lower median PSA level at baseline, less baseline pain, and less soft-tissue disease. A higher percentage of Japanese patients had an ECOG PS of zero, and a Gleason score of eight or higher, bone metastases, had received corticosteroids and had received at least three prior unique hormone therapies at baseline than patients in the overall study population. However, Japanese patients had fewer prior radical prostatectomies than the overall study population.

The HR (95% CI) of 0.43 for investigator assessed rPFS (0.18–1.04) (Fig. 24.1); 0.37 for updated OS (0.13–1.04) (Fig. 24.2) showed the treatment benefit of enzalutamide over placebo. As for the results of the secondary endpoints, the HR (95% CI) of 0.46 for time to chemotherapy (0.22–0.96) and 0.36 for time to PSA-PFS (0.17–0.75) showed the treatment benefit of enzalutamide over the placebo. PSA responses were observed in 60.7% in the enzalutamide group versus 21.2% in the placebo group.

The incidence of AEs and serious AEs was consistent between Japanese patients and the overall population. Treatment-related AEs grade ≥3 was reported in 3.6% in the enzalutamide group compared with 6.1% in the placebo group. Treatment discontinuation as a result of AE was reported in 3.6% of the enzalutamide group and 6.1% of the placebo group. Dose reductions as a result of AE were reported in 3.6% of enzalutamide-treated patients and no placebo-treated patients. The most common AEs reported in Japanese patients are presented in Table 24.1. AEs that occurred in at least 20% of Japanese patients (listed from highest to lowest incidence) were weight decrease, decreased appetite, constipation, and fatigue, with the majority being ≤ grade 2. No seizures were reported in Japanese patients.

The mean minimum concentrations of enzalutamide and the sum of enzalutamide and N-desmethyl enzalutamide, its active metabolite, in Japanese and non-Japanese patients at 5, 13, and 25 weeks were measured. The concentration of

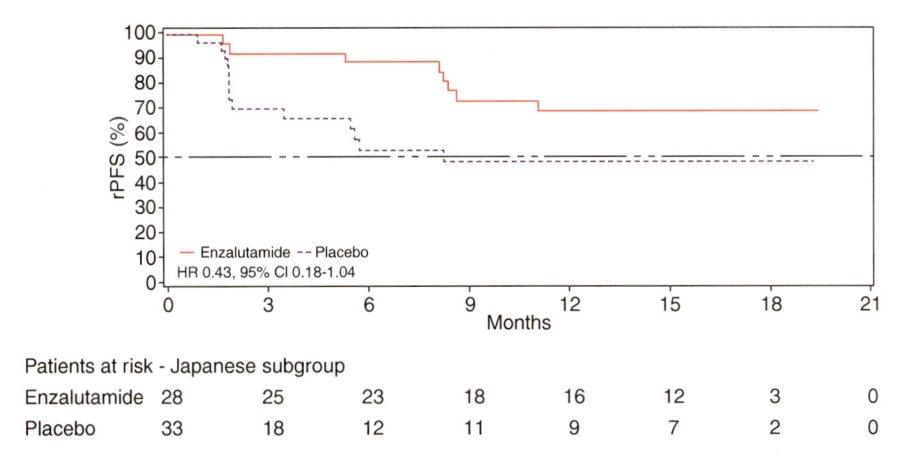

Fig. 24.1 Kaplan-Meier estimates of investigator-assessed rPFS for Japanese patients. The dashed horizontal lines indicate medians (data cutoff September 16, 2013). Hazard ratios are based on unstratified Cox regression models with treatment as the only covariate, with values <1.00 favoring enzalutamide. *CI* confidence interval, *HR* hazard ratio, *ITT* intent-to-treat, *NYR* not yet reached, *rPFS* radiographic progression-free survival. Reproductive from reference 14

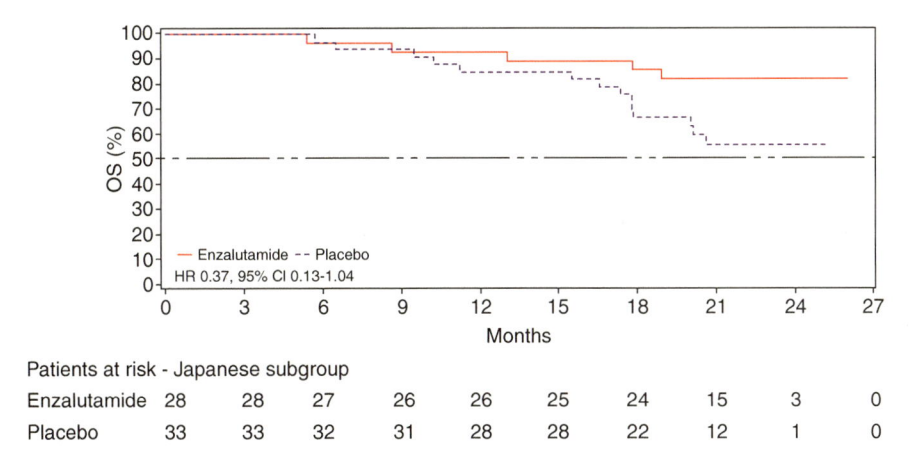

Fig. 24.2 Kaplan-Meier estimates of updated OS for Japanese patients. The dashed horizontal line indicates median (data cutoff January 15, 2014). Hazard ratios are based on unstratified Cox regression models with treatment as the only covariate, with values <1.00 favoring enzalutamide. *CI* confidence interval, *HR* hazard ratio, *OS* overall survival. Reproductive from reference 14

enzalutamide and its active metabolite were slightly higher in the Japanese population than in the non-Japanese population, with a geometric mean ratio (Japanese/non-Japanese) of 1.191 (90% CI 1.102–1.287), 1.063 (90% CI 0.982–1.150), and 1.137 (90% CI 1.017–1.271) at weeks 5, 13, and 25, respectively. Some differences in AEs might be related to the slightly higher concentrations of enzalutamide and its

Table 24.1 Overall adverse event summary

	Overall safety population (n = 1715), n (%)				Japanese subgroup (n = 61), n (%)			
	Enzalutamide (n = 871)		Placebo (n = 844)		Enzalutamide (n = 28)		Placebo (n = 33)	
	Any grade	Grade ≥ 3	Any grade	Grade ≥ 3	Any grade	Grade ≥ 3	Any grade	Grade ≥ 3
Weight decreased	100 (11.5)	5 (<1)	71 (8.4)	2 (<1)	7 (25.0)	1 (3.6)	6 (18.2)	0
Decreased appetite	158 (18.1)	2 (<1)	136 (16.1)	6 (<1)	7 (25.0)	0	5 (15.2)	1 (3.0)
Constipation	193 (22.2)	4 (<1)	145 (17.2)	3 (<1)	6 (21.4)	0	4 (12.1)	0
Fatigue	310 (35.6)	16 (1.8)	218 (25.8)	16 (1.9)	6 (21.4)	1 (3.6)	0	0
Bone pain	80 (9.2)	12 (1.4)	116 (13.7)	20 (2.4)	5 (17.9)	0	4 (12.1)	0
Fall	101 (11.6)	12 (1.4)	45 (5.3)	6 (<1)	5 (17.9)	0	1 (3.0)	0
Dysgeusia	66 (7.6)	1 (<1)	31 (3.7)	0	5 (17.9)	0	1 (3.0)	0
Pollakiuria	50 (5.7)	1 (<1)	37 (4.4)	0	5 (17.9)	0	0	0
Headache	91 (10.4)	2 (<1)	59 (7.0)	3 (<1)	4 (14.3)	1 (3.6)	2 (6.1)	0
Diarrhea	142 (16.3)	2 (<1)	119 (14.1)	3 (<1)	3 (10.7)	0	7 (21.2)	1 (3.0)
Cancer pain	10 (1.1)	4 (<1)	10 (1.2)	4 (<1)	3 (10.7)	0	6 (18.2)	0
Back pain	235 (27.0)	22 (2.5)	187 (22.2)	25 (3.0)	3 (10.7)	0	3 (9.1)	0
Upper respiratory tract infection	53 (6.1)	0	30 (3.6)	0	3 (10.7)	0	2 (6.1)	0
Pathological fracture	39 (4.5)	9 (1.0)	19 (2.3)	7 (1.0)	3 (10.7)	0	0	0

Occurring in ≥10% of Japanese patients in the enzalutamide-treated group. Results are from the September 16, 2013, data cutoff
Reproductive from reference 14

active metabolite in Japanese men compared with the overall population, which is likely related to their lower median weight at baseline.

It is concluded that treatment effects and safety in Japanese patients were generally consistent with the overall results from PREVAIL.

24.1.4 Phase I/II Study of Enzalutamide in Japanese Patients [15]

A multicenter phase I/II study was conducted to investigate safety, tolerability, PK, and antitumor activity of enzalutamide in post-docetaxel (TXT) Japanese patients with mCRPC. In phase I, patients received single, then multiple, ascending doses of enzalutamide at 80, 160, or 240 mg/day. Nine patients were enrolled in phase I and 38 in phase II. During phase I, enzalutamide was well tolerated in each cohort, and PK parameters were similar to those of non-Japanese populations in other studies. Overall radiographic response rate was 5.3%, and PSA response rate ($\geq$50% reduction from baseline) was 28.9%. These response rates were lower than the AFFIRM study (5.3 vs. 29%, 28.9 vs. 54%, respectively). It has been suggested that the differences in antitumor activity compared with the AFFIRM study may be attributed to the number of hormonal therapy lines prior to enzalutamide. In fact, with the exclusion of castration therapies, about 90% of patients in this study had received $\geq$3 prior hormonal therapy lines, whereas patients typically received $\leq$2 lines in AFFIRM.

The most frequent AEs with an incidence of $\geq$20% across both phases were weight decrease, decreased appetite, and constipation. Of the AEs reported in $\geq$10% of patients, those considered to be related to enzalutamide were hypertension, constipation, fatigue, decreased appetite, weight decrease, and prolonged electrocardiogram QT. No seizures were observed.

It was concluded that enzalutamide showed good tolerability in Japanese patients, with PK and safety profiles similar to those in non-Japanese populations included in other enzalutamide studies.

24.1.5 Retrospective Studies of Enzalutamide in Daily Practice with Japanese Patients

Retrospective studies on efficacy and safety of enzalutamide in real-world Japanese patients have been reported in Japan. Yamasaki et al. [16] compared the efficacy of enzalutamide between CRPC patients before (51 patients) and after (40 patients) TXT. The median PFS and OS for patients before TXT patients were 10.2 and 27.9 months, respectively. The median PFS for patients after TXT was 4.4, and OS was not reached. Among patients before and after TXT, 24% and 40% experienced AEs, respectively. Fatigue (15%) and appetite loss (13%) were the most common. Although they concluded that the treatment efficacy of enzalutamide might be worse in Japanese patients with CRPC, this might be due to higher numbers of prior treatment regimens including abiraterone acetate and a higher proportion of patients with

≥PS 2 in this study. Igarashi et al. [17] reported that a decline in the PSA level of 50% or more from baseline in CRPC patients before (44 cases) and after (29 cases) TXT were 61.4% and 24.1%, respectively. The most common AEs included fatigue (24.7%), anorexia (24.7%), and nausea (16.4%). Treatment discontinuation as a result of AEs was reported in five cases (6.8%). Although dose reductions as a result of AEs were seen in nine cases (12.3%), eight cases were able to continue the treatment.

Kato et al. [18] analyzed early PSA response to enzalutamide and oncological outcomes to study their prognostic significance in 51 Japanese patients, including 26 cases of pre-TXT and 25 of post-TXT. They showed that an early PSA response at 4 weeks to enzalutamide was significantly associated with a longer rPFS and OS. This information will aid in the management of patients treated with enzalutamide. Terada et al. [19] evaluated the factors predicting efficacy and AEs of enzalutamide in 345 Japanese CRPC patients, including 150 cases of pre-TXT and 195 of post-TXT. Gleason score >8, performance status ≥1, presence of bone metastasis, visceral metastasis, previous steroid treatment, and TXT treatment significantly predicted shorter PSA-PFS of enzalutamide. AEs, including fatigue or appetite loss, occurred in 169 patients (49%), 48 (18%) of whom stopped enzalutamide. Age > 75 years and lower enzalutamide dose were significantly associated with development of AEs.

From the results of both prospective and retrospective studies, some of the most common AEs of enzalutamide are fatigue and appetite loss. Such subjective AEs tend to be underestimated in clinical trials. Iguchi et al. [20] assessed 45 CRPC patients for the AEs of enzalutamide by using self-assessment questionnaire for subjective symptoms. In 12 cases, the dose reduction or discontinuation was needed due to fatigue and appetite loss. In eight cases, subjective symptoms improved after dose reduction. They concluded that self-assessment questionnaires for subjective symptoms are useful tools for finding the AEs of enzalutamide quickly, which may lead to better outcomes of enzalutamide for CRPC through the elimination of dropouts due to AEs.

Conclusions

A new AR signal inhibitor, enzalutamide, has shown high efficacy and a favorable safety profile irrespective of docetaxel use in both clinical trials and routine clinical practice in Japanese patients. It is highly convenient that enzalutamide can be taken as a single oral daily dose either before or after a meal and that there is no need to take additional steroids. However, in daily clinical practice, the patients often complaint of such difficulties as swallowing due to the size of the capsule, fatigue, and appetite loss. In order to continue this effective enzalutamide therapy without discontinuation due to these subjective symptoms, dose reduction seems to be the best way.

References

1. Huggins C, Hodges CV. Studies on prostate cancer 1: the effect of castration, of estrogen and of androgen injection on serum phosphatases in metastatic carcinoma of the prostate. Cancer Res. 1941;1:293–7.

2. Feldman BJ, Feldman D. The development of androgen-independent prostate cancer. Nat Rev Cancer. 2001;1:34–45.
3. Scher HI, Sawyers CL. Biology of progressive castration-resistant prostate cancer: directed therapies targeting the androgen- receptor signaling axis. J Clin Oncol. 2005;23:8253–61.
4. Montgomery RB, et al. Maintenance of intratumoral androgens in metastatic prostate cancer: a mechanism for castration-resistant tumor growth. Cancer Res. 2008;68:4447–54.
5. Cai C, et al. Intratumoral de novo steroid synthesis activates androgen receptor in castration-resistant prostate cancer and is upregulated by treatment with CYP17A1 inhibitors. Cancer Res. 2011;71:6503–13.
6. Linja MJ, et al. Amplification and overexpression of androgen receptor gene in hormone-refractory prostate cancer. Cancer Res. 2001;61:3550–5.
7. Chen CD, et al. Molecular determinants of resistance to antiandrogen therapy. Nat Med. 2004;10:33–9.
8. Scher HI, et al. Increased survival with enzalutamide in prostate cancer after chemotherapy. N Engl J Med. 2012;367:1187–97.
9. Beer TM, et al. Enzalutamide in metastatic prostate cancer before chemotherapy. N Engl J Med. 2014;371:424–33.
10. Jung ME, et al. Structure-activity relationship for thiohydantoin androgen receptor antagonists for castration-resistant prostate cancer (CRPC). J Med Chem. 2010;53:2779–96.
11. Tran C, et al. Development of a second-generation antiandrogen for treatment of advanced prostate cancer. Science. 2009;324:787–90.
12. Scher HI, et al. Antitumour activity of MDV3100 in castration- resistant prostate cancer: a phase 1-2 study. Lancet. 2010;375:1437–46.
13. Beer TM, et al. Enzalutamide in men with chemotherapy-naive metastatic castration-resistant prostate cancer: extended analysis of the phase 3 PREVAIL study. Eur Urol. 2017;71:151–4.
14. Kimura G, et al. Enzalutamide in Japanese patients with chemotherapy-naive, metastatic castration-resistant prostate cancer: a post-hoc analysis of the placebo-controlled PREVAIL trial. Int J Urol. 2016;23:395–403.
15. Akaza H, et al. A multicenter phase I/II study of enzalutamide in Japanese patients with castration-resistant prostate cancer. Int J Clin Oncol. 2016;21:773–82.
16. Yamasaki M, et al. Efficacy and safety profile of enzalutamide for Japanese patients with castration-resistant prostate cancer. Anticancer Res. 2016;36:361–5.
17. Igarashi A, et al. Initial experience of the enzalutamide treatment for castration-resistant prostate cancer. Jpn J Urol. 2016;107:155–61. (Japanese).
18. Kato H, et al. Consequences of an early PSA response to enzalutamide treatment for Japanese patients with metastatic castration-resistant prostate cancer. Anticancer Res. 2016;36:6141–50.
19. Terada N, et al. Factors predicting efficacy and adverse effects of enzalutamide in Japanese patients with castration-resistant prostate cancer: results of retrospective multi-institutional study. Int J Clin Oncol. 2016;21:1155–61.
20. Iguchi T, et al. Management of enzalutamide-related adverse events for castration resistant prostate cancer patients. Jpn J Urol Surg. 2015;28:1685–91. (Japanese).

Abiraterone Acetate Therapy for mCRPC in Japanese Men

25

Masaomi Ikeda and Takefumi Satoh

Abstract

Abiraterone acetate (AA) is a first-in-class CYP17 (17α-hydroxylase/C17, 20 lyase) inhibitor that is approved for the treatment of metastatic castration-resistant prostate cancer (mCRPC). AA prolonged overall survival in both mCRPC patients with or without previously chemotherapy by two randomized Phase III studies (COU-AA-301 and 302 trial). In Japan, AA approved in 2014, similar efficacy and safety of AA are demonstrated. Prostate-specific antigen (PSA) response rates were 60.4% in chemotherapy naïve mCRPC patients (JPN-201 study) and 28.3% in post-chemotherapy mCRPC patients (JPN-202 study), respectively. The most common were liver dysfunction and mineralocorticoid-related adverse events such as hypokalemia, hypertension, and edema. Majority of the adverse events were grade 1 or 2 in severity. PSA flare phenomenon observed approximately 10% during AA treatment, which is feature and different from that of enzalutamide. There is no clear answer to sequential androgen receptor-axis-targeted therapy. But, AA to enzalutamide sequence may be better outcome for PSA progression-free survival compared with reverse sequence. Even in elderly patients with mCRPC, if the patients can be treated, they can be safe and obtain the sufficient therapeutic effect. However, there is no report of AA treatment in Japanese elderly mCRPC patients. This review evaluated the use of AA for Japanese mCRPC patients in detail.

M. Ikeda, M.D., Ph.D. (✉)
Department of Urology, Kitasato University School of Medicine, Sagamihara, Kanagawa, Japan
e-mail: ikeda.masaomi@grape.plala.or.jp

T. Satoh, M.D., Ph.D.
Department of Urology, Kitasato University School of Medicine, Sagamihara, Kanagawa, Japan

Takefumi Satoh Prostate Clinic, Tokyo, Japan

Keywords

Abiraterone acetate · Castration-resistant prostate cancer · Chemotherapy naïve Post-chemotherapy · Japanese men

25.1 Introduction

Abiraterone acetate (AA), a prodrug of abiraterone, is a first-in-class CYP17 (17α-hydroxylase/C17, 20 lyase) inhibitor that selectively inhibits androgen synthesis in testis, adrenal glands, and prostate tumor tissues. The first inhuman dose escalation study of AA was published in 2004 [1]. After Phase II and III studies [2–4], oral AA in combination with prednisone 5 mg administered orally twice daily was approved by the USA in April 2011 for metastatic castration-resistant prostate cancer (mCRPC) patients who had received chemotherapy and that approval was expanded for chemotherapy-naïve patients in December 2012. In Japan, AA approved in July 2014, and clinical data of Japanese men are accumulating little by little.

25.2 Abiraterone in Chemotherapy-Naïve mCRPC

25.2.1 Efficacy

JPN-201 was a Phase II, multicenter, open-label, single-arm study conducted in Japan to evaluate the efficacy and safety of AA in chemotherapy-naïve mCRPC patients [5]. A total of 48 patients treated with AA, median age was 70 years (range, 46–89 years) and median baseline PSA level was 31.4 ng/mL (range, 6.0–469.0 ng/mL). Among them, 29 patients (60.4%) achieved a confirmed ≥50% prostate-specific antigen (PSA) response between baseline and week 12. On the other hand, COU-AA-302 was a global Phase III, double-blind, placebo-controlled study in chemotherapy-naïve mCRPC in which 1088 patients were randomly assigned at a 1:1 ratio to receive AA plus prednisone or placebo plus prednisone [6]. AA plus prednisone administered in 546 patients, median age was 71 years (range, 44–95 years), and median baseline PSA level was 42.0 ng/mL (range, 0.0–3927.4 ng/mL). Patients with decline of ≥50% in PSA level were 61.5%. The PSA response rate observed in JPN-201 study was consistent with the results of COU-AA-302 study in chemotherapy-naïve non-Japanese patients with median follow-up of 22.2 months (61.5%).

Recently, Miyake et al. retrospectively reported the data from 280 Japanese patients in real-world clinical practice who had been treated with either AA or enzalutamide (Enz) as first-line therapy for chemotherapy-naïve mCRPC [7]. Among them 113 patients received AA, median age was 76 years (range, 58–96 years), and median baseline PSA level was 24.3 ng/mL (range, 1.1–3402.7 ng/mL). PSA response rate was 53.1%, and the median time to PSA progression was 9.0 months. Although the median overall survival (OS) was not reached, the 1- and 2-year OS rates were 85.7% and 76.5%, respectively.

25.2.2 Toxicity

The most common adverse events reported in global studies for patients treated with AA plus prednisone were peripheral edema, hypokalemia, hypertension, and hepatic function abnormal [2, 6]. In JPN-201 study [5], all grade of edema was one patient (2%), hypokalemia was seven patients (15%), hypertension was three patients (6%), and hepatotoxicity was 21 patients (44%). Majority of the adverse events were grade 1 or 2 in severity. On the other hand, the percentage of patients with grade 3 or 4 was lower (40%) in JPN-201 study than in COU-AA-302 study in chemotherapy-naïve non-Japanese patients (48%) [5, 6]. Hepatotoxicity is a known risk of treatment with AA; grade 3 or 4 hepatotoxicity in JPN-201 study (10% vs. 8%) was similar compared with the global Phase III study. In addition, a well-known adverse event of AA is mineralocorticoid-related toxicities, and these toxicities are mostly grade 1 or 2. Among the 23% patients with mineralocorticoid-related adverse events in JPN-201 study, only one patient (2%) showed grade 3 hypertension, and these results were consistent with those observed in COU-AA-302 study in non-Japanese patients.

25.3 Abiraterone in Post-Chemotherapy mCRPC

25.3.1 Efficacy

JPN-202 Phase II study evaluated the efficacy and safety of AA in Japanese men with mCRPC who had received docetaxel-based chemotherapy [8]. A total of 47 patients were enrolled, and the median age of the patients was 72 years (range, 51–83 years), with 28% of patients ≥75 years of age. The median baseline PSA level was 143.0 ng/mL (range, 7.2–1450.0 ng/mL). In the full analysis set, 13 patients (28.3%) had a confirmed ≥50% PSA response by 12 weeks of therapy. The median OS was not reached, 6-month survival rate was estimated to be 89.1%, and the median PSA progression-free survival (PFS) and radiographic PFS were 3.6 months and 3.5 months, respectively. These results were comparable to those in the global Phase III trial. COU-AA-301 study randomly assigned, in a 2:1 ratio, 1195 patients who had previously received docetaxel to receive with either AA or placebo [4]. Of the 797 patients, the median age was 69 years (range, 42–95), and ≥75 years patients was 28%. The median baseline PSA level was 128.8 ng/mL (range, 0.4–9253.0). In the AA group, PSA response rate was 29.1%. In addition, the median OS, time to PSA progression, and median PFS were 14.8 months, 10.2 months, and 5.6 months, respectively.

25.3.2 Toxicity

In JPN-202 study, the expected adverse events with AA were reported in 20/47 (42.6%) patients. The most common were hepatic function abnormal (21.3%) followed by hypokalemia (8.5%), hypertension (6.4%), and edema (6.4%). Most of these adverse events were of grade <2 except four patients (8.5%) of grade 3 hepatic function abnormal. Although four patients required dose reduction or interruption, none of these adverse events led to study discontinuation.

Nineteen patients (40.4%) reported adverse events of grade ≥3. Grade 3 adverse events were reported for 17 patients, four patients (8.5%) were hepatic functional abnormal, three patients (6.4%) were hypermagnesemia, and each two patients (4.3%) were pneumonia, urinary tract infection, anemia, and disease progression. Two patients (4.3%) experienced grade 4 adverse events such as cerebral infection, subarachnoid hemorrhage, and disease progression.

The safety findings were consistent with those of other studies in men with mCRPC who had received docetaxel chemotherapy or not [4, 6]. The incidence of grade ≥3 adverse events in JPN-202 study was similar to the chemotherapy-naïve Japanese patients (40%). In particular, the most common grade 3 hepatic function abnormal (8.5%) was higher than COU-AA-301 study (3%) but similar to JPN-201 study (10%) and COU-AA-302 study (8%) [4–6].

25.4 PSA Flare

The PSA flare was defined as any initial increase in the PSA level, followed by a decrease, in accordance with that described in a previous report: (1) any decrease from the peak, (2) any decrease to less than baseline, and (3) a decrease of ≥30% from baseline [9]. We have sometimes observed the PSA flare phenomenon during AA treatment that consists of an early and transient rise in the PSA level, followed by a decline [10, 11]. However, all these reports were restricted to AA treatment after docetaxel-based chemotherapy, and data on chemotherapy-naïve patients were unavailable. Ueda et al. reported the incidence, characteristics, and clinical outcomes of the PSA flare in Japanese patients with mCRPC treated with first-line AA treatment before chemotherapy [12]. Of the 83 patients, using the various definitions of the PSA flare, the incidence ranged from 6.0 to 10.8%. This result was similar to that reported in post-chemotherapy patients during AA treatment (8.7%) [10]. In addition, the clinical outcomes of patients with the PSA flare did not significantly differ from those with an immediate PSA decline. The PSA flare phenomenon is not rare event during AA treatment; thus, AA should not be withdrawn early in patients with mCRPC in whom an initial, isolated PSA increase has been observed.

25.5 Sequential Androgen Receptor-Axis-Targeted Therapy

To date, there have been only small retrospective studies analyzing the outcomes of second-line androgen receptor-axis-targeted (ARAT) therapy for patients with in non-Japanese mCRPC following the failure of first-line therapy [13–15]. Miyake et al. retrospectively evaluated a total of 108 Japanese chemotherapy-naïve patients with mCRPC who sequentially received AA and Enz, in either order, to compare the clinical efficacies sequential ARAT therapy (AA-to-Enz vs. Enz-to-AA) [16]. Of these 108 patients, 49 (45.4%) and 59 (54.6%) were treated with ARAT therapy according to the AA-to-Enz sequence and reverse sequence (Enz-to-AA), respectively. The PSA response rate of the first-line ARAT agent (58.3%) was significantly higher than that of the second-line ARAT agent (21.3%). However, there was no significant difference in the PSA response rates of the first- or second-line ARAT therapy between the AA-to-Enz and Enz-to-AA. On the other hand, the median combined PSA PFS in the AA-to-Enz and Enz-to-AA groups were 18.4 and 12.8 months, respectively ($P = 0.0091$), and the treatment sequence was shown to be independently associated with combined PSA PFS on multivariate analysis. Although the study by Maughan et al. [13] included patients with mCRPC irrespective of the previous history of docetaxel treatment, both of these studies showed a significant difference in the combined PSA PFS favoring the AA-to-Enz sequence compared with the reverse sequence. Furthermore, the AA-to-Enz sequence was an independent predictive factor for the combined PSA PFS in both studies, but no significant difference in the OS was noted between the AA-to-Enz and Enz-to-AA. However, these studies have some limitations, using PSA PFS rather than radiographic PFS as the metric for comparison and imbalanced patient characteristics.

25.6 Efficacy and Safety of Abiraterone in Elderly Patient

Japan is one of the world's leading longevity countries. Prostate cancer is a typical elderly cancer, and recently it has been increasing in Japan. Even in elderly patients with mCRPC, if the patients can be treated, the therapeutic effect can be sufficiently obtained. The International Society of Geriatric Oncology recommends using the cumulative illness score rating-geriatrics [17, 18] and instrumental activities of daily living scale [19] indicators to determine treatment strategies for prostate cancer in the following four groups: (1) "Fit" or "healthy," (2) "vulnerable," (3) "frail," and (4) "too sick" with "terminal illness" [20]. "Fit" and "healthy" elderly patients should receive the same standard treatment as younger patients. In fact, post hoc analysis was investigated that efficacy and safety of AA in elderly (75 years or older) and younger patient subgroup in COU-AA-302 study [21]. Elderly patients treated with AA had significant improvements in radiographic PFS and OS versus those with prednisone alone (HR 0.63, $P = 0.0009$ and HR 0.71, $P = 0.0268$, respectively), similar to younger patients (HR 0.49, $P < 0.0001$ and HR 0.81 $P = 0.0841$, respectively). In addition, specific adverse events with AA such as fluid retention/edema, hypokalemia, hypertension, and hepatotoxicity were similar between the age subgroups. However, there is no report of AA treatment in Japanese elderly mCRPC patients and which is a future task.

Conclusions

AA approved from 2014 in Japan, and clinical data of Japanese CRPC patients are accumulating little by little. In particular, the JPN-201 and JPN-202 trials demonstrated efficacy and safety of AA treatment in chemotherapy-naïve and post-chemotherapy mCRPC. Efficacy and safety of AA treatment in Japanese men are similar compared to non-Japanese patients, but data collection is still necessary.

References

1. O'Donnell A, Judson I, Dowsett M, Raynaud F, Dearnaley D, Mason M, Harland S, Robbins A, Halbert G, Nutley B, Jarman M. Hormonal impact of the 17alpha-hydroxylase/C(17,20)-lyase inhibitor abiraterone acetate (CB7630) in patients with prostate cancer. Br J Cancer. 2004;90(12):2317–25. https://doi.org/10.1038/sj.bjc.6601879.
2. Ryan CJ, Shah S, Efstathiou E, Smith MR, Taplin ME, Bubley GJ, Logothetis CJ, Kheoh T, Kilian C, Haqq CM, Molina A, Small EJ. Phase II study of abiraterone acetate in chemotherapy-naive metastatic castration-resistant prostate cancer displaying bone flare discordant with serologic response. Clin Cancer Res. 2011;17(14):4854–61. https://doi.org/10.1158/1078-0432.CCR-11-0815.
3. Danila DC, Morris MJ, de Bono JS, Ryan CJ, Denmeade SR, Smith MR, Taplin ME, Bubley GJ, Kheoh T, Haqq C, Molina A, Anand A, Koscuiszka M, Larson SM, Schwartz LH, Fleisher M, Scher HI. Phase II multicenter study of abiraterone acetate plus prednisone therapy in patients with docetaxel-treated castration-resistant prostate cancer. J Clin Oncol. 2010;28(9):1496–501. https://doi.org/10.1200/JCO.2009.25.9259.
4. de Bono JS, Logothetis CJ, Molina A, Fizazi K, North S, Chu L, Chi KN, Jones RJ, Goodman OB Jr, Saad F, Staffurth JN, Mainwaring P, Harland S, Flaig TW, Hutson TE, Cheng T, Patterson H, Hainsworth JD, Ryan CJ, Sternberg CN, Ellard SL, Flechon A, Saleh M, Scholz M, Efstathiou E, Zivi A, Bianchini D, Loriot Y, Chieffo N, Kheoh T, Haqq CM, Scher HI, Investigators CA. Abiraterone and increased survival in metastatic prostate cancer. N Engl J Med. 2011;364(21):1995–2005. https://doi.org/10.1056/NEJMoa1014618.
5. Matsubara N, Uemura H, Satoh T, Suzuki H, Nishiyama T, Uemura H, Hashine K, Imanaka K, Ozono S, Akaza H. A phase 2 trial of abiraterone acetate in Japanese men with metastatic castration-resistant prostate cancer and without prior chemotherapy (JPN-201 study). Jpn J Clin Oncol. 2014;44(12):1216–26. https://doi.org/10.1093/jjco/hyu149.
6. Ryan CJ, Smith MR, de Bono JS, Molina A, Logothetis CJ, de Souza P, Fizazi K, Mainwaring P, Piulats JM, Ng S, Carles J, Mulders PF, Basch E, Small EJ, Saad F, Schrijvers D, Van Poppel H, Mukherjee SD, Suttmann H, Gerritsen WR, Flaig TW, George DJ, Yu EY, Efstathiou E, Pantuck A, Winquist E, Higano CS, Taplin ME, Park Y, Kheoh T, Griffin T, Scher HI, Rathkopf DE, Investigators CA. Abiraterone in metastatic prostate cancer without previous chemotherapy. N Engl J Med. 2013;368(2):138–48. https://doi.org/10.1056/NEJMoa1209096.
7. Miyake H, Hara T, Terakawa T, Ozono S, Fujisawa M. Comparative assessment of clinical outcomes between abiraterone acetate and enzalutamide in patients with docetaxel-naive metastatic castration-resistant prostate cancer: experience in real-world clinical practice in Japan. Clin Genitourin Cancer. 2017;15(2):313–9. https://doi.org/10.1016/j.clgc.2016.06.010.
8. Satoh T, Uemura H, Tanabe K, Nishiyama T, Terai A, Yokomizo A, Nakatani T, Imanaka K, Ozono S, Akaza H. A phase 2 study of abiraterone acetate in Japanese men with metastatic castration-resistant prostate cancer who had received docetaxel-based chemotherapy. Jpn J Clin Oncol. 2014;44(12):1206–15. https://doi.org/10.1093/jjco/hyu148.
9. Angelergues A, Maillet D, Flechon A, Ozguroglu M, Mercier F, Guillot A, Le Moulec S, Gravis G, Beuzeboc P, Massard C, Fizazi K, de La Motte Rouge T, Delanoy N, Elaidi RT, Oudard S. Prostate-specific antigen flare induced by cabazitaxel-based chemotherapy in patients with metastatic castration-resistant prostate cancer. Eur J Cancer. 2014;50(9):1602–9. https://doi.org/10.1016/j.ejca.2014.03.015.
10. Burgio SL, Conteduca V, Rudnas B, Carrozza F, Campadelli E, Bianchi E, Fabbri P, Montanari M, Carretta E, Menna C, De Giorgi U. PSA flare with abiraterone in patients with metastatic castration-resistant prostate cancer. Clin Genitourin Cancer. 2015;13(1):39–43. https://doi.org/10.1016/j.clgc.2014.06.010.
11. Narmala SK, Boulmay BC. PSA flare after initiation of abiraterone acetate. J Community Support Oncol. 2014;12(5):191–2.
12. Ueda Y, Matsubara N, Tabata KI, Satoh T, Kamiya N, Suzuki H, Kawahara T, Uemura H. Prostate-specific antigen flare phenomenon induced by abiraterone acetate in chemotherapy-

naive patients with metastatic castration-resistant prostate cancer. Clin Genitourin Cancer. 2017;15(2):320–5. https://doi.org/10.1016/j.clgc.2016.07.026.
13. Maughan BL, Luber B, Nadal R, Antonarakis ES. Comparing sequencing of abiraterone and enzalutamide in men with metastatic castration-resistant prostate cancer: a retrospective study. Prostate. 2017;77(1):33–40. https://doi.org/10.1002/pros.23246.
14. Noonan KL, North S, Bitting RL, Armstrong AJ, Ellard SL, Chi KN. Clinical activity of abiraterone acetate in patients with metastatic castration-resistant prostate cancer progressing after enzalutamide. Ann Oncol. 2013;24(7):1802–7. https://doi.org/10.1093/annonc/mdt138.
15. Azad AA, Eigl BJ, Murray RN, Kollmannsberger C, Chi KN. Efficacy of enzalutamide following abiraterone acetate in chemotherapy-naive metastatic castration-resistant prostate cancer patients. Eur Urol. 2015;67(1):23–9. https://doi.org/10.1016/j.eururo.2014.06.045.
16. Miyake H, Hara T, Tamura K, Sugiyama T, Furuse H, Ozono S, Fujisawa M. Comparative assessment of efficacies between 2 alternative therapeutic sequences with novel androgen receptor-axis-targeted agents in patients with chemotherapy-naive metastatic castration-resistant prostate cancer. Clin Genitourin Cancer. 2017;15(4):e591–7. https://doi.org/10.1016/j.clgc.2016.12.015.
17. Extermann M. Measuring comorbidity in older cancer patients. Eur J Cancer. 2000;36(4):453–71.
18. Linn BS, Linn MW, Gurel L. Cumulative illness rating scale. J Am Geriatr Soc. 1968;16(5):622–6.
19. Lawton MP, Brody EM. Assessment of older people: self-maintaining and instrumental activities of daily living. Gerontologist. 1969;9(3):179–86.
20. Droz JP, Balducci L, Bolla M, Emberton M, Fitzpatrick JM, Joniau S, Kattan MW, Monfardini S, Moul JW, Naeim A, van Poppel H, Saad F, Sternberg CN. Management of prostate cancer in older men: recommendations of a working group of the International Society of Geriatric Oncology. BJU Int. 2010;106(4):462–9. https://doi.org/10.1111/j.1464-410X.2010.09334.x.
21. Smith MR, Rathkopf DE, Mulders PF, Carles J, Van Poppel H, Li J, Kheoh T, Griffin TW, Molina A, Ryan CJ. Efficacy and safety of abiraterone acetate in elderly (75 years or older) chemotherapy naive patients with metastatic castration resistant prostate cancer. J Urol. 2015;194(5):1277–84. https://doi.org/10.1016/j.juro.2015.07.004.

Role of Estramustine Phosphate and Other Estrogens for Castration-Resistant Prostate Cancer

26

Takahiro Inoue

Abstract

The introduction of several expensive drugs, as abiraterone acetate and enzalutamide, and expansion of indication of these new drugs for prostate cancer patients resulted in dramatic increase in cancer treatment costs for castration-resistant prostate cancer. Estramustine phosphate and other estrogens such as ethinylestradiol are far less costly and might offer significant advantages over some of the new castration-resistant prostate cancer treatment, especially regarding bone health, cognition, and metabolic status for prostate cancer patients. Herein we discussed about mechanisms of estramustine phosphate and estrogen compounds for prostate cancer. Moreover, we reviewed several reports of efficacy of treatment with estramustine phosphate and other estrogens for castration-resistant prostate cancer. Furthermore, beneficial effects of estrogen compounds in comparison to luteinizing hormone-releasing hormone agonists during treatment for prostate cancer patients were discussed.

Keywords

Estramustine phosphate · Ethinylestradiol · Castration resistant · Prostate cancer Estrogens

---

T. Inoue, M.D., Ph.D.
Department of Urology, Kyoto University Graduate School of Medicine, Kyoto, Japan
e-mail: takahi@kuhp.kyoto-u.ac.jp

© Springer Nature Singapore Pte Ltd. 2018
Y. Arai, O. Ogawa (eds.), *Hormone Therapy and Castration Resistance of Prostate Cancer*, https://doi.org/10.1007/978-981-10-7013-6_26

26.1 Mechanisms of Estrogen or Estramustine Phosphate Therapy for Prostate Cancer

Estrogens had represented a key drug in the urological armamentarium against prostate cancer for more than half a decade since Huggins and Hodges reported in 1941 the clinical effects of serum testosterone suppression in prostate cancer by administration of estrogen, diethylstilbestrol (DES), as an alternative to surgical castration [1]. Because of high rate of cardiovascular events and thromboembolism receiving estrogen therapy, luteinizing hormone-releasing hormone (LHRH) agonists and nonsteroidal antiandrogen with equivalent oncological effect and lesser cardiovascular toxicity has replaced estrogen therapy for prostate cancer [2, 3]. The main mechanisms of the compound are primary steroidal effect of estrogen; negative feedback on the hypothalamus and anterior pituitary gland, which eventually reduce luteinizing hormone (LH) resulting in decrease in testosterone production to a castrate level by the Leydig cells of the testis [4]. In vitro investigations have shown antimitotic and proapoptotic effects as well as induction of cell cycle arrest in estrogens [5–7]. DES treatment reduce serum dehydroepiandrosterone sulfate (DHEA-S), a representative adrenal androgen, to approximately two-thirds of pretreatment levels [8]. Moreover, it induces increase in serum sex hormone binding globulin (SHBG), which also make decline in serum-free testosterone, bioavailable form of testosterone [8].

Estramustine phosphate (EMP) is a nitrogen mustard carbamate derivative of estratiol-17-β-phosphate, and it is a prodrug that is rapidly dephosphorylated to estramustine and estromustine in vivo [9, 10]. EMP was synthesized with the goal of selectively delivering the alkylating mustard moiety to estrogen-receptor positive cancer cells, but subsequent studies revealed that the dephosphorylated form estramustine and the derivative, estromustine showed very limited and slow dissociation of the molecule at the carbamate linkage and thus, it is atypical for an alkylating agent [11]. Estramustine and estromustine induce metaphase arrest and breakdown of interphase microtubules in vitro and in vivo [12, 13] and the effects of estramustine and estromustine on microtubules has been revealed to be through binding to tubulin [14, 15]. Estramustine can also induce cell death by interacting with nuclear matrix [16]. Estramustine and estromustine accumulate in prostate cancer tissues, and the concentrations were correlated with estramustine binding protein (EMBP: prostatin) [10]. Thus the levels of EMBP might be responsible for the efficacy against prostate cancer cells. The plasma concentrations of EMP metabolites, estrone and estradiol, exceeded normal endogenous plasma levels of them more than 1000-fold and 100-fold, respectively, and these metabolites indirectly suppress plasma testosterone levels [17].

26.2 Efficacy of Estramustine Phosphate in CRPC

EMP was introduced in the early 1970s and has been mainly evaluated as a second-line treatment for patients with CRPC, particularly in combination with other chemotherapy drugs [18]. In 2004, the randomized phase 3 trial revealed that a combination of docetaxel and EMP is superior to a regimen of mitoxantrone and prednisone [19]. Additionally, a meta-analysis assessed to reveal efficacy of addition of EMP to chemotherapy for CRPC patients showed that according to five randomized clinical trials, addition of EMP significantly improved PSA response and increased time to PSA progression and overall survival [20]. However, recent meta-analysis, including a total of 956 patients who received and divided into chemotherapy with or without EMP, revealed that chemotherapy with additional EMP increased the PSA response rate, but overall survival was not improved for the patients [21]. Several reports on oral EMP as a monotherapy against CRPC have shown a PSA response ranging from 24 to 48% with a median overall survival of about 9–42 months [22–26] (Table 26.1).

The tolerability and toxicology of EMP have been a cause for concern at the time of administration [27]. Major adverse events are the digestive system irritation, such as nausea and vomiting, which occur in about 40% of patients. Thromboembolic events are more severe adverse events associated with the use of EMP, and they may result in increased morbidity and mortality because of the increased risk of thromboembolic complications such as cardiovascular events, pulmonary embolism, and stroke [27]. All these issues resulted in rare utilization of EMP for CRPC treatment especially in Western countries nowadays [28].

To evaluate whether low-dose EMP can be administered with the same efficacy as higher dose of EMP with fewer side effects, Inoue et al. conducted a prospective study of low dose, 280 mg per day, of EMP administration to CRPC patients [23]. A total of 31 patients were enrolled and 32% of the patients had a PSA response, defined as a 50% decline in the serum PSA level and median overall survival was 42 months. Thus, the efficacy was comparable to that of higher dose EMP administration [22–26]. Moreover, low-dose EMP was well tolerated, and digestive system irritation occurred in 15% of patients but mostly grade 1 or 2. Only one patient discontinued the treatment because of grade 1 anorexia after 9 months of the administration. The rate of treatment discontinuation is lower than that of the previous higher dose administration studies [22, 24]. Furthermore, there was no severe cardiovascular or deep venous thrombus complications developed during the study protocol, suggesting that low dose, 280 mg/day, of EMP is a safe treatment option in CRPC patients.

Petrioli et al. showed the efficacy of 420 mg of oral EMP together with acetylsalicylic acid against heavily treated CRPC patients, who had been previously treated with docetaxel and abiraterone acetate, also including cabazitaxel in some patients. Among 31 patients enrolled, 9 patients (29.0%) had PSA response, and median overall survival was 7.6 months without grade 3/4 toxicity [29]. The results implicated that reduced dose EMP might also be partly effective and a safe regimen in advanced CRPC patients who failed and progressed after all recommended treatment options including docetaxel, abiraterone, and cabazitaxel.

26.3 Efficacy of Other Estrogens in CRPC

A large retrospective study to assess the efficacy and toxicity of DES at a dose of 1–3 mg daily with aspirin for CRPC was conducted at The Royal Marsden Hospital [30]. The total of 231 patients with large proportion of elderly patients

Table 26.1 Recent reports of oral EMP as a monotherapy against CRPC

Reference	No. of patients	Previous treatment	Age at EMP treatment	PSA value at EMP treatment	Dose	≥50% PSA reduction rate	Median overall survival	Termination rates due to toxicities
Matsumoto et al.	102	CAB + AAT	75.7	15.2	560	29.4	29.6 (prior HT≥3 years), 18.5 (prior HT <3 years)	10.8
Minato et al.	82	CAB + AAT	74	21.5	280 or 560	31.7	21 (good risk), 19 (intermediate risk), 9 (poor risk)	13.4
Naiki et al.	102	Various ADT	NA	NA	NA	48	NA	NA
Hirano et al.	34	CAB (85%) or LHRH agonist monotherapy (15%)	72	25.9	560	24	NA	15
Inoue et al.	31	LHRH agonist (29), antiandrogen (31), AAT (27), DOC(4)	75	19.6	280	32	42	3

with advanced disease including 173 patients with more than three previous hormone regimens and 150 patients with performance status 2 or more were included in the study. The PSA response rate (the PSA Working Group Criteria) was 28.9%, and the median time to PSA progression was 4.6 months. Among them, 68 patients (32%) showed a PSA response of up to 25 and 18% of them had an improvement in their pain score. Thromboembolic complications were seen in 9.9% of them. They concluded that DES has some activity in CRPC and can be of palliative benefit. Turo R et al. conducted retrospective study to investigate the efficacy of DES at a dose of 1 mg daily in 194 CRPC patients [31]. DES was the second-line treatment in 58 patients and the third-/fourth-line therapy in 136 patients. The PSA response rate was 48.9% and the median time to progression was 250 days. Among them, ten patients (5.1%) experienced thromboembolic events with uneventful recovery. Sciarra A et al. prospectively evaluated the efficacy of oral ethinylestradiol (EE) at a dose of 1 mg daily with aspirin for 116 CRPC patients [32]. They all had bone metastasis, ECOG score ≤ 2 (60.7% of the patients had at base line an ECOG score higher than 0), and progressed after at least two hormone therapy regimens. The PSA response rate was 70.5%, and the median time to PSA progression was 15.1 months. Thromboembolic events had occurred in 31 (27.7%) of the patients including 18 cases with grade 3. They concluded that EE provides a favorable PSA response rate against metastatic CRPC patients, and with accurate patient selection, cardiovascular toxicity can be manageable with concomitant anticoagulation therapy. The efficacy of oral EE at a dose of 1.5 mg daily was evaluated in 24 Japanese CRPC men retrospectively [33]. All patients received CAB followed by one or more other hormonal regimens, including three post-docetaxel patients. The PSA response rate was 70% and the median time to progression was 300 days. One patient experienced hearing failure and terminated the administration 56 days after with uneventful recovery. Onishi et al. reported the efficacy of oral EE treatment at a dose of 1.5 mg daily for 20 metastatic CRPC patients retrospectively [34]. After failure with LHRH agonist, PSA response of the first EE treatment was observed in 14 patients (70%) and the median time to progression was 7 months. Interestingly, after the first EE treatment failure they received median number of two other hormonal regimens including docetaxel, enzalutamide, and abiraterone acetate, and again they underwent rechallenge with EE. PSA response of rechallenge EE was 33.3% and the median time to progression was 4 months, including multiple rechallenges with EE. In terms of PSA response of first rechallenge with EE, it was 35% (7 out of 20) according to their report. A post hoc analysis of COU-AA-302 demonstrated that subsequent abiraterone acetate plus prednisone treatment following initial abiraterone acetate plus prednisone administration had limited efficacy; the PSA response rate was 44% and the median time to PSA progression was 3.9 months [35]. Therefore, although the efficacy of rechallenge with EE appeared to be less than that seen with initial EE treatment, oral EE might be a treatment choice for metastatic CRPC patients.

26.4 Benefit of Using Estrogen-Based Compounds as Therapeutic Options for CRPC

Cardiovascular events associated with administration of oral estrogen attributed to the effects of first-pass hepatic metabolism on coagulation molecules [3]. Therefore, parental administration of estrogen, avoiding the first-pass hepatic metabolism, might reduce the complications. Actually, PATCH trial conducted in UK revealed that the rate of cardiovascular events in men receiving estrogen patches was similar to that in men receiving LHRH agonist, although they were excluding patients with high baseline risks of cardiovascular events [36]. Moreover, they showed that parental estrogen administration by patches could lead to castrate testosterone concentrations like those achieved with LHRH agonist in men with locally advanced or metastatic prostate cancer [36]. Importantly, parental estrogen administration by patches could avoid the bone mineral density loss associated with LHRH agonist treatment. Mean fasting serum glucose levels and cholesterol concentration had increased in the LHRH agonist group but decreased in the estrogen patches group, showing that estrogen treatment has beneficial effects for metabolic status [36]. Hot flushes were more frequently seen in patients receiving LHRH agonist group than in the estrogen patch group [36, 37]. Whether the same beneficial effects can be seen by EMP used against CRPC has not yet been confirmed and reported. But recognition of considerable morbidity resulting in osteoporosis, hot flashes, cognitive dysfunction, and others by current conventional androgen deprivation therapies and the introduction and expanding indications of new potential hormone therapies, such as abiraterone acetate with prednisone and enzalutamide, led us to reconsider the old but still attractive compounds for the treatment not only CRPC but also every stage of prostate cancer.

References

1. Huggins C, Hodges CV. Studies on prostatic cancer. I. The effect of castration, of estrogen and of androgen injection on serum phosphatases in metastatic carcinoma of the prostate. Cancer Res. 1941;1:293–7.
2. Bailar JC 3rd, Byar DP. Estrogen treatment for cancer of the prostate. Early results with 3 doses of diethylstilbestrol and placebo. Cancer. 1970;26:257–61.
3. Ockrim J, Lalani El N, Abel P. Therapy insight: parenteral estrogen treatment for prostate cancer—a new dawn for an old therapy. Nat Clin Pract Oncol. 2006;3:552–63.
4. Cox RL, Crawford ED. Estrogens in the treatment of prostate cancer. J Urol. 1995;154:1991–8.
5. Hartley-Asp B, Deinum J, Wallin M. Diethylstilbestrol induces metaphase arrest and inhibits microtubule assembly. Mutat Res. 1985;143:231–5.
6. Robertson CN, Roberson KM, Padilla GM, O'brien ET, Cook JM, Kim CS, Fine RL. Induction of apoptosis by diethylstilbestrol in hormone-insensitive prostate cancer cells. J Natl Cancer Inst. 1996;88:908–17.
7. Schulz P, Link TA, Chaudhuri L, Fittler F. Role of the mitochondrial bc1-complex in the cytotoxic action of diethylstilbestrol-diphosphate toward prostatic carcinoma cells. Cancer Res. 1990;50:5008–12.

8. Kitahara S, Umeda H, Yano M, Koga F, Sumi S, Moriguchi H, Hosoya Y, Honda M, Yoshida K. Effects of intravenous administration of high dose-diethylstilbestrol diphosphate on serum hormonal levels in patients with hormone-refractory prostate cancer. Endocr J. 1999;46:659–64.
9. Saha P, Debnath C, Berube G. Steroid-linked nitrogen mustards as potential anticancer therapeutics: a review. J Steroid Biochem Mol Biol. 2013;137:271–300.
10. Walz PH, Bjork P, Gunnarsson PO, Edman K, Hartley-Asp B. Differential uptake of estramustine phosphate metabolites and its correlation with the levels of estramustine binding protein in prostate tumor tissue. Clin Cancer Res. 1998;4:2079–84.
11. Hudes G. Estramustine-based chemotherapy. Semin Urol Oncol. 1997;15:13–9.
12. Eklov S, Nilsson S, Larson A, Bjork P, Hartley-Asp B. Evidence for a non-estrogenic cytostatic effect of estramustine on human prostatic carcinoma cells in vivo. Prostate. 1992;20:43–50.
13. Hartley-Asp B. Estramustine-induced mitotic arrest in two human prostatic carcinoma cell lines DU 145 and PC-3. Prostate. 1984;5:93–100.
14. Laing N, Dahllof B, Hartley-Asp B, Ranganathan S, Tew KD. Interaction of estramustine with tubulin isotypes. Biochemistry. 1997;36:871–8.
15. Panda D, Miller HP, Islam K, Wilson L. Stabilization of microtubule dynamics by estramustine by binding to a novel site in tubulin: a possible mechanistic basis for its antitumor action. Proc Natl Acad Sci U S A. 1997;94:10560–4.
16. Pienta KJ, Lehr JE. Inhibition of prostate cancer growth by estramustine and etoposide: evidence for interaction at the nuclear matrix. J Urol. 1993;149:1622–5.
17. Norlen BJ, Andersson SB, Bjork P, Gunnarsson PO, Fritjofsson A. Uptake of estramustine phosphate (estracyt) metabolites in prostatic cancer. J Urol. 1988;140:1058–62.
18. Pienta KJ, Redman B, Hussain M, Cummings G, Esper PS, Appel C, Flaherty LE. Phase II evaluation of oral estramustine and oral etoposide in hormone-refractory adenocarcinoma of the prostate. J Clin Oncol. 1994;12:2005–12.
19. Petrylak DP, Tangen CM, Hussain MH, Lara PN Jr, Jones JA, Taplin M, Burch P, Berry D, Moinpour C, Kohli M, Benson M, Small E, Raghavan D, Crawford E. Docetaxel and estramustine compared with mitoxantrone and prednisone for advanced refractory prostate cancer. N Engl J Med. 2004;351:1513–20.
20. Fizazi K, Le Maitre A, Hudes G, Berry WR, Kelly WK, Eymard JC, Logothetis CJ, Pignon JP, Michiels S, Meta-analysis of Estramustine in Prostate Cancer (MECaP) Trialists' Collaborative Group. Addition of estramustine to chemotherapy and survival of patients with castration-refractory prostate cancer: a meta-analysis of individual patient data. Lancet Oncol. 2007;8:994–1000.
21. Qin Z, Li X, zhang J, Tang J, Han P, Xu Z, Yu Y, Yang C, Wang C, Xu T, Xu Z, Zou Q. Chemotherapy with or without estramustine for treatment of castration-resistant prostate cancer: a systematic review and meta-analysis. Medicine (Baltimore). 2016;95:e4801.
22. Hirano D, Minei S, Kishimoto Y, Yamaguchi K, Hachiya T, Yoshida T, Yoshikawa T, Endoh M, Yamanaka Y, Yamamoto T, Satoh Y, Ishida H, Okada K, Takimoto Y. Prospective study of estramustine phosphate for hormone refractory prostate cancer patients following androgen deprivation therapy. Urol Int. 2005;75:43–9.
23. Inoue T, Ogura K, Kawakita M, Tsukino H, Akamatsu S, Yamasaki T, Matsui Y, Segawa T, Sugino Y, Kamoto T, Kamba T, Tanaka S, Ogawa O. Effective and safe administration of low-dose estramustine phosphate for castration-resistant prostate cancer. Clin Genitourin Cancer. 2016;14:e9–e17.
24. Matsumoto K, Tanaka N, Hayakawa N, Ezaki T, Suzuki K, Maeda T, Ninomiya A, Nakamura S. Efficacy of estramustine phosphate sodium hydrate (EMP) monotherapy in castration-resistant prostate cancer patients: report of 102 cases and review of literature. Med Oncol. 2013;30:717.
25. Minato A, Fujimoto N, Kubo T, Harada S, Akasaka S, Matsumoto T. Efficacy of estramustine phosphate according to risk classification of castration-resistant prostate cancer. Med Oncol. 2012;29:2895–900.

26. Naiki T, Okamura T, Kawai N, Sakagami H, Yamada Y, Fujita K, Akita H, Hashimoto Y, Tozawa K, Kohri K. Advantages of second line estramustine for overall survival of hormone-refractory prostate cancer (HRPC) patients. Asian Pac J Cancer Prev. 2009;10:71–4.
27. Ravery V, Fizazi K, Oudard S, Drouet L, Eymard JC, Culine S, Gravis G, Hennequin C, Zerbib M. The use of estramustine phosphate in the modern management of advanced prostate cancer. BJU Int. 2011;108:1782–6.
28. Flaig TW, Potluri RC, Ng Y, Todd MB, Mehra M. Treatment evolution for metastatic castration-resistant prostate cancer with recent introduction of novel agents: retrospective analysis of real-world data. Cancer Med. 2016;5:182–91.
29. Petrioli R, Roviello G, Fiaschi AI, Laera L, Bianco V, Ponchietti R, Barbanti G, Francini E. Low-dose Estramustine phosphate and concomitant low-dose acetylsalicylic acid in heavily pretreated patients with advanced castration-resistant prostate cancer. Clin Genitourin Cancer. 2015;13:441–6.
30. Wilkins A, Shahidi M, Parker C, Gunapala R, Thomas K, Huddart R, Horwich A, Dearnaley D. Diethylstilbestrol in castration-resistant prostate cancer. BJU Int. 2012;110:E727–35.
31. Turo R, Tan K, Thygesen H, Sundaram SK, Chahal R, Prescott S, Cross WR. Diethylstilboestrol (1 mg) in the management of castration-resistant prostate cancer. Urol Int. 2015;94:307–12.
32. Sciarra A, Gentile V, Cattarino S, Gentilucci A, Alfarone A, D'eramo G, Salciccia S. Oral ethinylestradiol in castration-resistant prostate cancer: a 10-year experience. Int J Urol. 2015;22:98–103.
33. Izumi K, Kadono Y, Shima T, Konaka H, Mizokami A, Koh E, Namiki M. Ethinylestradiol improves prostate-specific antigen levels in pretreated castration-resistant prostate cancer patients. Anticancer Res. 2010;30:5201–5.
34. Onishi T, Shibahara T, Masui S, Sugino Y, Higashi S, Sasaki T. Efficacy of Ethinylestradiol re-challenge for metastatic castration-resistant prostate cancer. Anticancer Res. 2016;36:2999–3004.
35. Smith MR, Saad F, Rathkopf DE, Mulders PFA, de Bono JS, Small EJ, Shore ND, Fizazi K, Kheoh T, Li J, de Porre P, Todd MB, Yu MK, Ryan CJ. Clinical outcomes from androgen signaling-directed therapy after treatment with Abiraterone acetate and prednisone in patients with metastatic castration-resistant prostate cancer: post hoc analysis of COU-AA-302. Eur Urol. 2017;72:10–3.
36. Langley RE, Cafferty FH, Alhasso AA, Rosen SD, Sundaram SK, Freeman SC, Pollock P, Jinks RC, Godsland IF, Kockelbergh R, Clarke NW, Kynaston HG, Parmar MK, Abel PD. Cardiovascular outcomes in patients with locally advanced and metastatic prostate cancer treated with luteinising-hormone-releasing-hormone agonists or transdermal oestrogen: the randomised, phase 2 MRC PATCH trial (PR09). Lancet Oncol. 2013;14:306–16.
37. Gilbert DC, Duong T, Kynaston HG, Alhasso AA, Cafferty FH, Rosen SD, Kanaga-Sundaram S, Dixit S, Laniado M, Madaan S, Collins G, Pope A, Welland A, Nankivell M, Wassersug R, Parmar MK, Langley RE, Abel PD. Quality-of-life outcomes from the prostate adenocarcinoma: TransCutaneous hormones (PATCH) trial evaluating luteinising hormone-releasing hormone agonists versus transdermal oestradiol for androgen suppression in advanced prostate cancer. BJU Int. 2017;119:667–75.

Corticosteroid Therapy for CRPC

27

Kazuo Nishimura

Abstract

Corticosteroids have been used in the management of castration-resistant prostate cancer (CRPC) as a monotherapy or in combination with abiraterone acetate, docetaxel, or cabazitaxel. Several corticosteroids with varied potencies are used at different doses in daily medical practice. Although prednisolone or prednisone is the most commonly used corticosteroid in clinical trials, dexamethasone, coincident with its more intense glucocorticoid activity with less mineralocorticoid activity, has shown higher antitumor activity than prednisolone or prednisone without proven survival benefit.

In addition to the suppression of adrenal androgens, GR-mediated NF-κB inhibition is a potential mechanism of the action for dexamethasone in CRPC. Since long-term use of corticosteroids including dexamethasone is associated with multiple adverse events, a careful consideration of sequencing multiple therapies including corticosteroids is required. In this chapter, the biological antitumor activity, clinical benefits, and risks of corticosteroids in CRPC were discussed.

Keywords

Castration-resistant prostate cancer (CRPC) · Corticosteroid · Dexamethasone · Prednisone · Prednisolone · Glucocorticoid receptor (GR) · Nuclear factor-κB (NF-κB)

K. Nishimura
Department of Urology, Osaka International Cancer Institute,
Osaka, Japan
e-mail: nisimura-ka2@mc.pref.osaka.jp

Y. Arai, O. Ogawa (eds.), *Hormone Therapy and Castration Resistance of Prostate Cancer*, https://doi.org/10.1007/978-981-10-7013-6_27

27.1 Introduction

Corticosteroids have been widely used for advanced malignant tumors to palliate tumor-related symptoms such as pain and appetite loss. In prostate cancer, corticosteroids have been used as secondary hormonal treatment for patients with castration-resistant prostate cancer (CRPC) and are currently used to ameliorate toxic effects of abiraterone, docetaxel, or cabazitaxel in addition to managing tumor-related symptoms.

Regardless of these beneficial effects, the long-term use of corticosteroids has been associated with their own toxicities, including adrenal insufficiency, hyperglycemia, edema, osteoporosis, osteonecrosis, and immunosuppression.

In this chapter, the biological antitumor activity, clinical benefits, and risks of corticosteroids in CRPC were reviewed, and the treatment implications of corticosteroid use were discussed.

27.2 Biological Antitumor Activity of Corticosteroids in CRPC

It has been assumed that corticosteroids play a role in CRPC by suppression of the secretion of adrenocorticotrophic hormone (ACTH). The inhibition of ACTH leads to suppress adrenal androgen production. In a prospective study in 37patients with symptomatic metastatic CRPC (mCRPC), pain and quality of life were improved in 38% of patients treated with low-dose prednisone (7.5–10 mg daily) [1]. Symptomatic response was associated with a decrease in serum concentration of adrenal androgens. The results support the hypothesis that the inhibition of adrenal androgen secretion may be the part of the mechanism of action of prednisone in CRPC.

Abiraterone acetate, which is a selective inhibitor of cytochrome P450 c17 (CYP17) and blocks androgen biosynthesis, is approved for the treatment of mCRPC. In the use of abiraterone acetate, concomitant corticosteroids are required to manage the side effects of secondary mineralocorticoid excess that occurs as a result of loss of feedback inhibition of ACTH.

In addition to any effects that result from suppression of ACTH, corticosteroids can inhibit the growth of prostate cancer through the induction of growth-inhibitory cytokines or the inhibition of growth-stimulatory cytokines. In the androgen-independent prostate cancer cell line PC-3, dexamethasone showed the cell growth inhibition through the induction of transforming growth factor-β1 [2], whereas dexamethasone suppressed the production of several cytokines in DU145, androgen-independent prostate cancer cell line [3–5].

The biologic actions of corticosteroids occur in cells that express glucocorticoid receptors (GRs). In this regard, we checked mRNA and protein expression in the human prostate cancer cell lines LNCaP (androgen-sensitive cell line), DU145, and PC-3 by RT–PCR and Western blot analysis, respectively. GR-specific mRNA and protein were detected in DU145 and PC-3 cells but not in LNCaP cells (Fig. 27.1). However, in vitro GR levels are decreased by dexamethasone in a dose-dependent manner in DU145 and PC-3 cell lines (Fig. 27.2). The decrease in GR levels may explain the lack of an antitumor effect of high-dose dexamethasone in a previous

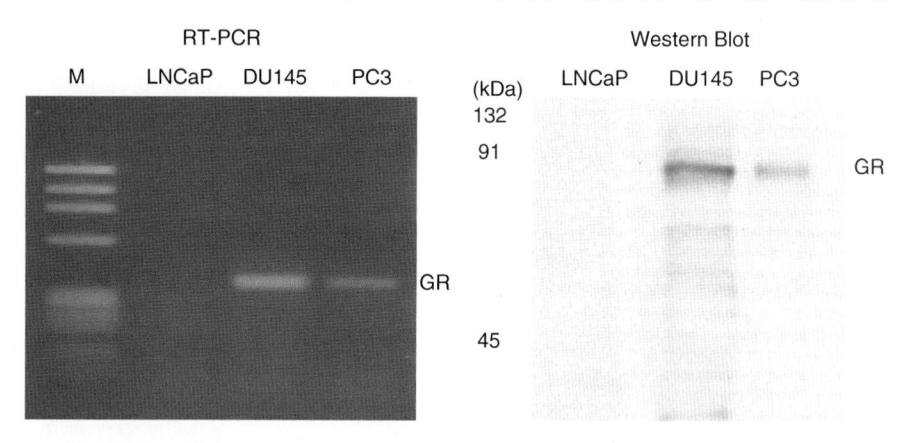

Fig. 27.1 GR expression in prostate cancer cell lines

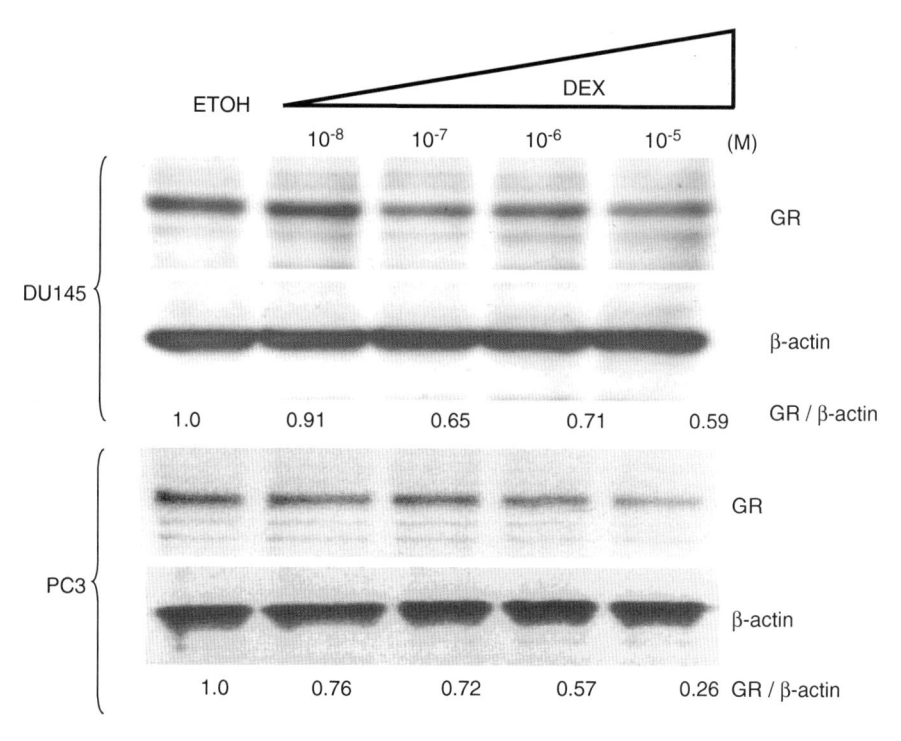

Fig. 27.2 GR protein levels are decreased by dexamethasone in a dose-dependent manner in DU145 and PC-3 cell lines. *ETOH* ethanol, *DEX* dexamethasone

clinical study [6, 7]. To determine whether dexamethasone (10^{-9} to 10^{-6} M) affects the growth of prostate cancer cells in vitro, we performed 5-day cell growth assays using LNCaP, DU145, and PC-3 cell lines. In accordance with GR expression, dexamethasone inhibited the growth of DU145 (10^{-8} to 10^{-6} M) and PC3 (10^{-7} M) but not LNCaP cells.

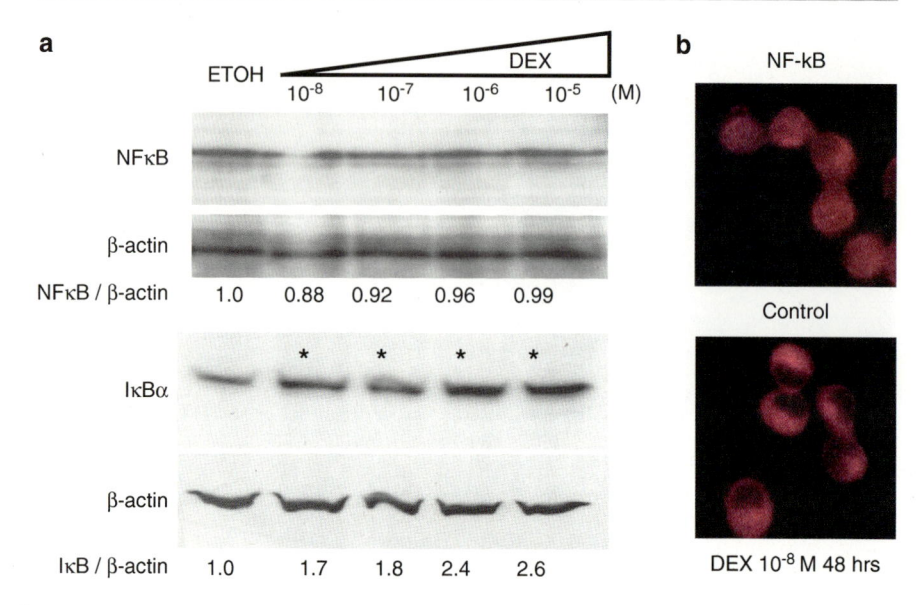

Fig. 27.3 Protein levels of NF-κB and IκB in dexamethasone treated DU-145 cells (**a**). Cellular localization of NF-κB in ethanol or dexamethasone treated DU-145 cells. Nuclear staining is attenuated in dexamethasone treated DU-145 cells (**b**). Ethanol was used as control. *DEX* dexamethasone

GR have been shown to crosstalk with other transcription factors in modulating gene expression [8]. One such transcription factor is NF-κB [9]. We assessed the effects of dexamethasone on the NF-κB activity in DU145 cells. DU145 cells were treated with dexamethasone (10^{-8} to 10^{-5} M) for 48 h, and the protein levels of p65, one of the components of NF-κB, and IκB, one of the natural cytoplasmic inhibitors of NF-κB, were analyzed by Western blot analyses. The levels of IκB, but not of NF-κB, increased in a dose-dependent manner in dexamethasone-treated cells (Fig. 27.3a).

Since IκB binds to NF-κB in cytosol to prevent nuclear localization of NF-κB, we tested the subcellular localization of NF-κB in DU145 cells by indirect immunofluorescence. In contrast to both the nuclear and cytoplasmic compartments in control ethanol-treated DU145 cells, NF-κB localized only to the cytoplasmic compartment, which was accompanied by a loss in localization to the nuclear compartment, in dexamethasone-treated DU145 cells (Fig. 27.3b).

NF-κB is a key regulator of several cytokine growth factors, including IL-6 [10], IL-8, and VEGF. IL-6 has been shown to be an autocrine growth factor for prostate cancer cells [11, 12]. IL-8 and VEGF are two major angiogenic factors which may promote prostate cancer growth [4]. We tested whether dexamethasone affects IL-6, IL-8, and VEGF production in DU145 cells. After 48 h, the mean secretory levels of IL-6, IL-8, and VEGF in conditioned medium from dexamethasone-treated DU145 cells were significantly lower than that in conditioned medium from ethanol-treated control cells (Fig. 27.4). These results suggest that corticosteroids act through GR in prostate cancer cells and suppress cytokine growth factors by inhibiting NF-κB activation.

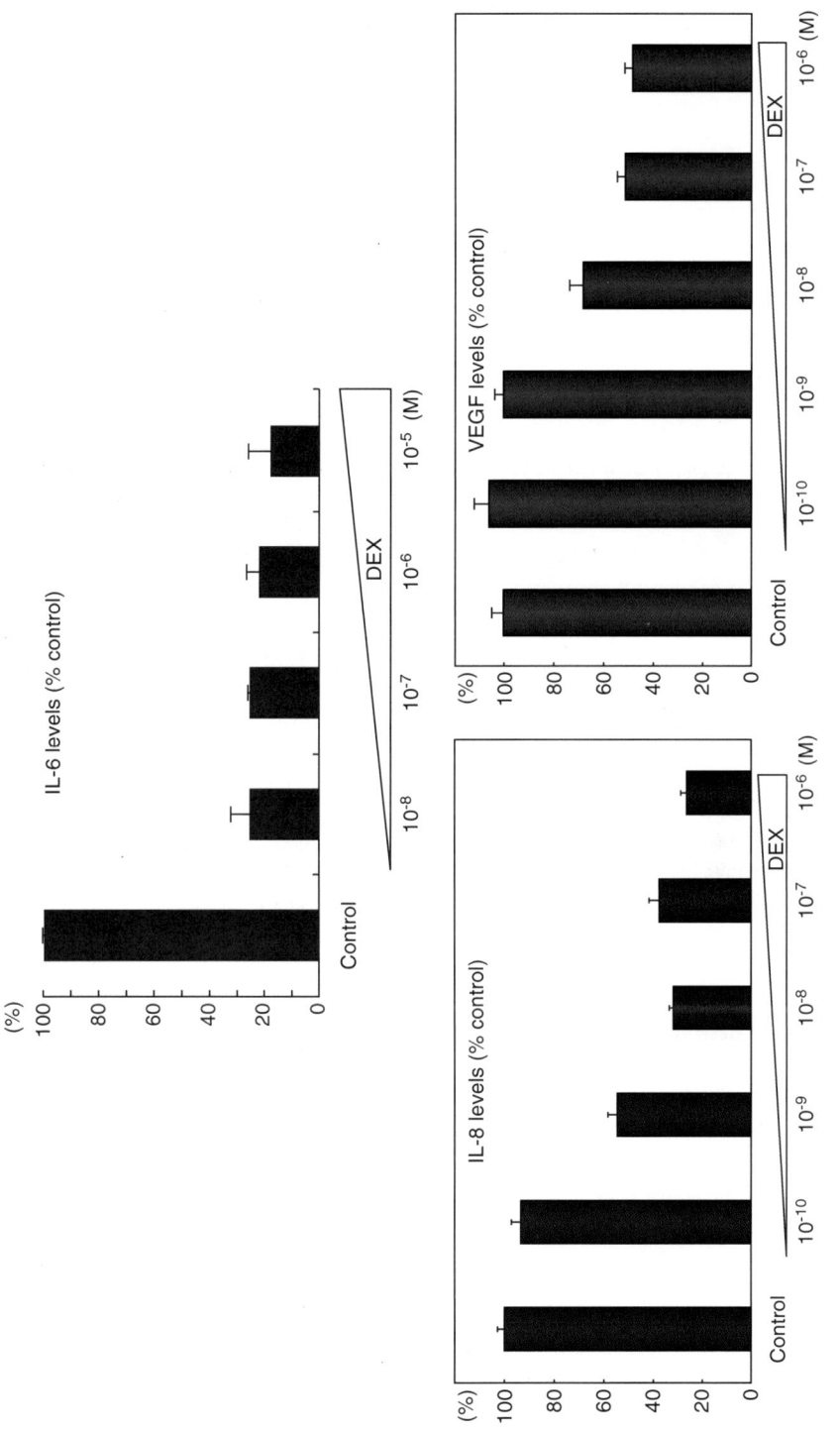

Fig. 27.4 Secretory levels of IL-6, IL-8, and VEGF in conditioned medium from dexamethasone or ethanol-treated DU145 cells. Ethanol was used as control. *DEX* dexamethasone

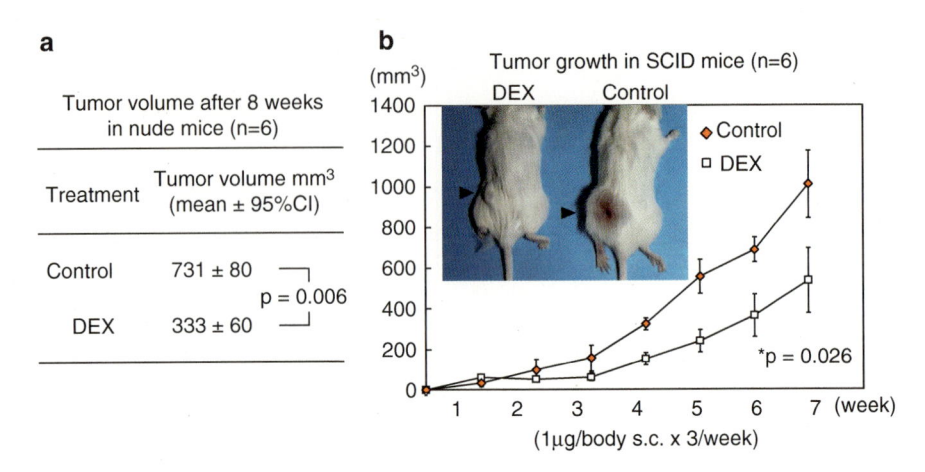

Fig. 27.5 DU145 xenograft tumors in athymic nude (**a**) and SCID mice (**b**) treated with ethanol (control) or dexamethasone. *DEX* dexamethasone

We next asked whether dexamethasone could also inhibit the growth of DU145 xenograft tumors in athymic nude and SCID mice. Since low-dose dexamethasone demonstrated clinical benefits in patients with CRPC [13], a dose of 1 μg per mouse three times per week was selected to mimic a similar low-dose dexamethasone regimen in these xenograft models. After 8 weeks, the mean tumor volume in the dexamethasone-treated nude mice was statistically significantly smaller ($P < 0.006$) than that in the control mice (Fig. 27.5a). After 7 weeks, the mean tumor volume in the dexamethasone-treated SCID mice was also statistically significantly smaller ($P < 0.026$) than that in the control mice (Fig. 27.5b). These results indicated that in vivo administration of low-dose dexamethasone inhibits the growth of androgen-independent prostate cancers. The levels of GR expression in these xenograft tumors were apparently unchanged. Thus, low-dose dexamethasone may continue to inhibit the proliferation of prostate cancer cells in vivo because GR expression is maintained.

27.3 Clinical Benefits of Corticosteroids in CRPC

Although corticosteroids have been used to treat patients with CRPC, there are several types of corticosteroids that have been used in different doses for clinical trials in prostate cancer.

The majority of studies used prednisolone, prednisone, or hydrocortisone to achieve suppression of adrenal androgen as a secondary hormonal therapy or as the control intervention in phase 3 trials of systemic chemotherapy in CRPC [3, 14–18]. According to these studies, a PSA decline of >50% was noted in 9–34% of patients [14, 15, 17, 18] and pain relief was noted in 12–38% [3, 15]. Overall median survivals were reported to be approximately 12 months [14, 17].

There have been fewer studies used dexamethasone for CRPC [13, 19–21]. In our prospective study, dexamethasone was chosen for its very intense glucocorticoid activity with little mineralocorticoid activity. In regard to dose of dexamethasone, no reports to date have shown a clear dose-response effect for dexamethasone. Furthermore, high doses of dexamethasone possibly produce adverse effects such as Cushing syndrome. Therefore, we administered low doses of dexamethasone starting from 0.5 mg to 1 mg/day for the treatment of CRPC. Thirty-two patients with metastatic CRPC typically received 0.5 mg twice daily, whereas five patients with non-metastatic CRPC received 0.5 mg once daily. The maximum doses varied from 0.5 mg/day in 2 patients to 1 mg/day in 13 patients, 1.5 mg/day in 19 patients, and 2 mg/day in 3 patients. The duration of dexamethasone treatment ranged from 1 to 22 months (median, 7 months).

Twenty-three patients (62%) have had a PSA decline of $\geq$ 50%, and the median response duration was 9 months. Among the 25 patients who were treated with dose escalation, 5 experienced additional PSA declines. Among the four patients who had experienced antiandrogen withdrawal syndrome, all had a PSA decline of $\geq$ 75% after dexamethasone therapy.

Among 32 patients assessable for a change in their hemoglobin level, 21 patients (65%) had an increase in their hemoglobin level of at least 1 g/dL and 10 patients (31%) had an increase of at least 2 g/dL, whereas only 2 patients (6%), including 1 patient with rectal bleeding, demonstrated a decrease in their hemoglobin level of >1 g/dL. The majority of patients with a change in their hemoglobin level of <1 g/dL had a hemoglobin level of $\geq$13 g/dL at baseline. Since anemia in patients with CRPC has been linked to both poor physical status and poor prognosis, improvement of anemia may be one of notable benefits of dexamethasone therapy.

To compare the activity of prednisolone and dexamethasone, a single-center, randomized, phase 2 trial was conducted in 82 men with chemotherapy-naive CRPC [21]. Prednisolone 5 mg twice daily versus dexamethasone 0.5 mg once daily versus intermittent dexamethasone 8 mg twice daily on days 1–3 every 3 week was assigned. The intermittent dexamethasone arm was stopped because of lack of antitumor activity. A PSA decline of $\geq$ 50% was noted in 47% of patients with dexamethasone versus 24% of patients with prednisolone, respectively (p = 0.05). Median time to PSA progression was 9.7 months on dexamethasone versus 5.1 months on prednisolone. Among 23 patients who crossed over to dexamethasone at PSA progression on prednisolone, 7 of the 19 evaluable patients (37%) achieved a PSA decline of $\geq$ 50% on dexamethasone. Among 43 patients with measurable disease, the response rate by RECIST was 15% (3 of 20) and 6% (1 of 18) for dexamethasone and prednisolone, respectively (p = 0.6). Clinically significant toxicities were rare. These results indicate the superiority of dexamethasone over prednisolone in the treatment of CRPC.

27.4 Adverse Events of Daily Use of Corticosteroids

Regardless of types and doses of corticosteroids, their long-term use has been associated with multiple adverse events, including hyperglycemia, infection, muscle weakness, insomnia, osteoporosis, necrosis of the jaw, edema, weight gain, cataract, immunosuppression, and adrenal insufficiency. Since the total dose exposure is reported to be associated with the increased risk of these adverse events, care should be taken for patients with mCRPC who may be treated with multiple lines of therapy including corticosteroids, either as a single agent or in combination.

Although a meta-analysis of randomized clinical trials comparing prednisone with other agents did not show significant differences in survival [22], the result was limited because the trials were not designed to assess the impact of prednisone on survival.

A retrospective analysis of patients treated with enzalutamide in the AFFIRM trial showed that men receiving corticosteroids at baseline had a significantly worse survival than those who did not [23]. Meanwhile, another retrospective analysis of patients treated with abiraterone acetate in the COU-AA-301 trial showed that corticosteroids at baseline did not impact on overall survival [24]. Since these results are inconsistent, further study is needed to elucidate the impact of corticosteroid use on survival in patients with CRPC.

Preclinical data have suggested that corticosteroids may promote the growth of prostate cancer. Enzalutamide resistance may occur through the upregulation of the GR by bypassing the androgen receptor (AR) blockade in prostatic cancer cells. In models of prostate cancer, GR expression is induced in the androgen-depleted state, and corticosteroid-GR complex induces the expression of tumor promoting genes, which overlap with genes promoted by AR activation [25]. These alterations of GR downstream may lead to tumor growth and enzalutamide resistance [26].

Conclusions

Corticosteroids have long played an important role in the management of prostate cancer as a monotherapy or in combination with abiraterone acetate, docetaxel, or cabazitaxel. Although prednisolone or prednisone is the most commonly used corticosteroid in clinical trials, dexamethasone has shown higher antitumor activity than prednisolone or prednisone without proven survival benefit. In addition to the suppression of adrenal androgens, GR-mediated NF-κB inhibition may be one the mechanism of the action for dexamethasone in CRPC. However, long-term use of corticosteroids including dexamethasone is associated with multiple adverse events including hyperglycemia, infection, and adrenal insufficiency. Therefore, a careful consideration of sequencing multiple therapies including corticosteroids is required. Further studies are needed to determine optimal use of corticosteroids for CRPC.

References

1. Tannock I, Gospodarowicz M, Meakin W, et al. Treatment of metastatic prostatic cancer with low-dose prednisone: evaluation of pain and quality of life as pragmatic indices of response. J Clin Oncol. 1989;7:590–7.
2. Reyes-Moreno C, Frenette G, Boulanger J, Lavergne E, Govindan MV, Koutsilieris M. Mediation of glucocorticoid receptor function by transforming growth factor beta I expression in human PC-3 prostate cancer cells. Prostate. 1995;26:260–9.

3. Nishimura K, Nonomura N, Satoh E, et al. Potential mechanism for the effects of dexamethasone on growth of androgen-independent prostate cancer. J Natl Cancer Inst. 2001;93:1739–46.
4. Yano A, Fujii Y, Iwai A, Kageyama Y, Kihara K. Glucocorticoids suppress tumor angiogenesis and in vivo growth of prostate cancer cells. Clin Cancer Res. 2006;12:3003–9.
5. Yano A, Fujii Y, Iwai A, Kawakami S, Kageyama Y, Kihara K. Glucocorticoids suppress tumor lymphangiogenesis of prostate cancer cells. Clin Cancer Res. 2006;12:6012–7.
6. Tuttle RM, Loop S, Jones RE, Meikle AW, Ostenson RC, Plymate SR. Effect of 5-alphareductase inhibition and dexamethasone administration on the growth characteristics and intratumor androgen levels of the human prostate cancer cell line PC-3. Prostate. 1994;24:229–36.
7. Weitzman AL, Shelton G, Zuech N, Owen CE, Judge T, Benson M, et al. Dexamethasone does not significantly contribute to the response rate of docetaxel and estramustine in androgen independent prostate cancer. J Urol. 2000;163:834–7.23.
8. Herrlich P. Cross-talk between glucocorticoid receptor and AP-1. Oncogene. 2001;20:2465–75.
9. De Bosscher K, Vanden Berghe W, Vermeulen L, Plaisance S, Boone E, Haegeman G. Glucocorticoids repress NF-kappaB-driven genes by disturbing the interaction of p65 with the basal transcription machinery, irrespective of coactivator levels in the cell. Proc Natl Acad Sci U S A. 2000;97:3919–24.
10. Yamamoto Y, Gaynor RB. Therapeutic potential of inhibition of the NF-κB pathway in the treatment of inflammation and cancer. J Clin Invest. 2001;107:135–42.
11. Chung TD, Yu JJ, Spiotto MT, Bartkowski M, Simons JW. Characterization of the role of IL-6 in the progression of prostate cancer. Prostate. 1999;38:199–207.
12. Okamoto M, Lee C, Oyasu R. Interleukin-6 as a paracrine and autocrine growth factor in human prostatic carcinoma cells in vitro. Cancer Res. 1997;57:141–6.
13. Nishimura K, Nonomura N, Yasunaga Y, et al. Low doses of oral dexamethasone for hormone-refractory prostate carcinoma. Cancer. 2000;89:2570–6.
14. Kantoff PW, Halabi S, Conaway M, Picus J, Kirshner J, Hars V, et al. Hydrocortisone with or without mitoxantrone in men with hormone-refractory prostate cancer: results of the cancer and leukemia group B 9182 study. J Clin Oncol. 1999;17:2506–13.
15. Tannock I, Osoba D, Stockler MR, Ernst DS, Neville AJ, Moore MJ, et al. Chemotherapy with mitoxantrone plus prednisone or prednisone alone for symptomatic hormoneresistant prostate cancer: a Canadian randomized trial with palliative endpoints. J Clin Oncol. 1996;14:1756–64.
16. Small EJ, Vogelzang NJ. Second-line hormonal therapy for advanced prostate cancer: a shifting paradigm. J Clin Oncol. 1997;15:382–8.
17. Sartor O, Weinberger M, Moore A, Li A, Figg WD. Effect of prednisone on prostate-specific antigen in patients with hormone-refractory prostate cancer. Urology. 1998;52:252–6.
18. Kelly WK, Curley T, Leibretz C, Dnistrian A, Schwartz M, Scher HI. Prospective evaluation of hydrocortisone and suramin in patients with androgen-independent prostate cancer. J Clin Oncol. 1995;13(9):2208–13.
19. Storlie JA, Buckner JC, Wiseman GA, Burch PA, Hartmann LC, Richardson RL. Prostate specific antigen level and clinical response to low dose dexamethasone for hormonerefractory metastatic prostate carcinoma. Cancer. 1995;76:96–100.
20. Venkitaraman R, Thomas K, Huddart RA, Horwich A, Dearnaley DP, Parker CC. Efficacy of low-dose dexamethasone in castration-refractory prostate cancer. BJU Int. 2008;101(4):440–3.
21. Venkitaraman R, Lorente D, Murthy V, et al. A randomised phase 2 trial of dexamethasone versus prednisolone in castration-resistant prostate cancer. Eur Urol. 2015;67:673–9.
22. Morgan CJ, WK O, Naik G, Galsky MD, Sonpavde G. Impact of prednisone on toxicities and survival in metastatic castration-resistant prostate cancer: a systematic review and meta-analysis of randomized clinical trials. Crit Rev Oncol Hematol. 2014;90:253–61.
23. Scher HI, Fizazi K, Saad F, et al. Association of baseline corticosteroid with outcomes in a multivariate analysis of the phase 3 Affirm study of enzalutamide (ENZA),an androgen receptor signaling inhibitor (ARSI). European Society for Medical Oncology meeting, Vienna, Austria; September 28–October 2, 2012.
24. Montgomery B, Kheoh T, Molina A, Li J, Bellmunt J, Tran N, Loriot Y, Efstathiou E, Ryan CJ, Scher HI, de Bono JS. Impact of baseline corticosteroids on survival and steroid androgens in

metastatic castration-resistant prostate cancer: exploratory analysis from COU-AA-301. Eur Urol. 2015;67(5):866–73.
25. Arora VK, Schenkein E, Murali R, et al. Glucocorticoid receptor confers resistance to antiandrogens by bypassing androgen receptor blockade. Cell. 2013;155:1309–22.
26. Sharifi N. Steroid receptors aplenty in prostate cancer. N Engl J Med. 2014;370:970–1.

microRNA Analysis in Prostate Cancer

Hideki Enokida

Abstract

microRNAs (miRNAs), a class of small noncoding RNAs, regulate protein-coding gene expression by repressing translation of RNA transcripts in a sequence-specific manner. Aberrantly expressed miRNAs contribute to cancer initiation, progression, metastasis, and drug resistance by targeting several cancer-related genes in various malignancies including prostate cancer (PCa). In the present review, we focused on 91 reliable papers investigating tumor-suppressive (TS) or oncogenic (Onco) miRNAs and their target genes. Several TS-miRNAs are located on different chromosomal regions, suggesting stable expression of TS-miRNAs might be warranted to prevent carcinogenesis in cases of inactivation of the miRNAs' expression due to genomic methylation, deletion, or mutation. On the other hand, several miRNAs are located in close proximity in the same genomic region; this is called a miRNA cluster. Because of their simultaneous expression, common target genes of miRNAs within a cluster may be important for PCa biology. We also discuss the functional significance of the differentially expressed miRNAs and the molecular pathways/targets through focusing androgen receptor (*AR*)-related miRNAs, bone metastasis-related miRNAs, and taxane-based chemotherapy resistance-related miRNAs in hormone-sensitive (HS) and castration-resistance PCa (CRPC). The miRNA-mediated tumor biology could provide important insights into the potential mechanisms of PCa oncogenesis and suggest novel therapeutic strategies for PCa.

Keywords

microRNA · Prostate cancer · Onco-miRNA · TS-miRNA · Tumor marker

H. Enokida, M.D., Ph.D.
Department of Urology, Graduate School of Medical and Dental Sciences, Kagoshima University, Kagoshima, Japan
e-mail: enokida@m.kufm.kagoshima-u.ac.jp

28.1 Introduction

Human DNA contains approximately three billion base pairs. Nonetheless, the Human Genome Project showed that only 2% of our genome encodes functional proteins [1]. Specifically, ~70% of the human genome is transcribed, but 98% of the transcripts are not translated into proteins. These transcripts are called noncoding RNAs (ncRNAs) [2]. These ncRNAs can be roughly classified into two groups based on their size. The first group includes short RNAs (shRNAs) that are less than 200 nucleotides (nt) in length; the second group consists of miRNAs that are around 18–22 nt in length. Other classes of sRNAs include piwi-interacting RNAs (piRNAs), around 23–30 nt [3]. Another group includes long ncRNAs [lncRNAs] of around 200 nt or more (Fig. 28.1).

miRNAs were first discovered as novel regulators of endogenous small ncRNA molecules in *Caenorhabditis elegans* in 1993 [4]. miRNAs are currently known to exist ubiquitously in animals and plants, and they negatively regulate the expression of protein-coding genes in a sequence-specific manner [5]. Recent bioinformatic analyses have shown that miRNAs regulate the expression of approximately 60% of all genes [6, 7]. Thus, miRNAs are used by cells to fine-tune gene expression. It is likely that they are involved in almost all biological processes where they maintain homeostasis in normal cells [8].

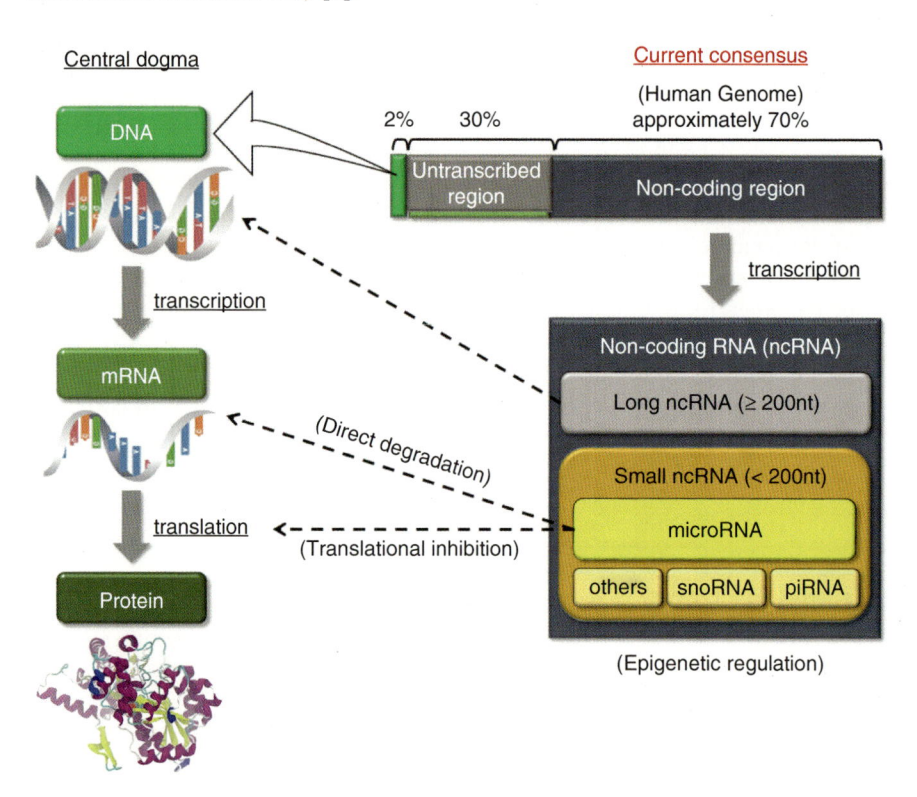

Fig. 28.1 Current consensus of epigenetic gene regulation by noncoding RNAs

With regard to cancer cells, it was first noted in 2002 that a specific miRNA cluster (miR-15 and miR-16) located at chromosome 13q14 was frequently deleted/downregulated in B-cell chronic lymphocytic leukemia. This was the first demonstration of the importance of miRNA in human cancer [9]. Since then, accumulating evidence has shown that aberrantly expressed miRNAs contribute to cancer initiation, progression, metastasis, and drug resistance through their targeting of cancer-related genes.

In the present review, a systematic search of the PubMed database was conducted, using the following terms: "prostate cancer" and "microRNA" or "microRNAs" or "miR" or "miRs." The search identified a total of 907 articles at the end of June 2017. Among them, luciferase reporter assays, which validate direct binding between a miRNA and its target gene, were performed in 91 of the articles. The highlights of those 91 articles were reviewed for their analyses of aberrant expression of the miRNAs and their specific target genes (Tables 28.1, 28.2, and 28.3). Note that in the tables, "GENE ID" referred to those used by the National Center for Biotechnology Information (NCBI) (https://www.ncbi.nlm.nih.gov/gene/) because the names of several genes were described by their alias.

Growing evidence has demonstrated that aberrantly expressed miRNAs can act as oncogenic miRNAs (Onco-miRNAs) or tumor-suppressive miRNAs (TS-miRNAs) in PCa. miRNAs participate in target gene networks that contribute to tumor initiation, survival, and invasion. Consequently, many investigators have focused on the genes targeted by aberrantly expressed miRNAs in PCa. In this review, the compelling roles of miRNAs as potential oncogenes or tumor suppressors are introduced and discussed. In addition, the possibility of using miRNAs as biomarkers for PCa is discussed.

28.2 miRNA Biogenesis

miRNAs are evolutionarily conserved and located either within the introns or exons of protein-coding genes (70%) or in intergenic regions (30%). Most intronic and exonic miRNAs are derived from their host genes, suggesting that they are transcribed concurrently with their host transcripts [10].

As shown in Figs. 28.2 and 28.3, transcripts containing primary miRNAs (pri-miRNAs), which can vary from 200 nt to several kb in length, are capped with a specially modified nucleotide at the 5′-terminus. Moreover, they are polyadenylated with multiple adenosines at the 3′-end. Pri-miRNA is cleaved into precursor-miRNA (pre-miRNA, 60–70 nt in length) by RNase III (also known as Drosha). Pre-miRNA is exported from the nucleus into the cytoplasm by exportin-5. In the cytoplasm, pre-miRNA is cleaved by another RNase III enzyme, known as Dicer, into miRNA duplexes approximately 19–22 nt in length. One miRNA duplex is then recruited into the RNA-induced silencing complex (RISC) and functions to recognize complementary sites within the target messenger RNA (mRNA), thereby regulating translation through mRNA cleavage, degradation, or transcriptional repression [10].

In normal cells, miRNAs are adequately expressed to maintain homeostasis. However, in cancer cells, several Onco-miRNAs are highly expressed, leading to

Table 28.1 miRNAs and their target genes validated by luciferase reporter assay

miRNAs	Stem-loop sequence	Locus	Clustered miRNAs	Type	Target	In vivo experiments	Validation in clinical PCa	References
7-5p	7-1	9q21.32		TS	KLF4	Yes	Yes	[19]
	7-2	15q26.1						
	7-3	19p13.3						
let-7a-5p	let-7a-1	9q22.32	let-7f-1, let-7d	TS	E2F2, CCND2	Yes	Yes	[44]
	let-7a-2	11q24.1	100					
	let-7a-3	22q13.31	4763, 7b					
let-7c-5p	let-7c	21q21.1	99a, 125b-2	TS	IL-6	Yes	No	[45]
					IGF1R	No	No	[26]
					EZH2	No	Yes	[27]
15a-5p	15a	13q14.2	16-1	TS	IHH	Yes	Yes	[32]
17-5p	17	13q31.3	18a, 19a, 20a, 19b-1, 92a-1	Onco	ZBTB4	Yes	No	[12]
19a-3p	19a	13q31.3	17, 18a, 20a, 19b-1, 92a-1	Onco	SUZ12	No	No	[28]
					RAB13	No	No	
					SC4MOL	No	No	
					PSAP	No	No	
					ABCA1	No	No	
19b-3p	19b-1	13q31.3	17, 18a, 19a, 20a, 92a-1	Onco	PTEN	No	No	[46]
	19b-2	Xq26.2	106a, 18b, 20b, 92a-1, 363					
20a-5p	20a	13q31.3	17, 18a, 19a, 19b-1, 92a-1	Onco	ZBTB4	Yes	No	[12]
21-5p	21	17q23.1		Onco	MARCKS	No	No	[47]
					PTCD4	No	No	[48]

22-3p	22	17p13.3		Onco	PTEN	Yes	Yes	[49]
				TS	IPO7	No	No	[50]
23b-3p	23b	9q22.32	27b, 3074, 24-1	Onco	PTEN	No	No	[46]
24-3p	24-1	9q22.32	23b, 27b, 3074	TS	ZNF217	No	No	[50]
	24-2	19p13.12	23a, 27a,					
26a-5p				TS	LOXL2	No	Yes	[51]
					LARP1	No	Yes	[52]
					WNT5A	No	Yes	[53]
	26a-1	3p22.2	153-3p320-3p		AMACR	No	Yes	[54]
	26a-2	12q14.1		Onco	PTEN	No	No	[46]
26b-5p	26b	2q35		TS	LOXL2	No	Yes	[51]
					LARP1	No	Yes	[52]
27a-3p	27a	19p13.12	23a, 24-2	Onco	ABCA1, PDS5B	No	No	[28]
27b-3p	27b	9q22.32	23b, 3074, 24-1	TS	GOLM1	No	Yes	[55]
29a-3p	29a	7q32.3	29b	TS	LOXL2	No	Yes	511
					LAMC1	No	Yes	[56]
					TRAF4	No	Yes	[57]
29b-3p				TS	LOXL2	No	Yes	[51]
	29b-1	7q32.3	29a		LAMC1	No	Yes	[56]
	29b-2	1q32.2	29c		VEGFA	No	No	[50]
29c-3p	29c	1q32.2	29b	TS	LOXL2	No	Yes	[51]
30a-5p	30a	6q13		TS	SOX4	No	Yes	[20]
30b-3p	30b	8q24.22	30d-5p	TS	AR	No	Yes	[24]
32-5p	32	9q31.3		Onco	BTG2	No	No	[29]
34a-5p	34a	1p36.22		TS	TCF7, BIRC5	Yes	Yes	[33]
					HOAIR	Yes	No	[58]
					MYC	Yes	Yes	[59]
					CD44	Yes	Yes	[18]

(continued)

Table 28.1 (continued)

miRNAs	Stem-loop sequence	Locus	Clustered miRNAs	Type	Target	In vivo experiments	Validation in clinical PCa	References
34c-5p	34c	11q23.1	34b	TS	MET	No	Yes	[60]
92a-3p	92a-1	13q31.3	17, 18a, 19a, 19b-1	Onco	PTEN	No	No	[46]
	92a-2	Xq26.2	106a, 18b, 20b, 92a-1, 363					
93-5p	93	7q22.1	106b, 25	Onco	ZBTB4	Yes	No	[12]
96-5p	96	7q32.2	182, 183	Onco	MTSS1	No	No	[61]
					FOXO1	No	Yes	[62]
					HZIP1	No	Yes	[13]
99a-5p	99a	21q21.1	let-7c, 125b-2	TS	IGF1R	No	No	[26]
100-5p	100	11q24.1	let-7a-2	TS	AGO2	No	Yes	[63]
103a-3p	103a-1	5q34	103b-1	TS	PDCD10	No	Yes	[64]
	103a-2	20p13	103b-2					
106b-5p	106b	7q22.1	93, 25	Onco	ZBTB4	Yes	No	[12]
124-3p	124-1	8p23.1		TS	AR	No	Yes	[25]
	124-2	8q12.3						
	124-3	20q13.33						
125a-3p	125a	19q13.41	99b, let-7e	TS	MTA1	No	No	[35]
125b-2-5p	125b-2	21q21.1	let-7c-5p, 99a-5p	TS	IGF1R	No	No	[26]
125b-5p	125b-1	11q24.1		TS	ERBB2	Yes	Yes	[49]
	125b-2	21q21.1		Onco	TP53, PUMA	Yes	No	[65]
129-5p	129-1	7q32.1		Onco	BECN1	No	No	[66]
	129-2	11p11.2						
130a-3p	130a	11q12.1		TS	SLAIN1	No	Yes	[36]
132-3p	132	17p13.3	212	TS	SOX4	No	Yes	[21]

133a-3p	133a-1	18q11.2		TS	EGFR	No	No	[14]
	133a-2	20q13.33						
133b-3p	133b	6p12.2	206	Onco	CDC2L5, PTPRK, RB1CC1, CPNE3	No	No	[28]
135-5p	135a-1	3p21.2		TS	ROCK1, ROCK2	Yes	Yes	[31]
	135a-2	12q23.1						
143-3p	143	5q32	145	TS	GOLM1	No	Yes	[11]
				Onco	FNDC3B	Yes	No	[67]
144-3p	144	17q11.2		TS	BECN1	No	Yes	[68]
145-5p	145	5q32	143	TS	GOLM1	No	Yes	[11]
					SWAP70	No	Yes	[69]
					FSCN1	No	No	[70]
146a-5p	146a	5q33.3		TS	ROCK1	No	Yes	[71]
148a-3p	148a	7p15.2		TS	MSK1	No	No	[38]
151a-5p	151	8q24.3		Onco	CASZ1, IL1RAPL1, SOX17, N4BP, ARHGDIA	No	Yes	[72]
152-3p	152	17q21.32		TS	TGFA	No	Yes	[73]
153-3p	153-1	2q35		Onco	PTEN	No	Yes	[74]
	153-2	7q36.3						
155-5p	155	21q21.3		Onco	GATA3	No	No	[75]
181b-5p	181b-1	1q32.1	181a	TS	HK2	No	Yes	[76]
	181b-2	9q33.3						
182-5p	182	7q32.2	183, 96	Onco	NDRG1	No	Yes	[77]
					FOXF2, RECK, MTSS1	Yes	Yes	[78]
					SLC39A1	No	Yes	[13]

(continued)

Table 28.1 (continued)

miRNAs	Stem-loop sequence	Locus	Clustered miRNAs	Type	Target	In vivo experiments	Validation in clinical PCa	References
183-5p	183	7q32.2	96, 182	Onco	DKK3, SMAD4	No	Yes	[79]
199a-3p	199a-1	19p13.2		TS	SLC39A1	No	Yes	[13]
	199a-2	1q24.3			CD44	Yes	Yes	[17]
199a-5p	199a-1	19p13.2	3120, 214	TS	HIF1A	No	No	[80]
	199a-2	1q24.3						
200c-3p	200c	12p13.31	141	TS	ZEB1	No	Yes	[81]
203a-3p	203	14q32.33	203b	TS	BIRC5, ZEB2, DLX5, RUNX2, SMAD4	Yes	Yes	[34]
205-5p	205	1q32.2		TS	AR	No	Yes	[23]
					HNRNPC	No	No	[50]
212-3p	212	17p13.3	132	TS	SOX4	No	Yes	[21]
218-5p	218-2	5q34		TS	LOXL2	No	Yes	[51]
	218-1	4p15.31			LASP1	No	Yes	[82]
221-3p	221	Xp11.3	222	Onco	CASP10	No	No	[83]
					TP27	No	No	[84]
222-3p	222	Xp11.3	221	Onco	CASP10	No	No	[83]
					TP27	No	No	[84]
301a-3p	301a	17q22		Onco	TP63	No	No	[85]
30d-5p	30d	8q24.22	30b	Onco	SOCS1	Yes	Yes	[86]
320-3p	320a	8p21.3		TS	CTNNB11	Yes	Yes	[87]
	320b-1	1p13.1						
	320b-2	1q42.11						
	320c-1	18q11.2						
	320c-2	18q11.2						
	320d-1	13q14.11						
	320d-2	Xq27.1						

28 microRNA Analysis in Prostate Cancer

328-3p	328	16q22.1		TS	PAK6	Yes	Yes	[37]
330-3p	330	19q13.32		TS	SP1	No	No	[88]
					E2F1	No	Yes	[89]
335-5p	335	7q32.2		TS	ENOS	No	Yes	[90]
370-3p	370	14q32.31		Onco	FOXO1	No	No	[91]
376c-3p	376c	14q32.31	1193, 543, 495, 376a-2, 654, 376b, 376a-1, 300, 1185-1, 1185-2, 381, 487b, 539, 889, 544a, 655	Onco	UGT2B15/17	No	No	[30]
382-5p	382	14q32.31		TS	NR2F2	No	Yes	[92]
421-3p	421	Xq13.2	374b/c	TS	NRAS, PRAME, CUL4B, PFKFB2	No	Yes	[93]
449a-5p	449a	5q11.2	449c, 449b	TS	CCND1	No	No	[94]
452-5p	452	Xq28	224	TS	WWP1	No	Yes	[95]
455-3p	455	9q32		TS	EIF4E	Yes	No	[96]
543-3p	543	14q32.31	379, 411, 299, 380, 1197, 323a, 758, 329-1, 329-2, 494, 1193, 495, 376c, 376a-2, 654, 376b, 376a-1, 300	TS	ENOS	No	Yes	[90]
573-5p	573	4p15.2		TS	FGFR3	No	Yes	[97]
]574-3p	574	4p14		TS	RAC1, EGFR, EP300	Yes	Yes	[15]
				Onco	REL	No	Yes	[98]

(continued)

Table 28.1 (continued)

miRNAs	Stem-loop sequence	Locus	Clustered miRNAs	Type	Target	In vivo experiments	Validation in clinical PCa	References
590-3p	590	7q11.23		Onco	INPP4B	Yes	Yes	[99]
613-3p	613	12p13.1		TS	FZD7	No	Yes	[100]
675-5p	675	11p15.5		TS	TGFB1	No	No	[101]
875-5p	875	8q22.2	599	TS	EGFR	Yes	Yes	[16]
1247-5p	1247	14q32.31		Onco	MYCBP2	No	Yes	[102]
1260-5p	1260a	14q24.3		Onco	SFRP1, SMAD4	No	Yes	[103]
	1260b	11q21						
1271-5p	1271	5q35.2		TS	DIXC1	No	Yes	[104]
1297-3p	1297	13q14.3		TS	MTDH	No	Yes	[105]
1301-3p	1301	2p23.3		TS	UBE4B	No	No	[106]
4638-5p	4638	5q35.3		TS	KIDINS220	Yes	Yes	[107]

Table 28.2 Tumor-suppressive microRNA in PCa

Annotation of target genes	Target genes	miRNAs	Validation in clinical PCa	References
Apoptosis inhibition	BIRC5	34a-5p, 203a-3p	Yes	[33, 34]
	PDCD10	103a-3p	Yes	[64]
Cell cycle	CCND1	449a-5p	No	[94]
	CCND2	let-7a-5p	Yes	[44]
	CUL4B	421-3p	Yes	[93]
	E2F1	330-3p	Yes	[89]
	E2F2	let-7a-5p	Yes	[44]
	MYC	34a-5p	Yes	[59]
Cytokine signaling	EGFR	133a/b-3p, 574-3p, 875-5p	Yes	[14, 15, 16]
	IGF1R	125b-2, 99a-5p, let7c-5p	No	[26]
	IL6	let-7c-5p	No	[45]
	MET	34c-5p	Yes	[60]
Drug resistance	BECN1	144-3p	Yes	[68]
	SLAIN1	130a-3p	Yes	[36]
Cancer stem cell features	CD44	34a-5p, 199a-3p	Yes	[18, 17]
	KLF4	7-5p	Yes	[19]
ECM remodeling	LAMC1	29a/b-3p	Yes	[56]
	LOXL2	218-5p, 26a-5p, 26b-5p, 29a/b/c-3p	Yes	[51]
	NR2F2	382-5p	Yes	[92]
EMT	AGO2	100-5p	Yes	[63]
	DLX5	203a-3p	Yes	[34]
	FSCN1	145-5p	No	[70]
	LASP1	218-5p	Yes	[82]
	ZEB1	200c-3p	Yes	[81]
	ZEB2	203a-3p	Yes	[34]
ERBB signaling	ERBB2	125b-5p	Yes	[49]
	PAK6	328-3p	Yes	[37]
	TGFA	152-3p	Yes	[73]
	ZNF217	24-3p	No	[50]
Glycolytic pathway	HK2	181b-5p	Yes	[76]
HIF-1 signaling	EP300	574-3p	Yes	[14]
	HIF1A	199a-5p	No	[80]
MAPK signaling	FGFR3	573-5p	Yes	[97]
	IPO7	22-3p	No	[50]
	MSK1	148a-3p	No	[38]
p53 pathway inhinition	UBE4B	1301-3p	No	[106]
PI3K/AKT signaling	EIF4E	455-3p	No	[96]
	KIDINS220	4638-5p	Yes	[107]

(continued)

Table 28.2 (continued)

Annotation of target genes	Target genes	miRNAs	Validation in clinical PCa	References
Proto-oncogene	NRAS	421-3p	Yes	[93]
	RAC1	574-3p	Yes	[14]
TGF-beta signaling	ROCK1	135a-5p, 146a-5p	Yes	[31, 71]
	ROCK2	135a-5p	Yes	[31]
	SOX4	30a, 132-3p, 212-3p	Yes	[20, 21]
	SP1	330-3p	No	[88]
	TRAF4	29a-3p	Yes	[57]
	TGFB1	675-5p	No	[101]
Transcription activation	AR	30b-3p, 30d-5p, 124-3p, 205-5p	Yes	[24, 25, 23]
	RUNX2	203a-3p	Yes	[34]
VEGF signaling	VEGFA	29b-3p	No	[50]
Wnt signaling	CTNNB11	320-3p	Yes	[87]
	DIXDC1	1271-5p	Yes	[104]
	FZD7	613-3p	Yes	[100]
	MTDH	1297-3p	Yes	[105]
	TCF7	34a-5p	Yes	[33]
	WNT5A	26a-5p	Yes	[53]
Others	AMACR	26a-5p	Yes	[54]
	ENOS	335-5p, 543-3p	Yes	[90]
	EZH2	Let-7c-5p	Yes	[27]
	GOLM1	27b-3p, 143-3p, 145-5p	Yes	[55, 11]
	HNRNPC	205-5p	No	[50]
	HOTAIR	34a-5p	No	[58]
	IHH	15a-5p, 16-5p	Yes	[32]
	LARP1	26a/b-5p	Yes	[52]
	MTA1	125a-3p	No	[35]
	PFKFB2	421-3p	Yes	[93]
	PRAME	421-3p	Yes	[93]
	SWAP70	145-5p	Yes	[69]
	WWP1	452-5p	Yes	[95]

Table 28.3 Oncogenic microRNA in PCa

Annotation of target genes	Target genes	miRNAs	Validation in clinical PCa	References
Apoptosis	BBC3	125b-5p	No	[65]
	CASP10	221-3p, 222-3p	No	[83]
	FOXO1	96-5p, 370-3p	Yes	[62, 91]
	MARCKS	21-5p	No	[47]
	NDRG1	182-5p	Yes	[77]
	TP53	125b-5p	No	[65]
	TP63	301a-3p	No	[85]

Table 28.3 (continued)

Annotation of target genes	Target genes	miRNAs	Validation in clinical PCa	References
Cell cycle inhibition	CDK13	133b-3p	No	[28]
	CDKN1B	221-3p, 222-3p	No	[84]
Cytocaine signaling inhibition	SOCS1	30d-5p	Yes	[86]
PI3K/AKT signaling inhibition	INPP4B	590-3p	Yes	[99]
	PTEN	22-3p, 153-3p, 19b-3p, 23b-3p, 26a-5p, 92a-5p	Yes	[49, 74, 46]
Proto-oncogene	REL	574-5p	Yes	[98]
TGF-beta signaling inhibition	SMAD4	183-5p, 203a-3p, 1260-5p	Yes	[79, 34, 103]
	ARHGDIA	151a-5p	Yes	[72]
Transcription activation	FOXF2	182-5p	Yes	[78]
Wnt signaling inhibition	SFRP1	1260-5p	Yes	[103]
	DKK3	183-5p	Yes	[79]
	SOX17	151a-5p	Yes	[72]
Zinc homeostasis	SLC39A1	96-5p, 182-5p, 183-5p	Yes	[13]
	ZBTB4	93-5p, 106b-5p, 17-5p, 20a-5p	No	[12]
Others	ABCA1	19a-3p, 27a-3p	No	[28]
	BTG2	32-5p	No	[29]
	CASZ1	151a-5p	Yes	[72]
	CPNE3	133b-3p	No	[28]
	FNDC3B	143-3p	No	[67]
	GATA3	155-5p	No	[75]
	IL1RAPL1	151a-5p	Yes	[72]
	MSMO1	19a-3p	No	[28]
	MTSS1	96-5p, 182-5p	Yes	[61, 78]
	MYCBP2	1247-5p	Yes	[102]
	N4BP1	151a-5p	Yes	[72]
	PDS5B	27a-3p	No	[28]
	PTPRK	133b-3p	No	[28]
	RAB13	19a-3p	No	[28]
	RB1CC1	133b-3p	No	[28]
	PTCD4	21-5p	No	[38]
	RECK	182-5p	Yes	[78]
	SUZ12	19a-3p	No	[28]
	UGT2B15	376c-3p	No	[30]
	UGT2B17	376c-3p	No	[30]

reduced expression of tumor suppressor genes (Fig. 28.2). On the other hand, tumor-suppressive miRNAs (TS-miRNAs) are downregulated in cancer cells, enhancing tumor development (Fig. 28.3). Therefore, different expression patterns of cancer-specific miRNAs are observed. Identification of aberrantly expressed miRNAs is an important first step toward elucidating miRNA-mediated oncogenic pathways.

Fig. 28.2 Biosynthesis of oncogenic miRNAs

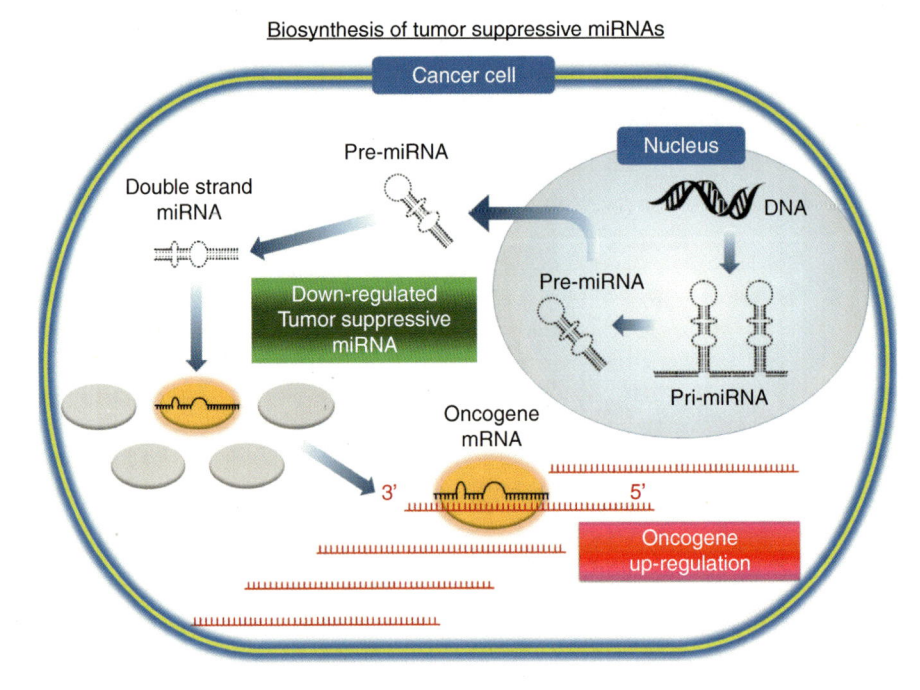

Fig. 28.3 Biosynthesis of tumor suppressive miRNAs

28.3 Features of miRNAs Studies in PCa

In Table 28.1, miRNAs are listed in order of miRNA number, and the validated target genes are indicated. Interestingly, among the 89 miRNAs examined, 56 were identified as TS-miRNAs, whereas 28 were Onco-miRNAs. Five miRNAs (*miR-22-3p*, *miR-26a-5p*, *miR-125b-5p*, *miR-143-3p*, and *miR-574-3p*) were reported as either TS or Onco-miRNAs. In our experience, we often encountered difficulties with the use of anti-miRNAs in in vitro studies; however, miRNA restoration systems using miRNA transfection are well established and commercially available. Accordingly, the latter system may be easier to use to examine the potential tumor-suppressive roles of the downregulated miRNAs, perhaps explaining why studies of TS-miRNAs are dominant.

Several TS-miRNAs, including *miR-7-5p*, *let-7a-5p*, *miR-24-3p*, *miR-26a-5p*, *miR-29b-3p*, *miR-103a-3p*, *miR-124-3p*, *miR-125b-5p*, *miR-133a-3p*, *miR-135a-5p*, *miR-181b-5p*, *miR-199a-3p*, *miR-199a-5p*, *miR-218-5p*, and *miR-320-3p*, are located in different chromosomal regions but have common sequences in their mature miRNAs (Table 28.1). This suggests that the expression of these TS-miRNAs may be maintained by another genomic region, even though one region may be functionally disordered because of methylation, deletion, or mutation. This type of backup system is thought to have important roles in protecting normal cells from carcinogenesis.

Several miRNAs are located in close proximity (within 10 kbp) of the same genomic region; this arrangement is called a miRNA cluster [218]. Clustered miRNAs in PCa are also listed in Table 28.1. Because of their simultaneous expression, common target genes of miRNAs within a cluster may be important for tumor biology. For example, the tumor-suppressive *miR-143/145* cluster was reported in other malignancies [11]. In PCa, it targets the Golgi membrane protein 1 (*GOLM1*), and low expression of the cluster in PCa might contribute to tumor aggressiveness through *GOLM1* upregulation [11]. Zinc finger and BTB domain containing 4 (*ZBTB4*) is a gene that represses transcription. It is targeted by both the *miR-17-92* cluster (*miRs-17-5p/20a*) on chromosome (chr.) 13q31.3 and *miR-106-25* cluster (*miRs-106b/93*) on chr. 7q22.1 in androgen-independent PCa cell lines. miRNAs-ZBTB4 interaction was disrupted by a synthetic triterpenoid methyl ester, glycyrrhetinic acid anti-methyl 2-cyano-3,11-dioxo-18b-olean-1,12-dien-30-oate (CDODA-Me) [12]. Epidemiological studies have suggested that high dietary zinc is associated with a decreased risk of advanced disease. Low zinc uptake into PC cells is caused by lower expression of the zinc transporters, including solute carrier family 39 member 1 (*SLC39A1*) (also known as *HZIP1*) in PCa cells. Overexpression of the entire *miR-183-96-182* cluster suppressed the expression levels of those zinc transporters [13].

28.4 Molecular Target of miRNAs in PCa

28.4.1 TS/Onco-miRNAs and Their Target Genes in PCa

Tables 28.2 and 28.3 show TS/Onco-miRNAs and their target genes in PCa. Among the 111 target genes examined, the expression levels in clinical PCa specimens were validated in 73 genes compared with those in normal bladder epithelium. Those target genes are arbitrarily classified into functional annotations associated with apoptosis, cell cycle, epithelial mesenchymal transition (EMT), drug resistance, and various signaling pathways including hypoxia inducible factor (HIF), mitogen-activated protein kinase (MAPK), phosphatidylinositol-4,5-bisphosphate 3-kinase catalytic subunit (PI3K)/AKT serine proteases (AKT), transforming growth factor beta (TGF-beta), RAS oncogenes (Ras), vascular endothelial growth factor (VEGF), WNT oncogenes (Wnt), and others.

Epidermal growth factor receptor (EGFR) is a critical part of the EGF cytokine signaling pathway. It has long been recognized as a key factor in cell growth, and its expression has been correlated with a high Gleason score, disease relapse, and hormone-refractory status in PCa [14, 15]. EGFR expression was directly repressed by TS-miRNAs, *miRs-133a/b-3p/-574-3p/-875-5p* [14–16]. Interestingly, Genistein, a phytoestrogenic isoflavonoid, showed antitumor effects through upregulation of *miR-574-3p* [14].

Cancer stem cells (CSCs) or tumor progenitor cells are involved in tumor progression and metastasis. CD44 is a cell surface adhesion receptor with pleiotropic signaling function and is highly enriched in CSCs in a variety of tumors, resulting in tumor development or metastasis. Several TS-miRNAs, including *miR-34a-5p* and *miR-199a-3p*, directly regulate CD44 and inhibit extracellular matrix (ECM) remodeling [17, 18]. *miR-7-5p* suppresses a stemness factor, the Kruppel-like factor 4 (*KLF4*), and its downregulation might induce prostate CSCs via activation of *KLF4*/PI3K/Akt/p21 pathway [19].

Metformin (1,1-Dimethylbiguanide) is one of the most commonly used drugs for type II diabetes. Recently, multiple epidemiological studies have shown that metformin may reduce cancer risk and/or improve cancer prognosis. Zhang et al. demonstrated that metformin could inhibit TGF-beta-induced EMT. Direct repression of SRY-box 4 (*SOX4*) was caused by metformin-mediated restoration of *miR-30a-5p* [20]. Also, Fu et al. suggested that *SOX4* is a key molecule targeted by other TS-miRNAs (*miR-132-3p* and *miR-212-3p*) [21].

28.4.2 Androgen Receptor (AR)-Related miRNAs

The androgen receptor (AR) plays a key role both in prostate biology and in the progression of PCa. *AR* gene amplification and overexpression have been observed in nearly one-third of PCa cases. *AR* is posttranscriptionally regulated by more than 20 miRNAs by direct binding to its 3′-untranslated region (UTR), and expressions of those miRNAs were markedly downregulated in clinical PCa samples [22–25].

On the other hand, *AR* itself transcriptionally represses several miRNAs by directly binding to activating transcription factors utilized by the promoter or competing for cofactors and thus interfering with their transcriptional activities. *AR* can also recruit corepressor complexes and histone modification enzymes [26]. *AR* represses *miRNAs-99a/let7c/125b-2* expression by directly binding to the host gene of the cluster in the presence of certain chromatin remodelers (enhancer of zeste 2 polycomb repressive complex 2 (*EZH2*) or lysine demethylase 6B (*KDM6B*)), resulting in upregulation of their target genes including insulin-like growth factor 1 receptor (*IGF1R*). *AR* stimulation of PCa growth involves genes directly induced/repressed by *AR* as well as genes indirectly induced by *AR* through the repression of key miRNAs [26]. Interestingly, a chromatin remodeler, *EZH2*, was also directly regulated by *miR-let7c* [27]. In contrast, *AR* directly activates transcription of *miR-19a*, *miR-27a*, and *miR-133b* by binding to their chromatin of androgen-responsive elements (AREs) and indirectly represses those miRNAs' target genes [28]. AREs are also found in the chromosomal regions of pre-miR-32 and pre-miR-148a that were markedly activated in clinical castration-resistant refractory PCa (CRPC) tissues. *miR-32* and *miR-148a* directly repress the expression levels of B-cell translocation gene 2 (*BTG2*) and phosphoinositide-3-kinase-interacting protein 1 (*PIK3IP1*). BTG2 is involved in cell cycle control and the induction of apoptosis; PIK3IP1 is a negative regulator of the PI3K/AKT pathway. These findings suggest that upregulation of these Onco-miRNAs might attenuate TS genes in CRPC through AR-Onco-miRNAs axes [29].

Other interesting AR-miRNAs axes are evident. For example, *miR-376c-3p*, an Onco-miRNA, represses expression of two UDP-glucuronosyltransferases (UGTs) that inactivate testosterone and dihydrotestosterone, resulting in activating AR signaling [30]. Moreover, AR activates *ROCK1* and *ROCK2* that belong to TGF-beta signaling through downregulation of *miR-135a-5p* that directly binds to these genes [31].

28.4.3 Bone Metastasis-Related miRNAs

Skeletal metastases occur in more than 80% of patients with advanced-stage PCa. Bonci et al. demonstrated that downregulation of miR-15a and miR-16 leads to bone metastasis via upregulating the Indian hedgehog (*IHH*) gene involved in hedgehog signaling [32]. Chen et al. reported that restoration of miR-34a5p expression inhibited bone metastasis through direct targeting of transcription factor 7 (*TCF7*), a key gene in the Wnt signaling pathway in Ras signaling-activated PCa cells [33]. Interestingly, a direct link between *miR-34a-5p* activity and the Ras signaling pathway was shown by p53-transactivated *miR-34a-5p*, where the pathway reduces the expression of p53, which in turn suppresses the posttranscriptional activity of *miR-34a-5p* [33]. Saini et al. found that *miR-203a-3p* directly regulated several EMT-related genes, including baculoviral IAP repeat containing 5 (*BIRC5*) (alias, Survivin), Distal-less homeobox 5 (*DLX5*), Runt-related transcription factor 2 (*RUNX2*), SMAD family member 4 (*SMAD4*), and zinc finger E-box binding homeobox 2 (*ZEB2*). *miR-203a-3p* markedly inhibited bone metastasis in mice following intravenous injection of *miR-203a-3p*-expressing PCa cells [34].

28.4.4 Taxane-Based Chemotherapy Resistance-Related miRNAs

Taxane-based regimens are considered by many to be the best chemotherapy and are believed to offer symptomatic and survival benefits in patients with metastatic CRPC [35]. However, the mechanisms of resistance to taxane chemotherapy remain largely unknown. Liu et al. reported that inhibition of *miR-125a-3p* significantly increased docetaxel resistance in PC-3 cells, whereas upregulation of *miR-125a-3p* effectively reduced docetaxel resistance in docetaxel-resistant PC-3R cells, suggesting that this miRNA may act as a tumor suppressor through regulating metastasis-associated protein 1(*MTA1*) that is associated with chromosomal acetylation [35]. *miR-130a* also activates apoptotic signaling in paclitaxel-resistant PCa cells via targeting of *SLAIN1*, which is one of the microtubule plus-end tracking proteins involved in the regulation of microtubule dynamics [36]. *miR-328* was upregulated in CRPC cells, and it could enhance docetaxel sensitivity through reducing p21 (*RAC1*)-activated kinase 6 (*PAK6*), a serine threonine kinase in the PAK family [37]. A famous Onco-miRNA, miR-21, is also associated with docetaxel resistance through targeting of programmed cell death protein 4 (*PDCD4*) that has been shown to be involved in the sensitivity to chemotherapy [38].

28.5 miRNAs as Potential Biomarkers in PCa

Currently, detection of prostate-specific antigen (PSA) in serum is the best available biomarker for diagnosis and response to treatment of PCa. In spite of that, identification of more sensitive and more specific biomarkers for early diagnosis of PCa is both important and necessary for patients to receive timely treatment. In that regard, certain circulating miRNAs appear in cell-free body fluids such as serum and plasma. Tumor cells release miRNAs into the circulation, and profiles of miRNAs are altered in the plasma and/or serum of patients with cancer, suggesting that it might be possible to use circulating miRNAs as novel noninvasive biomarkers in diagnosing and monitoring cancer patients. Yin et al. retrospectively analyzed ten publications, and the pooled results showed that circulating miRNAs (i.e., *miR-21, miR-26a, miR-32, miR-221*) have a relatively good diagnostic performance, with a sensitivity of 0.74, a specificity of 0.71, and an area under the bivariate summary receiver operator characteristic (SROC) curve (AUC) of 0.77 in indiscriminating PCa from controls [39]. Their results suggested the potential use of circulating miRNAs in the early diagnosis of PCa, especially the combination of multiple circulating miRNAs.

Recently, several studies shed light on exosomal miRNAs as biomarkers for PCa. Exosomes are membrane vesicles ranging in size from 30 to 100 nm. They are widely distributed in the blood, urine, and other bodily fluids. Stable miRNAs can be detected in exosomes, as well as in serum, and the majority of serum-circulating miRNAs are enriched in exosomes. In a retrospective study, Li et al. revealed that the level of serum exosomal miR-141 was significantly higher in PCa patients than in benign prostatic hypertrophy (BPH) patients or healthy controls. Moreover, ROC curve analysis showed that serum exosomal *miR-141* yielded an AUC of 0.8694, with 80% sensitivity and 87.1% specificity in discriminating patients with metastatic PCa from the patients with localized PCa [40]. Huang et al. demonstrated that the expression levels of plasma exosomal *miR-1290* and *miR-375* were significantly associated with overall survival in a follow-up cohort of 100 CRPC patients [41]. However, these studies were retrospectively performed with very small cohorts, and large-scale prospective studies are needed to further validate their findings.

28.6 Future Perspective: Clinical Application of miRNAs in PCa

Recent studies have shown that some miRNAs control the activity of major cancer-related signaling molecules. Thus, identification of instances of aberrant miRNA expression and oncogenic/tumor-suppressive molecular targets of miRNAs would greatly assist the clinical development of novel cancer therapeutics. Because many TS-miRNAs and their target oncogenes are components of complex molecular networks, treatment with multiple miRNAs may provide stronger anticancer effects than treatment with a single miRNA. In an interesting study by Liu et al., new vectors, termed "miRNA-mowers," which contained the entire sequence of the onco-*miR-183-96-182* cluster, were constructed. Transfection of the miRNA-mowers strongly inhibited cell growth and migration and induced apoptosis in vitro, suggesting the usefulness of targeting multiple Onco-miRNAs [42]. Chitosan, a biocompatible, low-immunogenic, and cytotoxic polymer, could be a useful candidate for various biomedical applications, including drug delivery. In fact, a recent study demonstrated that *miR-34a*-chitosan nanoparticles could be successfully delivered to PCa xenografts by in vivo tail vein injection. The nanoparticles inhibited prostate cancer growth in xenografts and showed tumor-suppressive effects on bone metastatic regions in mice [43]. However, the use of miRNA in a drug delivery system (DDS) has not yet been widely accepted. The development of an adequate DDS for TS-miRNAs could be a novel and useful approach to cancer therapeutics. Otherwise, it will be difficult to determine the value of miRNAs as a therapeutic modality in the future.

References

1. International Human Genome Sequencing Consortium. Finishing the euchromatic sequence of the human genome. Nature. 2004;431(7011):931–45. https://doi.org/10.1038/nature03001.
2. Huttenhofer A, Schattner P, Polacek N. Non-coding RNAs: hope or hype? Trends Genet. 2005;21(5):289–97. https://doi.org/10.1016/j.tig.2005.03.007.
3. Bushati N, Cohen SM. microRNA functions. Annu Rev Cell Dev Biol. 2007;23:175–205. https://doi.org/10.1146/annurev.cellbio.23.090506.123406.
4. Lee RC, Feinbaum RL, Ambros V. The C. elegans heterochronic gene lin-4 encodes small RNAs with antisense complementarity to lin-14. Cell. 1993;75(5):843–54.
5. Carthew RW, Sontheimer EJ. Origins and mechanisms of miRNAs and siRNAs. Cell. 2009;136(4):642–55. https://doi.org/10.1016/j.cell.2009.01.035.

6. Filipowicz W, Bhattacharyya SN, Sonenberg N. Mechanisms of post-transcriptional regulation by microRNAs: are the answers in sight? Nat Rev Genet. 2008;9(2):102–14. https://doi.org/10.1038/nrg2290.
7. Friedman RC, Farh KK, Burge CB, Bartel DP. Most mammalian mRNAs are conserved targets of microRNAs. Genome Res. 2009;19(1):92–105. https://doi.org/10.1101/gr.082701.108.
8. Bartel DP. MicroRNAs: target recognition and regulatory functions. Cell. 2009;136(2):215–33. https://doi.org/10.1016/j.cell.2009.01.002.
9. Adams BD, Kasinski AL, Slack FJ. Aberrant regulation and function of microRNAs in cancer. Curr Biol. 2014;24(16):R762–76. https://doi.org/10.1016/j.cub.2014.06.043.
10. Goto Y, Kurozumi A, Enokida H, Ichikawa T, Seki N. Functional significance of aberrantly expressed microRNAs in prostate cancer. Int J Urol. 2015;22(3):242–52. https://doi.org/10.1111/iju.12700.
11. Kojima S, Enokida H, Yoshino H, Itesako T, Chiyomaru T, Kinoshita T, et al. The tumor-suppressive microRNA-143/145 cluster inhibits cell migration and invasion by targeting GOLM1 in prostate cancer. J Hum Genet. 2014;59(2):78–87. https://doi.org/10.1038/jhg.2013.121.
12. Kim K, Chadalapaka G, Pathi SS, Jin UH, Lee JS, Park YY, et al. Induction of the transcriptional repressor ZBTB4 in prostate cancer cells by drug-induced targeting of microRNA-17-92/106b-25 clusters. Mol Cancer Ther. 2012;11(9):1852–62. https://doi.org/10.1158/1535-7163.mct-12-0181.
13. Mihelich BL, Khramtsova EA, Arva N, Vaishnav A, Johnson DN, Giangreco AA, et al. miR-183-96-182 cluster is overexpressed in prostate tissue and regulates zinc homeostasis in prostate cells. J Biol Chem. 2011;286(52):44503–11. https://doi.org/10.1074/jbc.M111.262915.
14. Chiyomaru T, Yamamura S, Fukuhara S, Hidaka H, Majid S, Saini S, et al. Genistein up-regulates tumor suppressor microRNA-574-3p in prostate cancer. PLoS One. 2013;8(3):e58929. https://doi.org/10.1371/journal.pone.0058929.
15. Tao J, Wu D, Xu B, Qian W, Li P, Lu Q, et al. microRNA-133 inhibits cell proliferation, migration and invasion in prostate cancer cells by targeting the epidermal growth factor receptor. Oncol Rep. 2012;27(6):1967–75. https://doi.org/10.3892/or.2012.1711.
16. El Bezawy R, Cominetti D, Fenderico N, Zuco V, Beretta GL, Dugo M, et al. miR-875-5p counteracts epithelial-to-mesenchymal transition and enhances radiation response in prostate cancer through repression of the EGFR-ZEB1 axis. Cancer Lett. 2017;395:53–62. https://doi.org/10.1016/j.canlet.2017.02.033.
17. Liu R, Liu C, Zhang D, Liu B, Chen X, Rycaj K, et al. miR-199a-3p targets stemness-related and mitogenic signaling pathways to suppress the expansion and tumorigenic capabilities of prostate cancer stem cells. Oncotarget. 2016;7(35):56628–42. https://doi.org/10.18632/oncotarget.10652.
18. Liu C, Kelnar K, Liu B, Chen X, Calhoun-Davis T, Li H, et al. The microRNA miR-34a inhibits prostate cancer stem cells and metastasis by directly repressing CD44. Nat Med. 2011;17(2):211–5. https://doi.org/10.1038/nm.2284.
19. Chang YL, Zhou PJ, Wei L, Li W, Ji Z, Fang YX, et al. MicroRNA-7 inhibits the stemness of prostate cancer stem-like cells and tumorigenesis by repressing KLF4/PI3K/Akt/p21 pathway. Oncotarget. 2015;6(27):24017–31. https://doi.org/10.18632/oncotarget.4447.
20. Zhang J, Shen C, Wang L, Ma Q, Xia P, Qi M, et al. Metformin inhibits epithelial-mesenchymal transition in prostate cancer cells: involvement of the tumor suppressor miR30a and its target gene SOX4. Biochem Biophys Res Commun. 2014;452(3):746–52. https://doi.org/10.1016/j.bbrc.2014.08.154.
21. Fu W, Tao T, Qi M, Wang L, Hu J, Li X, et al. MicroRNA-132/212 upregulation inhibits TGF-beta-mediated epithelial-mesenchymal transition of prostate cancer cells by targeting SOX4. Prostate. 2016;76(16):1560–70. https://doi.org/10.1002/pros.23241.
22. Ebron JS, Shukla GC. Molecular characterization of a novel androgen receptor transgene responsive to MicroRNA mediated post-transcriptional control exerted via 3′-untranslated region. Prostate. 2016;76(9):834–44. https://doi.org/10.1002/pros.23174.

23. Hagman Z, Haflidadottir BS, Ceder JA, Larne O, Bjartell A, Lilja H, et al. miR-205 negatively regulates the androgen receptor and is associated with adverse outcome of prostate cancer patients. Br J Cancer. 2013;108(8):1668–76. https://doi.org/10.1038/bjc.2013.131.
24. Kumar B, Khaleghzadegan S, Mears B, Hatano K, Kudrolli TA, Chowdhury WH, et al. Identification of miR-30b-3p and miR-30d-5p as direct regulators of androgen receptor signaling in prostate cancer by complementary functional microRNA library screening. Oncotarget. 2016;7(45):72593–607. https://doi.org/10.18632/oncotarget.12241.
25. Shi XB, Xue L, Ma AH, Tepper CG, Gandour-Edwards R, Kung HJ, et al. Tumor suppressive miR-124 targets androgen receptor and inhibits proliferation of prostate cancer cells. Oncogene. 2013;32(35):4130–8. https://doi.org/10.1038/onc.2012.425.
26. Sun D, Layer R, Mueller AC, Cichewicz MA, Negishi M, Paschal BM, et al. Regulation of several androgen-induced genes through the repression of the miR-99a/let-7c/miR-125b-2 miRNA cluster in prostate cancer cells. Oncogene. 2014;33(11):1448–57. https://doi.org/10.1038/onc.2013.77.
27. Kong D, Heath E, Chen W, Cher ML, Powell I, Heilbrun L, et al. Loss of let-7 up-regulates EZH2 in prostate cancer consistent with the acquisition of cancer stem cell signatures that are attenuated by BR-DIM. PLoS One. 2012;7(3):e33729. https://doi.org/10.1371/journal.pone.0033729.
28. Mo W, Zhang J, Li X, Meng D, Gao Y, Yang S, et al. Identification of novel AR-targeted microRNAs mediating androgen signalling through critical pathways to regulate cell viability in prostate cancer. PLoS One. 2013;8(2):e56592. https://doi.org/10.1371/journal.pone.0056592.
29. Jalava SE, Urbanucci A, Latonen L, Waltering KK, Sahu B, Janne OA, et al. Androgen-regulated miR-32 targets BTG2 and is overexpressed in castration-resistant prostate cancer. Oncogene. 2012;31(41):4460–71. https://doi.org/10.1038/onc.2011.624.
30. Wijayakumara DD, Hu DG, Meech R, McKinnon RA, Mackenzie PI. Regulation of human UGT2B15 and UGT2B17 by miR-376c in prostate cancer cell lines. J Pharmacol Exp Ther. 2015;354(3):417–25. https://doi.org/10.1124/jpet.115.226118.
31. Kroiss A, Vincent S, Decaussin-Petrucci M, Meugnier E, Viallet J, Ruffion A, et al. Androgen-regulated microRNA-135a decreases prostate cancer cell migration and invasion through downregulating ROCK1 and ROCK2. Oncogene. 2015;34(22):2846–55. https://doi.org/10.1038/onc.2014.222.
32. Bonci D, Coppola V, Patrizii M, Addario A, Cannistraci A, Francescangeli F, et al. A microRNA code for prostate cancer metastasis. Oncogene. 2016;35(9):1180–92. https://doi.org/10.1038/onc.2015.176.
33. Chen WY, Liu SY, Chang YS, Yin JJ, Yeh HL, Mouhieddine TH, et al. MicroRNA-34a regulates WNT/TCF7 signaling and inhibits bone metastasis in Ras-activated prostate cancer. Oncotarget. 2015;6(1):441–57. https://doi.org/10.18632/oncotarget.2690.
34. Saini S, Majid S, Yamamura S, Tabatabai L, Suh SO, Shahryari V, et al. Regulatory role of mir-203 in prostate cancer progression and metastasis. Clin Cancer Res. 2011;17(16):5287–98. https://doi.org/10.1158/1078-0432.ccr-10-2619.
35. Feng F, Wu J, Gao Z, Yu S, Cui Y. Screening the key microRNAs and transcription factors in prostate cancer based on microRNA functional synergistic relationships. Medicine (Baltimore). 2017;96(1):e5679. https://doi.org/10.1097/md.0000000000005679.
36. Fujita Y, Kojima T, Kawakami K, Mizutani K, Kato T, Deguchi T, et al. miR-130a activates apoptotic signaling through activation of caspase-8 in taxane-resistant prostate cancer cells. Prostate. 2015;75(14):1568–78. https://doi.org/10.1002/pros.23031.
37. Liu C, Zhang L, Huang Y, Lu K, Tao T, Chen S, et al. MicroRNA328 directly targets p21 activated protein kinase 6 inhibiting prostate cancer proliferation and enhancing docetaxel sensitivity. Mol Med Rep. 2015;12(5):7389–95. https://doi.org/10.3892/mmr.2015.4390.
38. Fujita Y, Kojima K, Ohhashi R, Hamada N, Nozawa Y, Kitamoto A, et al. MiR-148a attenuates paclitaxel resistance of hormone-refractory, drug-resistant prostate cancer PC3 cells by regulating MSK1 expression. J Biol Chem. 2010;285(25):19076–84. https://doi.org/10.1074/jbc.M109.079525.

39. Yin C, Fang C, Weng H, Yuan C, Wang F. Circulating microRNAs as novel biomarkers in the diagnosis of prostate cancer: a systematic review and meta-analysis. Int Urol Nephrol. 2016;48(7):1087–95. https://doi.org/10.1007/s11255-016-1281-4.
40. Li Z, Ma YY, Wang J, Zeng XF, Li R, Kang W, et al. Exosomal microRNA-141 is upregulated in the serum of prostate cancer patients. Onco Targets Ther. 2016;9:139–48. https://doi.org/10.2147/ott.s95565.
41. Huang X, Yuan T, Liang M, Du M, Xia S, Dittmar R, et al. Exosomal miR-1290 and miR-375 as prognostic markers in castration-resistant prostate cancer. Eur Urol. 2015;67(1):33–41. https://doi.org/10.1016/j.eururo.2014.07.035.
42. Liu Y, Han Y, Zhang H, Nie L, Jiang Z, Fa P, et al. Synthetic miRNA-mowers targeting miR-183-96-182 cluster or miR-210 inhibit growth and migration and induce apoptosis in bladder cancer cells. PLoS One. 2012;7(12):e52280. https://doi.org/10.1371/journal.pone.0052280.
43. Gaur S, Wen Y, Song JH, Parikh NU, Mangala LS, Blessing AM, et al. Chitosan nanoparticle-mediated delivery of miRNA-34a decreases prostate tumor growth in the bone and its expression induces non-canonical autophagy. Oncotarget. 2015;6(30):29161–77. https://doi.org/10.18632/oncotarget.4971.
44. Dong Q, Meng P, Wang T, Qin W, Qin W, Wang F, et al. MicroRNA let-7a inhibits proliferation of human prostate cancer cells in vitro and in vivo by targeting E2F2 and CCND2. PLoS One. 2010;5(4):e10147. https://doi.org/10.1371/journal.pone.0010147.
45. Sung SY, Liao CH, Wu HP, Hsiao WC, Wu IH, Jinpu, et al. Loss of let-7 microRNA upregulates IL-6 in bone marrow-derived mesenchymal stem cells triggering a reactive stromal response to prostate cancer. PLoS One. 2013;8(8):e71637. https://doi.org/10.1371/journal.pone.0071637.
46. Tian L, Fang YX, Xue JL, Chen JZ. Four microRNAs promote prostate cell proliferation with regulation of PTEN and its downstream signals in vitro. PLoS One. 2013;8(9):e75885. https://doi.org/10.1371/journal.pone.0075885.
47. Li T, Li D, Sha J, Sun P, Huang Y. MicroRNA-21 directly targets MARCKS and promotes apoptosis resistance and invasion in prostate cancer cells. Biochem Biophys Res Commun. 2009;383(3):280–5. https://doi.org/10.1016/j.bbrc.2009.03.077.
48. Shi GH, Ye DW, Yao XD, Zhang SL, Dai B, Zhang HL, et al. Involvement of microRNA-21 in mediating chemo-resistance to docetaxel in androgen-independent prostate cancer PC3 cells. Acta Pharmacol Sin. 2010;31(7):867–73. https://doi.org/10.1038/aps.2010.48.
49. Budd WT, Seashols-Williams SJ, Clark GC, Weaver D, Calvert V, Petricoin E, et al. Dual action of miR-125b as a tumor suppressor and OncomiR-22 promotes prostate cancer tumorigenesis. PLoS One. 2015;10(11):e0142373. https://doi.org/10.1371/journal.pone.0142373.
50. Szczyrba J, Nolte E, Hart M, Doll C, Wach S, Taubert H, et al. Identification of ZNF217, hnRNP-K, VEGF-A and IPO7 as targets for microRNAs that are downregulated in prostate carcinoma. Int J Cancer. 2013;132(4):775–84. https://doi.org/10.1002/ijc.27731.
51. Kato M, Kurozumi A, Goto Y, Matsushita R, Okato A, Nishikawa R, et al. Regulation of metastasis-promoting LOXL2 gene expression by antitumor microRNAs in prostate cancer. J Hum Genet. 2017;62(1):123–32. https://doi.org/10.1038/jhg.2016.68.
52. Kato M, Goto Y, Matsushita R, Kurozumi A, Fukumoto I, Nishikawa R, et al. MicroRNA-26a/b directly regulate La-related protein 1 and inhibit cancer cell invasion in prostate cancer. Int J Oncol. 2015;47(2):710–8. https://doi.org/10.3892/ijo.2015.3043.
53. Zhao S, Ye X, Xiao L, Lian X, Feng Y, Li F, et al. MiR-26a inhibits prostate cancer progression by repression of Wnt5a. Tumour Biol. 2014;35(10):9725–33. https://doi.org/10.1007/s13277-014-2206-4.
54. Erdmann K, Kaulke K, Thomae C, Huebner D, Sergon M, Froehner M, et al. Elevated expression of prostate cancer-associated genes is linked to down-regulation of microRNAs. BMC Cancer. 2014;14:82. https://doi.org/10.1186/1471-2407-14-82.
55. Goto Y, Kojima S, Nishikawa R, Enokida H, Chiyomaru T, Kinoshita T, et al. The microRNA-23b/27b/24-1 cluster is a disease progression marker and tumor suppressor in prostate cancer. Oncotarget. 2014;5(17):7748–59. https://doi.org/10.18632/oncotarget.2294.

56. Nishikawa R, Goto Y, Kojima S, Enokida H, Chiyomaru T, Kinoshita T, et al. Tumor-suppressive microRNA-29s inhibit cancer cell migration and invasion via targeting LAMC1 in prostate cancer. Int J Oncol. 2014;45(1):401–10. https://doi.org/10.3892/ijo.2014.2437.
57. Ahmed F, Shiraishi T, Vessella RL, Kulkarni P. Tumor necrosis factor receptor associated factor-4: an adapter protein overexpressed in metastatic prostate cancer is regulated by microRNA-29a. Oncol Rep. 2013;30(6):2963–8. https://doi.org/10.3892/or.2013.2789.
58. Chiyomaru T, Yamamura S, Fukuhara S, Yoshino H, Kinoshita T, Majid S, et al. Genistein inhibits prostate cancer cell growth by targeting miR-34a and oncogenic HOTAIR. PLoS One. 2013;8(8):e70372. https://doi.org/10.1371/journal.pone.0070372.
59. Yamamura S, Saini S, Majid S, Hirata H, Ueno K, Deng G, et al. MicroRNA-34a modulates c-Myc transcriptional complexes to suppress malignancy in human prostate cancer cells. PLoS One. 2012;7(1):e29722. https://doi.org/10.1371/journal.pone.0029722.
60. Hagman Z, Haflidadottir BS, Ansari M, Persson M, Bjartell A, Edsjo A, et al. The tumour suppressor miR-34c targets MET in prostate cancer cells. Br J Cancer. 2013;109(5):1271–8. https://doi.org/10.1038/bjc.2013.449.
61. Xu L, Zhong J, Guo B, Zhu Q, Liang H, Wen N, et al. miR-96 promotes the growth of prostate carcinoma cells by suppressing MTSS1. Tumour Biol. 2016;37(9):12023–32. https://doi.org/10.1007/s13277-016-5058-2.
62. Fendler A, Jung M, Stephan C, Erbersdobler A, Jung K, Yousef GM. The antiapoptotic function of miR-96 in prostate cancer by inhibition of FOXO1. PLoS One. 2013;8(11):e80807. https://doi.org/10.1371/journal.pone.0080807.
63. Wang M, Ren D, Guo W, Wang Z, Huang S, Du H, et al. Loss of miR-100 enhances migration, invasion, epithelial-mesenchymal transition and stemness properties in prostate cancer cells through targeting Argonaute 2. Int J Oncol. 2014;45(1):362–72. https://doi.org/10.3892/ijo.2014.2413.
64. Fu X, Zhang W, Su Y, Lu L, Wang D, Wang H. MicroRNA-103 suppresses tumor cell proliferation by targeting PDCD10 in prostate cancer. Prostate. 2016;76(6):543–51. https://doi.org/10.1002/pros.23143.
65. Shi XB, Xue L, Ma AH, Tepper CG, Kung HJ, White RW. miR-125b promotes growth of prostate cancer xenograft tumor through targeting pro-apoptotic genes. Prostate. 2011;71(5):538–49. https://doi.org/10.1002/pros.21270.
66. Xiao W, Dai B, Zhu Y, Ye D. Norcantharidin induces autophagy-related prostate cancer cell death through Beclin-1 upregulation by miR-129-5p suppression. Tumour Biol. 2015. https://doi.org/10.1007/s13277-015-4488-6.
67. Fan X, Chen X, Deng W, Zhong G, Cai Q, Lin T. Up-regulated microRNA-143 in cancer stem cells differentiation promotes prostate cancer cells metastasis by modulating FNDC3B expression. BMC Cancer. 2013;13:61. https://doi.org/10.1186/1471-2407-13-61.
68. Liu F, Wang J, Fu Q, Zhang X, Wang Y, Liu J, et al. VEGF-activated miR-144 regulates autophagic survival of prostate cancer cells against Cisplatin. Tumour Biol. 2015. https://doi.org/10.1007/s13277-015-4383-1.
69. Chiyomaru T, Tatarano S, Kawakami K, Enokida H, Yoshino H, Nohata N, et al. SWAP70, actin-binding protein, function as an oncogene targeting tumor-suppressive miR-145 in prostate cancer. Prostate. 2011;71(14):1559–67. https://doi.org/10.1002/pros.21372.
70. Fuse M, Nohata N, Kojima S, Sakamoto S, Chiyomaru T, Kawakami K, et al. Restoration of miR-145 expression suppresses cell proliferation, migration and invasion in prostate cancer by targeting FSCN1. Int J Oncol. 2011;38(4):1093–101. https://doi.org/10.3892/ijo.2011.919.
71. Xu B, Huang Y, Niu X, Tao T, Jiang L, Tong N, et al. Hsa-miR-146a-5p modulates androgen-independent prostate cancer cells apoptosis by targeting ROCK1. Prostate. 2015;75(16):1896–903. https://doi.org/10.1002/pros.23068.
72. Chiyomaru T, Yamamura S, Zaman MS, Majid S, Deng G, Shahryari V, et al. Genistein suppresses prostate cancer growth through inhibition of oncogenic microRNA-151. PLoS One. 2012;7(8):e43812. https://doi.org/10.1371/journal.pone.0043812.

73. Zhu C, Li J, Ding Q, Cheng G, Zhou H, Tao L, et al. miR-152 controls migration and invasive potential by targeting TGFalpha in prostate cancer cell lines. Prostate. 2013;73(10):1082–9. https://doi.org/10.1002/pros.22656.
74. Wu Z, He B, He J, Mao X. Upregulation of miR-153 promotes cell proliferation via downregulation of the PTEN tumor suppressor gene in human prostate cancer. Prostate. 2013;73(6):596–604. https://doi.org/10.1002/pros.22600.
75. Li B, Jin X, Meng H, Hu B, Zhang T, Yu J, et al. Morin promotes prostate cancer cells chemosensitivity to paclitaxel through miR-155/GATA3 axis. Oncotarget. 2017;8(29):47849–60. https://doi.org/10.18632/oncotarget.18133.
76. Tao T, Chen M, Jiang R, Guan H, Huang Y, Su H, et al. Involvement of EZH2 in aerobic glycolysis of prostate cancer through miR-181b/HK2 axis. Oncol Rep. 2017;37(3):1430–6. https://doi.org/10.3892/or.2017.5430.
77. Liu R, Li J, Teng Z, Zhang Z, Xu Y. Overexpressed microRNA-182 promotes proliferation and invasion in prostate cancer PC-3 cells by down-regulating N-myc downstream regulated gene 1 (NDRG1). PLoS One. 2013;8(7):e68982. https://doi.org/10.1371/journal.pone.0068982.
78. Hirata H, Ueno K, Shahryari V, Deng G, Tanaka Y, Tabatabai ZL, et al. MicroRNA-182-5p promotes cell invasion and proliferation by down regulating FOXF2, RECK and MTSS1 genes in human prostate cancer. PLoS One. 2013;8(1):e55502. https://doi.org/10.1371/journal.pone.0055502.
79. Ueno K, Hirata H, Shahryari V, Deng G, Tanaka Y, Tabatabai ZL, et al. microRNA-183 is an oncogene targeting Dkk-3 and SMAD4 in prostate cancer. Br J Cancer. 2013;108(8):1659–67. https://doi.org/10.1038/bjc.2013.125.
80. Zhong J, Huang R, Su Z, Zhang M, Xu M, Gong J, et al. Downregulation of miR-199a-5p promotes prostate adeno-carcinoma progression through loss of its inhibition of HIF-1alpha. Oncotarget. 2017;8(48):83523–38. https://doi.org/10.18632/oncotarget.18315.
81. Kim J, Wu L, Zhao JC, Jin HJ, Yu J. TMPRSS2-ERG gene fusions induce prostate tumorigenesis by modulating microRNA miR-200c. Oncogene. 2014;33(44):5183–92. https://doi.org/10.1038/onc.2013.461.
82. Nishikawa R, Goto Y, Sakamoto S, Chiyomaru T, Enokida H, Kojima S, et al. Tumor-suppressive microRNA-218 inhibits cancer cell migration and invasion via targeting of LASP1 in prostate cancer. Cancer Sci. 2014;105(7):802–11. https://doi.org/10.1111/cas.12441.
83. Wang L, Liu C, Li C, Xue J, Zhao S, Zhan P, et al. Effects of microRNA-221/222 on cell proliferation and apoptosis in prostate cancer cells. Gene. 2015;572(2):252–8. https://doi.org/10.1016/j.gene.2015.07.017.
84. Galardi S, Mercatelli N, Giorda E, Massalini S, Frajese GV, Ciafre SA, et al. miR-221 and miR-222 expression affects the proliferation potential of human prostate carcinoma cell lines by targeting p27Kip1. J Biol Chem. 2007;282(32):23716–24. https://doi.org/10.1074/jbc.M701805200.
85. Nam RK, Benatar T, Wallis CJ, Amemiya Y, Yang W, Garbens A, et al. MiR-301a regulates E-cadherin expression and is predictive of prostate cancer recurrence. Prostate. 2016;76(10):869–84. https://doi.org/10.1002/pros.23177.
86. Kobayashi N, Uemura H, Nagahama K, Okudela K, Furuya M, Ino Y, et al. Identification of miR-30d as a novel prognostic maker of prostate cancer. Oncotarget. 2012;3(11):1455–71. https://doi.org/10.18632/oncotarget.696.
87. Hsieh IS, Chang KC, Tsai YT, Ke JY, Lu PJ, Lee KH, et al. MicroRNA-320 suppresses the stem cell-like characteristics of prostate cancer cells by downregulating the Wnt/beta-catenin signaling pathway. Carcinogenesis. 2013;34(3):530–8. https://doi.org/10.1093/carcin/bgs371.
88. Mao Y, Chen H, Lin Y, Xu X, Hu Z, Zhu Y, et al. microRNA-330 inhibits cell motility by downregulating Sp1 in prostate cancer cells. Oncol Rep. 2013;30(1):327–33. https://doi.org/10.3892/or.2013.2452.
89. Lee KH, Chen YL, Yeh SD, Hsiao M, Lin JT, Goan YG, et al. MicroRNA-330 acts as tumor suppressor and induces apoptosis of prostate cancer cells through E2F1-mediated suppression of Akt phosphorylation. Oncogene. 2009;28(38):3360–70. https://doi.org/10.1038/onc.2009.192.

90. Fu Q, Liu X, Liu Y, Yang J, Lv G, Dong S. MicroRNA-335 and -543 suppress bone metastasis in prostate cancer via targeting endothelial nitric oxide synthase. Int J Mol Med. 2015;36(5):1417–25. https://doi.org/10.3892/ijmm.2015.2355.
91. Wu Z, Sun H, Zeng W, He J, Mao X. Upregulation of MircoRNA-370 induces proliferation in human prostate cancer cells by downregulating the transcription factor FOXO1. PLoS One. 2012;7(9):e45825. https://doi.org/10.1371/journal.pone.0045825.
92. Zhang W, Liu J, Qiu J, Fu X, Tang Q, Yang F, et al. MicroRNA-382 inhibits prostate cancer cell proliferation and metastasis through targeting COUP-TFII. Oncol Rep. 2016;36(6):3707–15. https://doi.org/10.3892/or.2016.5141.
93. Meng D, Yang S, Wan X, Zhang Y, Huang W, Zhao P, et al. A transcriptional target of androgen receptor, miR-421 regulates proliferation and metabolism of prostate cancer cells. Int J Biochem Cell Biol. 2016;73:30–40. https://doi.org/10.1016/j.biocel.2016.01.018.
94. Noonan EJ, Place RF, Basak S, Pookot D, Li LC. miR-449a causes Rb-dependent cell cycle arrest and senescence in prostate cancer cells. Oncotarget. 2010;1(5):349–58. https://doi.org/10.18632/oncotarget.167.
95. Goto Y, Kojima S, Kurozumi A, Kato M, Okato A, Matsushita R, et al. Regulation of E3 ubiquitin ligase-1 (WWP1) by microRNA-452 inhibits cancer cell migration and invasion in prostate cancer. Br J Cancer. 2016;114(10):1135–44. https://doi.org/10.1038/bjc.2016.95.
96. Zhao Y, Yan M, Yun Y, Zhang J, Zhang R, Li Y, et al. MicroRNA-455-3p functions as a tumor suppressor by targeting eIF4E in prostate cancer. Oncol Rep. 2017;37(4):2449–58. https://doi.org/10.3892/or.2017.5502.
97. Wang L, Song G, Tan W, Qi M, Zhang L, Chan J, et al. MiR-573 inhibits prostate cancer metastasis by regulating epithelial-mesenchymal transition. Oncotarget. 2015;6(34):35978–90. https://doi.org/10.18632/oncotarget.5427.
98. Lai X, Guo Y, Guo Z, Liu R, Wang X, Wang F. Downregulation of microRNA574 in cancer stem cells causes recurrence of prostate cancer via targeting REL. Oncol Rep. 2016;36(6):3651–6. https://doi.org/10.3892/or.2016.5196.
99. Chen H, Luo Q, Li H. MicroRNA-590-3p promotes cell proliferation and invasion by targeting inositol polyphosphate 4-phosphatase type II in human prostate cancer cells. Tumour Biol. 2017;39(3):1010428317695941. https://doi.org/10.1177/1010428317695941.
100. Ren W, Li C, Duan W, Du S, Yang F, Zhou J, et al. MicroRNA-613 represses prostate cancer cell proliferation and invasion through targeting Frizzled7. Biochem Biophys Res Commun. 2016;469(3):633–8. https://doi.org/10.1016/j.bbrc.2015.12.054.
101. Zhu M, Chen Q, Liu X, Sun Q, Zhao X, Deng R, et al. lncRNA H19/miR-675 axis represses prostate cancer metastasis by targeting TGFBI. FEBS J. 2014;281(16):3766–75. https://doi.org/10.1111/febs.12902.
102. Scaravilli M, Porkka KP, Brofeldt A, Annala M, Tammela TL, et al. MiR-1247-5p is overexpressed in castration resistant prostate cancer and targets MYCBP2. Prostate. 2015;75(8):798–805.
103. Hirata H, Hinoda Y, Shahryari V, Deng G, Tanaka Y, Tabatabai ZL, et al. Genistein downregulates onco-miR-1260b and upregulates sFRP1 and Smad4 via demethylation and histone modification in prostate cancer cells. Br J Cancer. 2014;110(6):1645–54. https://doi.org/10.1038/bjc.2014.48.
104. Zhong J, Liu Y, Xu Q, Yu J, Zhang M. Inhibition of DIXDC1 by microRNA-1271 suppresses the proliferation and invasion of prostate cancer cells. Biochem Biophys Res Commun. 2017;484(4):794–800. https://doi.org/10.1016/j.bbrc.2017.01.169.
105. Liang X, Li H, Fu D, Chong T, Wang Z, Li Z. MicroRNA-1297 inhibits prostate cancer cell proliferation and invasion by targeting the AEG-1/Wnt signaling pathway. Biochem Biophys Res Commun. 2016;480(2):208–14. https://doi.org/10.1016/j.bbrc.2016.10.029.
106. Wang B, Wu H, Chai C, Lewis J, Pichiorri F, Eisenstat DD, et al. MicroRNA-1301 suppresses tumor cell migration and invasion by targeting the p53/UBE4B pathway in multiple human cancer cells. Cancer Lett. 2017;401:20–32. https://doi.org/10.1016/j.canlet.2017.04.038.
107. Wang Y, Shao N, Mao X, Zhu M, Fan W, Shen Z, et al. MiR-4638-5p inhibits castration resistance of prostate cancer through repressing Kidins220 expression and PI3K/AKT pathway activity. Oncotarget. 2016;7(30):47444–64. https://doi.org/10.18632/oncotarget.10165.

AR Splice Variant in Prostate Cancer

29

Shinichi Yamashita and Yoichi Arai

Abstract

Androgen deprivation therapy has been the standard treatment for patients with advanced prostate cancer. Androgen deprivation therapy initially suppresses the growth of prostate cancer. However, most patients eventually progress to castration-resistant prostate cancer. Antiandrogens including enzalutamide and abiraterone acetate are recently able to be used for the patients with castration-resistant prostate cancer. Even so, the therapeutic options for castration-resistant prostate cancer are not enough. Androgen receptor splice variants have been attracted attention as one of the mechanisms for castration-resistant prostate cancer. Several androgen receptor splice variants lack the ligand-binding domain, and antiandrogens targeting the ligand-binding domain have little suppression on the growth of prostate cancer. Importantly, the androgen receptor splice variant lacking the ligand-binding domain functions as a constitutively active androgen receptor in the absence of androgen. In this chapter, androgen receptor splice variants are summarized.

Keywords

Androgen receptor · Splice variant · Castration-resistant prostate cancer

S. Yamashita (✉) · Y. Arai
Department of Urology, Tohoku University Graduate School of Medicine, Sendai, Miyagi, Japan
e-mail: yamashita@uro.med.tohoku.ac.jp

29.1 Androgen Receptor

Androgen deprivation therapy (ADT) has been the standard treatment for patients with advanced prostate cancer (PCa) since Huggins et al. reported the effects of castration on PCa [1]. ADT is initially effective for inhibiting the growth of androgen-dependent PCa, suppressing the progression of PCa. However, most patients treated with current ADT eventually progress to castration-resistant PCa (CRPC) [2, 3]. One of the recently proposed mechanisms for CRPC involves the androgen receptor (AR) splice variant [4–6].

AR plays a key role in the growth and progression of PCa. Complementary DNA encoding AR was first cloned by Chang et al. in 1988 [7]. The human AR gene comprises eight exons, and the AR protein is composed of several functional domains, including the NH2-terminal transactivation domain (NTD) encoded by exon 1, the central DNA-binding domain (DBD) encoded by exons 2 and 3, a hinge region encoded by exon 5, and a COOH-terminal ligand-binding domain (LBD) encoded by exons 6–8 [5, 6, 8]. The full-length AR is a 110-kDa steroid receptor. Androgen binds to the AR LBD in the cytoplasm, leading to entry into the nucleus and transcriptional activation of AR-targeted genes.

29.2 Truncated Androgen Receptor

In 2002, a truncated AR with a mass of 75–80 kDa was displayed in the CWR22Rv1 cell line. The origin of CWR22Rv1 cells differs from those of other CRPC cell lines, such as C4-2 or C81, which were derived from lymph node metastatic PCa (LNCaP) [9–12]. CWR22 xenografted tumor was established from a human primary prostate tumor obtained from a patient with bone metastases [13, 14]. CWR22Rv1 is a human castration-resistant PCa cell line derived from the CWR22R subline, which was isolated from a recurrent tumor comprising androgen-dependent CWR22 cells in castrated mice [15, 16]. The AR mutation occurred in a relapsed tumor and involved androgen-independent features.

29.3 Androgen Receptor Splice Variants Lacking the Ligand-Binding Domain

The truncated receptor has been suggested to be derived from the aberrant splicing. In 2008, an AR splice variant lacking a portion of the LBD was first reported [17]. Subsequently, a variety of AR splice variants lacking LBD have been discovered (Fig. 29.1). Although the specific truncation points differ, AR splice variants have been reported to be able to transactivate AR-targeted genes in the absence of androgens [17–21].

In 2008, Dehm et al. performed 3′ RACE with an exon 1-anchored primer and identified a novel AR exon (named "exon 2b") in intron 2 in the CWR22Rv1 cells [17]. Exon 2b included stop codons, and splicing of exon 2b generated two

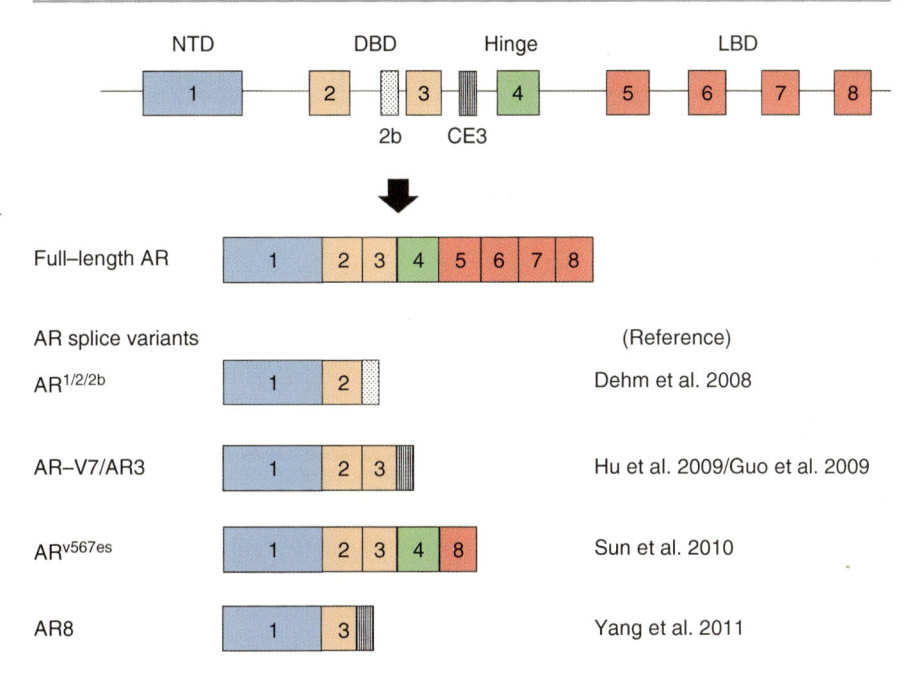

Fig. 29.1 Schema of androgen receptor splice variants. *AR* androgen receptor, *NTD* N-terminal transactivation domain, *DBD* DNA-binding domain, *LBD* ligand-binding domain

truncated ARs, termed "AR[1/2/2b]" and "AR[1/2/3/2b]." These new AR splice variants lacked the LBD but were found to promote AR-targeted transcriptional activities in the absence of androgen. Moreover, androgens had no effect on the activities of these AR splice variants.

In January 2009, Hu et al. identified several cryptic AR exons and reported seven AR splice variants (named AR-V1 to AR-V7) in cell lines and clinical specimens [19]. They confirmed that three cryptic exons (named CE1, CE2, and CE3) in intron 3 were joined to exon 3 and one cryptic exon (named CE4, identical to exon 2b as reported by Dehm et al. [17]) in intron 2 was contained in two splice variants (AR-V3 and AR-V4). Splicing of the intronic cryptic exons produced AR splice variants lacking the LBD. Importantly, AR-V1 and AR-V7 have been detected in specimens of human prostate tissue, with expressions under quantitative real-time PCR elevated by an average of 20-fold in CRPC compared with hormone-naive PCa. Polyclonal antibodies specific for AR-V7 have been established, and AR-V7 has been detected in both cell lines and human clinical specimens.

In March 2009, Guo et al. also demonstrated three AR splice variants lacking the LBD (named AR3, AR4, and AR5) in androgen-independent PCa cells [18]. Interestingly, the translated sequences of AR3, AR4, and AR5 are identical to those of AR-V7, AR-V1, and AR-V4 as identified by Hu et al. [19], respectively. AR-V7/AR3 has been confirmed as one of the major AR splice variants and is constitutively active in the absence of androgen. In addition, immunohistochemical analysis of human specimens showed that expression of AR-V7/AR3 was markedly changed in

CRPC. Antiandrogens targeting the LBD have shown little suppression of tumor cell growth for PCa with AR-V7/AR3 lacking the LBD [22].

AR-V7/AR3 by itself might be able to promote the cell growth of PCa, particularly in the absence of androgen [18, 22]. Furthermore, DHT-induced AR-targeted genes were obviously enhanced with the addition of AR-V7/AR3 in PCa cells, suggesting that AR-V7/AR3 might be able to cooperate with full-length AR to promote DHT-induced AR-targeted genes [21].

In 2010, Sun et al. found another AR splice variant (named AR^{v567es}) in LuCaP prostate cancer xenografts [20]. AR^{v567es} has sequences of exons 1–4 and exon 8 but lacks exons 5–7. AR^{v567es} was also found to be a constitutively active receptor, increasing expression of full-length AR and promoting the transcriptional activities of AR. Interestingly, expression of AR^{v567es} was frequently detected by PCR in 69 metastases collected from 13 PCa patients, compared with AR-V7/AR3.

In 2011, Yang et al. reported a membrane-associated AR splice variant (named AR8) [23]. AR8 was composed of exons 1, 3, and 3b identical to CE3 by Hu et al. [19]. This unique truncated AR splice variant had no DBD or LBD and was located on the plasma membrane. However, AR8 still cooperated with full-length AR to promote the transcriptional activities of AR.

29.4 Clinical Implications of Androgen Receptor Splice Variants

Antiandrogens targeting the LBD would theoretically provide little suppression of the growth and progression of PCa with AR splice variants lacking the LBD. In particular, clinical data regarding AR-V7 have been reported, and AR-V7 has the potential to provide a biomarker for CRPC. Expressions of AR-V7 have been shown to be increased in human specimens with CRPC [18, 19]. Yamashita et al. found no AR-V7/AR3 expression on most specimens of human benign prostate gland, weakly positive results in PCa cells before ADT, and increased results in PCa tissues obtained from the same patient after progression to CRPC [22]. In addition, patients with higher expression of AR-V7/AR3 show a risk of biochemical recurrence after radical prostatectomy [18].

In 2014, Antonarakis et al. reported detection of AR-V7 mRNA in circulating tumor cells (CTCs) from patients with CRPC [24]. AR-V7-positive patients showed little response to enzalutamide and abiraterone and shorter overall survival than AR-V7 negative patients. In contrast, PSA decrease during taxane treatment was seen in 7 of 17 AR-V7-positive patients (41%) and 13 of 20 AR-V7-negative patients (65%), showing no differences according to AR-V7 expression [25]. Onstenk et al. also demonstrated that PSA response rates to cabazitaxel did not differ in CTCs between patients with and without AR-V7 expression according to quantitative real-time PCR [26]. Liu et al. showed that AR-V7 and AR^{v567es} could be detected using a whole-blood assay in patients with CRPC [27].

AR-V7 may become a biomarker for therapeutic approaches in CRPC patients. However, larger prospective trials need to be conducted to clarify the efficacy of AR-V7 as a biomarker. Novel therapeutic approaches targeting not only full-length AR, but also AR splice variants may need to be established to overcome CRPC.

References

1. Huggins C, Hodges CV. Studies on prostatic cancer: I. The effect of castration, of estrogen and of androgen injection on serum phosphatases in metastatic carcinoma of the prostate. Cancer Res. 1941;1(1):293–7.
2. Eisenberger MA, Blumenstein BA, Crawford ED, Miller G, McLeod DG, Loehrer PJ, et al. Bilateral orchiectomy with or without flutamide for metastatic prostate cancer. N Engl J Med. 1998;339(15):1036–42. https://doi.org/10.1056/NEJM199810083391504.
3. Heidenreich A, Aus G, Bolla M, Joniau S, Matveev VB, Schmid HP, et al. EAU guidelines on prostate cancer. Eur Urol. 2008;53(1):68–80. https://doi.org/10.1016/j.eururo.2007.09.002.
4. Lu C, Luo J. Decoding the androgen receptor splice variants. Transl Androl Urol. 2013;2(3):178–86. https://doi.org/10.3978/j.issn.2223-4683.2013.09.08.
5. Wadosky KM, Koochekpour S. Androgen receptor splice variants and prostate cancer: from bench to bedside. Oncotarget. 2017;8(11):18550–76. https://doi.org/10.18632/oncotarget.14537.
6. Xu J, Qiu Y. Role of androgen receptor splice variants in prostate cancer metastasis. Asian J Urol. 2016;3(4):177–84. https://doi.org/10.1016/j.ajur.2016.08.003.
7. Chang CS, Kokontis J, Liao ST. Molecular cloning of human and rat complementary DNA encoding androgen receptors. Science. 1988;240(4850):324–6.
8. Lubahn DB, Brown TR, Simental JA, Higgs HN, Migeon CJ, Wilson EM, et al. Sequence of the intron/exon junctions of the coding region of the human androgen receptor gene and identification of a point mutation in a family with complete androgen insensitivity. Proc Natl Acad Sci U S A. 1989;86(23):9534–8.
9. Horoszewicz JS, Leong SS, Chu TM, Wajsman ZL, Friedman M, Papsidero L, et al. The LNCaP cell line—a new model for studies on human prostatic carcinoma. Prog Clin Biol Res. 1980;37:115–32.
10. Lin MF, Meng TC, Rao PS, Chang C, Schonthal AH, Lin FF. Expression of human prostatic acid phosphatase correlates with androgen-stimulated cell proliferation in prostate cancer cell lines. J Biol Chem. 1998;273(10):5939–47.
11. van Bokhoven A, Varella-Garcia M, Korch C, Johannes WU, Smith EE, Miller HL, et al. Molecular characterization of human prostate carcinoma cell lines. Prostate. 2003;57(3):205–25. https://doi.org/10.1002/pros.10290.
12. Wu HC, Hsieh JT, Gleave ME, Brown NM, Pathak S, Chung LW. Derivation of androgen-independent human LNCaP prostatic cancer cell sublines: role of bone stromal cells. Int J Cancer. 1994;57(3):406–12.
13. Pretlow TG, Wolman SR, Micale MA, Pelley RJ, Kursh ED, Resnick MI, et al. Xenografts of primary human prostatic carcinoma. J Natl Cancer Inst. 1993;85(5):394–8.
14. Wainstein MA, He F, Robinson D, Kung HJ, Schwartz S, Giaconia JM, et al. CWR22: androgen-dependent xenograft model derived from a primary human prostatic carcinoma. Cancer Res. 1994;54(23):6049–52.
15. Nagabhushan M, Miller CM, Pretlow TP, Giaconia JM, Edgehouse NL, Schwartz S, et al. CWR22: the first human prostate cancer xenograft with strongly androgen-dependent and relapsed strains both in vivo and in soft agar. Cancer Res. 1996;56(13):3042–6.
16. Sramkoski RM, Pretlow TG 2nd, Giaconia JM, Pretlow TP, Schwartz S, Sy MS, et al. A new human prostate carcinoma cell line, 22Rv1. In Vitro Cell Dev Biol Anim. 1999;35(7):403–9. https://doi.org/10.1007/s11626-999-0115-4.
17. Dehm SM, Schmidt LJ, Heemers HV, Vessella RL, Tindall DJ. Splicing of a novel androgen receptor exon generates a constitutively active androgen receptor that mediates prostate cancer therapy resistance. Cancer Res. 2008;68(13):5469–77. https://doi.org/10.1158/0008-5472.CAN-08-0594.

18. Guo Z, Yang X, Sun F, Jiang R, Linn DE, Chen H, et al. A novel androgen receptor splice variant is up-regulated during prostate cancer progression and promotes androgen depletion-resistant growth. Cancer Res. 2009;69(6):2305–13. https://doi.org/10.1158/0008-5472.CAN-08-3795.
19. Hu R, Dunn TA, Wei S, Isharwal S, Veltri RW, Humphreys E, et al. Ligand-independent androgen receptor variants derived from splicing of cryptic exons signify hormone-refractory prostate cancer. Cancer Res. 2009;69(1):16–22. https://doi.org/10.1158/0008-5472.CAN-08-2764.
20. Sun S, Sprenger CC, Vessella RL, Haugk K, Soriano K, Mostaghel EA, et al. Castration resistance in human prostate cancer is conferred by a frequently occurring androgen receptor splice variant. J Clin Invest. 2010;120(8):2715–30. https://doi.org/10.1172/JCI41824.
21. Watson PA, Chen YF, Balbas MD, Wongvipat J, Socci ND, Viale A, et al. Constitutively active androgen receptor splice variants expressed in castration-resistant prostate cancer require full-length androgen receptor. Proc Natl Acad Sci U S A. 2010;107(39):16759–65. https://doi.org/10.1073/pnas.1012443107.
22. Yamashita S, Lai KP, Chuang KL, Xu D, Miyamoto H, Tochigi T, et al. ASC-J9 suppresses castration-resistant prostate cancer growth through degradation of full-length and splice variant androgen receptors. Neoplasia. 2012;14(1):74–83.
23. Yang X, Guo Z, Sun F, Li W, Alfano A, Shimelis H, et al. Novel membrane-associated androgen receptor splice variant potentiates proliferative and survival responses in prostate cancer cells. J Biol Chem. 2011;286(41):36152–60. https://doi.org/10.1074/jbc.M111.265124.
24. Antonarakis ES, Lu C, Wang H, Luber B, Nakazawa M, Roeser JC, et al. AR-V7 and resistance to enzalutamide and abiraterone in prostate cancer. N Engl J Med. 2014;371(11):1028–38. https://doi.org/10.1056/NEJMoa1315815.
25. Antonarakis ES, Lu C, Luber B, Wang H, Chen Y, Nakazawa M, et al. Androgen receptor splice variant 7 and efficacy of taxane chemotherapy in patients with metastatic castration-resistant prostate cancer. JAMA Oncol. 2015;1(5):582–91. https://doi.org/10.1001/jamaoncol.2015.1341.
26. Onstenk W, Sieuwerts AM, Kraan J, Van M, Nieuweboer AJ, Mathijssen RH, et al. Efficacy of cabazitaxel in castration-resistant prostate cancer is independent of the presence of AR-V7 in circulating tumor cells. Eur Urol. 2015;68(6):939–45. https://doi.org/10.1016/j.eururo.2015.07.007.
27. Liu X, Ledet E, Li D, Dotiwala A, Steinberger A, Feibus A, et al. A whole blood assay for AR-V7 and ARv567es in patients with prostate cancer. J Urol. 2016;196(6):1758–63. https://doi.org/10.1016/j.juro.2016.06.095.

Detection of Circulating Tumor Cells in Castration-Resistant Prostate Cancer

30

Takatsugu Okegawa

Abstract

Metastasis from primary tumors is responsible for most cancer deaths. Several reports have suggested that early-stage cancer has the potential to begin shedding cancer cells into the circulation early in development. Several groups have noted that levels of circulating tumor cells (CTCs) in patients parallel the tumor burden and response to therapy. There are multiple approaches to detecting CTCs. CTCs at baseline are a strong, independent prognostic biomarker. In addition, measuring CTCs at any time point predicts the response to therapy. The goal of the present chapter is to provide an update on the advances in the clinical validation of CTCs as a surrogate biomarker in prostate cancer patients.

Keywords

Circulating tumor cells · Castration-resistant prostate cancer · Biomarker

30.1 Introduction

Prostate-specific antigen monitoring and imaging analysis have been the standards for detecting prostate cancer recurrence and progression. However, the identification of recurrence at earlier points would be extremely advantageous for immediate therapeutic intervention. In metastatic PCa treatments, predictors of response during treatment may allow for appropriate modifications. To address the need for prognostic markers, several groups have reported that the number and characteristics of circulating tumor cells (CTCs) in cancer patients parallel tumor burden and response to therapy [1–3]. CTCs are generally thought to detach from primary or

T. Okegawa, M.D.
Department of Urology, The University of Kyorin, Tokyo, Japan
e-mail: toke@ks.kyorin-u.ac.jp

secondary tumors of patients in advanced cancer prior to detection in the circulation. The developed CellSearch System (Veridex), which is approved by the Food and Drug Administration, was designed to detect CTCs in whole blood. Primary studies established that CTCs can be used in conjunction with other modalities for monitoring patients with several metastatic cancers [4, 5]. The malignant potential of CTCs has been suggested to be reflected in their morphological characteristics, and their attributes are thus starting to be evaluated in clinical studies in relation with outcome.

30.2 Prognostic Significance of CTCs in Patients with Castration-Resistant Prostate Cancer

Several investigators have demonstrated that CTCs predict survival pre-therapy, and changes in CTCs post-therapy are predictive of both PFS and OS in patients with CRPC [2, 3, 6–9]. de Bono et al. compared the reduction in CTCs versus reduction in PSA at earlier time points and revealed the limitations of PSA as a biomarker for survival and response to chemotherapy [2]. The persistence of CTCs after the initiation of therapy suggests that patients receive less than optimal benefits from treatment. Scher et al. found the CTC count to be a prognostic factor for survival in patients with progressive, metastatic CRPC receiving first-line chemotherapy [3]. At 4, 8, and 12 weeks after treatment, changes in CTC numbers were correlated with risk, whereas changes in the PSA titer were not. The most predictive factors for survival were the LDH concentration and the CTC count. Olmos D et al. evaluated the association of CTC counts, before and after commencing treatment, with OS in CRPC patients. Patients whose CTC counts reduced from ≥5 CTCs per 7.5 mL of blood at baseline to <5 CTCs/7.5 mL of blood following treatment had an improved OS than those who did not [9]. Our previous report as well as these reports found changes in CTC counts to be a reflection of treatment benefit in CRPC patients under several treatments [5].

30.3 CTCs as a Predictive Biomarker of Sensitivity in Castration-Resistant Prostate Cancer Patients Treated with Docetaxel Chemotherapy

Goldkorn et al. reported the correlation with CTCs and analyzed CTCs in patients with CRPC treated with first-line TXT-based therapy in SWOG S0421 [10]. Median OS was 26 months for <5 CTCs per 7.5 mL versus 13 months for ≥5 CTCs per 7.5 mL pre-docetaxel, and increasing CTCs at 3 weeks indicated significantly worse OS. We found CTCs in 62% of CRPC patients of pre-docetaxel using a cutoff of five cells per 7.5 mL of blood. A threshold of ≥5 CTCs per 7.5 mL blood was used to evaluate the suitability of CTCs to predict survival. We examined the usefulness of CTCs for predicting survival in 57 CRPC patients treated with docetaxel chemotherapy [11]. Patients with <5 CTCs per 7.5 mL of blood had a median OS time > 25.0 months compared with 10.5 months in patients with ≥5 CTCs ($p < 0.001$). The CTC levels accurately and reproducibly predicted clinical outcome, as previously reported [8]. Apart from CTC count ≥5, ALP > UNL was also independently associated with a poor OS. Changes may also offer additional prognostic information to that offered by CTCs because they had independent prognostic relevance in our study. As a response indicator of TXT efficacy, changes in CTC were more associated with survival than a decline in PSA measured after three cycles (Fig. 30.1). The prognostic factor for OS was ≥5 CTCs after three cycles. Together, CTCs at baseline are a strong, independent prognostic biomarker pre-docetaxel. In addition, measuring CTC after three cycles predicts the response to therapy.

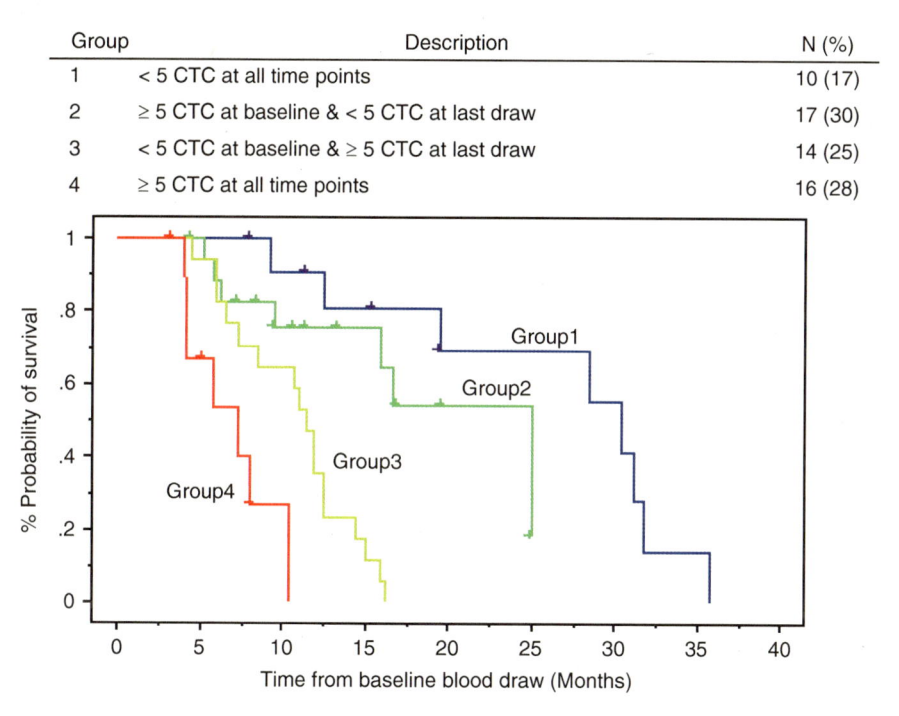

Group	Description	N (%)
1	< 5 CTC at all time points	10 (17)
2	≥ 5 CTC at baseline & < 5 CTC at last draw	17 (30)
3	< 5 CTC at baseline & ≥ 5 CTC at last draw	14 (25)
4	≥ 5 CTC at all time points	16 (28)

Fig. 30.1 Circulating tumor cells as a predictive biomarker of sensitivity to docetaxel chemotherapy in patients with CRPC. Kaplan–Meier curves for OS duration using the change in CTC count from baseline. Four different groups of patients were compared: group 1, patients with fewer than five CTCs/7.5 mL of blood at baseline and after three cycles; group 2, patients with five or more CTCs at baseline but fewer than five CTCs after three cycles of therapy; group 3, patients with fewer than five CTCs at baseline but five or more CTCs after three cycles; group 4, patients with five or more CTCs at baseline and after three cycles of therapy. The survival rates were calculated from the time of the baseline blood draw. Group 4 patients had a significantly shorter median OS (7.25 months) than did group 1 (30.5 months; $p < 0.001$) and group 2 (25 months; $p < 0.001$) patients. Patients of group 3 had a significantly shorter median OS (11.5 months) than those of group 1 ($p < 0.001$) and group 2 ($p = 0.003$). Differences between survival curves for group 1 and 2 ($p > 0.05$) and group 3 and 4 ($p > 0.05$) were not significant

30.4 CTCs as a Predictive Biomarker of Abiraterone Acetate and Enzalutamide Treatment in Castration-Resistant Prostate Cancer Patients

Phase I/II trials using CTC monitoring as an embedded end point studied CRPC patients progressing post-TXT being treated with abiraterone acetate or enzalutamide [12–15]. Two trials of abiraterone acetate demonstrated a CTC conversion (≥ 5 CTCs at baseline but <5 CTCs at the final blood draw) rate of 34% and 41%, respectively. A phase I/II trials of enzalutamide reported a CTC conversion rate of 49%. CTCs may reflect the effects of treatment on survival. In the COU-AA-301 trial comparing abiraterone plus prednisone versus prednisone alone for patients with mCRPC, Scher H et al. found that the combination of CTC number and LDH level was indicative of survival in individual patients [16]. However, PSA changes after treatment were not always prognostic in these studies and should not be used for selecting treatments.

30.5 AR-V7 in CTCs as a Predictive Biomarker of Abiraterone Acetate and Enzalutamide Treatment in Castration-Resistant Prostate Cancer Patients

The androgen receptor (AR) signaling axis has a critical role in CRPC. New drugs targeting the AR axis, abiraterone, and enzalutamide have been approved to treat metastatic CRPC based on survival improvements. However, primary resistance to enzalutamide or abiraterone has been observed in approximately 20–40% of patients with metastatic CRPC [17–20]. One mechanism of resistance to these new drugs is the presence of splice variants of AR that are devoid of a functional ligand-binding domain [21–24]. In particular, AR splice variant 7 (AR-V7) has been implicated in resistance to enzalutamide and abiraterone therapy [25]. In addition, AR-V7 is associated with more rapid disease progression and shorter survival in CRPC (Table 30.1) [25–28].

Antonarakis ES et al. prospectively evaluated AR-V7 messenger RNA in CTCs from CRPC patients receiving abiraterone and enzalutamide [25]. They focused on AR-V7 because it is the only known androgen receptor variant encoding a functional protein product that is detectable in clinical specimens [26]. They found that AR-V7 can be detected reliably from CTCs and that detection of AR-V7 in tumor cells appears to be associated with resistance to both abiraterone and enzalutamide. In a recent report, outcomes for the overall cohort (and separately for the first-line and second-line novel hormonal therapy cohorts) were best for CTC(−) patients, intermediate for CTC(+)/AR-V7(−) patients, and worse for CTC(+)/ARV7(+) patients. These correlations remained significant in multivariable models [27]. In a recent report, Scher HI et al. used 128 samples that were obtained before treatment with abiraterone and enzalutamide [28]. AR-V7-positive CTCs using the epic platform were detected in 18% of the samples. Presence of AR-V7-positive CTCs before treatment with abiraterone and enzalutamide was reduced on radiographic PFS and OS. Todenhofer T et al. reported the clinical importance of AR-V7 levels using RT-PCR detection of AR-V7 transcripts in whole blood as a marker of resistance to abiraterone [29].

Table 30.1 Response to treatment in AR-V7-expressing prostate cancer

Study	Therapeutic	Prevalence of AR-V7 (%)	PSA response in AR-V7 + vs. AR-V7 patients (%)	AR-V7 assay
Antonarakis et al. [25]	Abiraterone	19	0% vs. 68% ($P < 0.01$)	CTC-derived mRNA (AdnaTest; Qiagen, Hilden, Germany)
	Enzalutamide	39	0% vs. 53% ($P < 0.01$)	
Steinestel et al. [24]	Abiraterone or enzalutamide	64	7% vs. 63% ($P = 0.01$)	CTC-derived mRNA (AdnaTest; Qiagen, Hilden, Germany)
Todenhofer et al. [28]	Abiraterone	11	0% vs. 42% ($P = 0.04$)	Whole blood mRNA (PAXgene; PreAnalytiX, Hombrechtikon, Switzerland)
Antonarakis et al. [29]	Docetaxel or cabazitaxel	46	41% vs. 65% ($P = 0.19$)	CTC-derived mRNA (AdnaTest; Qiagen, Hilden, Germany)
Onstenck et al. [30]	Cabazitaxel	55	8% vs. 22% ($P = 0.70$)	CTC-derived mRNA (CellSearch; Janssen, Horsham, PA, USA)
Scher et al. [27]	Abiraterone, enzalutamide, or taxanes	18	0% vs. 64% 33% vs. 44%	CTC-derived mRNA

30.6 AR-V7 in CTCs and Efficacy of Taxane Chemotherapy in Castration-Resistant Prostate Cancer Patients

Antonarakis ES et al. reported a prospective study using a CTC-based RT-PCR assay on 37 patients who began treatment with docetaxel and cabazitaxel [30]. PSA responses were observed in both AR-V7-positive and AR-V7-negative men. Similarly, PSF was not significantly different in AR-V7-positive or AR-V7-negative men. They incorporated data from their priory study of 62 abiraterone or enzalutamide patients. They demonstrated that clinical outcomes appeared to improve with taxanes compared with abiraterone or enzalutamide in AR-V7-positive patients. In AR-V7-positive patients, PSA responses were higher with taxane therapy compared with abiraterone or enzalutamide therapy. Similarly, PSF was longer in taxane therapy. In agreement with this, a study from Onstenk W et al. did not observe differences in PSA response rates according to AR-V7 status in 29 patients treated with cabazitaxel [31]. Scher HI et al. reported a more favorable OS for AR-V7-positive patients receiving taxane chemotherapy compared with enzalutamide or abiraterone [28]. This implies that the presence of AR-V7 indicates a more favorable outcome for patients treated with taxanes compared with enzalutamide or abiraterone.

Conclusion

CTC analysis is a valuable fluid biopsy that provides information on PCa detection, prognosis, prediction, and treatment response. In the future, characterization of CTC molecules is necessary for development of novel anticancer compounds. It is important to enhance a knowledge of the mechanisms involved in metastatic development to predict therapeutic activity.

References

1. Allard WJ, Matera J, Miller MC, et al. Tumor cells circulate in the peripheral blood of all major carcinomas but not in healthy subjects or patients with nonmalignant diseases. Clin Cancer Res. 2004a;10:6897–904.
2. de Bono JS, Scher HI, Montgomery RB, et al. Circulating tumor cells predict survival benefit from treatment in metastatic castration-resistant prostate cancer. Clin Cancer Res. 2008;14:6302–9.
3. Scher HI, Jia X, de Bono JS, et al. Circulating tumour cells as prognostic markers in progressive, castration-resistant prostate cancer: a reanalysis of IMMC38 trial data. Lancet Oncol. 2009;10:233–9.
4. Allard WJ, Matera J, Miller MC, et al. Tumor cells circulate in the peripheral blood of all major carcinomas but not in healthy subjects or patients with nonmalignant diseases. Clin Cancer Res. 2004b;10:6897–904.
5. Okegawa T, Nutahara K, Higashihara E. Prognostic significance of circulating tumor cells in patients with hormone refractory prostate cancer. J Urol. 2009;181:1091–7.
6. Moreno JG, Miller MC, Gross S, et al. Circulating tumor cells predict survival in patients with metastatic prostate cancer. Urology. 2005;65:713–8.
7. Danila DC, Heller G, Gignac GA, et al. Circulating tumor cell number and prognosis in progressive castration-resistant prostate cancer. Clin Cancer Res. 2007;13:7053–8.
8. Chen BT, Loberg RD, Neeley CK, et al. Preliminary study of immunomagnetic quantification of circulating tumor cells in patients with advanced disease. Urology. 2005;65(3):616–21.
9. Olmos D, Arkenau HT, Ang JE, et al. Circulating tumour cell (CTC) counts as intermediate end points in castration-resistant prostate cancer (CRPC): a single-centre experience. Ann Oncol. 2009;20(1):27–33.
10. Goldkorn A, Ely B, Quinn DI, et al. Circulating tumor cell counts are prognostic of overall survival in SWOG S0421: a phase III trial of docetaxel with or without atrasentan for metastatic castration-resistant prostate cancer. J Clin Oncol. 2014;32(11):1136–42.
11. Okegawa T, Itaya N, Hara H, et al. Circulating tumor cells as a biomarker predictive of sensitivity to docetaxel chemotherapy in patients with castration-resistant prostate cancer. Anticancer Res. 2014;34(11):6705–10.
12. Danila DC, Fleisher M, Scher HI. Circulating tumor cells as biomarkers in prostate cancer. Clin Cancer Res. 2011a;17(12):3903–12.
13. Danila DC, Anand A, Sung CC, et al. TMPRSS2-ERG status in circulating tumor cells as a predictive biomarker of sensitivity in castration-resistant prostate cancer patients treated with abiraterone acetate. Eur Urol. 2011b;60(5):897–904.
14. Reid AH, Attard G, Danila DC, et al. Significant and sustained antitumor activity in post-docetaxel, castration-resistant prostate cancer with the CYP17 inhibitor abiraterone acetate. J Clin Oncol. 2010;28(9):1489–95.
15. Danila DC, Morris MJ, de Bono JS, et al. Phase II multicenter study of abiraterone acetate plus prednisone therapy in patients with docetaxel-treated castration-resistant prostate cancer. J Clin Oncol. 2010;28(9):1496–501.

16. Scher HI, Heller G, Molina A, et al. Circulating tumor cell biomarker panel as an individual-level surrogate for survival in metastatic castration-resistant prostate cancer. J Clin Oncol. 2015;33:1348–55.
17. Ryan CJ, Smith MR, de Bono JS, et al. Abiraterone in metastatic prostate cancer without previous chemotherapy. N Engl J Med. 2013;368:138–48.
18. Scher HI, Beer TM, Higano CS, et al. Antitumour activity of MDV3100 in castration-resistant prostate cancer: a phase 1–2 study. Lancet. 2010;375:1437–46.
19. Scher HI, Fizazi K, Saad F, et al. Increased survival with enzalutamide in prostate cancer after chemotherapy. N Engl J Med. 2012;367:1187–97.
20. de Bono JS, Logothetis CJ, Molina A, et al. Abiraterone and increased survival in metastatic prostate cancer. N Engl J Med. 2011;364:1995–2005.
21. Hu R, Lu C, Mostaghel EA, et al. Distinct transcriptional programs mediated by the ligand-dependent full-length androgen receptor and its splice variants in castration-resistant prostate cancer. Cancer Res. 2012;72:3457–62.
22. Li Y, Chan SC, Brand LJ, et al. Androgen receptor splice variants mediate enzalutamide resistance in castration-resistant prostate cancer cell lines. Cancer Res. 2013;73(2):483–9.
23. Nakazawa M, Antonarakis ES, Luo J. Androgen receptor splice variants in the era of enzalutamide and abiraterone. Horm Cancer. 2014;5(5):265–73.
24. Steinestel J, Luedeke M, Arndt A, et al. Detecting predictive androgen receptor modifications in circulating prostate cancer cells. Oncotarget. 2015. https://doi.org/10.18632/oncotarget.3925.
25. Antonarakis ES, Lu C, Wang H, et al. AR-V7 and resistance to enzalutamide and abiraterone in prostate cancer. N Engl J Med. 2014;371:1028–38.
26. Bryce AH, Antonarakis ES. Androgen receptor splice variant 7 in castration-resistant prostate cancer: clinical considerations. Int J Urol. 2016;23:646–53.
27. Antonarakis ES, Lu C, Luber B, et al. Clinical significance of androgen receptor splice variant-7 mRNA detection in circulating tumor cells of men with metastatic castration-resistant prostate cancer treated with first- and second-line abiraterone and enzalutamide. J Clin Oncol. 2017;35(19):2149–56.
28. Scher HI, Lu D, Schreiber NA, et al. Association of AR-V7 on circulating tumor cells as a treatment-specific biomarker with outcomes and survival in castration-resistant prostate cancer. JAMA Oncol. 2016;2:1441–9.
29. Todenhöfer T, Azad A, Stewart C, et al. AR-V7 transcripts in whole blood RNA of patients with metastatic castration resistant prostate cancer correlate with response to abiraterone acetate. J Urol. 2017;197(1):135–42.
30. Antonarakis ES, Lu C, Luber B, et al. Androgen receptor splice variant 7 and efficacy of taxane chemotherapy in patients with metastatic castration-resistant prostate cancer. JAMA. 2015;1(5):582–91.
31. Onstenk W, Sieuwerts AM, Kraan J, et al. Efficacy of cabazitaxel in castration-resistant prostate cancer is independent of the presence of AR-V7 in circulating tumor cells. Eur Urol. 2015;68(6):939–45.

New Biomarker for Castration-Resistant Prostate Cancer: A Glycobiological Perspective

31

Shingo Hatakeyama, Tohru Yoneyama, Hayato Yamamoto, Yuki Tobisawa, Shin-Ichiro Nishimura, and Chikara Ohyama

Abstract

Cancer-associated glycan aberrations are frequently observed in tumors. Glycan alterations are reported to have potential as cancer biomarkers. An aberrant glycosylation and glycosyl epitope have been known to be tumor-associated antigens. In addition, changes in glycosyltransferase could be associated with the signal pathways. Detecting in aberrant glycosylation on prostate-specific antigen (α2,3-linked sialylation) may improve specificity in detection of prostate cancer. However, a practical procedure to analyze a large number of glycan samples quickly is not available for serum due to methodological problems. Recent progress in mass spectrometry has led to new challenges in glycan analysis including a chemo-selective glycan enrichment technology called glycoblotting to purify oligosaccharides from a crude glycoprotein mixture. Previous study suggested that triand tetra-antennary *N*-glycans were significantly higher in CRPC patients than in non-CRPC patients, and the expression of *N*-glycan branching enzyme genes was significantly upregulated in CRPC cell lines. These results suggest that the overexpression of triand tetra-antennary *N*-glycans may be associated with the castration-resistant status in prostate cancer and may be a potential predictive biomarker for CRPC. The incorporation of glycan biomarkers appears to be a promising approach for improving CRPC detection.

S. Hatakeyama, M.D. (✉) · T. Yoneyama · H. Yamamoto · Y. Tobisawa · C. Ohyama
Department of Urology, Hirosaki University Graduate School of Medicine, Hirosaki, Japan
e-mail: shingoh@hirosaki-u.ac.jp; tohruyon@hirosaki-u.ac.jp; tobisawa@hirosaki-u.ac.jp; coyama@hirosaki-u.ac.jp

S.-I. Nishimura
Graduate School of Life Science, Frontier Research Centre for Advanced Material and Life Science, Hokkaido University, Sapporo, Japan
e-mail: shin@sci.hokudai.ac.jp

Keywords

Prostate cancer · Castration-resistant prostate cancer · N-glycan · Glycobiology

31.1 Introduction

Although serum prostate-specific antigen (PSA) has been used as a prostate cancer (PC) biomarker for several decades, PSA lacks the ability to predict aggressive potential in castration-resistant prostate cancer (CRPC). Several clinicopathological prognostic biomarkers (Gleason score, metastatic volume, circulating tumor cell enumeration, lactate dehydrogenase levels, and pain) exist in CRPC, but only a few glycan-based biomarkers have been reported [1].

Cancer-associated glycan aberrations are frequently observed in tumors [2–8]. Many tumor markers, including PSA, are glycoproteins that have glycosylation sites in their amino acid sequence. Although cancer-associated glycan alterations represent potential cancer biomarkers, glycan analysis has not been incorporated into clinical use because the protocols for preparing glycan derivatives vary depending on the analytical method and conducting these protocols requires specialized expertise. Therefore, a practical procedure for analyzing many glycan samples in biological materials such as serum had not been available. Recently, an approach that combines high-throughput, quantitative N-glycomics with mass spectrometry analysis was developed [9–11]. The technique is based on a chemoselective glycan enrichment technology that enables the purification of oligosaccharides from 10 μL of crude glycoproteins. Previous results indicate that serum N-glycan analysis is a promising approach for screening diagnostic and prognostic markers associated with multiple types of cancer [1, 4, 7, 8]. This chapter provides general information regarding to glycobiology for PC and future perspectives for a glycomics approach to the discovery of potential PC biomarkers.

31.2 Glycobiology in Prostate Cancer

Since the correlation between certain structures of glycans and a clinical prognosis in cancer was first suggested a decade ago [12], the interest in structural studies of glycans has increased substantially. In PC, aberrant glycosylation and glycosyl epitope have been known to be tumor-associated antigens [13]. In addition, changes in glycosyltransferase could be associated with the signal pathways [2]. Core3 O-glycan synthase suppresses tumor formation and metastasis of PC cell lines through downregulation of α2β1 integrin complex [14]. On the other hand, Core2 O-glycan synthase facilitates prostate cancer progression [15]. Because glycan biosynthesis depends on several highly competitive processes, detecting in glycosylation may be a specific and sensitive approach to biomarker discovery and possibly disease diagnosis.

A PSA is a glycoprotein that has glycosylation sites in its amino acid sequence. After the report of glycan analysis of PSA [16], an attempt to identify the carbohydrate structure difference between PC and non-PC was made in several studies. Ohyama et al.

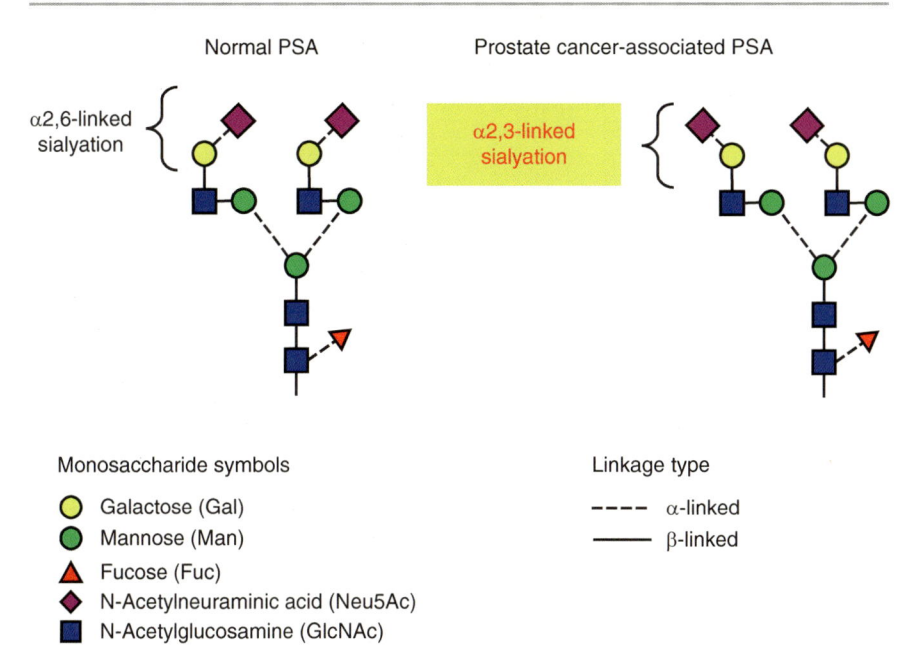

Fig. 31.1 Prostate cancer-associated aberrant glycosylation of *N*-glycan on PSA (S2, 3PSA). In normal PSA, the terminal sialic acids link to galactose residues with α2,6 linkages. In prostate cancer-associated PSA, the linkage between the terminal sialic acid and galactose residues changes to α2,3 linkages

reported that a glycan structure of PSA in the serum of PC patients is different from that of patients with benign prostate hyperplasia (Fig. 31.1) [17–19]. The different glycan structure of PSA is expected to be useful for differential diagnosis between malignant and benign prostate diseases. Recent studies suggested the measurement of aberrant glycosylation of PSA (α2,3-linked sialylation is an additional terminal *N*-glycan on free PSA) can improve specificity in detection of PC [20]. More recently, an automated micro-total immunoassay system (μTAS system) for measuring PC-associated α2,3-linked sialyl *N*-glycan on PSA may improve the accuracy of PC detection [21].

31.3 Serum Glycan Analysis (Glycoblotting and Mass Spectrometry)

A practical procedure to analyze a large number of glycan samples quickly is not available for serum due to methodological problems. Recent progress in mass spectrometry has led to new challenges in glycan analysis including a chemo-selective glycan enrichment technology called glycoblotting to purify oligosaccharides from a crude glycoprotein mixture (Fig. 31.2) [22, 23]. Serum *N*-glycan was quantitatively measured from 10 μL of serum samples using glycoblotting and matrix-assisted laser desorption/ionization-time of flight (MALDI-TOF) mass spectrometry. High-throughput *N*-glycan analysis

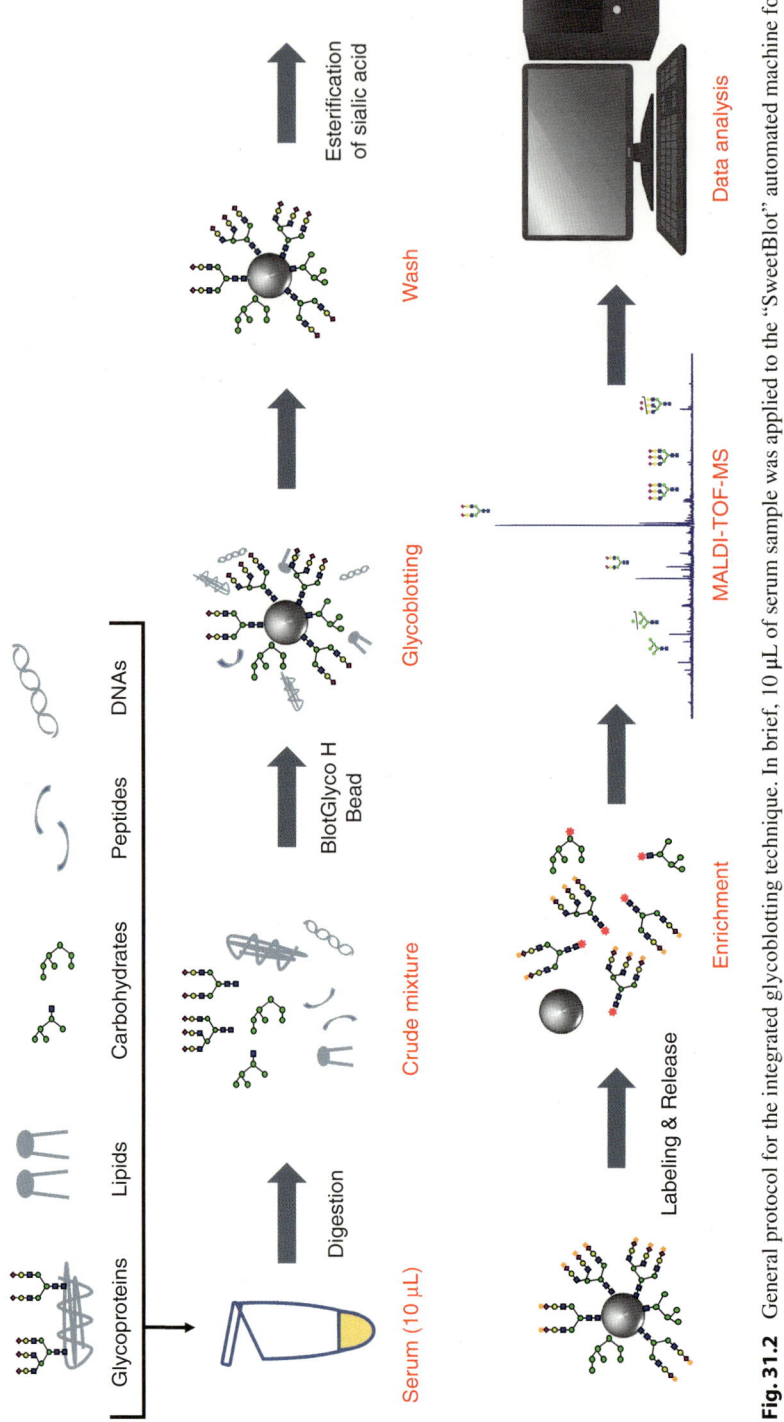

Fig. 31.2 General protocol for the integrated glycoblotting technique. In brief, 10 μL of serum sample was applied to the "SweetBlot" automated machine for glycoblotting. After enzymatic cleavage from serum proteins, total serum N-glycans released in the digest mixture were directly used for glycoblotting with BlotGlyco H beads (Sumitomo Bakelite, Co., Tokyo, Japan). Sialic acid was methyl esterified after washing the beads. The processed N-glycans were labeled with benzyloxiamine (BOA) and released from the BlotGlyco H beads. Mass spectra of BOA-labeled N-glycans were acquired with an UltraFlex III instrument (Bruker Daltonics)

combined with mass spectrometry analysis enables serum glycan profiling in a simple, highly effective, and quantitative procedure. A novel glycan biomarker for PC can be detected using glycoblotting and mass spectrometry.

31.4 Glycan-Associated Biomarkers (Tri and Tetra-Antennary Serum *N*-Glycans) in CRPC

Ishibashi et al. [1] reported a comprehensive *N*-glycan structural analysis of sera from 80 healthy volunteers, 286 patients with benign prostatic hyperplasia (BPH), 258 patients with early-stage PC, 46 patients with PC that had been treated with androgen deprivation therapy (ADT), and 68 patients with CRPC. They found that tri and tetra-antennary *N*-glycans (*m/z* 3049 and 3414) were significantly enriched in patients with CRPC compared with the other groups (Fig. 31.3a, b). The longitudinal follow-up of highly branched *N*-glycan (*m/z* 3049 and 3414) levels predicted CRPC despite castrate levels of testosterone. Quantitative qRT-PCR of *N*-glycan

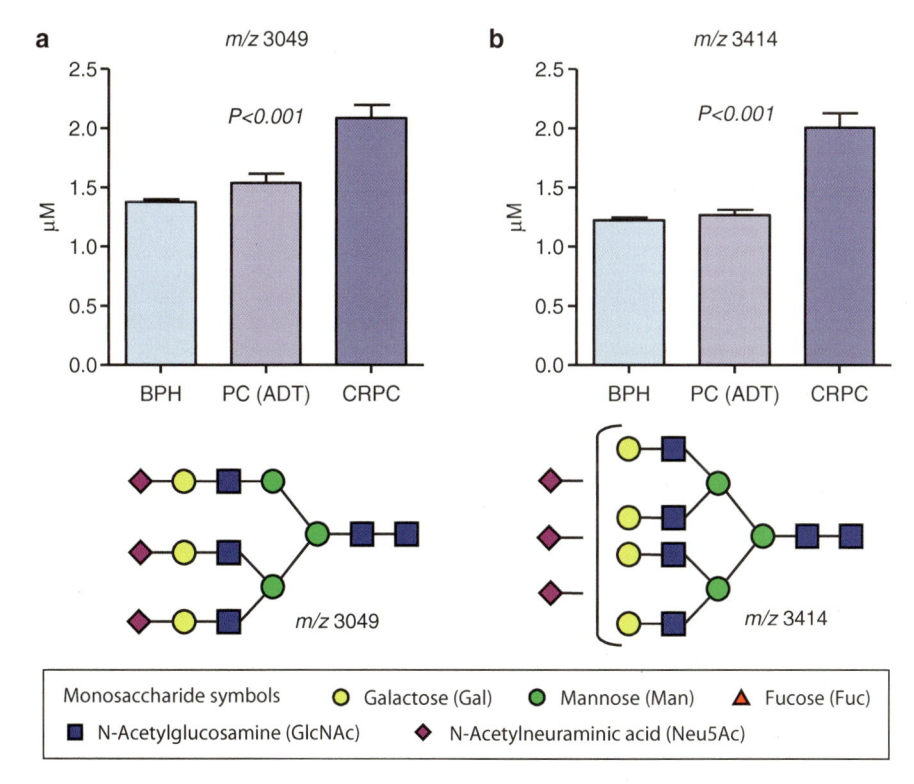

Fig. 31.3 The difference in *N*-glycan concentration. The difference in *N*-glycan concentration (*m/z* 3049 and 3414) among the BPH, PC with ADT, and CRPC patients. There was a significant difference in the serum *N*-glycan levels between non-CRPC patients and CRPC patients in *m/z* 3049 (**a**) and *m/z* 3414 (**b**)

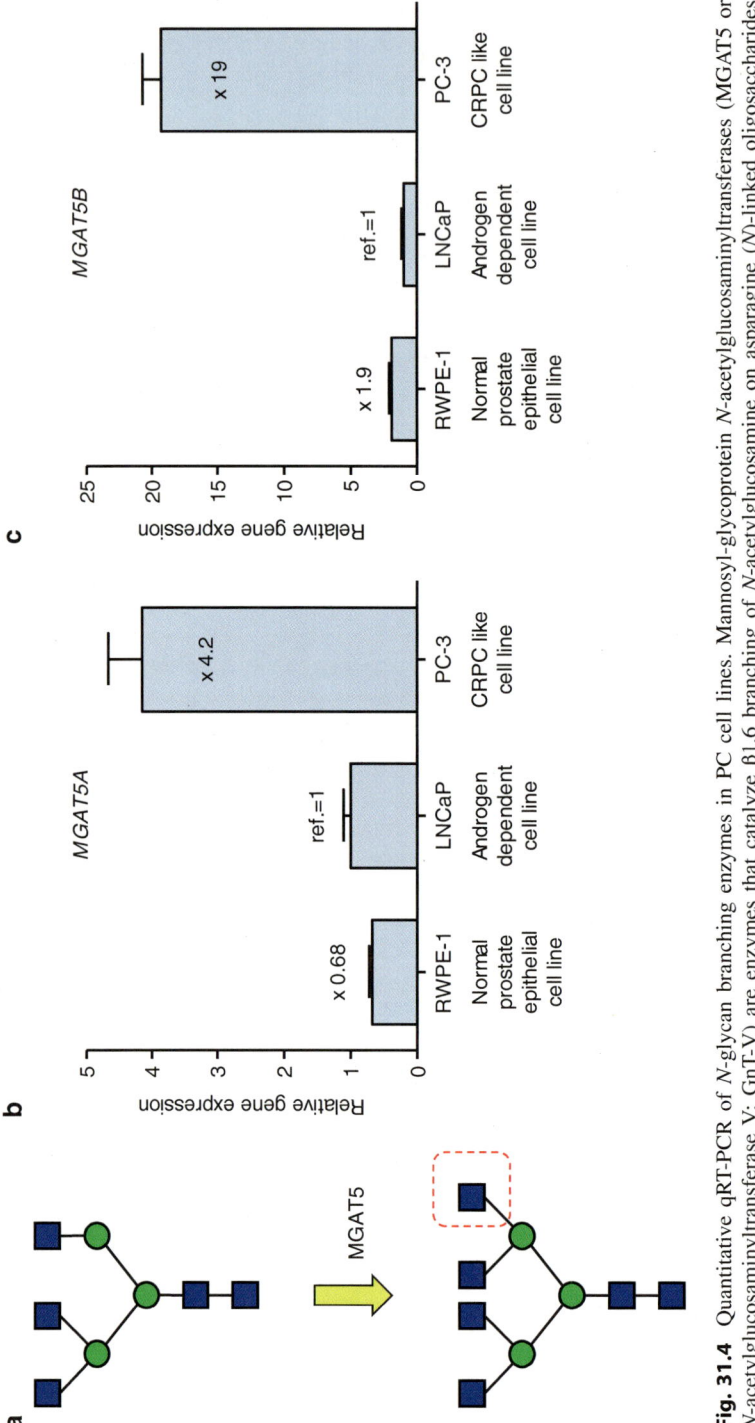

Fig. 31.4 Quantitative qRT-PCR of *N*-glycan branching enzymes in PC cell lines. Mannosyl-glycoprotein *N*-acetylglucosaminyltransferases (MGAT5 or *N*-acetylglucosaminyltransferase V: GnT-V) are enzymes that catalyze β1,6 branching of *N*-acetylglucosamine on asparagine (*N*)-linked oligosaccharides (*N*-glycan) of cell proteins (**a**). We examined the transcription levels of *MGAT* families. The relative expression levels of *MGAT* genes were normalized to the expression of the GAPDH gene in each cell line. The expression of the *MGAT5A* and *B* genes in androgen-dependent PC cells (LNCaP) was used as the control and was defined as 1.0. The expression of *MGAT5A* (**b**) and *B* (**c**) genes in the CRPC-like cell line (PC-3) was significantly higher than that in the normal prostate epithelial cell line (RWPE-1) and LNCaP

branching enzyme (mannosyl-glycoprotein *N*-acetylglucosaminyltransferases: MGAT) genes, which are medial Golgi enzymes that initiate the β1,6GlcNAc branching in tetra-branched *N*-glycans, revealed that the CRPC-like PC-3 cell lines had significantly increased transcription of *MGAT5A* and *MGAT5B* genes compared to androgen-dependent LNCaP cells and normal prostate epithelial RWPE-1 cells (Fig. 31.4a–c). The levels of MGAT5 glycan products are typically increased in many malignancies, and several reports have suggested that MGAT5 may play an important role in the metastasis of PC [24, 25]. In addition, MGAT5 *N*-glycosylation was associated with cancer progression, metastasis [26], and negative regulation for T-cell activation [27]. Therefore, these results suggest that the overexpression of specific *N*-glycans might be associated with CRPC and that it might represent a predictive CRPC biomarker [1].

31.5 Conclusion and Perspectives

Currently, qualified predictive biomarkers for CRPC are largely lacking, and predictive biomarkers are needed to match each patient to the optimal therapy. The incorporation of glycan biomarkers appears to be a promising approach for improving CRPC detection. Further large-scale prospective studies can help evaluate the utility of these new approaches, as well as to improve risk assessment strategies and outcomes in patients with CRPC.

Acknowledgments This work was supported by a Grant-in-Aid for Scientific Research (No. 15H02563 15 K15579, 17 K11118, 17 K11119, 17 K16768, 17 K16770, and 17 K16771) from the Japan Society for the Promotion of Science.

References

1. Ishibashi Y, Tobisawa Y, Hatakeyama S, Ohashi T, Tanaka M, Narita S, et al. Serum triand tetra-antennary N-glycan is a potential predictive biomarker for castration-resistant prostate cancer. Prostate. 2014;74(15):1521–9. https://doi.org/10.1002/pros.22869.
2. Tsuboi S, Hatakeyama S, Ohyama C, Fukuda M. Two opposing roles of O-glycans in tumor metastasis. Trends Mol Med. 2012;18(4):224–32. https://doi.org/10.1016/j.molmed.2012.02.001.
3. Kyan A, Kamimura N, Hagisawa S, Hatakeyama S, Koie T, Yoneyama T, et al. Positive expressions of N-acetylglucosaminyltransferase-V (GnT-V) and beta1-6 branching N-linked oligosaccharides in human testicular germ cells diminish during malignant transformation and progression. Int J Oncol. 2008;32(1):129–34.
4. Hatakeyama S, Amano M, Tobisawa Y, Yoneyama T, Tsushima M, Hirose K, et al. Serum N-glycan profiling predicts prognosis in patients undergoing hemodialysis. ScientificWorldJournal. 2013;2013:268407. https://doi.org/10.1155/2013/268407.
5. Sato T, Yoneyama T, Tobisawa Y, Hatakeyama S, Yamamoto H, Kojima Y, et al. Core 2 beta-1, 6-N-acetylglucosaminyltransferase-1 expression in prostate biopsy specimen is an indicator of prostate cancer aggressiveness. Biochem Biophys Res Commun. 2016;470(1):150–6. https://doi.org/10.1016/j.bbrc.2016.01.011.

6. Hatakeyama S, Yoneyama T, Tobisawa Y, Ohyama C. Recent progress and perspectives on prostate cancer biomarkers. Int J Clin Oncol. 2017;22(2):214–21. https://doi.org/10.1007/s10147-016-1049-y.
7. Narita T, Hatakeyama S, Yoneyama T, Narita S, Yamashita S, Mitsuzuka K, et al. Clinical implications of serum N-glycan profiling as a diagnostic and prognostic biomarker in germ-cell tumors. Cancer Med. 2017;6(4):739–48. https://doi.org/10.1002/cam4.1035.
8. Oikawa M, Hatakeyama S, Narita T, Yoneyama T, Tobisawa Y, Yamamoto H, et al. Significance of serum N-glycan profiling as a diagnostic biomarker in urothelial carcinoma. Eur Urol Focus. 2017. https://doi.org/10.1016/j.euf.2016.11.004.
9. Kita Y, Miura Y, Furukawa J, Nakano M, Shinohara Y, Ohno M, et al. Quantitative glycomics of human whole serum glycoproteins based on the standardized protocol for liberating N-glycans. Mol Cell Proteomics. 2007;6(8):1437–45. https://doi.org/10.1074/mcp.T600063-MCP200.
10. Furukawa J, Shinohara Y, Kuramoto H, Miura Y, Shimaoka H, Kurogochi M, et al. Comprehensive approach to structural and functional glycomics based on chemoselective glycoblotting and sequential tag conversion. Anal Chem. 2008;80(4):1094–101. https://doi.org/10.1021/ac702124d.
11. Miura Y, Hato M, Shinohara Y, Kuramoto H, Furukawa J, Kurogochi M, et al. BlotGlycoABCTM, an integrated glycoblotting technique for rapid and large scale clinical glycomics. Mol Cell Proteomics. 2008;7(2):370–7. https://doi.org/10.1074/mcp.M700377-MCP200.
12. Hakomori S. Tumor malignancy defined by aberrant glycosylation and sphingo(glyco)lipid metabolism. Cancer Res. 1996;56(23):5309–18.
13. Kyselova Z, Mechref Y, Al Bataineh MM, Dobrolecki LE, Hickey RJ, Vinson J, et al. Alterations in the serum glycome due to metastatic prostate cancer. J Proteome Res. 2007;6(5):1822–32. https://doi.org/10.1021/pr060664t.
14. Lee SH, Hatakeyama S, Yu SY, Bao X, Ohyama C, Khoo KH, et al. Core3 O-glycan synthase suppresses tumor formation and metastasis of prostate carcinoma PC3 and LNCaP cells through down-regulation of alpha2beta1 integrin complex. J Biol Chem. 2009;284(25):17157–69. https://doi.org/10.1074/jbc.M109.010934.
15. Hagisawa S, Ohyama C, Takahashi T, Endoh M, Moriya T, Nakayama J, et al. Expression of core 2 beta1,6-N-acetylglucosaminyltransferase facilitates prostate cancer progression. Glycobiology. 2005;15(10):1016–24. https://doi.org/10.1093/glycob/cwi086.
16. Prakash S, Robbins PW. Glycotyping of prostate specific antigen. Glycobiology. 2000;10(2):173–6.
17. Ohyama C, Hosono M, Nitta K, Oh-eda M, Yoshikawa K, Habuchi T, et al. Carbohydrate structure and differential binding of prostate specific antigen to Maackia Amurensis lectin between prostate cancer and benign prostate hypertrophy. Glycobiology. 2004;14(8):671–9. https://doi.org/10.1093/glycob/cwh071.
18. Tsuchiya N, Ohyama C, Habuchi T. Tumor markers in prostate cancer—clinical significance and future prospect of prostate specific antigen (PSA). Gan To Kagaku Ryoho. 2005;32(2):275–80.
19. Tajiri M, Ohyama C, Wada Y. Oligosaccharide profiles of the prostate specific antigen in free and complexed forms from the prostate cancer patient serum and in seminal plasma: a glycopeptide approach. Glycobiology. 2008;18(1):2–8. https://doi.org/10.1093/glycob/cwm117.
20. Yoneyama T, Ohyama C, Hatakeyama S, Narita S, Habuchi T, Koie T, et al. Measurement of aberrant glycosylation of prostate specific antigen can improve specificity in early detection of prostate cancer. Biochem Biophys Res Commun. 2014;448(4):390–6. https://doi.org/10.1016/j.bbrc.2014.04.107.
21. Ishikawa T, Yoneyama T, Tobisawa Y, Hatakeyama S, Kurosawa T, Nakamura K, et al. An automated micro-total immunoassay system for measuring cancer-associated alpha2,3-linked Sialyl N-Glycan-carrying prostate-specific antigen may improve the accuracy of prostate cancer diagnosis. Int J Mol Sci. 2017;18(2):E470. https://doi.org/10.3390/ijms18020470.
22. Nishimura S, Niikura K, Kurogochi M, Matsushita T, Fumoto M, Hinou H, et al. High-throughput protein glycomics: combined use of chemoselective glycoblotting and MALDI-TOF/TOF mass spectrometry. Angew Chem Int Ed Engl. 2004;44(1):91–6. https://doi.org/10.1002/anie.200461685.

23. Hatakeyama S, Amano M, Tobisawa Y, Yoneyama T, Tsuchiya N, Habuchi T, et al. Serum N-glycan alteration associated with renal cell carcinoma detected by high throughput glycan analysis. J Urol. 2014;191(3):805–13. https://doi.org/10.1016/j.juro.2013.10.052.
24. Tsui KH, Chang PL, Feng TH, Chung LC, Sung HC, Juang HH. Evaluating the function of matriptase and N-acetylglucosaminyltransferase V in prostate cancer metastasis. Anticancer Res. 2008;28(4A):1993–9.
25. Bennun SV, Yarema KJ, Betenbaugh MJ, Krambeck FJ. Integration of the transcriptome and glycome for identification of glycan cell signatures. PLoS Comput Biol. 2013;9(1):e1002813. https://doi.org/10.1371/journal.pcbi.1002813.
26. Taniguchi N, Kizuka Y. Glycans and cancer: role of N-glycans in cancer biomarker, progression and metastasis, and therapeutics. Adv Cancer Res. 2015;126:11–51. https://doi.org/10.1016/bs.acr.2014.11.001.
27. Demetriou M, Granovsky M, Quaggin S, Dennis JW. Negative regulation of T-cell activation and autoimmunity by Mgat5 N-glycosylation. Nature. 2001;409(6821):733–9. https://doi.org/10.1038/35055582.

Bone-Targeted Treatment in CRPC Management

32

Tomomi Kamba

Abstract

Prostate cancer frequently metastasizes to bone, and progression of advanced prostate cancer is parallel to progression of bone metastases. Metastatic bone disease often causes skeletal-related events (SREs). SREs lead to deterioration of patients' quality of life and even their prognosis. SREs also have significant impacts on health resource utilization and financial burden. Ironically, androgen deprivation therapy (ADT) itself induces osteoporosis and may affect the incidence of SREs. Thus, preventing SREs is considered as one of major issues in the management of patients with prostate cancer and bone metastases, and bone-targeted treatment combined with systemic therapy against prostate cancer is a rational approach.

The usefulness of zoledronic acid and denosumab has been established for the prevention of SREs in men with CRPC and bone metastases. These agents are also proved to be effective for the prevention of ADT-induced bone loss. Alpha-emitter radium-223 demonstrates a survival benefit as well as a preventive effect for SSEs in men with bony metastatic CRPC patients without visceral metastases. The survival benefit or SRE-preventive effect of bisphosphonates or denosumab for men with CSPC is controversial and routine use of these agents for these purposes is not currently recommended. Bone-metastasis-directed SBRT is a new and aggressive treatment approach for patients with oligometastatic prostate cancer recurrence, but is still under investigation.

Keywords

Prostate cancer · SRE · SSE · Bone-targeted therapy

T. Kamba, M.D., Ph.D.
Department of Urology, Kumamoto University Graduate School of Medical Sciences, Kumamoto, Japan
e-mail: kamba@kumamoto-u.ac.jp

© Springer Nature Singapore Pte Ltd. 2018
Y. Arai, O. Ogawa (eds.), *Hormone Therapy and Castration Resistance of Prostate Cancer*, https://doi.org/10.1007/978-981-10-7013-6_32

32.1 Introduction

Prostate cancer frequently metastasizes to bone, and progression of advanced prostate cancer is parallel to progression of bone metastases. We reported that among 151 patients with advanced prostate cancer the prevalence of bone metastasis was 62.9% at initial diagnosis and 83.8% at the diagnosis of so-called hormone-refractory prostate cancer (HRPC) [1]. HRPC was previously used as a synonym of castration-resistant prostate cancer (CRPC), but currently CRPC is recommended as the preferred term by the Prostate Cancer Working Group 2 (PCWG2) [2]. Furthermore, an autopsy series demonstrated that 90% of patients with metastatic prostate cancer had bone metastases at the end-stage of prostate cancer [3].

Metastatic bone disease often causes skeletal complications, namely skeletal-related events (SREs). A population-based cohort study in Denmark demonstrated that 43.6% of the patients presented with bone metastasis at prostate cancer diagnosis experienced SREs during follow-up [4]. In a placebo-controlled randomized clinical trial (RCT) examining the preventive effect of zoledronic acid against SREs in patients with HRPC, 49% of the patients in the placebo arm had at least one SRE during the entire 24-month study period [5]. It is well known that SRE leads to deterioration of patients' quality of life [6, 7] and even their prognosis [1, 4, 8]. SREs also have significant impacts on health resource utilization and financial burden [9–11]. Ironically, androgen deprivation therapy (ADT) itself can induce osteoporosis and bone fracture [12, 13]. Moreover, a history of bone fracture negatively impacts the survival of prostate cancer patients [14]. Thus, preventing SREs is considered as one of major issues in the management of patients with prostate cancer and bone metastases, and bone-targeted treatment combined with systemic therapy against prostate cancer is a rational approach.

32.2 Prevention of ADT-Induced Bone Loss

In general, ADT is thought to be still mandatory in order to maintain castrated status in men with CRPC, which means that most CRPC patients have substantially long-term ADT and face to the risk of ADT-induced bone loss. Unfortunately, there have been no RCT examining whether or not osteoclast-targeted agents, such as bisphosphonate or anti-receptor activator of nuclear factor κB ligand (RANKL) monoclonal antibody, can prevent bone loss in patients with CRPC. However, several RCTs demonstrated anti-osteopenic effect of such agents in patients with nonmetastatic or metastatic prostate cancer under or initiating ADT [15].

Among bisphosphonates, zoledronic acid, a third-generation nitrogen-containing bisphosphonate, had most vigorously been investigated on its preventive effect of ADT-induced bone loss. In a double-blind randomized placebo-controlled trial enrolling 106 men with nonmetastatic prostate cancer beginning ADT, zoledronic acid 4 mg i.v. every 3 months for 1 year increased bone mineral density (BMD) at 1 year from baseline in lumbar spine, femoral neck, trochanter, and total hip (mean percent change from baseline; +5.6%, +1.2%, +2.2%, +1.2%, respectively), but placebo decreased (mean percent change from baseline; −2.2%, −2.1%, −2.7%, −2.8%, respectively). The mean difference in percent change from baseline differed significantly between zoledronic acid and placebo ($p < 0.001$) [16]. In another randomized controlled trial, 44 men with nonmetastatic prostate cancer receiving ADT and with T scores more than −2.5 were randomly assigned to a single treatment of zoledronic acid (4 mg i.v.) or placebo. BMD of the posteroanterior lumbar spine decreased by 3.1% in the placebo group and increased by 4.0% in the annual zoledronic acid group with a significant between-group difference of 7.1% in percent change from baseline to 12 months ($p < 0.001$). Similar between-group differences favoring annual zoledronic acid were observed for the femoral neck and trochanter [17]. In a randomized pilot study over 12 months, 40 men with hormone-naive prostate cancer and bone metastasis were assigned to either ADT plus a single dose of zoledronic acid (4 mg, i.v.) or ADT alone. The between-group difference in percent BMD change of posteroanterior lumbar spine from baseline to 12 months was statistically significant (+3.5% versus −8.2%, $p = 0.0004$). Similar significant between-group differences were also observed for the total hip and femoral neck, indicating zoledronic acid preserved BMD during 1-year ADT [18].

A large-scale RCT by Denosumab HALT Prostate Cancer Study Group demonstrated the anti-osteopenic efficacy of denosumab, a human monoclonal anti-RANKL antibody, in patients with nonmetastatic prostate cancer receiving ADT. Patients were randomly assigned to either denosumab at a dose of 60 mg subcutaneously every 6 months or placebo (734 patients in each group). At 24 months, denosumab treatment increased BMD of the lumbar spine by 5.6% compared with a decrease by 1.0% with placebo treatment ($p < 0.001$). Significant between-group differences were observed through 36-month study period. Similar significant increases in BMD were demonstrated in the total hip, femoral neck, and distal radius. Moreover, the incidence of new vertebral fractures was decreased in the denosumab group compared with the placebo group (1.5% versus 3.9%, $p = 0.006$) [19].

32.3 Prevention of SRE

Most studies have defined skeletal-related events (SREs) as a composite of local skeletal complications mainly consisting of pathological fracture, spinal cord compression, radiotherapy to bone, and surgery to bone. Some older studies considered malignant hypercalcemia or change of anti-neoplastic therapy due to bone pain as SRE. Some of latest trials use only symptomatic skeletal events (SSEs) as an endpoint [20]. Such trials have proved that zoledronic acid, denosumab, radiopharmaceuticals, and new generation hormonal agents such as abiraterone and enzalutamide are effective for the prevention of SREs or SSEs in CRPC patients.

Zoledronic acid was the first agent demonstrating an SRE-preventing efficacy in patients with CRPC. In a placebo-controlled randomized trial, zoledronic acid (4 mg i.v. every 3 weeks for up to 24 months) significantly reduced the incidence of SREs in men with HRPC by 11.0% compared with placebo (38% versus 49%,

$p = 0.028$). In addition, zoledronic acid significantly prolonged the median time to first on-study SRE (488 days versus 321 days, $p = 0.009$) and reduced on-going risk of SREs (hazard ratio [HR] = 0.64, $p = 0.002$) compared with placebo [5]. Similarly, another RCT demonstrated the significant effect of zoledronic acid on SRE-free interval in bony metastatic CRPC patients under docetaxel chemotherapy. The median SRE-free interval was significantly prolonged in the zoledronic acid arm compared with the control arm (13.6 months versus 11.2 months, HR = 0.78, $p = 0.01$). Total number of SREs at the time of analysis (median follow-up 22 months) decreased by 30% in patients allocated to the zoledronic acid arm. In addition, the proportion of patients experiencing ≥2 SREs decreased from 40% to 27% and the number of patients experiencing no SREs increased from 39% to 46% in the zoledronic acid arm compared with the control arm. In this trial, zoledronic acid was administered intravenously at a dose of 4 mg every 3 weeks up to the end of chemotherapy and thereafter every 4 weeks as clinically indicated, or until disease progression or other discontinuation criteria, and thus the results suggested a role of zoledronic acid as post-chemotherapy maintenance therapy [21].

Recently, a randomized trial was conducted to determine the optimal dosing interval for zoledronic acid, in which the non-inferiority of the longer dosing interval (every 12 weeks) to the standard interval (every 4 weeks) was examined in 1822 patients with metastatic breast cancer, metastatic prostate cancer, or multiple myeloma who had at least one site of bone involvement. The proportions of patients experiencing at least one SRE within 2 years were not different between the longer interval group and standard interval group (29% versus 28%, $p < 0.001$ for non-inferiority). In the subgroup analysis in 689 patients with bony metastatic prostate cancer, the probability of experiencing at least one SRE was not statistically different (32% versus 30%, $p = 0.58$). There were not significant differences in pain scores, performance status, incidence of osteonecrosis of the jaw, and kidney dysfunction between the treatment groups, indicating that the longer interval may be an acceptable option [22].

The effect of bisphosphonates on preventing SREs or SSEs was also tested in patients with castration sensitive prostate cancer (CSPC) in several trials [23–26]. However, the results were contradictory among the trials, and the routine use of bisphosphonates for this purpose is not currently recommended.

Denosumab (120 mg s.c.) was compared with zoledronic acid (4 mg i.v.) for prevention of SREs in men with bony metastatic CRPC in a randomized, double-blind trial. The median time to first on-study SRE was significantly longer in the patients allocated to denosumab than in those to zoledronic acid (20.7 months versus 17.1 months, HR = 0.82, $p = 0.008$). The between-group difference was observed consistently from 3 months after initiation of study treatment. Denosumab also significantly delayed the time to first and subsequent on-study SREs [27]. A subsequent exploratory analysis demonstrated similar results on the time to first SSE or on the time to first and subsequent SSEs in favor of denosumab [28].

Bone-seeking radiopharmaceuticals such as strontium-89, samarium-153, rhenium-186, and radium-223 were also examined on the effect of palliating malignant bone pain from prostate cancer, especially due to multifocal osteoblastic metastases in many studies. Overall, each radiopharmaceutical demonstrated pain response greater than 50–60% [29]. To date, alpha-emitter radium-223 is the only radionuclide demonstrating the preventive effect for SSEs in patients with bony metastatic CRPC without visceral metastases. In a randomized, double-blind, placebo-controlled trial, radium-223 significantly prolonged the time to the first on-study SSE (15.6 months versus 9.8 months, HR = 0.66, p = 0.00037). Among SSEs, radium-223 significantly reduced the risks of radiotherapy for bone pain (HR = 0.67) and spinal cord compression (HR = 0.52) [30].

32.4 Improvement of Survival Outcome

To date, several studies have investigated whether bone-targeted therapy can improve the survival outcome of patients with bony metastatic or nonmetastatic CRPC, patients with bony metastatic CSPC, or patients with high-risk localized or locally advanced prostate cancer.

In men with CRPC and bone metastases, the survival benefit of zoledronic acid, denosumab, or radium-223 was also evaluated in the aforementioned landmark trial of each agent. The median time of survival was numerically longer in patients treated with zoledronic acid 4 mg than in patients with placebo (546 days versus 464 days), but this difference was not statistically significant (p = 0.091) [31]. Denosumab did not significantly prolong overall survival (19.4 months versus 19.8 months, HR = 1.03, p = 0.65) or progression-free survival (8.4 months versus 8.4 months, HR = 1.06, p = 0.30), compared with zoledronic acid [27]. On the contrary, radium-223 significantly prolonged overall survival compared with placebo (14.9 months versus 11.3 months, HR = 0.70, p < 0.001), demonstrating a 30% reduction in the risk of death [32].

In men with nonmetastatic CRPC, denosumab was assessed for prevention of bone metastasis or death in a phase 3, randomized, placebo-controlled trial. Compared with placebo, denosumab significantly prolonged bone-metastasis-free survival (29.5 months versus 25.2 months, HR = 0.85, p = 0.028), but not overall survival (49.3 months versus 44.8 months, HR = 1.01, p = 0.91) [33].

In men with CSPC, bisphosphonates were investigated on the effect for survival outcome in several RCTs. In men with metastatic CSPC starting ADT, sodium clodronate demonstrated a survival benefit with an HR of 0.77 compared with placebo (p = 0.032). The estimated 5-year and 10-year survivals were 30% and 17%, respectively, with clodronate versus 21% and 9%, respectively, with placebo. However, such a benefit of clodronate was not seen in men with nonmetastatic CSPC [34]. In CALGB 90202 trial, early zoledronic acid combined with ADT did not yield a significant improvement either in progression-free survival (10.6 months versus 9.2 months, p = 0.22) or in overall survival (37.9 months versus 36.0 months, p = 0.29) compared with ADT alone in men with bony metastatic CSPC [24]. In STAMPEDE trial recruiting men with high-risk locally advanced, metastatic or recurrent prostate cancer starting first-line ADT, zoledronic acid plus ADT failed to show a survival benefit compared with ADT alone with HR of 0.94 (not reached versus 71 months, $p = 0.45$) [25]. In ZAPCA trial, zoledronic acid plus ADT demonstrated a marginal benefit for time to treatment failure compared with ADT alone (12.4 months versus 9.7 months, HR = 0.75, $p = 0.051$), but did not affect overall survival (not reached versus 60.2 months, HR = 0.78, $p = 0.28$) [26]. ZEUS study examined whether zoledronic acid can prevent bone metastases in men with high-risk localized prostate cancer or not, demonstrating that zoledronic acid 4 mg every 3 months was ineffective for the prevention of bone metastases in this population [35].

32.5 Bone Metastasis-Directed Therapy for Oligometastatic Prostate Cancer

Recently, retrospective studies suggest that aggressive treatment approaches including local therapy and metastasis-directed therapy could be beneficial with minimal risk of toxic effects in patients with oligometastatic prostate cancer. Stereotactic body radiotherapy (SBRT) to bone metastatic sites is one of such aggressive approaches [36]. A multi-institutional analysis pooled data of SBRT for prostate cancer patients with three or fewer metachronous metastases after radical local therapy from small retrospective studies. The primary endpoint was distant progression-free survival (DPFS), defined as the absence of new metastatic lesions. Out of 119 patients, 43 patients had bone metastases. The median DPFS was 21 months, and the 3-year and 5-year DPFS were 31% and 15%, respectively. These results suggest that SBRT for oligometastatic prostate cancer recurrence could result in a substantial ADT-free period [37]. Definitive conclusions on this issue should be awaited after the completion of several prospective RCTs [36].

Conclusion

The usefulness of zoledronic acid and denosumab has been established for the prevention of SREs in men with CRPC and bone metastases. These agents are also proved to be effective for the prevention of ADT-induced bone loss. Alpha-emitter radium-223 demonstrates a survival benefit as well as a preventive effect for SSEs in men with bony metastatic CRPC patients without visceral metastases. The survival benefit or SRE-preventive effect of bisphosphonates or denosumab for men with CSPC is controversial and routine use of these agents for these purposes are not currently recommended. Bone-metastasis-directed SBRT is a new and aggressive treatment approach for patients with oligometastatic prostate cancer recurrence, but is still under investigation.

References

1. Inoue T, Segawa T, Kamba T, Yoshimura K, Nakamura E, Nishiyama H, et al. Prevalence of skeletal complications and their impact on survival of hormone refractory prostate cancer patients in Japan. Urology. 2009;73:1104–9. https://doi.org/10.1016/j.urology.2008.07.062.

2. Scher HI, Halabi S, Tannock I, Morris M, Sternberg CN, Carducci MA, et al. Design and end points of clinical trials for patients with progressive prostate cancer and castrate levels of testosterone: recommendations of the Prostate Cancer Clinical Trials Working Group. J Clin Oncol. 2008;26:1148–59. https://doi.org/10.1200/JCO.2007.12.4487.
3. Bubendorf L, Schöpfer A, Wagner U, Sauter G, Moch H, Willi N, et al. Metastatic patterns of prostate cancer: an autopsy study of 1,589 patients. Hum Pathol. 2000;31:578–83.
4. Nørgaard M, Jensen AØ, Jacobsen JB, Cetin K, Fryzek JP, Sørensen HT. Skeletal related events, bone metastasis and survival of prostate cancer: a population based cohort study in Denmark (1999 to 2007). J Urol. 2010;184:162–7. https://doi.org/10.1016/j.juro.2010.03.034.
5. Saad F, Gleason DM, Murray R, Tchekmedyian S, Venner P, Lacombe L, et al. Long-term efficacy of zoledronic acid for the prevention of skeletal complications in patients with metastatic hormone-refractory prostate cancer. J Natl Cancer Inst. 2004;96:879–82.
6. Weinfurt KP, Li Y, Castel LD, Saad F, Timbie JW, Glendenning GA, et al. The significance of skeletal-related events for the health-related quality of life of patients with metastatic prostate cancer. Ann Oncol. 2005;16:579–84.
7. DePuy V, Anstrom KJ, Castel LD, Schulman KA, Weinfurt KP, Saad F. Effects of skeletal morbidities on longitudinal patient-reported outcomes and survival in patients with metastatic prostate cancer. Support Care Cancer. 2007;15:869–76.
8. Sathiakumar N, Delzell E, Morrisey MA, Falkson C, Yong M, Chia V, et al. Mortality following bone metastasis and skeletal-related events among men with prostate cancer: a population-based analysis of US Medicare beneficiaries, 1999-2006. Prostate Cancer Prostatic Dis. 2011;14:177–83. https://doi.org/10.1038/pcan.2011.7.
9. Bahl A, Hoefeler H, Duran I, Hechmati G, Garzon-Rodriguez C, Ashcroft J, et al. Health resource utilization associated with skeletal-related events in patients with advanced prostate cancer: a European subgroup analysis from an observational, multinational study. J Clin Med. 2014;3:883–96. https://doi.org/10.3390/jcm3030883.
10. Hagiwara M, Delea TE, Saville MW, Chung K. Healthcare utilization and costs associated with skeletal-related events in prostate cancer patients with bone metastases. Prostate Cancer Prostatic Dis. 2013;16:23–7. https://doi.org/10.1038/pcan.2012.42.
11. Krupski TL, Foley KA, Baser O, Long S, Macarios D, Litwin MS. Health care cost associated with prostate cancer, androgen deprivation therapy and bone complications. J Urol. 2007;178:1423–8.
12. Morote J, Morin JP, Orsola A, Abascal JM, Salvador C, Trilla E, et al. Prevalence of osteoporosis during long-term androgen deprivation therapy in patients with prostate cancer. Urology. 2007;69:500–4.
13. Shahinian VB, Kuo YF, Freeman JL, Goodwin JS. Risk of fracture after androgen deprivation for prostate cancer. N Engl J Med. 2005;352:154–64.
14. Oefelein MG, Ricchiuti V, Conrad W, Resnick MI. Skeletal fractures negatively correlate with overall survival in men with prostate cancer. J Urol. 2002;168:1005–7.
15. Bienz M, Saad F. Androgen-deprivation therapy and bone loss in prostate cancer patients: a clinical review. Bonekey Rep. 2015;4:716. https://doi.org/10.1038/bonekey.2015.85.
16. Smith MR, Eastham J, Gleason DM, Shasha D, Tchekmedyian S, Zinner N. Randomized controlled trial of zoledronic acid to prevent bone loss in men receiving androgen deprivation therapy for nonmetastatic prostate cancer. J Urol. 2003;169:2008–12.
17. Michaelson MD, Kaufman DS, Lee H, McGovern FJ, Kantoff PW, Fallon MA, et al. Randomized controlled trial of annual zoledronic acid to prevent gonadotropin-releasing hormone agonist-induced bone loss in men with prostate cancer. J Clin Oncol. 2007;25:1038–42.
18. Satoh T, Kimura M, Matsumoto K, Tabata K, Okusa H, Bessho H, et al. Single infusion of zoledronic acid to prevent androgen deprivation therapy-induced bone loss in men with hormone-naive prostate carcinoma. Cancer. 2009;115:3468–74. https://doi.org/10.1002/cncr.24404.
19. Smith MR, Egerdie B, Hernández Toriz N, Feldman R, Tammela TL, Saad F, et al. Denosumab in men receiving androgen-deprivation therapy for prostate cancer. N Engl J Med. 2009;361:745–55. https://doi.org/10.1056/NEJMoa0809003.

20. Vignani F, Bertaglia V, Buttigliero C, Tucci M, Scagliotti GV, Di Mario M. Skeletal metastases and impact of anticancer and bone-targeted agents in patients with castration-resistant prostate cancer. Cancer Treat Rev. 2016;44:61–73. https://doi.org/10.1016/j.ctrv.2016.02.002.
21. James ND, Pirrie SJ, Pope AM, Barton D, Andronis L, Goranitis I, et al. Clinical outcome and survival following treatment of metastatic castrate-refractory prostate cancer with docetaxel alone or with strontium-89, zoledronic acid, or both: the TRAPEZE randomized clinical trial. JAMA Oncol. 2016;2:493–9. https://doi.org/10.1001/jamaoncol.2015.5570.
22. Himelstein AL, Foster JC, Khatcheressian JL, Roberts JD, Seisler DK, Novotny PJ, et al. Effect of longer-interval vs standard dosing of zoledronic acid on skeletal events in patients with bone metastases: a randomized clinical trial. JAMA. 2017;317:48–58. https://doi.org/10.1001/jama.2016.19425.
23. Dearnaley DP, Sydes MR, Mason MD, Stott M, Powell CS, Robinson AC, et al. A double-blind, placebo-controlled, randomized trial of oral sodium clodronate for metastatic prostate cancer (MRC PR05 trial). J Natl Cancer Inst. 2003;95:1300–11.
24. Smith MR, Halabi S, Ryan CJ, Hussain A, Vogelzang N, Stadler W, et al. Randomized controlled trial of early zoledronic acid in men with castration-sensitive prostate cancer and bone metastases: results of CALGB 90202 (alliance). J Clin Oncol. 2014;32:1143–50. https://doi.org/10.1200/JCO.2013.51.6500.
25. James ND, Sydes MR, Clarke NW, Mason MD, Dearnaley DP, Spears MR, et al. Addition of docetaxel, zoledronic acid, or both to first-line long-term hormone therapy in prostate cancer (STAMPEDE): survival results from an adaptive, multiarm, multistage, platform randomised controlled trial. Lancet. 2016;387:1163–77. https://doi.org/10.1016/S0140-6736(15)01037-5.
26. Kamba T, Kamoto T, Maruo S, Kikuchi T, Shimizu Y, Namiki S, et al. A phase III multicenter, randomized, controlled study of combined androgen blockade with versus without zoledronic acid in prostate cancer patients with metastatic bone disease: results of the ZAPCA trial. Int J Clin Oncol. 2017;22:166–73. https://doi.org/10.1007/s10147-016-1037-2.
27. Fizazi K, Carducci M, Smith M, Damião R, Brown J, Karsh L, et al. Denosumabu versus zoledronic acid for treatment of bone metastases in men with castration-resistant prostate cancer: a randomised, double-blind study. Lancet. 2011;377:813–22. https://doi.org/10.1016/S0140-6736(10)62344-6.
28. Smith MR, Coleman RE, Klotz L, Pittman K, Milecki P, Ng S, et al. Denosumab for the prevention of skeletal complications in metastatic castration-resistant prostate cancer: comparison of skeletal-related events and symptomatic skeletal events. Ann Oncol. 2015;26:368–74. https://doi.org/10.1093/annonc/mdu519.
29. Jong JM, Oprea-Lager DE, Hooft L, de Klerk JM, Bloemendal HJ, Verheul HM, et al. Radiopharmaceuticals for palliation of bone pain in patients with castration-resistant prostate cancer metastatic to bone: a systematic review. Eur Urol. 2016;70:416–26. https://doi.org/10.1016/j.eururo.2015.09.005.
30. Sartor O, Coleman R, Nilsson S, Heinrich D, Helle SI, O'Sullivan JM, et al. Effect of radium-223 dichloride on symptomatic skeletal events in patients with castration-resistant prostate cancer and bone metastases: results from a phase 3, double-blind, randomised trial. Lancet Oncol. 2014;15:738–46. https://doi.org/10.1016/S1470-2045(14)70183-4.
31. Saad F, Gleason DM, Murray R, Tchekmedyian S, Venner P, Lacombe L, et al. A randomized, placebo-controlled trial of zoledronic acid in patients with hormone-refractory metastatic prostate carcinoma. J Natl Cancer Inst. 2002;94:1458–68.
32. Parker C, Nilsson S, Heinrich D, Helle SI, O'Sullivan JM, Fosså SD, et al. Alpha emitter radium-223 and survival in metastatic prostate cancer. N Engl J Med. 2013;369:213–23. https://doi.org/10.1056/NEJMoa1213755.
33. Smith MR, Saad F, Coleman R, Shore N, Fizazi K, Tombal B, et al. Denosumab and bone-metastasis-free survival in men with castration-resistant prostate cancer: results of a phase 3, randomised, placebo-controlled trial. Lancet. 2012;379:39–46. https://doi.org/10.1016/S0140-6736(11)61226-9.
34. Dearnaley DP, Mason MD, Parmar MK, Sanders K, Sydes MR. Adjuvant therapy with oral sodium clodronate in locally advanced and metastatic prostate cancer: long-term overall

survival results from the MRC PR04 and PR05 randomised controlled trials. Lancet Oncol. 2009;10:872–6. https://doi.org/10.1016/S1470-2450(09)70201-3.
35. Wirth M, Tammela T, Cicalese V, Gomez Veiga F, Delaere K, Miller K, et al. Prevention of bone metastases in patients with high-risk non metastatic prostate cancer treated with zoledronic acid: efficacy and safety results of the Zometa European Study (ZEUS). Eur Urol. 2015;67:482–91. https://doi.org/10.1016/j.eururo.2014.02.014.
36. Tosoian JJ, Gorin MA, Ross AE, Pienta KJ, Tran PT, Schaeffer EM. Oligometastatic prostate cancer: definitions, clinical outcomes, and treatment considerations. Nat Rev Urol. 2017;14:15–25. https://doi.org/10.1038/nrurol.2016.175.
37. Ost P, Jereczek-Fossa BA, As NV, Zilli T, Muacevic A, Olivier K, et al. Progression-free survival following stereotactic body radiotherapy for oligometastatic prostate cancer treatment-naive recurrence: a multi-institutional analysis. Eur Urol. 2016;69:9–12. https://doi.org/10.1016/j.eururo.2015.07.004.

Skeletal Complications in Patients with CRPC

33

Takamitsu Inoue and Tomonori Habuchi

Abstract

Skeletal complications in patients with prostate cancer can result in significant morbidity. There is a relatively high prevalence of bone metastasis and reduction of bone mineral density due to androgen deprivation therapy, and together, these can result in the development of multiple skeletal complications in patients with prostate cancer. The relatively long survival (median, 3–4 years) after bone metastases with multiple skeletal complications makes a significant negative impact on patients' functional status, quality of life, and social resource utilization. To evaluate skeletal complications, the term "skeletal-related events (SREs)" has frequently been used in most randomized trials conducted previously. SREs usually include pathological bone fracture, spinal cord compression, surgery to bone, and radiotherapy to the bone. Recently, symptomatic skeletal events (SSEs), including only symptomatic events, is the recommended term for use in clinical trials. Local therapies for skeletal complications, such as radiation and surgery, are usually performed to reduce local symptoms, such as bone pain or neurological deficits, leading to improvement of the health-related quality of life. Systemic therapies, such as radiopharmaceuticals, bisphosphonates, and monoclonal antibodies against the receptor activator of the nuclear factor-kappa B ligand, are administered to reduce presymptomatic and symptomatic skeletal complications.

Keywords

Skeletal-related events · Symptomatic skeletal events · Bone mineral density Pathological bone fracture · Spinal cord compression

T. Inoue, M.D. (✉) · T. Habuchi, M.D.
Department of Urology, Akita University Graduate School of Medicine, Akita, Japan
e-mail: takamitu@doc.med.akita-u.ac.jp

© Springer Nature Singapore Pte Ltd. 2018
Y. Arai, O. Ogawa (eds.), *Hormone Therapy and Castration Resistance of Prostate Cancer*, https://doi.org/10.1007/978-981-10-7013-6_33

33.1 Introduction

Skeletal complications can lead to significant morbidity in patients with prostate cancer by two viewpoints: first, the prevalence of bone metastasis in patients with prostate cancer is relatively higher than that in other cancers [1]; second, androgen deprivation therapy (ADT) for the treatment of prostate cancer reduces bone mineral density (BMD), leading to an acceleration of osteoporosis and bone metastases [2, 3]. These two factors closely interact with each other, leading to the development of multiple skeletal complications in patients with prostate cancer. The relatively long survival (median, 3–4 years) after bone metastases with multiple skeletal complications in patients with prostate cancer makes a significant negative impact on patients' functional status, quality of life, and social resource utilization [4].

33.2 Skeletal-Related Events and Symptomatic Skeletal Events

To assess the incidence of skeletal complications as endpoints of clinical trials, the term "skeletal-related events (SREs)" was previously defined by the Food and Drug Administration of the United States and has been used in several trials [5]. In most clinical studies, SREs included four factors: pathological bone fracture, spinal cord compression, surgery to bone, and radiotherapy to the bone; thus, SREs have been defined as a composite endpoint, mostly including the need for local treatments of radiation or orthopedic surgery ([6–9]; Table 33.1). Radiotherapy is usually indicated for the treatment of uncontrolled pain, pathologic fractures, and spinal cord compression. Surgery usually includes procedures to stabilize or prevent pathologic fractures or spinal cord compression. The definition of SRE, however, is different in several randomized trials. In a broad sense, SREs include a change of antineoplastic therapy to treat bone pain [6, 9]. A reduction in the frequency of SREs has been used in several phase III trials to support the approval of zoledronic acid (ZOL) and denosumab [6, 7]. The definition of SREs includes asymptomatic nonclinical fractures ascertained by serial imaging. Recently, the Prostate Cancer Clinical Trial Working Group 3 [10] stated that they did not consider SREs and instead they recommended using "symptomatic skeletal events (SSEs)" that include only symptomatic events of clear clinical significance. In phase III clinical trial for radium-223, SSEs were defined as symptomatic fracture, radiation or surgery to bone, or spinal cord compression [11].

33.3 Incidence and Prevalence of Skeletal Complications in Patients with CRPC

According to data in the placebo arm of the randomized phase III trials evaluating the effectiveness of ZOL, the incidence of SREs was reported to be 44.2% in patients with castration-resistant prostate cancer (CRPC) during approximately 9 months

Table 33.1 Definitions of skeletal-related events (SREs) and symptomatic skeletal events (SSEs) in selected randomized clinical trials conducted in patients with metastatic castration-resistant prostate cancer

| Drug | References | Endpoints | Definition of skeletal complications ||||||
			Radiation Therapy	Surgery to bone	Pathological bone fracture	Symptomatic bone fracture	Spinal cord compression	Change of antineoplastic therapy to treat bone pain
Zoledronic acid	J Natl Cancer Inst 94:1458–68 (2002) [6]	Primary: proportion of patients with at least one SRE	O	O	O	–	O	O
		Exploratory: proportion of patients with at least one SSE	O	O	–	O	O	O
Denosumab	Lancet 377:813–22 (2011) [7]	Primary: time to first SRE	O	O	O	–	O	–
		Exploratory: time to first SSE	O	O	–	O	O	–
Abiraterone	Lancet Oncol 13:1210–7 (2012) [8]	Secondary: time to first SRE	O	O	O	–	O	–
Enzalutamide	Lancet Oncol 15: 1147–56 (2014) [9]	Secondary: time to first SRE	O	O	O	–	O	O
Radium-223	Lancet Oncol 15:738–46 (2014) [11]	Secondary: time to first SSE	O	O	–	O	O	–

(median) of observation in the study [6]. Furthermore, all types of pathologic fractures were observed in 22.1%, vertebral fractures in 8.2%, non-vertebral fractures in 15.9%, radiation therapy in 29.3%, bone surgery in 3.4%, and spinal cord compression in 6.7% of patients in the placebo arm. In another study comparing the incidence of SREs in patients with bone metastases in the breast, lung, or prostate cancer, the incidence of SREs in patients with prostate cancer was approximately 20% and 30% at 6 and 12 months after the diagnosis of bone metastasis, respectively, which was less than that in patients with breast and lung cancer. However, the incidence eventually reached approximately 45%, which is comparable to the incidence of lung cancer at 36 months when using ZOL in 48.9% of the prostate cancer patients [12] (Fig. 33.1).

Conversely, the prevalence of bone metastasis and bone pain at the time of CRPC diagnosis was 84% and 45%, respectively, in a Japanese study [13]. In the present study, the medical charts of the enrolled patients with CRPC were retrospectively reviewed at a single institute, and the patients were not using bone-modifying agents, such as ZOL or denosumab. During a median 18 months of follow-up, the incidences of bone pain, neurological deficits, and pathologic fractures were 80%, 44%, and 14%, respectively. The incidences of taking nonsteroidal anti-inflammatory drugs and opioids were 74% and 43%, respectively, and those of radiation therapies for bone pain and laminectomy for paraplegia were 51% and 10% during the follow-up period, respectively (Fig. 33.2).

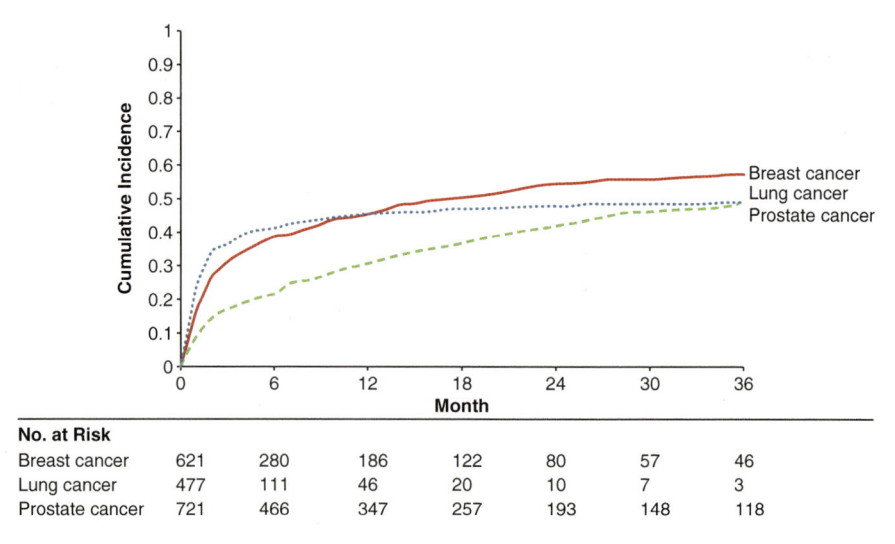

Fig. 33.1 Cumulative incidence of skeletal-related events (SREs) in patients with breast, lung, and prostate cancers after the diagnosis of bone metastasis

33 Skeletal Complications in Patients with CRPC 331

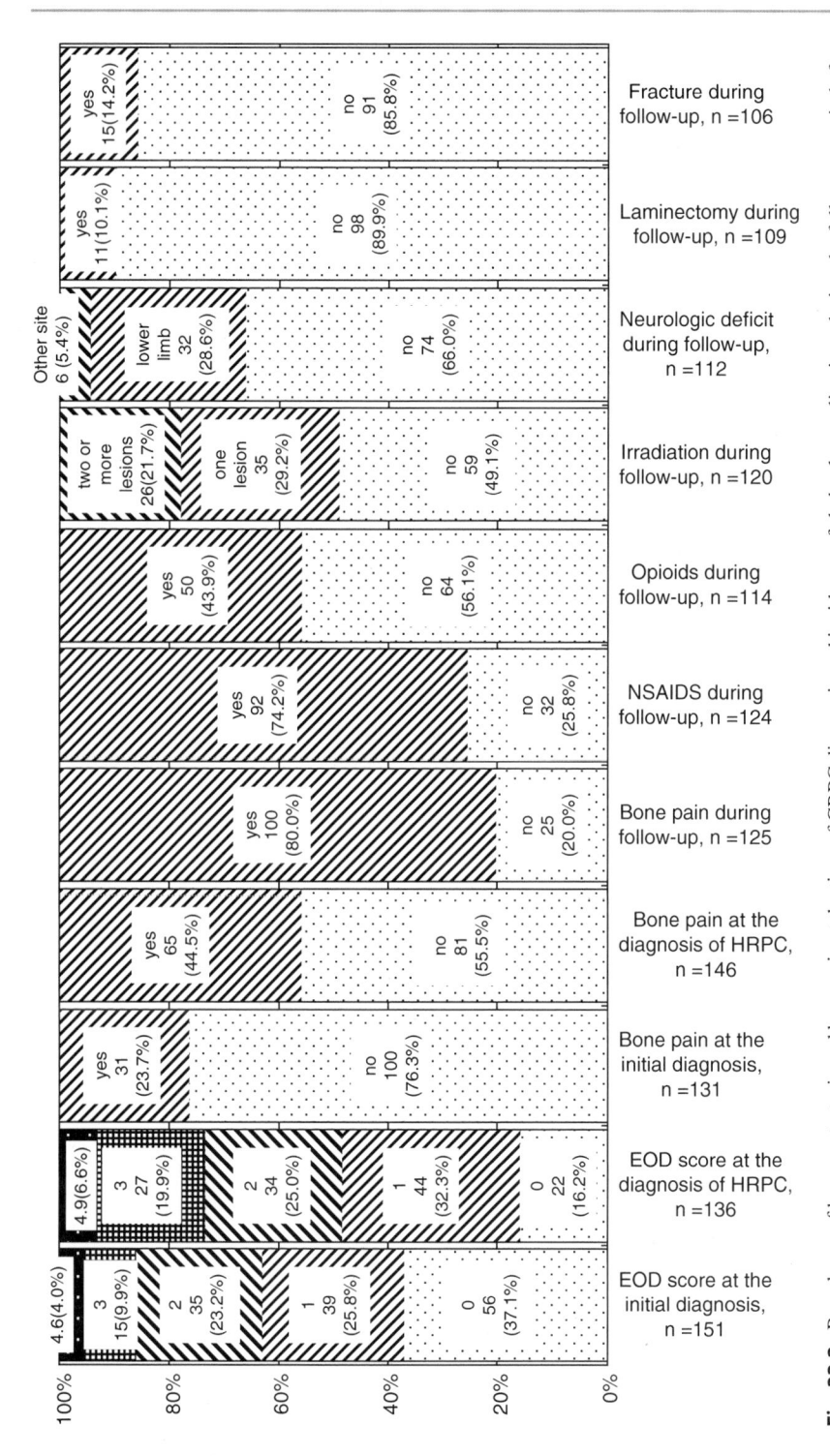

Fig. 33.2 Prevalence of bone metastasis and bone pain at the time of CRPC diagnosis and incidence of skeletal complications during the follow-up period after diagnosis of CRPC

33.4 Pathophysiology of Bone Metastases in Prostate Cancer

The metastasizing mechanism of prostate cancer cells to bone involves colonization of the skeletal microenvironment by circulating tumor cells (CTCs). Reportedly, only 0.2% of experimentally introduced CTCs were estimated to colonize distant sites [14]. According to Paget's well-established "seed and soil" hypothesis published in 1889, a bone microenvironment is ideal "soil" for circulating prostate cancer cells [15]. The three steps of metastatic seeding include survival of CTCs in circulation, homing to skeletal tissue, and attachment to bone parenchyma [16].

Platelets play an important role in the survival of CTCs in that they shield CTCs from NK cell-mediated lysis [17]. In the homing process of CTCs into skeletal tissue, chemotactic factors responsible for the migration of hematopoietic stem cells into bone marrow have been investigated as key molecules [18]. One of these chemotactic factors is stromal-derived factor-1 (SDF-1), also called CXCL12, which is predominantly produced by osteoblasts. C-X-C motif chemokine receptor 4, expressed on the surface of hematopoietic stem cells as well as prostate cancer CTCs, interacts with SDF-1 to induce homing to the bone marrow [19, 20]. In the attachment and invading process of CTCs to bone parenchyma, integrin- and lectin-mediated attachment or protease-dependent invasion has been characterized. Three major integrins, including $\alpha v \beta 3$, $\alpha 2 \beta 1$, and $\alpha 4 \beta 1$, have demonstrated instructive roles in metastatic bone seeding [21].

The activation of osteoclast-mediated bone resorption is one of the most investigated areas in this field. Induction of the receptor activator of nuclear factor-kappa B ligand (RANKL), granulocyte macrophage colony stimulating factor (GM-CSF), and macrophage colony-stimulating factor (M-CSF) from the tumor cells results in maturation of osteoclast precursor cells into multinucleated osteoclasts. Enhanced osteoclast-mediated lysis of the bone matrix releases various cytokines, such as GM-CSF, M-CSF, tumor growth factor beta, insulin-like growth factors, epidermal growth factors, fibroblast growth factors, and interleukin 6 stored in the bone matrix. These growth factors stimulate the expression of pro-metastatic factors, such as Jagged 1 [22], parathyroid hormone-related peptide [23], or cathepsin K [24] from tumor cells, which then stimulate the osteoblasts to release RANKL to promote osteoclast activation [25]. These cycles are called "vicious cycles" in the bone microenvironment in that they promote bone metastasis [23, 26].

Prostate cancer typically presents as osteoblastic lesions, and reportedly 43%, 21%, and 36% of the prostate cancer metastases studied in one report were osteoblastic, osteolytic, and mixed, respectively [27]. The transcription factor runt-related transcription factor 2 (RUNX2) is a promising molecule involved in the osteoblastic lesion formation mechanism and is normally expressed by mesenchymal progenitor cells to differentiate osteoblasts. In the microenvironment of prostate cancer bone metastases, RUNX2 is also expressed by prostate cancer cells [28] and activates bone matrix protein transcription, such as bone sialoprotein and osteocalcin. Serin protease Endothelin-1 (ET-1), which is also secreted from prostate cancer cells in the bone microenvironment, is a well-established osteoblast mitogen that promotes osteoblastic bone metastasis by binding ET_A receptor on the osteoblast [29, 30]. The randomized phase III trial for the ET-1 antagonist Atrasentan did not decrease the risk of disease progression in patients with metastatic prostate cancer [31].

33.5 Reduction of BMD Due to ADT and Its Interaction with Bone Metastasis

ADT has been demonstrated to have various adverse effects, including the reduction of BMD. Reportedly, around 45% of patients with prostate cancer receiving ADT develop osteoporosis [32]. The reduction of BMD was maximal in the first year after the initiation of ADT, peaking at 2%–5% [33, 34].

Androgen receptor (AR) is expressed in osteoblasts, osteoclasts, and osteocytes [35–37]. ADT has been shown to increase the levels of RANKL in rat serum and bone marrow [38], which caused a reduction in BMD due to osteoclast activation [39]. Moreover, bone-marrow RANKL mRNA levels have been shown to be up-regulated in mice lacking AR [36, 40] and down-regulated in mice overexpressing AR [37]. Conversely, glucocorticoid promotes the production of RANKL by osteoblasts [41, 42]. Previous reports have suggested that AR regulates RANK/RANKL signaling in the bone microenvironment and that ADT enhances this pathway, inducing osteoclast precursors to mature into osteoclasts, leading to a reduced BMD.

The high prevalence of bone metastases in patients with prostate cancer and reduction of BMD due to ADT together make skeletal complications in these patients more common. In a murine model, Ottewell et al. showed that ADT triggered the growth of disseminated PC3 cells to form bone metastases and that this was prevented with ZOL [2]. Takayama et al. also illustrated the ADT-induced acceleration of bone metastases and involvement of the RANK/RANKL signaling in this interaction [3]. These findings suggest that osteoclast suppression by RANK/RANKL signaling from the initiation of ADT is required to prevent the accelerated establishment of new bone metastases in patients with organ-confined or locally advanced high-risk prostate cancer with a high possibility of the existence of CRPC CTCs at the time of ADT initiation.

In the contemporary oncological strategy for patients with CRPC, relatively long-term ADT (median, 3–4 years) after bone metastasis is usually required. The interactions among the high incidence of bone metastases, reduction of BMD due to ADT, and acceleration of bone metastases due to ADT may together lead to frequent skeletal complications resulting in a poorer health-related quality of life (HRQOL) and survival in patients with CRPC despite the anticancer effect of ADT.

33.6 Prognosis, HRQOL, and Health Resource Utilization in Patients with Prostate Cancer Who Have Skeletal Complications

The presence of SREs is significantly associated with a worse survival and poorer HRQOL. Patients who developed a pathologic fracture had a 32% increased risk of death relative to patients without a fracture in an adjusted analysis, with comparable results observed for both vertebral and non-vertebral fractures [43]. Increasing SRE

Table 33.2 Annual costs of skeletal-related events (SREs)

Variable	No.	Mean (95% Confidence Interval), $
Total SRE costs		
All patients	342	12,469 (10,007–14,861)
Patients with 1 SRE	266	8484 (6810–10,177)
Patients with >1 SREs	76	26,384 (17,959–34,809)
Costs of SREs		
By component		
Therapeutic radiology	342	5930 (4829–7032)
Pathologic fracture	342	3179 (1745–4614)
Bone surgery	342	2218 (1059–3378)
Spinal cord compression	342	460 (116–803)
Other	342	681 (316–1047)
Inpatient vs. outpatient		
Inpatient	342	5641 (3738–7543)
Outpatient	342	5951 (4849–7052)

intensity shows a pattern of poorer survival and HRQOL [44, 45]. In patients with SREs, a significantly worse outcome was observed compared with those without SREs in validated assessment instruments, such as the functional assessment of cancer therapy-general and the brief pain inventory [44]. Complications of osteoporosis and fractures in men undergoing ADT have important economic consequences: there is an associated $22,000 cost per person during the 36 months of treatment [46]. All SREs are associated with health resource utilization, including both inpatient hospitalizations and outpatient or emergency room visits, of $12,469 per year per person [47, 48] (Table 33.2). Furthermore, those studies may have underestimated their impact because of the exclusion of patients with a short life expectancy and health resource with bone pain management [49].

33.7 Treatments for Skeletal Complications

Treatments for skeletal complications include local and systemic therapies. Local therapies include radiation and surgical therapies that are usually performed to reduce local symptoms and improve HRQOL regarding bone pain or neurological deficits. Radiation therapy for local lesions reportedly improves mobility, daily life activity, and sphincter control in patients with metastatic spinal cord compression [50]. Moreover, in one study, radiation therapy significantly improved HRQOL of patients suffering from bone pain [45]. It was reported that functional outcomes after radiation therapy were significantly influenced by the amount of time taken to develop motor deficits before radiation therapy and the number of involved vertebrae. Local control was significantly better after long-course radiation, such as 2 Gy × 20 times, than after short courses, such as 8 Gy × 1 time or 4 Gy × 5 times [51].

Surgical treatments for neurological deficits due to spinal cord compression usually consist of posterior decompression and stabilization with pedicle screws or with pedicle screws and hooks. There have only been a few studies that specifically addressed the surgical treatment of metastatic spinal cord compression in patients with prostate cancer [52–54]. Furthermore, the criteria for which patient may benefit from the surgical therapy of spinal cord compression are poorly defined; in selected patients, however, aggressive surgical decompression and spinal reconstruction is a useful treatment option [54]. Patients with hormone-naive disease and those with the hormone-refractory disease with good performance status and lacking visceral metastases may benefit from surgery for metastatic spinal cord compression [52].

Systemic therapies, including bisphosphonates, a monoclonal antibody against RANKL, and radiopharmaceuticals, are administered to prevent and reduce presymptomatic and symptomatic SREs. The first agent approved for the management of bone metastases in patients with CRPC was ZOL, a third-generation bisphosphonate. A phase III trial comparing ZOL vs. placebo demonstrated a significant reduction of at least one SRE with ZOL from 49% to 38% during the 24-month study period [6]. Denosumab is a fully humanized monoclonal antibody against RANKL that prevents the activation of its receptor RANK leading to inhibition of osteoclast maturation and bone resorption. In a phase III trial comparing denosumab vs. ZOL in patients with CRPC who have bone metastases, there was a significant improvement in median time (3.6 months) to the first SRE in the denosumab arm [7].

Regarding radiopharmaceuticals, strontium-89 is a pure beta-emitter with a long half-life, whereas samarium-153 is a gamma-emitter with a shorter half-life. Multiple randomized trials have been conducted with strontium-89 and samarium-153 in men with metastatic CRPC that have shown no improvement in OS, but palliative benefits have been demonstrated with both agents [55, 56]. The alpha-emitter radium-223 causes breaks in double-stranded DNA with less irradiation of healthy adjacent bone marrow and normal tissues. In a randomized phase III trial, radium-223 significantly prolonged the median OS in 3.8 months and significantly delayed the time to all SRE components, particularly the components of external-beam radiation therapy and spinal cord compression [11].

References

1. Coleman RE. Metastatic bone disease: clinical features, pathophysiology and treatment strategies. Cancer Treat Rev. 2001;27:165–76.
2. Ottewell PD, Wang N, Meek J, Fowles CA, Croucher PI, Eaton CL, Holen I. Castration-induced bone loss triggers growth of disseminated prostate cancer cells in bone. Endocr Relat Cancer. 2014;21:769–81.
3. Takayama K, Inoue T, Narita S, Maita S, Huang M, Numakura K, Tsuruta H, Saito M, Maeno A, Satoh S, Tsuchiya N, Habuchi T. Inhibition of the RANK/RANKL signaling with osteoprotegerin prevents castration-induced acceleration of bone metastasis in castration-insensitive prostate cancer. Cancer Lett. 2017;397:103–10.

4. Vignani F, Bertaglia V, Buttigliero C, Tucci M, Scagliotti GV, Di Maio M. Skeletal metastases and impact of anticancer and bone-targeted agents in patients with castration-resistant prostate cancer. Cancer Treat Rev. 2016;44:61–73.
5. Clinical Trials Endpoints for the Approval of Cancer Drugs and Biologics, US Department of Health and Human Services, Food and Drug Administration, Center for Drug Evaluation and Research (CDER), Center for Biologics Evaluation and Research (CBER). 2007.
6. Saad F, Gleason DM, Murray R, Tchekmedyian S, Venner P, Lacombe L, Chin JL, Vinholes JJ, Goas JA, Chen B, Zoledronic Acid Prostate Cancer Study Group. A randomized, placebo-controlled trial of zoledronic acid in patients with hormone-refractory metastatic prostate carcinoma. J Natl Cancer Inst. 2002;94:1458–68.
7. Fizazi K, Carducci M, Smith M, Damião R, Brown J, Karsh L, Milecki P, Shore N, Rader M, Wang H, Jiang Q. Denosumab versus zoledronic acid for treatment of bone metastases in men with castration-resistant prostate cancer: a randomised, double-blind study. Lancet. 2011;377:813–22.
8. Logothetis CJ, Basch E, Molina A, Fizazi K, North SA, Chi KN, Jones RJ, Goodman OB, Mainwaring PN, Sternberg CN, Efstathiou E, Gagnon DD, Rothman M, Hao Y, Liu CS, Kheoh TS, Haqq CM, Scher HI, de Bono JS. Effect of abiraterone acetate and prednisone compared with placebo and prednisone on pain control and skeletal-related events in patients with metastatic castration-resistant prostate cancer: exploratory analysis of data from the COU-AA-301 randomized trial. Lancet Oncol. 2012;13:1210–7.
9. Fizazi K, Scher HI, Miller K, Basch E, Sternberg CN, Cella D, Forer D, Hirmand M, de Bono JS. Effect of enzalutamide on time to first skeletal-related event, pain, and quality of life in men with castration-resistant prostate cancer: results from the randomized, phase 3 AFFIRM trial. Lancet Oncol. 2014;15:1147–56.
10. Scher HI, Morris MJ, Stadler WM, Higano C, Basch E, Fizazi K, Antonarakis ES, Beer TM, Carducci MA, Chi KN, Corn PG. Trial design and objectives for castration-resistant prostate cancer: updated recommendations from the Prostate Cancer Clinical Trials Working Group 3. J Clin Oncol. 2016;34:1402–18.
11. Sartor O, Coleman R, Nilsson S, Heinrich D, Helle SI, O'Sullivan JM, Fosså SD, Chodacki A, Wiechno P, Logue J, Widmark A, Johannessen DC, Hoskin P, James ND, Solberg A, Syndikus I, Vogelzang NJ, O'Bryan-Tear CG, Shan M, Bruland ØS, Parker C. Effect of radium-223 dichloride on symptomatic skeletal events in patients with castration-resistant prostate cancer and bone metastases: results from a phase 3, double-blind, randomised trial. Lancet Oncol. 2014;15:738–46.
12. Oster G, Lamerato L, Glass AG, Richert-Boe KE, Lopez A, Chung K, Richhariya A, Dodge T, Wolff GG, Balakumaran A, Edelsberg J. Natural history of skeletal-related events in patients with breast, lung, or prostate cancer and metastases to bone: a 15-year study in two large US health systems. Support Care Cancer. 2013;21:3279–86.
13. Inoue T, Segawa T, Kamba T, Yoshimura K, Nakamura E, Nishiyama H, Ito N, Kamoto T, Habuchi T, Ogawa O. Prevalence of skeletal complications and their impact on survival of hormone refractory prostate cancer patients in Japan. Urology. 2009;73:1104–9.
14. Chambers AF, Groom AC, MacDonald IC. Dissemination and growth of cancer cells in metastatic sites. Nat Rev Cancer. 2002;2:563–72.
15. Paget S. The distribution of secondary growths in cancer of the breast. 1889. Cancer Metastasis Rev. 1989;8:98–101.
16. Esposito M, Kang Y. Targeting tumor-stromal interactions in bone metastasis. Pharmacol Ther. 2014;141:222–33.
17. Nieswandt B, Hafner M, Echtenacher B, Männel DN. Lysis of tumor cells by natural killer cells in mice is impeded by platelets. Cancer Res. 1999;59:1295–300.
18. Weilbaecher KN, Guise TA, McCauley LK. Cancer to bone: a fatal attraction. Nat Rev Cancer. 2011;11:411–25.
19. Sun YX, Wang J, Shelburne CE, Lopatin DE, Chinnaiyan AM, Rubin MA, Pienta KJ, Taichman RS. Expression of CXCR4 and CXCL12 (SDF-1) in human prostate cancers (PCa) in vivo. J Cell Biochem. 2003;89:462–73.

20. Sun YX, Fang M, Wang J, Cooper CR, Pienta KJ, Taichman RS. Expression and activation of alpha v beta 3 integrins by SDF-1/CXC12 increases the aggressiveness of prostate cancer cells. Prostate. 2007;67:61–73.
21. Schneider JG, Amend SR, Weilbaecher KN. Integrins and bone metastasis: integrating tumor cell and stromal cell interactions. Bone. 2011;48:54–65.
22. Sethi N, Dai X, Winter CG, Kang Y. Tumor-derived JAGGED1 promotes osteolytic bone metastasis of breast cancer by engaging notch signaling in bone cells. Cancer Cell. 2011;19:192–205.
23. Roodman GD. Mechanisms of bone metastasis. N Engl J Med. 2004;350:1655–64.
24. Brubaker KD, Vessella RL, True LD, Thomas R, Corey E. Cathepsin K mRNA and protein expression in prostate cancer progression. J Bone Miner Res. 2003;18:222–30.
25. Hauschka PV, Mavrakos AE, Iafrati MD, Doleman SE, Klagsbrun M. Growth factors in bone matrix. Isolation of multiple types by affinity chromatography on heparin-Sepharose. J Biol Chem. 1986;261:1266574.
26. Mundy GR. Metastasis to bone: causes, consequences and therapeutic opportunities. Nat Rev Cancer. 2002;2:584–93.
27. Reddington JA, Mendez GA, Ching A, Kubicky CD, Klimo P Jr, Ragel BT. Imaging characteristic analysis of metastatic spine lesions from breast, prostate, lung, and renal cell carcinomas for surgical planning: osteolytic versus osteoblastic. Surg Neurol Int. 2016;7:S361–5.
28. Akech J, Wixted JJ, Bedard K, van der Deen M, Hussain S, Guise TA, van Wijnen AJ, Stein JL, Languino LR, Altieri DC, Pratap J, Keller E, Stein GS, Lian JB. Runx2 association with progression of prostate cancer in patients: mechanisms mediating bone osteolysis and osteoblastic metastatic lesions. Oncogene. 2010;29:811–21.
29. Nelson JB, Hedican SP, George DJ, Reddi AH, Piantadosi S, Eisenberger MA, Simons JW. Identification of endothelin-1 in the pathophysiology of metastatic adenocarcinoma of the prostate. Nat Med. 1995;1(9):944.
30. Yin JJ, Mohammad KS, Käkönen SM, Harris S, Wu-Wong JR, Wessale JL, Padley RJ, Garrett IR, Chirgwin JM, Guise TA. A causal role for endothelin-1 in the pathogenesis of osteoblastic bone metastases. Proc Natl Acad Sci U S A. 2003;100:10954–9.
31. Carducci MA, Saad F, Abrahamsson PA, Dearnaley DP, Schulman CC, North SA, Sleep DJ, Isaacson JD, Nelson JB, Atrasentan Phase III Study Group Institutions. A phase 3 randomized controlled trial of the efficacy and safety of atrasentan in men with metastatic hormone-refractory prostate cancer. Cancer. 2007;110:1959–66.
32. Morote J, Morin JP, Orsola A, Abascal JM, Salvador C, Trilla E, Raventos CX, Cecchini L, Encabo G, Reventos J. Prevalence of osteoporosis during long-term androgen deprivation therapy in patients with prostate cancer. Urology. 2007;69:500–4.
33. Greenspan SL, Coates P, Sereika SM, Nelson JB, Trump DL, Resnick NM. Bone loss after initiation of androgen deprivation therapy in patients with prostate cancer. J Clin Endocrinol Metab. 2005;90:6410–7.
34. Morote J, Orsola A, Abascal JM, Planas J, Trilla E, Raventos CX, Cecchini L, Encabo G, Reventos J. Bone mineral density changes in patients with prostate cancer during the first 2 years of androgen suppression. J Urol. 2006;175:1679–83.
35. Colvard DS, Eriksen EF, Keeting PE, Wilson EM, Lubahn DB, French FS, Riggs BL, Spelsberg TC. Identification of androgen receptors in normal human osteoblast-like cells. Proc Natl Acad Sci U S A. 1989;86:854–7.
36. Russell PK, Clarke MV, Skinner JP, Pang TP, Zajac JD, Davey RA. Identification of gene pathways altered by deletion of the androgen receptor specifically in mineralizing osteoblasts and osteocytes in mice. J Mol Endocrinol. 2012;49:1–10.
37. Wiren KM, Zhang XW, Toombs AR, Kasparcova V, Gentile MA, Harada S, Jepsen KJ. Targeted overexpression of androgen receptor in osteoblasts: unexpected complex bone phenotype in growing animals. Endocrinology. 2004;145:3507–22.
38. Proell V, Xu H, Schüler C, Weber K, Hofbauer LC, Erben RG. Orchiectomy upregulates free soluble RANKL in bone marrow of aged rats. Bone. 2009;45:677–81.
39. Li X, Ominsky MS, Stolina M, Warmington KS, Geng Z, Niu QT, Asuncion FJ, Tan HL, Grisanti M, Dwyer D, Adamu S. Increased RANK ligand in bone marrow of orchiectomized

rats and prevention of their bone loss by the RANK ligand inhibitor osteoprotegerin. Bone. 2009;45:669–76.
40. Kawano H, Sato T, Yamada T, Matsumoto T, Sekine K, Watanabe T, Nakamura T, Fukuda T, Yoshimura K, Yoshizawa T, Aihara K, Yamamoto Y, Nakamichi Y, Metzger D, Chambon P, Nakamura K, Kawaguchi H, Kato S. Suppressive function of androgen receptor in bone resorption. Proc Natl Acad Sci U S A. 2003;100:9416–21.
41. Humphrey EL, Williams JH, Davie MW, Marshall MJ. Effects of dissociated glucocorticoids on OPG and RANKL in osteoblastic cells. Bone. 2006;38:652–61.
42. Swanson C, Lorentzon M, Conaway HH, Lerner UH. Glucocorticoid regulation of osteoclast differentiation and expression of receptor activator of nuclear factor-kappaB (NF-kappaB) ligand, osteoprotegerin, and receptor activator of NF-kappaB in mouse calvarial bones. Endocrinology. 2006;147:3613–22.
43. Saad F, Lipton A, Cook R, Chen YM, Smith M, Coleman R. Pathologic fractures correlate with reduced survival in patients with malignant bone disease. Cancer. 2007;110:1860–7.
44. DePuy V, Anstrom KJ, Castel LD, Schulman KA, Weinfurt KP, Saad F. Effects of skeletal morbidities on longitudinal patient-reported outcomes and survival in patients with metastatic prostate cancer. Support Care Cancer. 2007;15:869–76.
45. Weinfurt KP, Li Y, Castel LD, Saad F, Timbie JW, Glendenning GA, Schulman KA. The significance of skeletal-related events for the health-related quality of life of patients with metastatic prostate cancer. Ann Oncol. 2005;16:579–84.
46. Krupski TL, Foley KA, Baser O, Long S, Macarios D, Litwin MS. Health care cost associated with prostate cancer, androgen deprivation therapy and bone complications. J Urol. 2007;178:1423–8.
47. Hagiwara M, Delea TE, Saville MW, Chung K. Healthcare utilization and costs associated with skeletal-related events in prostate cancer patients with bone metastases. Prostate Cancer Prostatic Dis. 2013;16:23–7.
48. Lage MJ, Barber BL, Harrison DJ, Jun S. The cost of treating skeletal-related events in patients with prostate cancer. Am J Manag Care. 2008;14:317–22.
49. Hechmati G, Cure S, Gouépo A, Hoefeler H, Lorusso V, Lüftner D, Duran I, Garzon-Rodriguez C, Ashcroft J, Wei R, Ghelani P, Bahl A. Cost of skeletal-related events in European patients with solid tumours and bone metastases: data from a prospective multinational observational study. J Med Econ. 2013;16:691–700.
50. Aass N, Fosså SD. Pre- and post-treatment daily life function in patients with hormone resistant prostate carcinoma treated with radiotherapy for spinal cord compression. Radiother Oncol. 2005;74:259–65.
51. Rades D, Stalpers LJ, Veninga T, Rudat V, Schulte R, Hoskin PJ. Evaluation of functional outcome and local control after radiotherapy for metastatic spinal cord compression in patients with prostate cancer. J Urol. 2006;175:552–6.
52. Crnalic S, Hildingsson C, Wikström P, Bergh A, Löfvenberg R, Widmark A. Outcome after surgery for metastatic spinal cord compression in 54 patients with prostate cancer. Acta Orthop. 2012;83:80–6.
53. Shoskes DA, Perrin RG. The role of surgical management for symptomatic spinal cord compression in patients with metastatic prostate cancer. J Urol. 1989;142:337–9.
54. Williams BJ, Fox BD, Sciubba DM, Suki D, Tu SM, Kuban D, Gokaslan ZL, Rhines LD, Rao G. Surgical management of prostate cancer metastatic to the spine. J Neurosurg Spine. 2009;10:414–22.
55. Lewington VJ, McEwan AJ, Ackery DM, Bayly RJ, Keeling DH, Macleod PM, Porter AT, Zivanovic MA. A prospective, randomized double-blind crossover study to examine the efficacy of strontium-89 in pain palliation in patients with advanced prostate cancer metastatic to bone. Eur J Cancer. 1991;27:954–8.
56. Serafini AN, Houston SJ, Resche I, Quick DP, Grund FM, Ell PJ, Bertrand A, Ahmann FR, Orihuela E, Reid RH, Lerski RA, Collier BD, McKillop JH, Purnell GL, Pecking AP, Thomas FD, Harrison KA. Palliation of pain associated with metastatic bone cancer using samarium-153 lexidronam: a double-blind placebo-controlled clinical trial. J Clin Oncol. 1998;16:1574–81.

Urological Complications in Men Dying from Prostate Cancer

34

Takashi Kobayashi

Abstract

Most of advanced prostate cancers (PCa) are incurable and disease-specific mortality rate becomes much higher once PCa has progressed to metastatic disease. Almost all patients who die from PCa had developed castration-resistant disease (CRPC) since the standard of care for unresectable PCa is androgen deprivation therapy.

As the disease progressed to CRPC, patients often experience various debilitating symptoms from non-urological and urological complications. Non-urological complications include bone metastasis causing pain, pathological fracture and spinal compression as well as anemia, fatigue, lymphedema, and psychiatric problems such as delirium. In addition to these non-urological complications, various problems caused by urological complications also impact patient survival and quality of life. The incidence of urological complications that require palliative intervention in men dying from PCa is unexpectedly high. This chapter highlights incidence and management of urological complications that occur in men dying from PCa.

Keywords

Prostate cancer · End of life · Quality of life · Urinary retention · Ureteral obstruction · Hematuria · Palliative therapy · Surgical intervention

T. Kobayashi, M.D., Ph.D.
Department of Urology, Kyoto University Graduate School of Medicine, Kyoto, Japan
e-mail: selecao@kuhp.kyoto-u.ac.jp

34.1 Introduction

Prostate cancer (PCa) is the most common non-skin cancer in males and its estimated mortality exceeds 300,000 worldwide [1]. It was reported that patients who were dying of PCa had more impaired physical function compared to patients who were dying of other causes, while there were no significant differences in other health-related quality-of-life (QOL) items [2]. Some patients dying of PCa are suffered from urological complications due to involvement of the upper and lower urinary tract by progressing cancer lesions [3]. There is little evidence for the incidence and management of those urological complications towards the end of life. Although almost all patients dying of PCa develop castration-resistant PCa (CRPC), guidelines for CRPC describe little about the management of those painful complications comprehensively [4]. According to previous studies, an appropriate intervention to end-of-life adverse events improves QOL of the patients [5–8]. Therefore, it is important for clinicians to understand the incidence of urological complications and its risk factors to improve the management of patients with lethal PCa. We previously focused on urological complications that suffered patients who were dying of PCa [9]. The previous study showed that more than 30% of men dying from PCa were suffered from CaP-related urological complications and needed subsequent palliative interventions.

34.2 Incidence of Urological Complications in Men Dying from PCa

In the previous study, 3552 individuals diagnosed with PCa were identified based on institutional registry [9]. Among them, 240 PCa patients who died of the disease and 144 PCa patients who died of other cause were retrospectively reviewed with regard to the incidence of PCa-related urological complications and subsequent palliative interventions. As a result, major urological complications that required therapeutic intervention were observed in 30.8% of PCa patients dying of the disease, whereas it was much less frequent (4%) in PCa patients dying of other cause. Urological complication was associated with local recurrence in men who underwent prostatectomy, lower irradiation dose in men who underwent radiotherapy, and pretreatment higher T stage and absence of metastasis in men who underwent androgen deprivation therapy (ADT) as the primary treatment. Patients who received long-term ADT for localized disease had the highest risk for urological complication. Therapeutic intervention was highly effective for palliation.

Thus, it was demonstrated that patients with lethal prostate cancer were at high risk for urological complications. The incidence of each complication was much higher than those who were diagnosed with prostate cancer and dying of other cause. This indicates that urological complication is associated with PCa progression to lethal disease. Indeed, most of the urological complications in our series were recorded after disease progression to CRPC. Incidence of any urological complications and major urological complication that required therapeutic intervention in our series was 55.0% and 30.4%, respectively. Khafagy and colleagues reported that 46% of men with lethal PCa had cancer-related complications and 25% required intervention [10]. Considering that Khafagy's report included all cancer-related complications such as anemia and bony pain, our incidence of urological complication was considerably higher than the previous study. This seemed to be partly because our institute is an academic hospital and therefore a large part of the patients were referred with advanced, complicated disease. Additionally, management of CRPC progressed rapidly in this decade and survival of CRPC patients have dramatically improved, which could jeopardize patients at higher risk for urological complications that require palliative intervention.

It is also attributable to the difference in the observation period during a patient's life; we included those that occurred more than 1 year prior to PCa death, whereas the previous study included only those that occurred within the final year of life. In this regard, practice guidelines from the World Health Organization advocates a model of comprehensive palliative care that is introduced from the point of diagnosis of life-threatening illness [11]. Indeed, early palliative care was reported to improve survival of patients with lethal malignant disease [12], presumably by enabling oncologists to focus on cancer treatment and managing medical complications, by improving patient's QOL, by assisting with treatment decision-making, and by increasing social support [13].

34.3 Management of Urological Complications

Urinary retention and hematuria were the most frequently observed urological complications [9]. Both were associated with poorly controlled local disease and may require therapeutic intervention such as external beam radiotherapy (EBRT) and transurethral resection of prostate (TURP). A previous study showed that 5% and 14% of patients with lethal PCa needed EBRT and TURP, respectively, in the final year of their life [10]. In our series, EBRT (16.3%) was even more frequent compared to TURP (10.8%), which is presumably because we usually recommend EBRT for early palliative care for lower urinary tract symptom related to local progression of PCa. Crain and colleagues reported their experience of 24 palliative TURPs for refractory PCa, which were performed safely and resulted in significant improvement in urinary symptoms although it was associated with higher rates of postoperative urinary retention and reoperation compared to those performed for the management of benign prostatic enlargement [6]. EBRT is also effective to relieve advanced PCa patients from cancer-related urinary symptoms as evidenced by a previous report by Din and colleagues [7] demonstrating a high rate (89%) of complete or partial resolution of symptoms in advanced prostate cancer, which was equivalent to our data. However, it is sometimes very difficult to control symptoms caused by local relapse of PCa with EBRT or a transurethral approach. In such cases, open palliative surgery was reported to provide effective palliation [14]. Indeed, three patients in our series needed bilateral ileal conduit ($n = 1$) or ureterocutaneostomy ($n = 2$) urinary diversion, which were very effective for symptom relief.

Upper urinary tract obstruction is also a burdensome complication by refractory growth of PCa, which eventually leads to obstructive renal failure. A population-based study showed that 16% of prostate cancer patients experience ureteral obstruction, which was significantly associated with PCa mortality [15]. Although it is unknown whether PNS improves survival of advanced prostate cancer, previous reports and the present study show that considerable improvement in serum creatinine was obtained in 67–91% of the patients [10, 16].

34.4　Factors Associated with Urological Complications

Our study demonstrated similar complication rates among patients with lethal prostate cancer who received different primary treatment [9]. This was slightly surprising since a previous study by Won and colleagues [8] showed that radical prostatectomy (RP) or EBRT as a primary treatment resulted in local palliation in men who ultimately develop CRPC. The discrepancy could stem from a difference in patient population. The study by Won et al. targeted CRPC patients and included patients who were alive at the time of analysis. Ours included only patients who were dying of PCa and all subjects were followed up until the end of life. It could be also attributable to the retrospective nature of the two studies. Higher rates of complicated referrals of patients who underwent RP and developed local relapse could result in a higher incidence of local recurrence in RP patients, which was significantly associated with urological complication in our series.

In patients who received EBRT as a primary treatment, lower dose of radiation was significantly associated with urological complication. Moreover, higher cT stage was significantly associated with urological complication in patients who were treated with ADT as the primary treatment. In addition to the findings from the patients treated by RP, these findings clearly indicate that local relapse is responsible for urological adverse event at the time of disease progression. Better control of primary prostate tumor burden is a key factor for the improvement palliation of urological complication, which is basically consistent with the previous study by Won and colleagues [8]. Recently published results from a population-based outcome study were also very implicative. Culp and colleagues analyzed survival of stage IV (M1a-c) PCa patients using Surveillance Epidemiology and End Results (SEER) and found survival benefit of definitive therapy (RP or RT) in those patients [17]. The results of our study provide another rationale for local therapy in selected metastatic prostate cancer.

It is also intriguing that presence of metastasis at diagnosis was inversely correlated with higher incidence of urological complication. This seems to be associated with longer survival of patients without metastasis at diagnosis compared to those with disseminated disease. Indeed, the cumulative complication rate showed a steady increase over time until 5–7 years and patients who achieved longer survival after diagnosis were more likely to eventually develop urological complications [9]. In this regard, patients who received ADT for locally advanced but nonmetastatic PCa were at highest risk for urological complication. These findings suggest that specific attention should be paid to prevention or early diagnosis of urological complications, and even more so in patients with good treatment response and potentially longer life expectancy.

Conclusion

Taken together, these evidences heighten the clinical awareness for early therapeutic palliative intervention for high-risk patients, although it should be examined by prospective clinical study whether it can improve treatment outcome and overall patient well-being.

References

1. Ferlay J, Shin H, Bray F, Forman D, Mathers C, Parkin DM. GLOBOCAN 2012 Estimated Cancer Incidence, Mortality and Prevalence Worldwide in 2012. 2012. http://globocan.iarc.fr/Pages/fact_sheets_cancer.aspx. Accessed 4 Feb 2014.
2. Litwin MS, Lubeck DP, Stoddard ML, Pasta DJ, Flanders SC, Henning JM. Quality of life before death for men with prostate cancer: results from the CaPSURE database. J Urol. 2001;165(3):871–5.
3. Ok JH, Meyers FJ, Evans CP. Medical and surgical palliative care of patients with urological malignancies. J Urol. 2005;174(4 Pt 1):1177–82.
4. Heidenreich A, Bastian PJ, Bellmunt J, Bolla M, Joniau S, van der Kwast T, et al. EAU guidelines on prostate cancer. Part II: treatment of advanced, relapsing, and castration-resistant prostate cancer. Eur Urol. 2014;65(2):467–79. https://doi.org/10.1016/j.eururo.2013.11.002.
5. Anast JW, Andriole GL, Grubb RL 2nd. Managing the local complications of locally advanced prostate cancer. Curr Urol Rep. 2007;8(3):211–6.
6. Crain DS, Amling CL, Kane CJ. Palliative transurethral prostate resection for bladder outlet obstruction in patients with locally advanced prostate cancer. J Urol. 2004;171(2 Pt 1):668–71. https://doi.org/10.1097/01.ju.0000104845.24632.92.
7. Din OS, Thanvi N, Ferguson CJ, Kirkbride P. Palliative prostate radiotherapy for symptomatic advanced prostate cancer. Radiother Oncol. 2009;93(2):192–6. https://doi.org/10.1016/j.radonc.2009.04.017.
8. Won AC, Gurney H, Marx G, De Souza P, Patel MI. Primary treatment of the prostate improves local palliation in men who ultimately develop castrate-resistant prostate cancer. BJU Int. 2013;112(4):E250–5. https://doi.org/10.1111/bju.12169.
9. Kobayashi T, Kamba T, Terada N, Yamasaki T, Inoue T, Ogawa O. High incidence of urological complications in men dying from prostate cancer. Int J Clin Oncol. 2016;21(6):1150–4. https://doi.org/10.1007/s10147-016-0993-x.
10. Khafagy R, Shackley D, Samuel J, O'Flynn K, Betts C, Clarke N. Complications arising in the final year of life in men dying from advanced prostate cancer. J Palliat Med. 2007;10(3):705–11. https://doi.org/10.1089/jpm.2006.0185.
11. World Health Organization. WHO Definition of Palliative Care. http://www.who.int/cancer/palliative/definition/en/. Accessed 17 Feb 2014.
12. Temel JS, Greer JA, Muzikansky A, Gallagher ER, Admane S, Jackson VA, et al. Early palliative care for patients with metastatic non-small-cell lung cancer. N Engl J Med. 2010;363(8):733–42. https://doi.org/10.1056/NEJMoa1000678.
13. Irwin KE, Greer JA, Khatib J, Temel JS, Pirl WF. Early palliative care and metastatic non-small cell lung cancer: potential mechanisms of prolonged survival. Chron Respir Dis. 2013;10(1):35–47. https://doi.org/10.1177/1479972312471549.
14. Leibovici D, Pagliaro L, Rosser CJ, Pisters LL. Salvage surgery for bulky local recurrence of prostate cancer following radical prostatectomy. J Urol. 2005;173(3):781–3. https://doi.org/10.1097/01.ju.0000152394.32858.14.

15. Spencer BA, Insel BJ, Hershman DL, Benson MC, Neugut AI. Racial disparities in the use of palliative therapy for ureteral obstruction among elderly patients with advanced prostate cancer. Support Care Cancer. 2013;21(5):1303–11. https://doi.org/10.1007/s00520-012-1666-6.
16. Chiou RK, Chang WY, Horan JJ. Ureteral obstruction associated with prostate cancer: the outcome after percutaneous nephrostomy. J Urol. 1990;143(5):957–9.
17. Culp SH, Schellhammer PF, Williams MB. Might men diagnosed with metastatic prostate cancer benefit from definitive treatment of the primary tumor? A SEER-based study. Eur Urol. 2014;65(6):1058–66. https://doi.org/10.1016/j.eururo.2013.11.012.

Prediction of Optimal Number of Cycles in Docetaxel Regimen for Patients with mCRPC

35

Hideyasu Matsuyama, Tomoyuki Shimabukuro, Isao Hara, Kazuhiro Suzuki, Hirotsugu Uemura, Munehisa Ueno, Yoshihiko Tomita, and Nobuaki Shimizu

H. Matsuyama (✉)
Department of Urology, Yamaguchi University Graduate School of Medicine, Yamaguchi, Japan
e-mail: hidde@yamaguchi-u.ac.jp

T. Shimabukuro
Department of Urology, Ube-kohsan Central Hospital Corp., Ube, Japan
e-mail: shimaube@siren.ocn.ne.jp

I. Hara
Department of Urology, Wakayama Medical University, Wakayama, Japan
e-mail: hara@wakayama-med.ac.jp

K. Suzuki
Department of Urology, Gunma University Graduate School of Medicine, Maebashi, Japan
e-mail: kazu@gunma-u.ac.jp

H. Uemura
Department of Urology, Kinki University Faculty of Medicine, Osakasayama, Japan
e-mail: huemura@med.kindai.ac.jp

M. Ueno
Department of Uro-Oncology, Saitama Medical University International Medical Center, Hidaka, Japan
e-mail: m-ueno@shunjinkai.or.jp

Y. Tomita
Department of Urology, Yamagata University Faculty of Medicine, Yamagata, Japan

Department of Urology, Molecular Oncology, Graduate School of Medical and Dental Sciences, Niigata University, Niigata, Japan
e-mail: ytomita@med.niigata-u.ac.jp

N. Shimizu
Division of Urology, Gunma Prefectural Cancer Center, Ota, Japan
e-mail: nshimizu@gunma-cc.jp

© Springer Nature Singapore Pte Ltd. 2018
Y. Arai, O. Ogawa (eds.), *Hormone Therapy and Castration Resistance of Prostate Cancer*, https://doi.org/10.1007/978-981-10-7013-6_35

Abstract

Although 75 mg/m^2 docetaxel (DTX) with 10 mg prednisolone regimen is a gold standard of the first-line chemotherapy for patients with metastatic castration-resistant prostate cancer (mCRPC), optimal number of the cycles remains controversial. Most guidelines recommend DTX regimen should be terminated up to 10 cycles, but the optimal number is controversial. We retrospectively analyzed 279 CRPC patients who received DTX regimen. Patients having more than 10 cycles of DTX had significantly better overall survival (OS) than those having 10 or less, and prediction model of optimal number of cycles in DTX regimen was constructed based on the risk table employing the combination of three factors (ALP [cutoff 189 IU/L], hemoglobin [11.3 g/dL], and age [65 years] at the start of DTX therapy), and scoring based on the hazard ratio of each risk factor (ALP 4, hemoglobin 2, age 3). The prediction model could effectively predict the probability of the length of DTX therapy, with the c-index of 0.7274. Since the new drugs are clinically available, optimal number of cycles should be determined based on the PS, toxicities, or patients' wish. Our predicting model may help in patients' consultation before starting DTX regimen, or in selecting potential patients with intolerant DTX regimen.

Keywords

Docetaxel cycle · OS · mCRPC

35.1 Introduction

Since the approval of docetaxel (DTX) regimen (75 mg/m^2 every 3 weeks with 10 mg/day prednisolone) for castration-resistant prostate cancer (CRPC), DTX remains one of the most important therapeutic options for metastatic prostate cancer patients not only with CRPC [1], but also with hormone-sensitive (HSPC) status [2]. Maximal cycle number of docetaxel is set up to 10 cycles based on the tax 327 trial. The number of docetaxel, however, was arbitrarily set to 10 cycles with actual median administration of 9.5 cycles [1]. Thus, the optimal number of cycles remains controversial. To reject the possibility of lead-time bias of DTX regimen, we retrospectively compared overall survival (OS) from the initiation of ADT to death in 117 CRPC patients who received ADT followed by DTX regimen to 118 counterparts without DTX. Significant survival benefit was found in DTX group (94 vs. 70 months, Hazard ratio: 0.57 [0.37–0.87], $p = 0.0077$), and more than 3 cycles of DTX therapy (50–75 mg/m^2) was one of the independent prognostic factors for OS [3]. Several investigators reported no benefit of DTX regimen beyond 10, while others emphasized treatment should be continued 10 or more if they tolerate their treatment well. To enjoy the maximal benefit from DTX regimen, simple query must be addressed that what is the optimal cycle number of DTX regimen. In this chapter, prediction model of the optimal number of cycles in each patient, and risk and benefit of longer DTX regimen are discussed.

35.2 Definition of Regular Number of Cycles of Docetaxel Regimen

Recommended dose and interval of DTX regimen was determined by the two large prospective randomized trials (SWOG99-16 and TAX 327) [1, 4].

In SWOG99-16 trial [4], DTX (60 mg/m^2 on day 2, every 3 weeks) with dexamethasone (60 mg/day on day 2) plus estramustine (840 mg/day on day 1–5, every 3 weeks) were given to 338 eligible patients with mCRPC, and OS was compared with 336 counterpart who were treated with mitoxantrone (12 mg/m^2 on day 1, every 3 weeks) plus prednisolone (10 mg/day). Dose escalation of DTX and mitoxantrone was permitted up to 70 mg/m^2 and 14 mg/m^2, respectively, provided no grade 3 or 4 toxicities in the first cycle. Statistically significant improvement of median OS in DTX plus estramustine arm was observed (17.5 vs. 15.6 months). In this regimen, maximal cycle number was arbitrary defined to 12. In TAX327 trial [1], 1006 patients with mCRPC were divided into three arms: mitoxantrone (12 mg/m^2 on day 1, every 3 weeks), DTX (75 mg/m^2, every 3 weeks), or DTX (30 mg/m^2 once in each 5 of 6-week interval) with adding prednisolone (10 mg/day) in all arm, and OS was compared as a primary endpoint. As compared with mitoxantrone group, a hazard ratio (HR) of death was 0.76 (95% Confidence Interval [95% CI]: 0.62–0.94, $p = 0.009$) in 3-week DTX group, 0.91 (95%CI: 0.75–1.11, $p = 0.36$) in weekly DTX group. In this regimen, maximal cycle number was arbitrary defined to 10 with a median number of cycles was 9.5 ranging from 1 to 11. Forty-six percent of patients with 3-week DTX group had stopped treatment due to completion of planned 10 cycles.

Based on these trials, most guidelines recommend standard DTX regimen as 75 mg/m^2 3 weekly with prednisone 5 mg BID, up to 10 cycles [5]. Whereas, no theoretical background or explanation has been established why 10 cycles is an optimal number of DTX regimen.

35.3 Extended Cycles of DTX Regimen: Pro

To determine whether the number of docetaxel cycles is an independent prognostic factor for OS, de Morree et al. retrospectively analyzed data of 1059 patients with mCRPC [6] who were enrolled in the Mainsail trial [7]. In this trial, patients were randomized to receive DTX with or without lenalidomide. Although this study had early termination due to inferior OS of lenalidomide plus DTX group, the investigator paid attention to relation between cycle number of DTX and OS. Patients who received eight or more cycles of the therapy had significant improvement of OS than those with less than seven regardless of lenalidomide treatment. When OS was compared among three groups (more than 10, 8–10, or 5–7 cycles), median OS was 33.0, 26.9, and 22.8 months, respectively ($p < 0.001$). The investigators concluded that patients who may have clinical benefit from DTX regimen should continue six or more regimens if they tolerate their treatment well.

Kawahara et al. studied 52 Japanese prostate cancer patients who received 55 mg/m^2 DTX plus 8 mg dexamethasone, every 3 or 4 weeks. The median duration of OS from starting DTX therapy was 11.2 months in the short-term (9 or lower cycles) group and 28.5 months in the long-term (10 or more cycles) group. They found four risk factors (presence of anemia, bone metastases, significant pain, and visceral metastases), and constructed the risk group classification. They concluded that 10 or more cycles of DTX regimen can significantly prolong survival in Japanese men with CRPC [8].

35.4 Extended Cycle of DTX Regimen: Cons

No survival advantage of more than 10 cycles of DTX regimen has been reported. Pond et al. concluded that the 6- and 12-month estimated survival in patients with prolonged number (median: 15 cycles) were similar to those who received up to 10 cycles of DTX regimen from two clinical trials. The lack of survival benefit of prolonged cycles may be attributable to the small cohort (37.4%) receiving longer treatment and different characteristics such as a lower median ALP value at baseline of cohorts with up to 10 cycles [9].

35.5 Risk Table Deciding Optimal Cycle Determination

To address the simple clinical question that what is the optimal number of cycles in DTX regimen, we retrospectively collected 279 CRPC patients who received DTX regimen (50–75 mg/m^2 every 3–4 weeks) from 7 institutions, and constructed a risk table predicting the optimal number of cycles of DTX regimen [10]. Patient background is listed in Table 35.1. The median age, median OS from starting DTX, initial DTX dose, relative dose intensity, and interval of the regimen was 71 years, 26 months, 70 mg/m^2, 0.8, and 4 weeks. The median number of cycles was 8 ranging from 1 to 62. One hundred one patients (36.2%) received more than 10 cycles (extended-cycle group), while 178 (63.7%) received 10 or less cycles (regular-cycle group). In this study, we found that the extended-cycle group had a significantly longer median OS from the start of DTX than the regular-cycle group (40 [32–49] vs. 18 months [14–22], $p < 0.0001$). PSA response ($\geq$50% decline) was significantly higher in extended-cycle group than in regular-cycle group (67.1 vs. 52.3%, $p = 0.0214$), while time to CRPC or best response was not different between two groups. Figure 35.1 shows the Kaplan-Meier's plots comparing OS between extended- and regular-cycle groups.

Multivariate analysis for OS proved PSA decline $\geq$50%, serum markers at the start of DTX therapy [PSA, alkaline phosphatase (ALP), and C-reactive protein (CRP)], and the number of DTX cycles were independent predictors. Notably, hazard ratio with 95% confidence interval of the number of DTX cycles was 0.91 (0.87–0.95), meaning 9% risk reduction of OS per cycle (data not shown). Except for cycle number, most of these factors have been reported by several investigators [11–15].

Table 35.1 Patient backgrounds of the study

Factors[a]	Variables	
Age, Median years (Range)		71 (48–91)
	<65	65 (23.4)
	>65	213 (76.6)
ECOG PS	0	200
	1	53
	≥2	13
Gleason Score	≤6	13
	7	54
	≥8	186
Clinical stage, No. (%)	II	0
	III	60 (21.5)
	IV	219 (78.5)
Laboratory data[b], Median (Range)		
PSA ng/mL		35.2 (0.05–3134)
CRP, mg/dL		0.3 (0–22)
corrected Ca, mg/dL		8.7 (6.9–10.2)
LDH, IU/L		192 (92–1160)
	<215	143 (61.1)
	>215	91 (38.9)
ALP, IU/L		271 (102–6130)
	<189	50 (20.1)
	>189	198 (79.8)
Hemoglobin, g/dL		11.8 (6–15.8)
	≤11.2	87 (34.7)
	>11.3	164 (65.3)
Metastases, No. (%)		
Bone		169 (60.5)
Lymphnode		89 (31.9)
Visceral organs		22 (7.9)
	FT	2
Docetaxel treatment, Median(Range)		
Initial dose, mg/m²		70 (50–85)
Interval, weeks		4 (3–8)
Total dose, mg/m²		525 (60–3720)
Relative dose intensiy		0.8 (0.4–1.1)
DTX course		8 (1–62)
	≤10	178 (63.7)
	>10	101 (36.2)

[a]Values are at the initiation of docetaxel treatment except Gleason score
[b]Missing data: Age: 1, ECOG PS: 13, Gleason score:26, PSA 15, LDH: 45, ALP: 31, Hemoglobin: 28 (Permission of reprint from Int J Clin Oncol. 2014;19: 946–54)

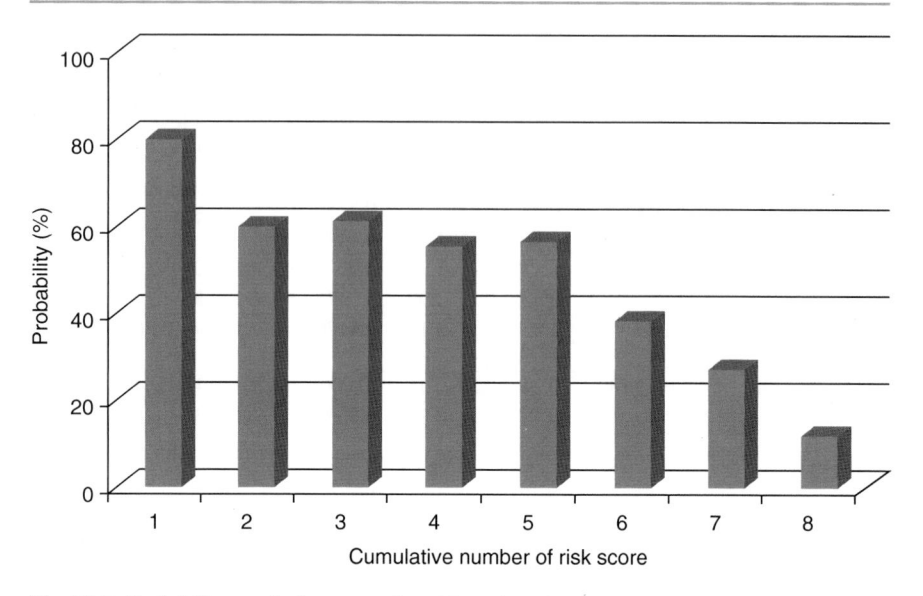

Fig. 35.2 Probability predicting more than 10 cycles of docetaxel regimen according to risk score. Probability predicting more than 10 cycles of DTX regimen was proportionally decreased to increasing risk score

Fig. 35.3 Receiver Operator Characteristic curve of risk factor predicting for extended cycle (>10) of DTX regimen

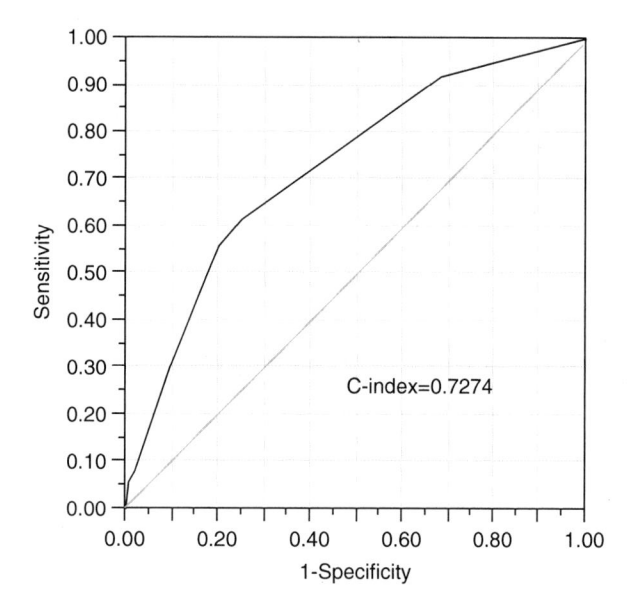

C-index=0.7274

respectively [14]. Their risk table may help to predict the prognosis of DTX within regular cycle, since their model was based on the cohort of TAX 327 trial. Since an optimal number of DTX cycles is controversial, optimal number should individually be decided considering patients' baseline (pre-DTX) physical and oncological conditions. Reasons for the discontinuation due to AE or patient refusal were only

Table 35.4 Adverse events

	DTX cycle						
	≤10 (n = 178)			>10 (n = 101)			
	G1–2	≥G3	(%)	G1–2	≥G3	(%)	p value[a]
Blood/Bone Marrow (%)	41	108	(60.7)	27	58	(57.4)	0.6136
Cardiovascular	6	0	(0)	4	0	(0)	–
Gastrointestinal	36	2	(1.1)	20	3	(3.0)	0.356
Hepatic	7	2	(1.1)	6	0	(0)	0.5364
Pulmonary	8	4	(2.2)	8	1	(1.0)	0.7566
Bone Pain	8	1	(5.6)	7	1	(1.0)	1.0000
Infection	39	8	(4.5)	24	2	(2.0)	0.5561
Others	6	7	(3.9)	5	6	(5.9)	0.3375
Any event	–	114	(64)	–	59	(58.4)	0.3710

[a]Comparison of ≥G3 event between ordinal and longer course group (Permission of reprint from Int J Clin Oncol. 2014;19: 946–54)

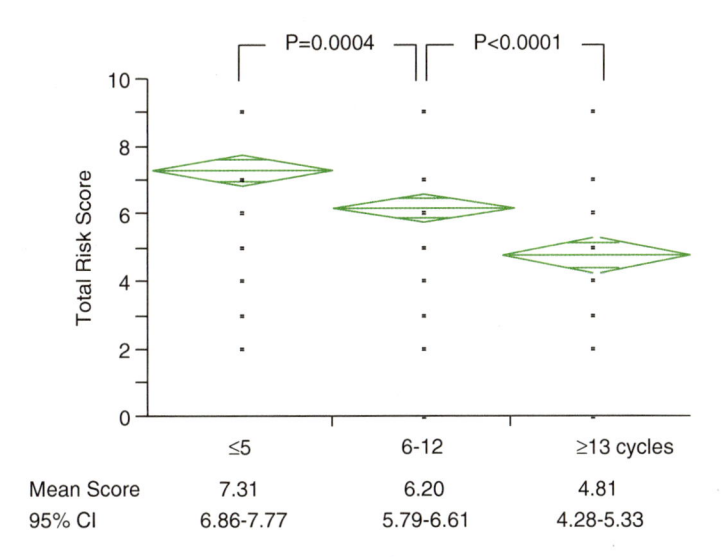

Fig. 35.4 Total risk score and the number of docetaxel regimen. Number of cycles was classified with lower quartile (≤5), 25–75 percentile (6–12), and upper quartile (≥13 cycles), risk score was significantly different among three groups ($p = 0.0004$: ≤5 vs. 6–12 cycle; $p < 0.0001$: 6–12 cycle vs. (≥13 cycles). Permission of reprint from Int J Clin Oncol. 2014;19: 946–54

2.4 and 1.2%, respectively [10]. The data suggest our DTX regimen including 36% of extended-cycle cohort is feasible, and tolerant for the Japanese patients. Our risk table model includes both physical (age, Hb) and oncological (ALP) factors. These factors may be appropriate for the estimation of global condition of CRPC patients. However, how do we utilize, if possible, this model in the context of the replacing of the extended DTX regimen with many attractive options, such as new AR signal blockade, cabazitaxel, or Ra-223? One possibility is to predict DXT unfit patient and avoid the treatment. Risk score is significantly associated with decreasing number of cycles (Fig. 35.4), 58 patients (12.1%) with highest risk score 9, i.e., higher age, lower Hb, and higher ALP, are at risk of DTX intolerant cases. Preferential use of the new AR signal blockade or Ra-223 may be suitable for such patients.

There are limitations of this model, most of which were inherited from retrospective study design.

Conclusion

Although optimal number of cycles remains controversial in DTX regimen, the number should individually be decided considering patients' baseline (pre-DTX) physical and oncological conditions. Our risk table may help in patients' consultation before starting DTX regimen, or in selecting potential patients with intolerant DTX regimen.

References

1. Tannock IF, de Wit R, Berry WR, Horti J, Pluzanska A, Chi KN, Oudard S, Théodore C, James ND, Turesson I, Rosenthal MA, Eisenberger MA, TAX 327 Investigators. Docetaxel plus prednisone or mitoxantrone plus prednisone for advanced prostate cancer. N Engl J Med. 2004;351(15):1502–12.
2. Sweeney CJ, Chen YH, Carducci M, Liu G, Jarrard DF, Eisenberger M, Wong YN, Hahn N, Kohli M, Cooney MM, Dreicer R, Vogelzang NJ, Picus J, Shevrin D, Hussain M, Garcia JA, DiPaola RS. Chemohormonal therapy in metastatic hormone-sensitive prostate cancer. N Engl J Med. 2015;373(8):737–46.
3. Shimabukuro T, Sakano S, Matsuda K, Kamiryo Y, Yamamoto N, Kaneda Y, Nasu T, Baba Y, Suga A, Yamamoto M, Aoki A, Takai K, Yoshihiro S, Konishi M, Imoto K, Matsuyama H. Can docetaxel therapy improve overall survival from primary therapy compared with androgen-deprivation therapy alone in Japanese patients with castration-resistant prostate cancer? A multi-institutional cooperative study. Int J Clin Oncol. 2013;18(1):62–7.
4. Petrylak DP, Tangen CM, Hussain MH, Lara PN Jr, Jones JA, Taplin ME, Burch PA, Berry D, Moinpour C, Kohli M, Benson MC, Small EJ, Raghavan D, Crawford ED. Docetaxel and estramustine compared with mitoxantrone and prednisone for advanced refractory prostate cancer. N Engl J Med. 2004;351(15):1513–20.
5. Cornford P, Bellmunt J, Bolla M, Briers E, De Santis M, Gross T, Henry AM, Joniau S, Lam TB, Mason MD, van der Poel HG, van der Kwast TH, Rouvière O, Wiegel T, Mottet N. EAU-ESTRO-SIOG guidelines on prostate cancer. Part II: treatment of relapsing, metastatic, and castration-resistant prostate cancer. Eur Urol. 2017;71(4):630–42.
6. de Morrée ES, Vogelzang NJ, Petrylak DP, Budnik N, Wiechno PJ, Sternberg CN, Doner K, Bellmunt J, Burke JM, Ochoa de Olza M, Choudhury A, Gschwend JE, Kopyltsov E, Flechon A, van As N, Houede N, Barton D, Fandi A, Jungnelius U, Li S, Li JS, de Wit R. Association of survival benefit with docetaxel in prostate cancer and total number of cycles administered: a post hoc analysis of the mainsail study. JAMA Oncol. 2017;3(1):68–75.
7. Petrylak DP, Vogelzang NJ, Budnik N, Wiechno PJ, Sternberg CN, Doner K, Bellmunt J, Burke JM, de Olza MO, Choudhury A, Gschwend JE, Kopyltsov E, Flechon A, Van AN, Houede N, Barton D, Fandi A, Jungnelius U, Li S, de Wit R, Fizazi K. Docetaxel and prednisone with or without lenalidomide in chemotherapy-naive patients with metastatic castration-resistant prostate cancer (MAINSAIL): a randomised, double-blind, placebo-controlled phase 3 trial. Lancet Oncol. 2015;16(4):417–25.
8. Kawahara T, Miyoshi Y, Sekiguchi Z, Sano F, Hayashi N, Teranishi J, Misaki H, Noguchi K, Kubota Y, Uemura H. Risk factors for metastatic castration-resistant prostate cancer (CRPC) predict long-term treatment with docetaxel. PLoS One. 2012;7(10):e48186.

9. Pond GR, Armstrong AJ, Wood BA, Brookes M, Leopold L, Berry WR, de Wit R, Eisenberger MA, Tannock IF, Sonpavde G. Evaluating the value of number of cycles of docetaxel and prednisone in men with metastatic castration-resistant prostate cancer. Eur Urol. 2012;61(2):363–9.
10. Matsuyama H, Shimabukuro T, Hara I, Kohjimoto Y, Suzuki K, Koike H, Uemura H, Hayashi T, Ueno M, Kodaira K, Tomita Y, Sakurai T, Shimizu N. Combination of hemoglobin, alkaline phosphatase, and age predicts optimal docetaxel regimen for patients with castration-resistant prostate cancer. Int J Clin Oncol. 2014;19(5):946–54.
11. Smaletz O, Scher HI, Small EJ, Verbel DA, McMillan A, Regan K, Kelly WK, Kattan MW. Nomogram for overall survival of patients with progressive metastatic prostate cancer after castration. J Clin Oncol. 2002;20(19):3972–82.
12. Halabi S, Small EJ, Kantoff PW, Kattan MW, Kaplan EB, Dawson NA, Levine EG, Blumenstein BA, Vogelzang NJ. Prognostic model for predicting survival in men with hormone-refractory metastatic prostate cancer. J Clin Oncol. 2003;21(7):1232–7.
13. Armstrong AJ, Garrett-Mayer ES, Yang YC, de Wit R, Tannock IF, Eisenberger M. A contemporary prognostic nomogram for men with hormone-refractory metastatic prostate cancer: a TAX327 study analysis. Clin Cancer Res. 2007;13(21):6396–403.
14. Armstrong AJ, Garrett-Mayer E, de Wit R, Tannock I, Eisenberger M. Prediction of survival following first-line chemotherapy in men with castration-resistant metastatic prostate cancer. Clin Cancer Res. 2010;16(1):203–11.
15. Pond GR, Armstrong AJ, Wood BA, Leopold L, Galsky MD, Sonpavde G. Ability of C-reactive protein to complement multiple prognostic classifiers in men with metastatic castration resistant prostate cancer receiving docetaxel-based chemotherapy. BJU Int. 2012;110(11 Pt B):E461–8.

Intermittent Chemotherapy with Docetaxel for Metastatic Castration-Resistant Prostate Cancer

36

Shintaro Narita and Tomonori Habuchi

Abstract

The optimal schedule of docetaxel chemotherapy for castration-resistant prostate cancer is unknown, although continuous administration is accepted as the standard. However, several disadvantages, including side effects, costs, and development of resistant clones, need to be considered during continuous administration of docetaxel. Intermittent docetaxel therapy represents an appealing option to address these issues. Previous studies have reported that intermittent docetaxel therapy is associated with favorable outcomes, with successful chemotherapy holidays and maintained Quality of Life (QOL). However, limitations of these studies include a wide variation in study design and schedule and a lack of randomized trials comprising a large number of patients allowing comparison of outcomes with continuous administration. This chapter summarizes current data on intermittent docetaxel therapy in androgen-independent and castration-resistant prostate cancer from previous literature and examines future directions regarding the use of this strategy as a therapeutic option for advanced prostate cancer.

Keywords

Castration-resistant prostate cancer · Chemotherapy · Docetaxel · Intermittent · Metastasis

---

S. Narita, M.D. (✉) · T. Habuchi, M.D.
Department of Urology, Akita University School of Medicine, Akita, Japan
e-mail: narishin@doc.med.akita-u.ac.jp; nari6202@gipc.akita-u.ac.jp

36.1 Background

Docetaxel is one of the standard treatment options as first-line therapy in patients with metastatic castration-resistant prostate cancer (mCRPC) since the demonstration of survival benefits of docetaxel over mitoxantrone in two consecutive phase III trials [1–3]. The TAX 327 study, a three-arm phase III trial to compare two schedules of docetaxel/prednisone with mitoxantrone/prednisone, demonstrated a significant survival advantage in patients treated with a docetaxel/prednisone regimen every 3 weeks over those treated with a mitoxantrone/prednisone regimen [1, 3]. The SWOG 9916 trial was another phase III study conducted to assess the impact of the combination of docetaxel/estramustine phosphate versus mitoxantrone/prednisone, which also reported a significant survival benefit in mCRPC [2]. In recent years, even in patients with castration-sensitive metastatic prostate cancer, several studies have demonstrated that early administration of docetaxel combined with androgen deprivation therapy (ADT) has clear survival benefits compared with ADT alone, with a meta-analysis confirming these results [4–6]. Although new classes of drugs, such as CYP17 inhibitors, second-generation antiandrogens, immunotherapy, and internal radiotherapy, have become available for the treatment of advanced prostate cancer, chemotherapy with docetaxel remains a mainstay in the treatment of mCRPC.

However, the appropriate schedule of docetaxel administration remains controversial. Based on the treatment protocols used in the two phase III trials described above, continuous administration with up to 10–12 cycles is currently the standard schedule for docetaxel therapy in mCRPC [1, 5]. In more recent years, continuous administration of docetaxel with >12 cycles has been introduced into clinical practice in the treatment of mCRPC [7]. Although docetaxel is continuously administered in actual clinical practice, the side effects, costs, and development of resistant clones should be considered. In addition to the expanding applications of docetaxel for advanced prostate cancer, it may be possible to minimize and avoid the disadvantages of continuous administration with the use of multiple cycles in patients with advanced prostate cancer who have a plan to receive docetaxel therapy.

One strategy to solve the problems mentioned above is the use of intermittent administration of chemotherapeutic drugs. Intermittent chemotherapy is based on the concept of treatment holidays, when no chemotherapy agents are administered, which may allow patients to minimize side effects, maintain QOL, delay the emergence of drug-resistant clones, and activate angiogenesis and/or antitumor immunity [8]. However, in basic research fields, the benefit of the intermittent administration of chemotherapeutic drugs has been controversial. A previous in vivo study reported by De Souza et al. concluded that continuous chemotherapy with docetaxel resulted in greater antitumor efficacy and lesser upregulation of drug resistance-related genes than intermittent administration in ovarian cancer xenografts [9], whereas studies using xenografts in brain tumors have demonstrated that intermittent administration of cyclophosphamide induces an innate antitumor immune response and tumor regression [10]. In the clinical treatment of breast and colorectal cancer, intermittent chemotherapy has been shown to provide equivalent survival rates with less toxicity and good QOL in randomized phase III trials when compared with continuous schedules [11, 12]. However, there has been considerable controversy regarding the benefit of continuous and maintenance chemotherapy after the first response to cancer treatment [8, 13].

In prostate cancer, intermittent administration of ADT is known to provide comparable survival with continuous ADT with some improvements in QOL scores [14]. Although, there has been no randomized trial involving a large number of patients to indicate the superiority of intermittent docetaxel in patients with prostate cancer over continuous therapy, several previous trials of intermittent docetaxel in patients with prostate cancer have been published [8, 15–25]. However, the optimal protocol and timing for the intermittent administration of docetaxel in patients with prostate cancer remains largely unknown. This chapter provides a review of previous studies of intermittent docetaxel therapy in advanced prostate cancer and also examines future directions in the use of this strategy as a therapeutic option for advanced prostate cancer.

36.2 Intermittent Chemotherapy for mCRPC

36.2.1 Design and Schedule of Intermittent Administration of Docetaxel

Ten studies of intermittent docetaxel in patients with advanced prostate cancer have previously been published [15–19, 22–27]. The eligibility criteria were mCRPC in 4, CRPC in 3, and metastatic androgen-independent prostate cancer (AIPC) which was previously defined as evidence of disease progression despite standard hormone management with serum PSA $\geq$5.0 ng/mL [15] in 3, respectively. The protocols of all studies are described in Table 36.1. All studies except one retrospective study [19] were conducted as a prospective study, although no randomized study to compare the efficacy of intermittent therapy over continuous therapy has been reported. A representative image of intermittent administration of docetaxel without progression is shown in Fig. 36.1 [25]. A wide variation in the design and schedule of intermittent administration was observed among the studies. The dose and the frequency of docetaxel administration varied with the range of 35–75 mg/m^2 and weekly to monthly, respectively. On the other hand, recent trials tended to offer standard administration of docetaxel at 70–75 mg/m^2 triweekly in light of the results of the TAX327 study. The use of additional drugs also differed greatly between studies, which applied prednisone/prednisolone (3), estramustine phosphate (3), bicalutamide (1), dexamethasone (1), and other drugs (2). In addition, so far, the timing of suspension and re-administration of docetaxel during intermittent therapy has not been standardized.

In general, two strategies of "on- and off-chemotherapy" have been considered, which include efficacy-dependent and a duration-dependent protocols. The "efficacy-dependent" protocol involves continuing docetaxel until a response, which has previously been defined based on the level of serum PSA and/or

Table 36.1 Design and schedule of previous intermittent docetaxel series in patients with prostate cancer

No.	Author	Year	Dosage of DOC (mg/m^2)	Schedule for administration of DOC	Combination	Timing to suspend chemotherapy	Timing to resume chemotherapy
1	Beer et al.	2003	36	Weekly (3 of every 4 weeks)	High-dose calcitriol	≥50% reduction of PSA or PSA <4	≥50% increase of PSA or PSA ≥1 or any progression
2	Beer et al.	2008	36	Weekly (3 of every 4 weeks)	High-dose calcitriol	≥50% reduction of PSA or PSA <4	≥50% increase of PSA or PSA ≥2 or any progression
3	Soga et al.	2009	70	Triweekly	EMP 560 mg (5 days)	After 3 or 6 cycles	PSA elevation from nadir occurred three times
4	Mountzios et al.	2011	45	Biweekly	Prednisone 10 mg	≥50% reduction of PSA	≥25% increase of PSA or radiographic progression
5	Narita et al.	2012	60	Monthly	EMP 560 mg + carboplatin AUC5	After 2 cycles	PSA increase above baseline
6	Li et al.	2013	75	Triweekly	Bicalutamide 50 mg	≥50% reduction of PSA	≥25% increase of PSA or radiographic progression
7	Kume et al.	2015	75	Triweekly	Dexamethasone 1.0–2.0 mg	PSA <4 and >50% reduction of PSA	PSA >2 and >50% increase of PSA
8	Caffo et al.	2015	70	Triweekly	EMP or not	After 4 cycle	After 3 m (pre-defined)
9	Aggarwal et al.	2015	60–75	Triweekly	Prednisone 10 mg (± GM-CSF in holiday)	After 6 cycles and ≥50% reduction of PSA	Progression based on PSA or RECIST (PCWG1 criteria)
10	Narita et al.	2015	70	Monthly	Prednisolone 10 mg	After 3 cycles	PSA increase above baseline

DOC docetaxel, *PSA* prostate specific antigen, *EMP* estramustine phosphate, *GM-CSF* granulocyte-macrophage colony-stimulating factor, *m* month, *RECIST* Response Evaluation Criteria in Solid Tumor, *PCWG1* prostate cancer working group 1

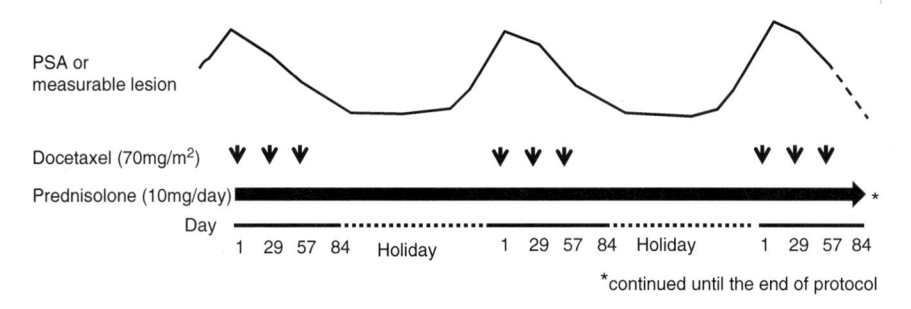

Fig. 36.1 Representative image of intermittent docetaxel therapy (Narita S et al. Jpn J Clin Oncol, 2016) [20]

radiographic response based on the RECIST criteria. The "duration-dependent" protocol involves the administration of docetaxel for pre-defined cycles before suspension of treatment. Half of the trials have applied the duration-dependent approach, while the other half have applied the efficacy-dependent approach. The number of pre-defined cycles in the duration-dependent studies was between two and four cycles. One study allowed three additional cycles after three cycles of docetaxel [18]. In the efficacy-dependent protocol, >50% reduction from baseline or a serum PSA level <4 ng/mL were the most commonly used cutoff points for the suspension of chemotherapy.

Regarding the timing of resuming chemotherapy, there was a wide variation observed among studies. Patients in our two studies took a treatment holiday until the PSA levels returned to baseline levels recorded at the initiation of each cycle in patients achieving a PSA decline with or without radiographic response during a course of chemotherapy [20, 25]. In other trials, each study established original cutoff points using different percentage changes in PSA levels from the nadir, PSA levels, and signs of disease progression as described in Table 36.1.

The only trial to compare outcomes with continuous treatment of docetaxel was reported by Li et al., which was conducted in a matched historical cohort of patients with prostate cancer treated with ADT alone [21]. Caffo et al. conducted a unique randomized 2 × 2 factorial phase II trial to assess the impact of intermittent chemotherapy and combination therapy with estramustine phosphate on QOL over continuous therapy [23]. In this study, patients received four cycles of 70 mg/m^2 docetaxel every 3 weeks and took a pre-defined 3-month treatment holiday [23]. In a further intriguing study, Aggarwal et al. reported a randomized trial to assess the efficacy of granulocyte-macrophage colony-stimulating factor (GM-CSF) during docetaxel holidays, which indicates the potential utility of therapies during the holiday period to extend drug holiday duration [22]. These studies describe multiple potential regimens of intermittent docetaxel administration.

In summary, the design and the schedule of intermittent docetaxel in CRPC and AIPC varies between trials and has yet to be standardized. Therefore, bias due to differences in background characteristics and methods of intermittent docetaxel induction should be considered when interpreting the results of each trial.

36.2.2 Outcomes of Intermittent Chemotherapy

The major results of studies evaluating intermittent docetaxel therapies in prostate cancer are summarized in Table 36.2. In the first study of intermittent docetaxel for prostate cancer, Beer et al. investigated the detailed outcomes of 11 patients using an intermittent protocol in a phase II trial that was conducted to assess the efficacy of docetaxel plus high-dose calcitriol [15]. Even in this limited number of patients, their intermittent chemotherapy regimen achieved a median treatment holiday of 20 weeks, retained sensitivity to re-treatment, and improved QOL during the chemotherapy holiday. The authors also reported long follow-up data including after the use of multiple cycles of intermittent docetaxel administration in a consecutive study [16]. Subsequently, Soga et al. evaluated 15 patients who received intermittent chemotherapy comprising docetaxel (70 mg/m^2 on day 1) and estramustine phosphate (560 mg on days 1–5). Nine patients with a response in the first three cycles of chemotherapy took a chemotherapy holiday, while three patients suspended treatment after six cycles of chemotherapy. Of the 15 patients, 8 received a second course of chemotherapy, with a 25% response rate achieved [18]. The median overall survival (OS) in the study was 21 months with a median follow-up of 16 months. In a retrospective study from Greece, Mountzios et al. reported the first trial to assess combination therapy of docetaxel with prednisone with a mean interval of "off-chemotherapy" of 4.5 months and a median interval to treatment failure of 8.2 months [19]. However, the schedule of docetaxel administration was biweekly at 45 mg/m^2, which has not been the standard administration schedule in recent years. In 2012, we conducted a phase II trial to assess the efficacy and feasibility of docetaxel-based combination chemotherapy with carboplatin and estramustine phosphate (DEC therapy) in patients with metastatic AIPC. After two consecutive administrations of DEC, the treatment was repeated until progression of disease, severe adverse events, or withdrawal of consent. We achieved a median total time of chemotherapy holiday of 7.7 months, and a median OS following DEC of 17.8 months with a median follow-up of 11.1 months, although the median number of DEC cycles was 3 (range 1–9). More recently, Li et al. conducted a retrospective study comparing the outcomes of intermittent triweekly docetaxel (75 mg/m^2) plus bicalutamide in CRPC with a historical control group consisting of patients treated with continuous docetaxel plus prednisone [21]. Although the study was retrospective and the number of enrolled patients was small ($n = 42$ for tested patients, and $n = 60$ for historical controls), they reported the first results to compare the outcome of intermittent docetaxel over continuous therapy and showed that there were no significant differences in progression-free survival and OS between the two groups [21]. A further Japanese study reported by Kume et al. enrolled 51 patients treated with continuous docetaxel administration of 75 mg/m^2 every 3 weeks and allowed a chemotherapy holiday after serum PSA levels were reduced to <4 ng/mL with a reduction rate of >50%[24]. Twenty-seven (52.9%) patients qualified for intermittent treatment, including 17 patients treated with two courses and 10 patients treated with three courses. The median off-treatment interval was 266 days for the first chemotherapy holiday, 129.5 days for the second, and

Table 36.2 Outcomes of previous intermittent docetaxel series in patients with prostate cancer

No.	Author	Year	No. of Pts who received ID	Median follow-up	Median duration of 1st CH	No. of Pts who received 2nd ID	Median duration of 2nd CH	QOL results	OS
1	Beer et al.	2003	11	10.1 m	20 w	8	21 w	Improved: Fatigue	NA
2	Beer et al.	2008	45	NA	18 w	33	12 w (at least)	NA	NA
3	Soga et al.	2009	15	16 m	NA	8	NA	Improved: Nausea, vomiting	21 m
4	Mountzios et al.	2011	35	NA	4.5 m	18	NA	Improved: 6 domains, general condition	NA
5	Narita et al.	2012	35	11.1 m	7.7 m	14	NA	NA	17.8 m
6	Li et al.	2013	42	20 m	5.3 m	11	2.8 m	Improved: Global health, fatigue	19 m
7	Kume et al.	2015	51	19.9 m	266 d	17	129.5 d	NA	NA
8	Caffo et al.	2015	73	21 m	3 m (pre-defined)	56	NA	No difference between intermittent vs. continuous	24 m
9	Aggarwal et al.	2015	125	NA	2.3–2.6 m	26	NA	NA	15.6 m
10	Narita et al.	2015	120	17 m	18.6 m	60	11.0 w	No change	35 m

ID intermittent docetaxel, *Pts* patients, *CH* chemotherapy holiday, *QOL* quality of life, *OS* overall survival, *m* month, *w* week, *d* day, *NA* not assessed

146.5 days for the third. They also indicated that a low baseline PSA and a low Gleason score at diagnosis were significant indicators for the resumption of intermittent docetaxel. In a recent study reported by Aggarwal et al. assessing the impact of GM-CSF during chemotherapy holidays, 52 (42%) of the 125 patients enrolled achieved a >50% decline in serum PSA level. Patients were divided into a GM-CSF group and an observation group based on drug administration during chemotherapy holidays. The median durations of chemotherapy holiday after the first course of docetaxel were 2.6 months in the GM-CSF group and 2.3 months in the observation group, respectively. The median OS from the start of the first "off-chemotherapy" interval was 28.4 months in the GM-CSF group and 14.0 months in the observation group (log-rank test, $p = 0.08$). The difference in OS observed in this study was not significant; however, the findings indicate the impact of maintenance therapies on cancer progression during chemotherapy holidays in patients treated with intermittent docetaxel. Recently, we reported the largest single-arm study to evaluate outcomes of intermittent docetaxel in patients with CRPC, including 6 (5%) patients without metastasis. Of the 120 patients enrolled in this study, sixty (50.0%) patients resumed chemotherapy, and a maximum of six courses were administered to four patients. The median period of the first, second, and third to fifth holiday was 18.6, 11.0, and 4.9 weeks, respectively. The median times to treatment failure and OS from the initiation of docetaxel were 17.5 and 35.0 months, which were comparable to previous Japanese studies assessing outcomes in prostate cancer among Japanese patients treated with continuous docetaxel [7, 28]. As it is not possible to compare OS and other oncological outcomes between previous reports and our study due to the substantial difference in patient background and treatment regimens, intermittent docetaxel may have the potential to achieve equivalent outcomes compared with continuous docetaxel.

The delicate balance between survival benefit and QOL is extremely important in advanced cancer patients, and intermittent docetaxel therapy is expected to maintain QOL in patients with CRPC. Six (60%) of the 10 studies of intermittent docetaxel described above evaluated QOL scores using the QLQ-C30 questionnaire [29]. Three studies reported predominantly unchanged QOL scores between pre- and posttreatment, except for improvement in some scores (fatigue, nausea, vomiting, and global health) [15, 18, 21]. Mountzios et al. compared the QOL scores of 17 patients during the "off-chemotherapy" period with during the "on-chemotherapy" period. They reported that several domains of symptom report (fatigue and diarrhea), cognition (mental focus and distraction), and daily activities (ability to take a long walk and perform hobbies), as well as general condition assessments, were significantly improved during the "off-chemotherapy" period [19]. We found that there were no significant differences among three time points with QOL data available in 45 (37.5%) patients at baseline, 42 (35%) patients 12 weeks after the initiation of chemotherapy, and 15 (25%) patients at the beginning of chemotherapy after the first chemotherapy holiday. In our study, all QOL functional domains except the emotional score were improved at the beginning of the second course chemotherapy compared to baseline in patients with CRPC treated with intermittent docetaxel and prednisolone therapy. In a randomized trial reported by Caffo et al. comparing QOL scores between intermittent and continuous administration of docetaxel in mCRPC every two treatment courses, assessable QOL data were available for 111 (75%) patients. This study found no statistically significant difference in general health status between the continuous and intermittent arms at any assessment time. Although the number and percentage of patients who responded to the QOL survey was relatively small in some studies, the results of QOL surveys administered to patients receiving intermittent chemotherapy indicate this protocol has the potential to maintain QOL during treatment.

In summary, the results of previous studies support the benefit of intermittent docetaxel in patients with CRPC (including AIPC) without compromising OS or oncological outcomes. However, differences in patient background, such as pre-treatment PSA levels, the extent of metastatic spread, performance status, and the length of ADT therapy, may influence OS in CRPC patients. In addition, sequential treatments after intermittent docetaxel may also influence OS. Therefore, randomized trials are warranted to confirm evidence from previous studies of intermittent docetaxel in advanced prostate cancer.

36.3 Future Directions

As the intermittent approach to chemotherapy is considered to be inappropriate in a proportion of patients with mCRPC, the detection of appropriate candidates for intermittent docetaxel is of increasing clinical importance. In advanced cases, the discontinuation of chemotherapy may result in cancer progression during chemotherapy holidays. In recent univariate and multivariate analyses in patients with CRPC who received intermittent docetaxel, a low performance status and a high PSA level before intermittent docetaxel plus prednisolone therapy were significant prognostic factors for OS [25]. However, these factors were reported to be significant risk factors for OS in previous trials of patients treated using the continuous administration of docetaxel [7]. It remains unknown whether these factors have utility in identifying an appropriate population for intermittent chemotherapy. Furthermore, the identification of clinicopathological factors, including pain, anemia, or bone scan index values, to better characterize suitable patients for intermittent chemotherapy may be an important clinical issue in the future.

Appropriate candidates for intermittent docetaxel can be screened by direct comparison between continuous and intermittent in randomized studies. One of the important issues in this field is a lack of randomized trials comparing outcomes between intermittent therapy and continuous therapy. A German group conducted a randomized phase II trial called the PRINCE study [30, 31], and the early results of this study have been reported [32]. The study randomly assigned patients with mCRPC to either intermittent ($n = 78$) or continuous ($n = 78$) docetaxel therapy. Patients in the intermittent therapy arm were treated with either four cycles of docetaxel (70 mg/m^2) triweekly or three cycles of docetaxel (30 mg/m^2) weekly, with chemotherapy suspended until disease progression. The median duration of chemotherapy holiday was 15 weeks. One-year survival was similar between the intermittent and continuous treatment arms (75.8% vs. 72.6%) and met the non-inferiority criteria. However, the difference in median OS (18.3 months vs. 19.3 months) did not meet the non-inferiority criteria, according to a post hoc analysis. Differences in progression-free survival and time to treatment failure were not significant between the two groups and the safety profiles of both study arms were comparable. However, the results of the PRINCE study have yet to be published in a peer-reviewed journal, and the study was limited by poor recruitment, resulting in a power of only 39% of the planned study.

Lastly, cabazitaxel is a second-generation taxane chemotherapy indicated for the treatment of patients with mCRPC pretreated with castration and docetaxel [33]. Intermittent cabazitaxel may represent an appropriate treatment option as the incidence of QOL-related toxic adverse events, such as alopecia, nail changes, peripheral neuropathy, and dysgeusia, in patients who received cabazitaxel have been known to be comparatively lower than those with docetaxel [34, 35]. However, there has been no previous study assessing the clinical impact of intermittent cabazitaxel.

Conclusion

Herein, we review the results of previous studies of intermittent docetaxel therapy in patients with CRPC and AIPC. Intermittent docetaxel therapy achieved a favorable outcome with successful chemotherapy holidays and maintained QOL. Therefore, intermittent docetaxel therapy may be a promising option for the treatment of CRPC, even in the new treatment era of prostate cancer as it allows reasonable oncological outcomes with less toxicity and a high QOL. However, as study designs and baseline characteristics have varied among previous studies, the true effect of intermittent chemotherapy over continuous chemotherapy and the superiority of each treatment regimen remains unclear due to lack of randomized studies in this field. Further evaluation using a large-scale randomized trial and selection of appropriate candidates for intermittent docetaxel is strongly warranted.

References

1. Tannock IF, de Wit R, Berry WR, Horti J, Pluzanska A, Chi KN, et al. Docetaxel plus prednisone or mitoxantrone plus prednisone for advanced prostate cancer. N Engl J Med. 2004;351(15):1502–12.
2. Petrylak DP, Tangen CM, Hussain MH, Lara PN Jr, Jones JA, Taplin ME, et al. Docetaxel and estramustine compared with mitoxantrone and prednisone for advanced refractory prostate cancer. N Engl J Med. 2004;351(15):1513–20.
3. Berthold DR, Pond GR, Soban F, de Wit R, Eisenberger M, Tannock IF. Docetaxel plus prednisone or mitoxantrone plus prednisone for advanced prostate cancer: updated survival in the TAX 327 study. J Clin Oncol. 2008;26(2):242–5.
4. Sweeney CJ, Chen YH, Carducci M, Liu G, Jarrard DF, Eisenberger M, et al. Chemohormonal therapy in metastatic hormone-sensitive prostate cancer. N Engl J Med. 2015;373(8):737–46.
5. James ND, Sydes MR, Clarke NW, Mason MD, Dearnaley DP, Spears MR, et al. Addition of docetaxel, zoledronic acid, or both to first-line long-term hormone therapy in prostate cancer

(STAMPEDE): survival results from an adaptive, multiarm, multistage, platform randomised controlled trial. Lancet. 2016;387(10024):1163–77.
6. Klil-Drori AJ, Azoulay L, Pollak MN. Cancer, obesity, diabetes, and antidiabetic drugs: is the fog clearing? Nat Rev Clin Oncol. 2017;14(2):85–99.
7. Miyake H, Sakai I, Terakawa T, Harada K, Fujisawa M. Oncological outcome of docetaxel-based chemotherapy for Japanese men with metastatic castration-resistant prostate cancer. Urol Oncol. 2013;31(6):733–8.
8. Gyawali B, Koomulli-Parambil S, Iddawela M. Continuous versus intermittent docetaxel for metastatic castration resistant prostate cancer. Crit Rev Oncol Hematol. 2016;102:118–24.
9. De Souza R, Zahedi P, Moriyama EH, Allen CJ, Wilson BC, Piquette-Miller M. Continuous docetaxel chemotherapy improves therapeutic efficacy in murine models of ovarian cancer. Mol Cancer Ther. 2010;9(6):1820–30.
10. Chen CS, Doloff JC, Waxman DJ. Intermittent metronomic drug schedule is essential for activating antitumor innate immunity and tumor xenograft regression. Neoplasia. 2014;16(1):84–96.
11. Muss HB, Case LD, Richards F 2nd, White DR, Cooper MR, Cruz JM, et al. Interrupted versus continuous chemotherapy in patients with metastatic breast cancer. The piedmont oncology association. N Engl J Med. 1991;325(19):1342–8.
12. Maughan TS, James RD, Kerr DJ, Ledermann JA, Seymour MT, Topham C, et al. Comparison of intermittent and continuous palliative chemotherapy for advanced colorectal cancer: a multicentre randomised trial. Lancet. 2003;361(9356):457–64.
13. Gerber DE, Schiller JH. Maintenance chemotherapy for advanced non-small-cell lung cancer: new life for an old idea. J Clin Oncol. 2013;31(8):1009–20.
14. Magnan S, Zarychanski R, Pilote L, Bernier L, Shemilt M, Vigneault E, et al. Intermittent vs continuous androgen deprivation therapy for prostate cancer: a systematic review and meta-analysis. JAMA Oncol. 2015;1(9):1261–9.
15. Beer TM, Garzotto M, Henner WD, Eilers KM, Wersinger EM. Intermittent chemotherapy in metastatic androgen-independent prostate cancer. Br J Cancer. 2003;89(6):968–70.
16. Beer TM, Garzotto M, Henner WD, Eilers KM, Wersinger EM. Multiple cycles of intermittent chemotherapy in metastatic androgen-independent prostate cancer. Br J Cancer. 2004;91(8):1425–7.
17. Beer TM, Ryan CW, Venner PM, Petrylak DP, Chatta GS, Ruether JD, et al. Intermittent chemotherapy in patients with metastatic androgen-independent prostate cancer: results from ASCENT, a double-blinded, randomized comparison of high-dose calcitriol plus docetaxel with placebo plus docetaxel. Cancer. 2008;112(2):326–30.
18. Soga N, Kato M, Nishikawa K, Hasegawa Y, Yamada Y, Kise H, et al. Intermittent docetaxel therapy with estramustine for hormone-refractory prostate cancer in Japanese patients. Int J Clin Oncol. 2009;14(2):130–5.
19. Mountzios I, Bournakis E, Efstathiou E, Varkaris A, Wen S, Chrisofos M, et al. Intermittent docetaxel chemotherapy in patients with castrate-resistant prostate cancer. Urology. 2011;77(3):682–7.
20. Narita S, Tsuchiya N, Yuasa T, Maita S, Obara T, Numakura K, et al. Outcome, clinical prognostic factors and genetic predictors of adverse reactions of intermittent combination chemotherapy with docetaxel, estramustine phosphate and carboplatin for castration-resistant prostate cancer. Int J Clin Oncol. 2012;17(3):204–11.
21. Li YF, Zhang SF, Zhang TT, Li L, Gan W, Jia HT, et al. Intermittent tri-weekly docetaxel plus bicalutamide in patients with castration-resistant prostate cancer: a single-arm prospective study using a historical control for comparison. Asian J Androl. 2013;15(6):773–9.
22. Aggarwal RR, Beer TM, Weinberg VK, Higano C, Taplin ME, Ryan CJ, et al. Intermittent chemotherapy as a platform for testing novel agents in patients with metastatic castration-resistant prostate cancer: a department of defense prostate cancer clinical trials consortium randomized phase II trial of intermittent docetaxel with prednisone with or without maintenance GM-CSF. Clin Genitourin Cancer. 2015;13(3):e191–8.
23. Caffo O, Lo Re G, Sava T, Buti S, Sacco C, Basso U, et al. Intermittent docetaxel chemotherapy as first-line treatment for metastatic castration-resistant prostate cancer patients. Future Oncol. 2015;11(6):965–73.

24. Kume H, Kawai T, Nagata M, Azuma T, Miyazaki H, Suzuki M, et al. Intermittent docetaxel chemotherapy is feasible for castration-resistant prostate cancer. Mol Clin Oncol. 2015;3(2):303–7.
25. Narita S, Koie T, Yamada S, Orikasa K, Matsuo S, Aoki H, et al. A prospective multicenter study of intermittent chemotherapy with docetaxel and prednisolone for castration-resistant prostate cancer. Jpn J Clin Oncol. 2016;46(6):547–53.
26. Huang M, Narita S, Numakura K, Tsuruta H, Saito M, Inoue T, et al. A high-fat diet enhances proliferation of prostate cancer cells and activates MCP-1/CCR2 signaling. Prostate. 2012;72(16):1779–88.
27. Abdollah F, Sood A, Sammon JD, Hsu L, Beyer B, Moschini M, et al. Long-term cancer control outcomes in patients with clinically high-risk prostate cancer treated with robot-assisted radical prostatectomy: results from a multi-institutional study of 1100 patients. Eur Urol. 2015;68(3):497–505.
28. Matsuyama H, Shimabukuro T, Hara I, Kohjimoto Y, Suzuki K, Koike H, et al. Combination of hemoglobin, alkaline phosphatase, and age predicts optimal docetaxel regimen for patients with castration-resistant prostate cancer. Int J Clin Oncol. 2014;19(5):946–54.
29. Aaronson NK, Ahmedzai S, Bergman B, Bullinger M, Cull A, Duez NJ, et al. The European Organization for Research and Treatment of Cancer QLQ-C30: a quality-of-life instrument for use in international clinical trials in oncology. J Natl Cancer Inst. 1993;85(5):365–76.
30. Rexer H. AUO study in hormone-refractory prostate cancer. Phase III study on treatment of hormone-refractory prostate cancer (HRPC) with docetaxel: continuous treatment vs. intermittent repetition of treatment after renewed progression—PRINCE. Urologe A. 2006;45(7):872.
31. Kapoor A, Hotte SJ. Chemotherapy research for metastatic prostate cancer. Can Urol Assoc J. 2016;10(7-8Suppl3):S140–3.
32. Cash H, Steiner U, Heidenreich A. PRINCE: a phase 3 study comparing intermittent docetaxel therapy vs. continuous docetaxel therapy in patients with castration-resistant prostate cancer. J Clin Oncol. 2016;34:Abstr 5005.
33. de Bono JS, Oudard S, Ozguroglu M, Hansen S, Machiels JP, Kocak I, et al. Prednisone plus cabazitaxel or mitoxantrone for metastatic castration-resistant prostate cancer progressing after docetaxel treatment: a randomised open-label trial. Lancet. 2010;376(9747):1147–54.
34. Nozawa M, Mukai H, Takahashi S, Uemura H, Kosaka T, Onozawa Y, et al. Japanese phase I study of cabazitaxel in metastatic castration-resistant prostate cancer. Int J Clin Oncol. 2015;20(5):1026–34.
35. Omlin A, Sartor O, Rothermundt C, Cathomas R, De Bono JS, Shen L, et al. Analysis of side effect profile of alopecia, nail changes, peripheral neuropathy, and dysgeusia in prostate cancer patients treated with docetaxel and cabazitaxel. Clin Genitourin Cancer. 2015;13(4):e205–8.

Chemotherapy with Cabazitaxel for mCRPC in Japanese Men

37

Masahiro Nozawa and Hirotsugu Uemura

Abstract

Efficacy and safety of cabazitaxel in Japanese patients with docetaxel-failure castration-resistant prostate cancer were largely identical with Western population based on a phase I study. However, febrile neutropenia among treatment-emergent adverse events can occur more commonly in Japanese, especially in patients who administered a relatively high total dose of previous docetaxel, and an aggressive prophylaxis may be important using granulocyte colony-stimulating factor for those patients.

Keywords

Cabazitaxel · Castration · Chemotherapy · Prostate · Taxane

37.1 Cabazitaxel as Second-Line Chemotherapy for mCRPC

Cabazitaxel is called as a second-generation taxane. Cabazitaxel has shown an antitumor effect against docetaxel-resistant prostate cancer cells in a preclinical system [1–3]. In a pivotal global phase III clinical trial, named TROPIC, cabazitaxel demonstrated a benefit to elongate overall survival of patients with docetaxel-failure castration-resistant prostate cancer [4]. TROPIC study targeted mainly Caucasians, containing only 7% of Asian, and no Japanese medical center participated to it.

A phase I study coded as NCT01324583 was only one prospective of cabazitaxel that targeted Japanese population, in which were evaluated mainly safety but also a certain impact of efficacy in its expansion cohort [5]. In this study, enrolled were patients with histologically confirmed prostate adenocarcinoma with metastasis

M. Nozawa (✉) · H. Uemura
Faculty of Medicine, Department of Urology, Kindai University, Osaka-Sayama, Japan
e-mail: nozawa06@med.kindai.ac.jp

whose diseases were failure to androgen-deprivation therapy and docetaxel regardless of antiandrogen treatment. And excluded were patients with an age of 75 years or older or with less than 225 mg/m^2 of total dose of previous docetaxel.

37.2 Efficacy of Cabazitaxel in Japanese Patient Population

In this Japanese phase I study, cabazitaxel was administered triweekly with a dose of 25 mg/m^2 per time into a total of 44 patients, including 41 from an expanding cohort and 3 from a dose-escalation cohort.

No complete response (CR), two (16.7%) partial response (PR), 10 (83.3%) stable disease (SD), and no disease progression were found as the best RECIST response in 12 evaluable among 41 patients from the expansion cohort. Twelve (29.3%) among those 41 patients acquired PSA response defined as the decline of PSA level of 50% or greater from baseline. The median time to PSA progression was 3.68 months with 95% confidence interval of 1.35–4.63.

RECIST evaluation was one PR and one SD in two evaluable patients among three from the dose-escalation cohort. PSA decline of 50% or greater from baseline was detected in two among three of those patients.

37.3 Safety of Cabazitaxel in Japanese

Cabazitaxel treatment had been discontinued at the time of analysis in 28 patients among 44 patients treated with a dose of triweekly 25 mg/m^2. The reasons for discontinuation were disease progression (57%), adverse events (32%), and withdrawal of consent (11%). The number of treatment cycles with cabazitaxel was median of 7.5 and maximum of 29. Among total of 338 cycles, dose reduction was needed in 9.5% of cycles. Dose retardation of more than 3 days was detected in 37.4% of cycles. Dose-limiting toxicity, defined as grade 4 of neutropenia continuing for more than 7 days, grade 4 of thrombocytopenia, grade 4 of febrile neutropenia, or grade 3 or 4 of nausea, vomiting, diarrhea, hypersensitivity, fatigue, or hyponatremia, was detected in two (4.7%) patients. Of those two patients, one developed grade 4 of necrotizing fasciitis and septic shock and the other grade 3 of otitis media and bronchopneumonia, respectively.

Neutropenia was the most common one among all treatment-emergent adverse events and occurred in all of patients with grade 4 but one with grade 3. Other adverse events included anemia (100%), lymphocytopenia (88.6%), thrombocytopenia (72.7%), febrile neutropenia (54.5%), fatigue (54.5%), nausea (52.3%), diarrhea (50.0%), appetite loss (40.9%), constipation (29.5%), dysgeusia (27.3%), peripheral neuropathy (25.0%), stomatitis (22.7%), vomiting (22.7%), nasopharyngitis (20.5%), and insomnia (20.5%) in order of the frequency at all grade. As to adverse events at grade 3 or more, the order was as follows: neutropenia (100%), febrile neutropenia (54.5%), lymphocytopenia (52.3%), anemia (47.7%), thrombocytopenia (6.8%), fatigue (6.8%), nausea (6.8%), and appetite loss (6.8%). Serious treatment-emergent adverse events occurred in 25 (56.8%) patients, including neutropenia (20.5%) and febrile neutropenia (15.9%). No fatal treatment-emergent adverse event was detected.

Twenty-eight (63.6%) patients needed dose modification due to treatment-emergent adverse events, including neutropenia (15.9%), febrile neutropenia (13.6%), anemia (11.4%), serum aspartate aminotransferase increase (11.4%), and serum alanine aminotransferase increase (9.1%). Dose modification contributed to the improvement of their adverse events for 25 among 28 patients; however, other three patients eventually discontinued the treatment due to their adverse events regardless of dose modification. A total of nine patients discontinued cabazitaxel treatment due to adverse events, including fatigue for two patients and necrotizing fasciitis, septic shock, anemia, appetite loss, paralysis, and nausea for one each. No patients quitted the treatment by cause of neutropenia or febrile neutropenia, suggesting these adverse events can be controlled by adding appropriate granulocyte colony-stimulating factor (G-CSF) and antibiotics. Three out of nine patients who discontinued cabazitaxel due to adverse events eventually received more than nine cycles of cabazitaxel, whereas four patients underwent only less than four cycles.

No association was found between the occurrence of neutropenia or febrile neutropenia by cabazitaxel and the incidence of previous neutropenia of grade 3 or greater due to docetaxel. All patients developed grade 3 or greater neutropenia by cabazitaxel regardless of the past history, and the incidence of febrile neutropenia due to cabazitaxel in the patient group with or without the previous neutropenia by docetaxel was 57.1% or 53.3%, respectively, that indicated no significant difference. Febrile neutropenia triggered by cabazitaxel was all grade 3 and no grade 4 one was observed.

Administration of G-CSF was not permitted at cycle 1 of each patient based on the protocol in this Japanese phase I study, and that seems one of the reasons for such a high incidence of neutropenia, that is 100% of patients. Indeed, the incidence of neutropenia of grade 3 or greater decreased to 16 (53.3%) among 30 cycles in patients who underwent G-CSF prophylaxis at cycle 2 or later. Time from administration of cabazitaxel to the nadir of neutrophil count was about 7 to 14 days (median, 9 days). Duration until recovering of neutrophil count took about 2 to 14 days (median, 3–4 days) even if G-CSF was used. In some patient, it took as long as 28 days.

37.4 Signature of Cabazitaxel in Japanese Clinical Practice

In the global pivotal phase III trial TROPIC, objective response rate (CR + PR) was 14.4% and PSA response rate (50% or more decrease of PSA level from baseline) was 39.2% [1]. Objective response rate 16.7% was almost equal but PSA response rate 29.3% was relatively low in Japanese population compared to the results of TROPIC trial. This trend could have been caused by the difference in patient characteristics between the two studies. For example, the median total dose of previous docetaxel was 752.8 mg/m^2 in the Japanese phase I study, obviously higher than

576.6 mg/m^2 in TROPIC trial. Patients administered with a total dose of previous docetaxel of 750 mg/m^2 or lower, compared to those with higher than 750 mg/m^2, responded at PSA level numerically more in the number and had a longer treatment period and a longer time to PSA progression with cabazitaxel. However, such tendency was not statistically significant because of the lack of enough patient number.

The impact of total dose of previous docetaxel may be associated with treatment-emergent adverse events, especially febrile neutropenia, due to cabazitaxel. Neutropenia itself commonly occurred also in global TROPIC trial, that is, in 94% of patients at any grade and in 82% at grade 3 or greater, however the incidence of febrile neutropenia was obviously lower (8.0%) in TROPIC trial compared to that (54.5%) in the Japanese phase I study. One of the reasons for this gap may be the difference of total dose of previous docetaxel. The difference of incidence of G-CSF prophylaxis also can cause the gap. G-CSF prophylaxis has a potential to reduce the incidence of febrile neutropenia [6]. No patient received G-CSF prophylaxis at the first cycle and as small as 18.2% of patients did even at the second or later cycles in the Japanese phase I study, whereas 24.7% of patients underwent G-CSF prophylaxis in TROPIC trial. Asian ethnicity can also cause a severe myelosuppression due to anticancer agents [7, 8]. Pharmacokinetics of cabazitaxel were almost identical between Japanese and Caucasian populations based on phase I studies, suggesting that the racial difference itself may have an impact on incidence of febrile neutropenia regardless of pharmacokinetics of cabazitaxel [9–12].

References

1. Bouchet BP, Galmarini CM. Cabazitaxel, a new taxane with favorable properties. Drugs Today (Barc). 2010;46:735–42.
2. Vrignaud P, Semiond D, Lejeune P, Bouchard H, Calvet L, Combeau C, Riou JF, Commercon A, Lavelle F, Bissery MC. Preclinical antitumor activity of cabazitaxel, a semisynthetic taxane active in taxane-resistant tumors. Clin Cancer Res. 2013;19:2973–83.
3. Paller CJ, Antonarakis ES. Cabazitaxel: a novel second-line treatment for metastatic castration-resistant prostate cancer. Drug Des Devel Ther. 2011;10:117–24.
4. de Bono JS, Oudard S, Ozguroglu M, Hansen S, Machiels JP, Kocak I, Gravis G, Bodrogi I, Mackenzie MJ, Shen L, Roessner M, Gupta S, Sartor AO. Prednisone plus cabazitaxel or mitoxantrone for metastatic castration-resistant prostate cancer progressing after docetaxel treatment: a randomized open-label trial. Lancet. 2010;376:1147–54.
5. Nozawa M, Mukai H, Takahashi S, Uemura H, Kosaka T, Onozawa Y, Miyazaki J, Suzuki K, Okihara K, Arai Y, Kamba T, Kato M, Nakai Y, Furuse H, Kume H, Ide H, Kitamura H, Yokomizo A, Kimura T, Tomita Y, Ohno K, Kakehi Y. Japanese phase I study of cabazitaxel in metastatic castration-resistant prostate cancer. Int J Clin Oncol. 2015;20:1026–34.
6. Di Lorenzo G, D'Aaniello C, Buonerba C, Federico P, Rescigno P, Puglia L, Ferro M, Bosso D, Cavaliere C, Palmieri G, Sonpavde G, De Placido S. Peg-filgrastim and cabazitaxel in prostate cancer patients. Anti-Cancer Drugs. 2013;24:84–9.
7. Lee JL, Park SH, Koh SJ, Lee SH, Kim YJ, Choi YJ, Lee J, Lim HY. Effectiveness and safety of cabazitaxel plus prednisolone chemotherapy for metastatic castration-resistant prostatic carcinoma: data on Korean patients obtained by the cabazitaxel compassionate-use program. Cancer Chemother Pharmacol. 2014;74(5):1005–13.

8. Heidenreich A, Scholz HJ, Rogenhofer S, Arsov C, Retz M, Muller SC, Albers P, Gschwend J, Wirth M, Steiner U, Miller K, Heinrich E, Trojan L, Volkmer B, Honecker F, Bokemeyer C, Keck B, Otremba B, Ecstein-Fraisse E, Pfister D. Cabazitaxel plus prednisone for metastatic castration-resistant prostate cancer progressing after docetaxel: results from the German compassionate-use programme. Eur Urol. 2013;63:977–82.
9. Mukai H, Takahashi S, Nozawa M, Onozawa Y, Miyazaki J, Ohno K, Suzuki K, Investigators TED. Phase I dose escalation and pharmacokinetic study (TED 11576) of cabazitaxel in Japanese patients with castration-resistant prostate cancer. Cancer Chemother Pharmacol. 2014;73:703–10.
10. Mita AC, Denuis LJ, Rowinsky EK, de Bono JS, Goez AD, Ochoa L, Forouzesh B, Beeram M, Patnaik A, Molpus K, Semiond D, Besenval M, Tolcher AW. Phase I and pharmacokinetic study of XRP6258 (RPR116258A), a novel taxane, administered as a 1-hour infusion every 3 weeks in patients with advanced solid tumors. Clin Cancer Res. 2009;15:723–30.
11. Dieras V, Lortholary A, Lawrence V, Delva R, Girre V, Livartowski A, Assadourian S, Semiond D, Pierga Y. Cabazitaxel in patients with advanced solid tumors: results of a phase I and pharmacokinetic study. Eur J Cancer. 2013;49:25–34.
12. Ferron GM, Dai Y, Semiond D. Population pharmacokinetics of cabazitaxel in patients with advanced solid tumors. Cancer Chemother Pharmacol. 2013;71:681–92.

New Targeted Approach to CRPC

Takeo Kosaka and Mototsugu Oya

Abstract

Our understanding of the heterogeneity and genetic characteristics of CRPC demonstrates underlying their complexity, which has been thought to be associated with their intractability. Recent advance of integrative next generation sequencing unveiled the extensive mutational landscape of metastatic CRPC, many of which can be a targetable mutation and been linked to ongoing clinical trials. Molecular stratification of patient groups will clearly be critical to successful drug development and clinical trials from the view point of precision medicine. In this review, we discuss the potential of new targeted approach to impact the clinical management of CRPC.

Keywords

CRPC · AR signaling pathway · PI3K-PTEN-AKT-mTOR pathway · DNA repair pathway · WNT pathway · Liquid biopsy · Circulating tumor cells · Cell-free DNA · Precision medicine

38.1 Introduction

Recent advance of integrative whole-exome sequencing and whole transcriptome sequencing unveiled the extensive mutational landscape of metastatic CRPC in contrast to primary prostate cancers. These mutations have been thought to be defined as predicting response or resistance to a targeted therapy, as well as prognostic indications. Many of which can be a targetable mutation and been linked to ongoing clinical trials.

T. Kosaka, M.D., Ph.D. (✉) · M. Oya
Department of Urology, Keio University School of Medicine, Tokyo, Japan

© Springer Nature Singapore Pte Ltd. 2018
Y. Arai, O. Ogawa (eds.), *Hormone Therapy and Castration Resistance of Prostate Cancer*, https://doi.org/10.1007/978-981-10-7013-6_38

Precision cancer medicine: The use of genomic profiling at the point-of-care testing to inform treatment decisions for patients is changing cancer care and expected to provide more accurate prediction and efficient therapies for individual patients.

In this review, we discuss the potential of genomics to impact the clinical management of CRPC.

38.2 Androgen Receptor and Androgen Production in Prostate Cancer Tissues

The results of studies using cell lines and those on AR expression in patients with prostate cancer showed that AR expression was maintained or enhanced despite reduced androgen circulation in CRPC [1–3] (Fig. 38.1). AR is still activated through various mechanisms, including AR amplification or overexpression, activating AR mutations, elevated expression of co-activators enhancing AR transcriptional activity, and indirect androgen receptor activation through STAT3/MAPK-mediated phosphorylation [4, 5]. It has been reported that one-third of CRPC patients have as a clinically significant mutation of AR, indicating different sensitivity to novel AR-directed therapies [6–9]. However, the clinical significance of these AR mutations for predicting response or resistance to these agents remains to be determined. Although several drugs have demonstrated inhibitory activity of AR signaling, the clinical significance of these AR mutations for predicting response or resistance to these agents remains to be determined [10–12]. Unfortunately, most patients eventually develop resistance to these agents.

Regarding androgen production in prostate cancer tissues, intratumoral conversion of adrenal androgens and de novo steroid synthesis have been proposed as potential causes of PCa progression [2, 13]. The results of these studies provide the molecular basis for the inhibition of androgen production in CRPC tissues, leading to actual drug discovery and development of CYP17A1 inhibitor: such as abiraterone and clinical trials [14–18].

In relation to 5AR activity and the use of 5AR inhibitors to prevent development and progression of PCA, the findings of two large randomized, placebo-controlled trials: the Prostate Cancer Prevention Trial (PCPT) with finasteride [19] and the Reduction by Dutasteride of Prostate Cancer Events (REDUCE) trial [20] were interesting. The FDA reanalyzed these two major trials and intriguingly cited the fact that the absolute incidence of tumors with Gleason scores between 8 and 10 was significantly increased by 0.7% with finasteride and by 0.5% with dutasteride. FDA Advisory Committee voted against recommending 5-ARI for the indication to reduce PCa risk, because the risk of more aggressive tumors outweighed their potential for chemoprevention.

We previously reported the reduced 5-AR activity and the suppressive effect of DHT in CRPC cells [21]. The suppressive effect of androgens on PCa cells is not limited to these in vitro results [22–24]. Some recent clinical reports showed that CRPC could be treated with androgens due to the inhibitory action of excess androgens [25, 26]. Accumulating evidence has suggested that AR has a finite ability to

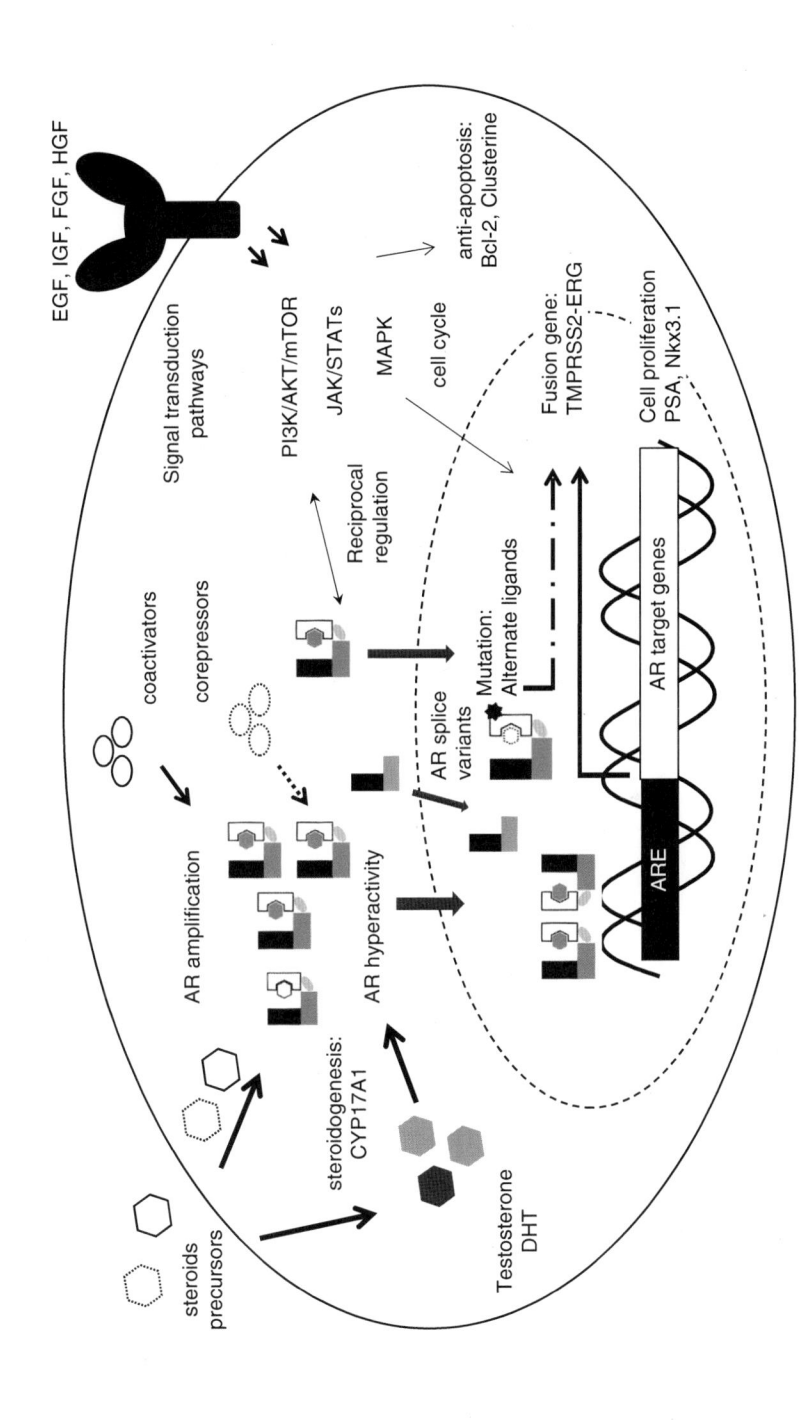

Fig. 38.1 DDR: PARP1/ and BRCA1/2

bind to T or DHT and that at higher concentrations T or DHT has no further effect on prostate growth when all ARs are bound to T or DHT, which was proposed to be termed the saturation point. Due to this saturation point, excess DHT may result in the suppression of androgenic-induced proliferation of CRPC cells.

CRPC may have an unknown regulation system to protect themselves from the androgenic suppressive effect.

38.3 The PI3K-PTEN-AKT-mTOR Pathway

Phosphatidylinositol (PI), a phospholipid constructing the cell membrane, and its phosphorylated product, phosphatidylinositol-3-phosphate, play important roles in the intracellular signal transduction pathway. Phosphatidylinositol 3-kinase (PI3K) is activated by growth factors and receptor tyrosine kinases. PI3K activation transmits to the AKT signaling pathway, which, in turn, regulates many downstream factors and is involved in various signaling pathways, such as cell growth, inhibition of apoptosis, and metabolism control. Phosphatase and tensin homolog deleted on chromosome 10 (PTEN) is a lipid phosphatase that negatively regulates PI3K by catalyzing dephosphorylation, the reverse reaction of PI3K-induced phosphorylation. PI3K-PTEN-AKT-mTOR pathway was altered in a half of the patients, making it the second most frequently altered pathway after androgen receptor, commonly through loss of PTEN, amplification of PIK3CA/B, and activating mutation of PIK3CA/B and AKT1 [4, 6].

Loss of PTEN function is considered to induce AKT phosphorylation and further augment constitutive activation of the AKT signaling pathway. mTOR kinase is a serine-threonine kinase involved in cell growth, proliferation, and survival. It forms mTOR complex1 (mTORC1) and mTOR complex2 (mTORC2). mTORC1 is one of the AKT signaling pathways. Consequently, the PI3K/Akt signaling pathway is an important target in CRPC (Fig. 38.2). Consequently, the PI3K-PTEN-AKT-mTOR signaling pathway is attracting attention as a mechanism of oncogenesis in prostate cancer and as a therapeutic target [27, 28]. In prostate cancer cells lacking PTEN, activated AKT phosphorylates FOXO1, resulting in its nuclear exclusion. FOXO1 binds to AR in the nucleus and inhibits transcriptional activity of AR splice variants, thereby inducing androgen-independent activation of the AR [29]. The targeting intracellular networks of PTEN–AKT–FOXO1 axis could be a potential strategy for inhibiting aberrant AR activation and androgen-independent tumor growth. In the past, many inhibitors targeting PI3K-PTEN-AKT-mTOR signaling by monotherapies have had a lack of efficacy leading to failure of clinical study [27, 28].

This is thought to be due to lack of specificity, coexisting alterations, and reciprocal signaling feedback [30–32]. Recently, multiple inhibitors of specific PI3K isoforms have begun testing in clinical trials, potentially increasing the specificity of these agents. In CRPC, there are recurrent mutations in PIK3CB and frequent loss of PTEN, which may activate PIK3CB over PIK3CA, suggesting the need for these specific PI3K isoforms inhibitors to effectively clinically target these signaling pathways [33].

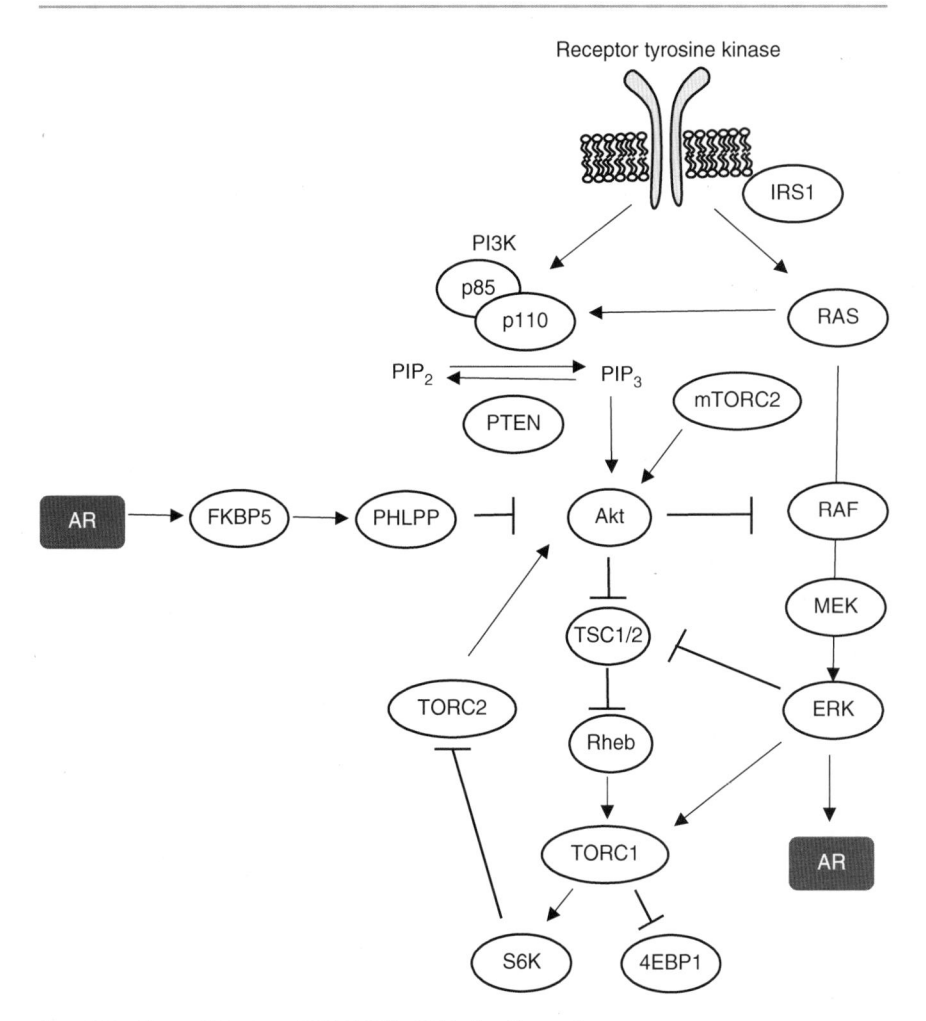

Fig. 38.2 Crosstalk between PI3k/AKT/mTOR signaling pathways

38.4 DNA Repair Defects

The most common aberrant gene is a germ line mutation of BRCA2 with 12.7% of PCa patients [6, 34]. Other somatic and germ line DNA repair alterations were found in ATM, BRCA1, FANCA, RAD51B, etc. Those DNA repair alterations are involved in homologous recombination (HR) DNA repair, mismatch repair (MMR), and nucleotide excision repair (NER). Alterations in these genes that are involved in HR occur in up to 30% of CRPC cases. These results indicate the implications for PARP inhibitors, which revealed significant efficacy in patients with BRCA2 mutations or other DNA repair alterations in CRPC and other tumor types (Fig. 38.3). A

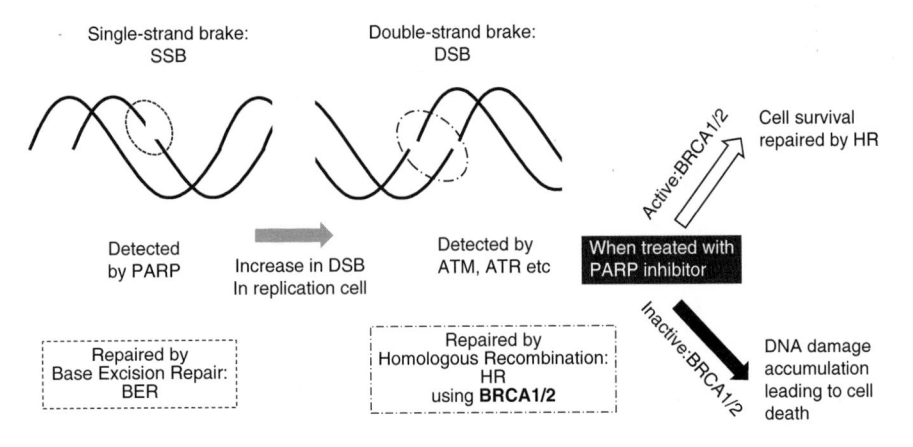

Fig. 38.3 PARP and BRCA1/2

phase II trial of olaparib, one of PARP inhibitors, was conducted for CRPC patients: TOPARP study [35]. Sixteen of the 50 patients harbored DNA repair gene alterations, and 14 out of those 16 patients responded to olaparib, highlighting potential therapy for mCRPC with DNA repair gene alterations. Based on these promising findings, multiple clinical trials using PARP inhibitors are ongoing in conjunction with genetic characteristics of DNA repair gene alterations.

Notably, recent studies have reported that 12.9% metastatic prostate cancers have germline mutations in DNA repair genes [36]. These results suggest the change of the clinical care of patient with advanced prostate cancer irrespective of family history. Higher rate of germline mutations in DNA repair genes than expected will provide the change of clinical practice of germline testing of DDR-related genes for CRPC patients.

Other studies have reported that PARP was significantly correlated with ETS family, AR signaling pathways or PI3K/AKT signaling pathways [37–43], suggesting the broader efficacy of targeting DNA repair pathways including PARP inhibitor more than expected.

38.5 WNT Pathway

The WNT pathway has many biologic functions from embryonic development and differentiations. WNT pathway, including activating CTNNB1, APC, RNF43 mutations, or rearrangements of R-spondin family members, have been identified in metastatic CRPC [6, 44]. These mutations have consisted of 18% of metastatic CRPC patient. Recent study demonstrated an upregulation of WNT signaling pathways in CRPC patients' circulating tumor cells. The WNT pathway has been known to be extremely difficult to target by inhibitors because of the multiple and complexities of ligands and downstream pathways [45, 46]. The WNT pathway activated by proteins secreted by tumor cells or stromal cells as part of an autocrine loop resulted in the difficulty of targeting this pathway [47–49]. It is controversial and unknown whether an agonists or antagonists would work better to inhibit tumor growth in CRPC [45, 46].

38.6 Liquid Biopsy

Genomic profiling of tissue biopsies can be used to investigate genomic alteration. There is also the reality that not all patients can get a safety biopsy. Moreover, specimens got by biopsy may not capture the precise extent of disease due to the heterogeneity in a CRPC patient.

Recent research have focused on several noninvasive strategies, including the use of liquid biopsy techniques, which include the use of circulating tumor cells (CTCs) and cell-free DNA (cfDNA) to identify genomic alterations of CRPC [50–60]. These methods avoid the problem of accessibility and the safety of tumor biopsy, as well as the heterogeneity (Fig. 38.4).

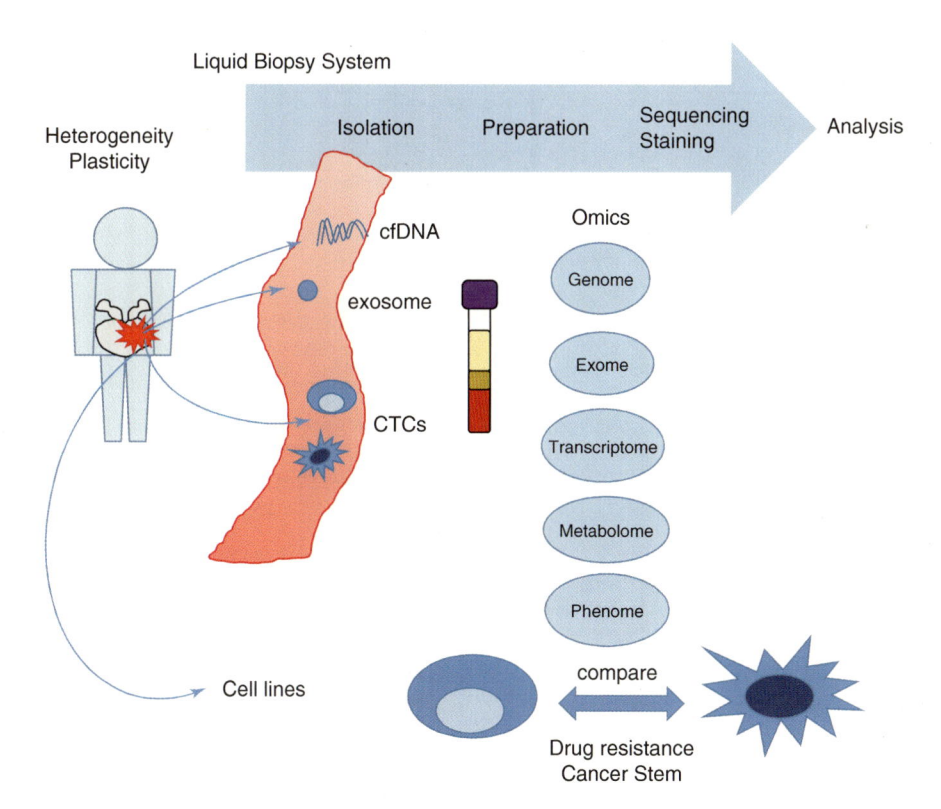

Fig. 38.4 Liquid biopsy system and precision medicine

Although studies of CTCs in CRPC have focused on CTC enumeration or count in the past, the topics have shifted towards the molecular characterization of CTCs. Recent studies have also developed primary cell cultures from CTCs, which may lead to investigate the drug sensitivity or genome analysis.

Genomic profiling of CTCs and cfDNA can be used to investigate the sequential monitoring of molecular dynamics and to overcome resistance and select adaptive drug administration [51, 55, 57, 60].

From a clinical viewpoint, early detection of drug resistance is critical issue. These Liquid Biopsy systems may also help us identify patients who are developing resistance earlier than imaging modalities near future.

Conclusion

This review refers to a large number of genetic studies, drug development, and clinical trial of CRPC, especially focusing on targeted approach to CRPC. Our understanding of the heterogeneity and genetic characteristics of CRPC demonstrates underlying their complexity. Molecular stratification of patient groups will clearly be critical to successful drug development and clinical trials. Future trials may take into account the genotypic characteristics of CRPC by selecting patients who are optimized to respond the trial drugs.

References

1. Chen CD, Welsbie DS, Tran C, et al. Molecular determinants of resistance to antiandrogen therapy. Nat Med. 2004;10:33–9.
2. Montgomery RB, Mostaghel EA, Vessella R, et al. Maintenance of intratumoral androgens in metastatic prostate cancer: a mechanism for castration-resistant tumor growth. Cancer Res. 2008;68:4447–54.
3. Nishiyama T, Ikarashi T, Hashimoto Y, Wako K, Takahashi K. The change in the dihydrotestosterone level in the prostate before and after androgen deprivation therapy in connection with prostate cancer aggressiveness using the Gleason score. J Urol. 2007;178:1282–8; discussion 8–9
4. Taylor BS, Schultz N, Hieronymus H, et al. Integrative genomic profiling of human prostate cancer. Cancer Cell. 2010;18:11–22.
5. Ueda T, Bruchovsky N, Sadar MD. Activation of the androgen receptor N-terminal domain by interleukin-6 via MAPK and STAT3 signal transduction pathways. J Biol Chem. 2002;277:7076–85.
6. Robinson D, Van Allen EM, YM W, et al. Integrative clinical genomics of advanced prostate cancer. Cell. 2015;161:1215–28.
7. Beer TM, Armstrong AJ, Rathkopf DE, et al. Enzalutamide in metastatic prostate cancer before chemotherapy. N Engl J Med. 2014;371:424–33.
8. Scher HI, Fizazi K, Saad F, et al. Increased survival with enzalutamide in prostate cancer after chemotherapy. N Engl J Med. 2012;367:1187–97.
9. Tran C, Ouk S, Clegg NJ, et al. Development of a second-generation antiandrogen for treatment of advanced prostate cancer. Science. 2009;324:787–90.
10. Ferraldeschi R, Welti J, Luo J, Attard G, de Bono JS. Targeting the androgen receptor pathway in castration-resistant prostate cancer: progresses and prospects. Oncogene. 2015;34:1745–57.
11. Wong YN, Ferraldeschi R, Attard G, de Bono J. Evolution of androgen receptor targeted therapy for advanced prostate cancer. Nat Rev Clin Oncol. 2014;11:365–76.

12. Romanel A, Gasi Tandefelt D, Conteduca V, et al. Plasma AR and abiraterone-resistant prostate cancer. Sci Transl Med. 2015;7:312re10.
13. Nishiyama T, Hashimoto Y, Takahashi K. The influence of androgen deprivation therapy on dihydrotestosterone levels in the prostatic tissue of patients with prostate cancer. Clin Cancer Res. 2004;10:7121–6.
14. Basch E, Autio K, Ryan CJ, et al. Abiraterone acetate plus prednisone versus prednisone alone in chemotherapy-naive men with metastatic castration-resistant prostate cancer: patient-reported outcome results of a randomised phase 3 trial. Lancet Oncol. 2013;14:1193–9.
15. de Bono JS, Logothetis CJ, Molina A, et al. Abiraterone and increased survival in metastatic prostate cancer. N Engl J Med. 2011;364:1995–2005.
16. Fizazi K, Scher HI, Molina A, et al. Abiraterone acetate for treatment of metastatic castration-resistant prostate cancer: final overall survival analysis of the COU-AA-301 randomised, double-blind, placebo-controlled phase 3 study. Lancet Oncol. 2012;13:983–92.
17. Ryan CJ, Smith MR, de Bono JS, et al. Abiraterone in metastatic prostate cancer without previous chemotherapy. N Engl J Med. 2013;368:138–48.
18. Ryan CJ, Smith MR, Fong L, et al. Phase I clinical trial of the CYP17 inhibitor abiraterone acetate demonstrating clinical activity in patients with castration-resistant prostate cancer who received prior ketoconazole therapy. J Clin Oncol. 2010;28:1481–8.
19. Thompson IM, Goodman PJ, Tangen CM, et al. The influence of finasteride on the development of prostate cancer. N Engl J Med. 2003;349:215–24.
20. Andriole GL, Bostwick DG, Brawley OW, et al. Effect of dutasteride on the risk of prostate cancer. N Engl J Med. 2010;362:1192–202.
21. Kosaka T, Miyajima A, Nagata H, Maeda T, Kikuchi E, Oya M. Human castration resistant prostate cancer rather prefer to decreased 5alpha-reductase activity. Sci Rep. 2013;3:1268.
22. Chuu CP, Kokontis JM, Hiipakka RA, et al. Androgens as therapy for androgen receptor-positive castration-resistant prostate cancer. J Biomed Sci. 2011;18:63.
23. Kokontis JM, Lin HP, Jiang SS, et al. Androgen suppresses the proliferation of androgen receptor-positive castration-resistant prostate cancer cells via inhibition of Cdk2, CyclinA, and Skp2. PLoS One. 2014;9:e109170.
24. Umekita Y, Hiipakka RA, Kokontis JM, Liao S. Human prostate tumor growth in athymic mice: inhibition by androgens and stimulation by finasteride. Proc Natl Acad Sci U S A. 1996;93:11802–7.
25. Schweizer MT, Wang H, Luber B, et al. Bipolar androgen therapy for men with androgen ablation naive prostate cancer: results from the Phase II BATMAN Study. Prostate. 2016;76:1218–26.
26. Schweizer MT, Antonarakis ES, Wang H, et al. Effect of bipolar androgen therapy for asymptomatic men with castration-resistant prostate cancer: results from a pilot clinical study. Sci Transl Med. 2015;7:269ra2.
27. Statz CM, Patterson SE, Mockus SM. mTOR inhibitors in castration-resistant prostate cancer: a systematic review. Target Oncol. 2017;12:47–59.
28. Edlind MP, Hsieh AC. PI3K-AKT-mTOR signaling in prostate cancer progression and androgen deprivation therapy resistance. Asian J Androl. 2014;16:378–86.
29. Mediwala SN, Sun H, Szafran AT, et al. The activity of the androgen receptor variant AR-V7 is regulated by FOXO1 in a PTEN-PI3K-AKT-dependent way. Prostate. 2013;73:267–77.
30. Carver BS, Chapinski C, Wongvipat J, et al. Reciprocal feedback regulation of PI3K and androgen receptor signaling in PTEN-deficient prostate cancer. Cancer Cell. 2011;19:575–86.
31. Yasumizu Y, Miyajima A, Kosaka T, Miyazaki Y, Kikuchi E, Oya M. Dual PI3K/mTOR inhibitor NVP-BEZ235 sensitizes docetaxel in castration resistant prostate cancer. J Urol. 2014;191:227–34.
32. Kosaka T, Miyajima A, Shirotake S, Suzuki E, Kikuchi E, Oya M. Long-term androgen ablation and docetaxel up-regulate phosphorylated Akt in castration resistant prostate cancer. J Urol. 2011;185:2376–81.
33. Schwartz S, Wongvipat J, Trigwell CB, et al. Feedback suppression of PI3Kalpha signaling in PTEN-mutated tumors is relieved by selective inhibition of PI3Kbeta. Cancer Cell. 2015;27:109–22.

34. Beltran H. DNA mismatch repair in prostate cancer. J Clin Oncol. 2013;31:1782–4.
35. Mateo J, Carreira S, Sandhu S, et al. DNA-repair defects and Olaparib in metastatic prostate cancer. N Engl J Med. 2015;373:1697–708.
36. Pritchard CC, Mateo J, Walsh MF, et al. Inherited DNA-repair gene mutations in men with metastatic prostate cancer. N Engl J Med. 2016;375:443–53.
37. Brenner JC, Ateeq B, Li Y, et al. Mechanistic rationale for inhibition of poly(ADP-ribose) polymerase in ETS gene fusion-positive prostate cancer. Cancer Cell. 2011;19:664–78.
38. Han S, Brenner JC, Sabolch A, et al. Targeted radiosensitization of ETS fusion-positive prostate cancer through PARP1 inhibition. Neoplasia (New York, NY). 2013;15:1207–17.
39. Feng FY, Brenner JC, Hussain M, Chinnaiyan AM. Molecular pathways: targeting ETS gene fusions in cancer. Clin Cancer Res. 2014;20:4442–8.
40. Schiewer MJ, Goodwin JF, Han S, et al. Dual roles of PARP-1 promote cancer growth and progression. Cancer Discov. 2012;2:1134–49.
41. Wang D, Li C, Zhang Y, et al. Combined inhibition of PI3K and PARP is effective in the treatment of ovarian cancer cells with wild-type PIK3CA genes. Gynecol Oncol. 2016;142:548–56.
42. Wang D, Wang M, Jiang N, et al. Effective use of PI3K inhibitor BKM120 and PARP inhibitor Olaparib to treat PIK3CA mutant ovarian cancer. Oncotarget. 2016;7:13153–66.
43. Ciccarese C, Massari F, Iacovelli R, et al. Prostate cancer heterogeneity: discovering novel molecular targets for therapy. Cancer Treat Rev. 2017;54:68–73.
44. Grasso CS, YM W, Robinson DR, et al. The mutational landscape of lethal castration-resistant prostate cancer. Nature. 2012;487:239–43.
45. Kahn M. Can we safely target the WNT pathway? Nat Rev Drug Discov. 2014;13:513–32.
46. Takebe N, Miele L, Harris PJ, et al. Targeting Notch, Hedgehog, and Wnt pathways in cancer stem cells: clinical update. Nat Rev Clin Oncol. 2015;12:445–64.
47. Kypta RM, Waxman J. Wnt/beta-catenin signalling in prostate cancer. Nat Rev Urol. 2012;9:418–28.
48. Cristobal I, Rojo F, Madoz-Gurpide J, Garcia-Foncillas J. Cross talk between Wnt/beta-catenin and CIP2A/Plk1 signaling in prostate cancer: promising therapeutic implications. Mol Cell Biol. 2016;36:1734–9.
49. Terry S, Yang X, Chen MW, Vacherot F, Buttyan R. Multifaceted interaction between the androgen and Wnt signaling pathways and the implication for prostate cancer. J Cell Biochem. 2006;99:402–10.
50. Pantel K, Alix-Panabieres C. The potential of circulating tumor cells as a liquid biopsy to guide therapy in prostate cancer. Cancer Discov. 2012;2:974–5.
51. Frenel JS, Carreira S, Goodall J, et al. Serial next-generation sequencing of circulating cell-free DNA evaluating tumor clone response to molecularly targeted drug administration. Clin Cancer Res. 2015;21:4586–96.
52. Jiang R, YT L, Ho H, et al. A comparison of isolated circulating tumor cells and tissue biopsies using whole-genome sequencing in prostate cancer. Oncotarget. 2015;6:44781–93.
53. Punnoose EA, Ferraldeschi R, Szafer-Glusman E, et al. PTEN loss in circulating tumour cells correlates with PTEN loss in fresh tumour tissue from castration-resistant prostate cancer patients. Br J Cancer. 2015;113:1225–33.
54. Hegemann M, Stenzl A, Bedke J, Chi KN, Black PC, Todenhofer T. Liquid biopsy: ready to guide therapy in advanced prostate cancer? BJU Int. 2016;118:855–63.
55. Lallous N, Volik SV, Awrey S, et al. Functional analysis of androgen receptor mutations that confer anti-androgen resistance identified in circulating cell-free DNA from prostate cancer patients. Genome Biol. 2016;17:10.
56. McDaniel AS, Ferraldeschi R, Krupa R, et al. Phenotypic diversity of circulating tumour cells in patients with metastatic castration-resistant prostate cancer. BJU Int. 2017;120(5B):E30–44.
57. Wyatt AW, Azad AA, Volik SV, et al. Genomic alterations in cell-free DNA and enzalutamide resistance in castration-resistant prostate cancer. JAMA Oncol. 2016;2:1598–606.

58. Yap TA, Smith AD, Ferraldeschi R, Al-Lazikani B, Workman P, de Bono JS. Drug discovery in advanced prostate cancer: translating biology into therapy. Nat Rev Drug Discov. 2016;15:699–718.
59. Barbieri CE, Chinnaiyan AM, Lerner SP, Swanton C, Rubin MA. The emergence of precision urologic oncology: a collaborative review on biomarker-driven therapeutics. Eur Urol. 2017;71:237–46.
60. Goodall J, Mateo J, Yuan W, et al. Circulating free DNA to guide prostate cancer treatment with PARP inhibition. Cancer Discov. 2017;7:1006.

Molecular Basis of Neuroendocrine Prostate Cancer

39

Shusuke Akamatsu

Abstract

Although de-novo neuroendocrine prostate cancer (NEPC) is rare, with increasing use of potent androgen receptor (AR) pathway inhibitors, the incidence of treatment-related NEPC (t-NEPC) is rapidly rising. Since NEPC is an aggressive disease with poor prognosis, novel therapeutic strategies are urgently needed. Recent genomic and molecular analysis have identified key oncogenes (*MYCN, AURKA*) and tumor suppressor genes (*TP53, RB1*) to play key roles in driving NEPC. Novel in vivo and in vitro research models of NEPC were developed to serve as valuable resource to study functional relevance of the key genes in NEPC development. Upon AR pathway inhibition, these genomic alterations seem to facilitate epithelial plasticity by upregulating the genes implicated in maintaining pluripotency (*SOX2, EZH2*), resulting in development of divergent tumor including NEPC from castration resistant prostate cancer. Further understanding of the molecular biology is required to identify novel molecular targets and biomarkers that would help rescue patients from this lethal variant.

Keywords

Neuroendocrine prostate cancer · Anaplastic prostate cancer · Aggressive variant prostate cancer · Epithelial plasticity

39.1 Introduction

Neuroendocrine prostate cancer (NEPC) is a rare form of aggressive prostate cancer which grows independently of androgen receptor (AR) signaling pathway. Typically, the tumor shows small cell carcinoma morphology, expresses neuroendocrine(NE)

S. Akamatsu
Department of Urology, Graduate School of Medicine, Kyoto University, Kyoto, Japan
e-mail: akamats@kuhp.kyoto-u.ac.jp

© Springer Nature Singapore Pte Ltd. 2018
Y. Arai, O. Ogawa (eds.), *Hormone Therapy and Castration Resistance of Prostate Cancer*, https://doi.org/10.1007/978-981-10-7013-6_39

markers such as Chromogranin A, Synaptophysin, NCAM1, and NSE, and does not express AR or PSA. Clinically, it is characterized by exclusive visceral or predominantly lytic bone metastases, bulky tumor masses, sensitivity to platinum containing chemotherapy regimen, and poor survival [1]. The incidence of *de-novo* NEPC was reported to be 0.5–2% [2]. However, NEPC is also known to arise in patients who have been heavily treated with AR pathway targeting therapy [3]. This form of NEPC is known as treatment-related neuroendocrine prostate cancer (t-NEPC) [4]. The incidence of t-NEPC has been rising rapidly due to increasing use of potent AR pathway inhibitors such as Abiraterone and Enzalutamide. A recent autopsy series showed that up to 25% of the patients dying from CRPC demonstrated some signs of t-NEPC [5]. With its increasing incidence and lack of appropriate treatment, NEPC is emerging as an imminent threat to treatment of prostate cancer patients, and it is imperative to understand its disease biology and develop novel treatment strategy for this lethal disease [6].

39.2 Classification of NEPC

In 2013, a working group assembled by Prostate Cancer Foundation proposed a new pathologic classification of NEPC [7]. The new classification consisted of (1) usual prostate adenocarcinoma with NE differentiation, (2) adenocarcinoma with Paneth cell NE differentiation, (3) carcinoid tumor, (4) small cell carcinoma (SCC), (5) large cell neuroendocrine carcinoma (LCNEC), and (6) mixed NE carcinoma-acinar adenocarcinoma. In addition, CRPC with small cell carcinoma-like clinical presentation was defined as an independent entity. The word "treatment-related neuroendocrine prostate cancer (t-NEPC)" has been used interchangeably with "anaplastic prostate carcinoma" [1] and "aggressive variant prostate carcinoma (AVPC)" [6]; however, the latter two are defined entirely based on clinical factors and may encompass a broader range of AR independent CRPC. Prior to the proposal of the new pathologic classification, the clinical impact of NEPC was confounded by contradictory results [8, 9]. Since the clinical implication of NEPC other than SCC and t-NEPC is unclear, the working group recommended against routine IHC examination of prostate cancer specimen for NE markers. Currently, it is recommended that PCa mixed with NE marker positive cells be treated with androgen deprivation therapy unless the tumor shows morphologically distinct SCC [6].

39.3 Cell of Origin of NEPC

Normal prostate gland contains foci of NE cells scattered within the prostatic epithelium [7]. These cells are known to release various peptide hormones including chromogranin A, calcitonin, and NSE and affect the surrounding cells. However, in normal prostate gland, these cells are quiescent. Whether NEPC arises from these NE cells or from epithelial cells has been under long debate. Although the origin of de-novo NEPC is still not clear, recent genomic and molecular studies have shown that t-NEPC arises from adenocarcinoma by transdifferentiation [6, 10–13]. *TMPRSS-ERG* gene fusion is the most frequent structural variation seen in prostate cancer, and is reported to be observed in nearly half of PCa cases [14]. *TMPRSS-ERG* translocation is known to be an early event in PCa carcinogenesis [15]. Intriguingly, the reported frequency of the translocation is similar in t-NEPC compared to that in adenocarcinoma [16], and a recent study reported that there was a large overlap in the overall somatic copy-number landscape between CRPC and t-NEPC [13]. Epithelial plasticity is a phenomenon in which cells treated with specific molecular targeting therapy acquire phenotypic characteristics of a cell lineage whose survival no longer depends on the targeted pathway [17]. A recent molecular study has shown that *MYCN* and *AKT1* could transform human epithelial cells to both PCa and NEPC [18], and another study demonstrated that *TP53* and *RB1* silenced prostate cancer cells could give rise to both CRPC and NEPC [19, 20]. Supported by these robust genetic and molecular biology data, it is now considered that upon potent AR pathway inhibition, NEPC develops from adenocarcinoma as a result of epithelial plasticity [13].

39.4 Research Models of NEPC

Until recently, LNCaP cell line has been studied extensively as a model of NEPC transdifferentiation, since the cells start to take "neuronal" cell morphology and express NE markers under various stress including androgen depletion [21, 22] and treatments with cAMP [23–25], cytokines [26, 27], and growth factors [28]. However, the morphology of the cells is completely distinct from those of SCC, and the cells are generally slower growing than the untreated cells [29]. Even though some researchers have claimed that these cells promote growth of the surrounding cells in a paracrine manner [30], it is more likely that these cells represent quiescent NE cells seen in some CRPC specimen and not the clinically aggressive NEPC. It has recently been reported that dual knockdown of *TP53* and *RB1* in LNCaP cells facilitates lineage plasticity and some of the cells transdifferentiate into NEPC. Considering the critical role of these major tumor suppressors discussed later in this chapter, this may be a more appropriate model to study NEPC development in vitro.

To date, only one cell line has been established from clinical NEPC. NCI-H660 was initially described as a small cell lung carcinoma [31], however, later corrected to be derived from the prostate, and the cell line harbors *TMPRSS-ERG* translocation [32]. The cell line also harbors *TP53* mutation and *RB1* deletion. Interestingly, the cell line grows as floating cells similar to most other cell lines derived from SCC of the lung, and is easier to grow in vivo than in vitro. Considering the origin of the cell line, NCI-H660 represents the best model to study t-NEPC; however, its slow growth in vitro and difficulty of transfection raises the bar in terms of its use in many molecular biology experiments.

Several patient-derived xenograft (PDX) models of NEPC have been reported [33–35]. Of those, LTL-331/LTL-331R is a unique model of transdifferentiation [11].

LTL-331, which was established by grafting a Gleason score 9 adenocarcinoma from a patient into mouse sub-renal capsule, regresses upon castration, however, later regrows as a PSA negative NEPC (LTL-331R). Even though LTL-331 shows normal adenocarcinoma morphology and expresses AR and PSA, LTL-331R is consistent with SCC, does not express AR or PSA, and expresses NE markers including Chromogranin A and Synaptophysin. The rapid growth of LTL-331R is consistent with aggressive behavior of clinical NEPC, and at the transcriptome level, LTL-331R is highly similar to clinical NEPC. At the DNA level, LTL-331 and LTL-331R show very similar copy-number profile and fusion gene profile, suggesting transdifferentiation from adenocarcinoma to NEPC rather than clonal selection of preexisting minor NEPC cells. Even though the transdifferentiation from LTL-331 to LTL-331R is highly reproducible, the exact mechanism or genetic signature that predispose to NEPC transdifferentiation is unclear. Intriguingly, the LTL-331 harbors a single-copy loss of *TP53* and functional C277G mutation in the remaining allele [10]. In addition, there is a single-copy loss of *RB1*. Since dual alteration of *TP53* and *RB1* is known to facilitate lineage plasticity, and there is significant alteration in the Rb pathway genetic signature upon transdifferentiation from LTL-331 to LTL-331R, these baseline alterations of *TP53* and *RB1* may be one of the factors which predispose to transdifferentiation. To date, LTL-331 model serves as the only model of transdifferentiation.

With recent identification of key oncogenes and tumor suppressor genes in NEPC development, several genetically engineered mouse models of NEPC have been developed. Next generation sequencing studies have identified amplification of *MYCN* in NEPC [2], and a murine model expressing N-myc specifically in the prostate was generated [36]. In the model, N-myc overexpression, in cooperation with Pten knockout, resulted in large invasive prostate tumors with a variety of morphologies including foci of AR positive adenocarcinoma and SCC. This likely represents the NEPC formation as a result of lineage plasticity. Another genomic hallmark of NEPC is aberration of p53 and Rb pathway, which is also common in SCC of the lung. Conditional double knockout of Pten and Rb1 in the murine prostate resulted in development of heterogenous tumor, and additional p53 knockout conferred de-novo resistance to hormone therapy [19]. The double and triple knockout models showed gene signature similar to clinical NEPC. Overall, these genetically engineered mouse models could serve as ideal models to study development of NEPC which occurs as a result of epithelial plasticity.

A classic murine model of spontaneous prostate carcinogenesis is transgenic adenocarcinoma mouse prostate (TRAMP) [37]. TRAMP model is a genetically engineered murine model driven by conditional expression of SV40 large T antigen in the prostate, and p53 and Rb pathways are inactivated. TRAMP male mouse develops PCa with distant metastasis by 24–30 weeks of age, and subsequently some tumors progresses to NEPC, in line with lineage plasticity [38]. Cell lines have also been established from TRAMP tumors for in vitro use [39].

The research models discussed in this section are mainly for studies of t-NEPC. Currently, there is no specific model for de-novo NEPC, and whether the research models for t-NEPC could also be used to study de-novo NEPC is not clear.

39.5 Molecular Basis of NEPC

Next generation sequencing of clinical NEPC samples have opened the door to understanding the genomic and molecular features of NEPC. Here we specifically focus on the major pathways and genes involved in t-NEPC development, and how these findings contributed to the current concept that t-NEPC develops from adenocarcinoma as a result of epithelial plasticity.

39.5.1 *MYCN, AURKA,* and NEPC

MYCN and *AURKA* amplifications were among the first genomic aberrations identified using next generation sequencing of NEPC [2]. These alterations were discovered by RNA-sequencing and oligonucleotide array of a cohort of NEPC and PCa clinical samples followed by validation using a large patient cohort. The study showed *MYCN* and *AURKA* overexpression/ gene amplification in 40% of NEPC and 5% of PCa. *MYCN* and *AURKA* are oncogenes that are known to interact with each other. Interestingly, in nearly all *AURKA* amplification positive case of NEPC, there was concurrent amplification of *MYCN*. Aurora kinase A and N-myc protein interacted in vitro and enhanced Aurora kinase A stability. N-myc overexpressed LNCaP cells were sensitive to Aurora kinase A inhibitor in vitro. In vivo, NCI-H660 xenograft model was sensitive to Auroka kinase A inhibitor in contrast to LNCaP xenograft which showed no response. These findings have led to an ongoing multicenter phase II clinical trial using Auroka kinase A inhibitor MLN8237 in NEPC patients (ClinicalTrials.gov Identifier: NCT01799278). Early results showed modest response; however, two patients achieved exceptional response with complete resolution of liver metastasis. Additional biomarker to predict responders is likely to be required.

The critical role of *MYCN* in NEPC development has prompted generation of the murine model discussed above. Gene set enrichment analysis of the tumor that developed in the model showed enrichment of PRC2/EZH2 targets and suppression of AR signaling [36]. EZH2 is a component of PRC2 complex that primarily methylates H3K27 to suppress transcription and is implicated in maintaining pluripotency. EZH2 cooperatively suppress expression of N-Myc targets including AR and drives NEPC. EZH2 silencing as well as EZH2 inhibition using GSK503 restored Enzalutamide sensitivity of *PTEN* and *RB1* double knockout mouse in vivo. Another EZH2 inhibitor (GSK343) preferentially decreased the viability of NCI-H660 cells, as compared to that in other non-neuroendocrine prostate cancer cells. EZH2 inhibition may be a novel approach for NEPC treatment.

Another study showed that in primary human prostate basal epithelium, overexpression of *MYCN* and *AKT1* was sufficient to transform the cells to grow tumors in mice, and the tumor that developed showed mixed NEPC and adenocarcinoma, which also supports the concept that *MYCN* facilitates epithelial plasticity [18].

39.5.2 p53, Rb Pathway, and NEPC

p53 mutation and RB1 inactivation have been known to be one of the most common genomic aberrations in lung SCC [40, 41]. In prostate SCC, strongly positive p53 staining by IHC was observed in 56% of SCC with 60% of the cases showing TP53 mutation. Rb protein loss was seen in 90% of SCC with *RB1* allelic loss in 85% of the cases [42]. In addition, *RB1* copy number loss was identified to be the strongest discriminator between "aggressive variant prostate cancer" and unselected CRPC [43]. However, in routine clinical practice, it is difficult to examine *RB1* copy number. Therefore, the usefulness of p16 and cyclin D1 expression by IHC as surrogates for Rb pathway activity was tested [44]. As a result, expression of Cyclin D1 paralleled with loss of Rb signature, and overall, 88% of SCC showed Cyclin D1 loss by IHC compared with less than 10% in high grade PCa, confirming the usefulness of Cyclin D1 IHC as a marker of Rb pathway aberration.

Functionally, p53 and Rb inactivation collaborate to enhance epithelial plasticity, which eventually lead to development of NEPC. In vitro, dual knockdown or knockout of *TP53* and *RB1* in LNCaP resulted in increase of basal cell and NE markers and reduction of luminal cell markers [20]. Dual knockdown of *TP53* and *RB1* was sufficient to confer resistance to Enzalutamide. The study also identified that dual knockdown of *TP53* and *RB1* results in *SOX2* elevation, and that the increased expression of NE and basal markers as well as Enzalutamide resistance in these cells can be rescued with *SOX2* knockdown. These results indicate that *SOX2* overexpression upon p53 and Rb inactivation is one of the major mechanisms of enhanced lineage plasticity. Another study, using the previously discussed in vivo model of conditional knockout mouse, similarly showed that increased lineage plasticity observed upon *RB1* and *TP53* loss is conferred by increased expression of *SOX2* and *EZH2* [19]. Even though direct relationship between *MYCN/AURKA* amplification and p53/ Rb inactivation has not been clarified yet, both pathways seem to drive NEPC by upregulating genes implicated in maintenance of pluripotency and facilitating lineage plasticity.

39.5.3 AR Inhibition and NEPC

Another area of intensive research is how AR inhibition drives NEPC. A recent study identified a neural transcription factor *BRN2* to be one of the major genes that link AR inhibition to NEPC development [45]. The gene was identified using a unique panel of Enzalutamide resistant cell lines derived from serial in vivo selection of LNCaP xenografts. The panel consisted of heterogenous clones with different AR and PSA expression levels. One of the clones, 42D^{ENZR} represented NEPC, and by comparing the whole transcriptome of the panel of cells, *BRN2* was identified to be specifically upregulated in 42D^{ENZR}. *BRN2* was directly repressed by *AR*, and *BRN2* expression induced NE marker expression and promoted cell growth. Furthermore, *BRN2* regulated expression and activity of *SOX2*, again showing association between NEPC and increased lineage plasticity.

Paternally Expressed 10 (PEG10) is another gene directly repressed by *AR* that is implicated development of NEPC [10]. PEG10 is a unique retrotransposon derived gene that retains gag and pol domain [46]. Structurally, PEG10 resembles HIV virus, and has a unique −1 ribosomal frameshift sequence which enables balanced expression of gag (RF1) and pol (RF1/2) protein [47]. PEG10 integrated into the therian mammalian genome after the split with prototherians and is indispensable for placental development [48]. PEG10 RF1 promotes cell invasion through TGF-β pathway, and PEG10 RF1/2 promotes cell cycle progression in the absence of *TP53* and *RB1* [10]. The expression and function of PEG10 is tightly regulated by p53, Rb, and N-myc. Since PEG10 is a testicular antigen whose expression in normal cells is restricted to embryonal organs and neurons [49], and it has domains similar to HIV, PEG10 is potentially targetable [50].

39.5.4 Clonal Evolution of NEPC

The mode of clonal evolution of NEPC has been recently studied by whole-exome sequencing of sequential biopsies from the same patients during treatment [13]. Divergent clonal evolution, in which CRPC and NEPC cells could arise from the same CRPC clone in a divergent manner, was the most compatible mode of evolution. A recent report from SU2C/PCF/AACR West Coast Prostate Cancer Dream Team reported another distinct subtype of CRPC which histologically shows intermediate pattern between SCC and adenocarcinoma. These results are consistent with in vivo and in vitro data which supports the concept that t-NEPC arises as a result of enhanced epithelial plasticity upon potent AR pathway inhibition and additional aberrations in major oncogenes and tumor suppressor genes.

39.6 Future Perspective

Due to the rarity of NEPC and lack of suitable in vitro and in vivo models that represents clinical NEPC, NEPC was understudied until quite recently. However, next generation sequencing of NEPC samples have opened the door to understanding the genetic hallmarks of NEPC, and novel in vivo models are now at hand to study molecular mechanisms underlying its disease biology. With increasing threat of NEPC, further efforts are required to identify novel therapeutic targets and biomarkers that would lead to effective treatment of this lethal variant.

References

1. Aparicio AM, Harzstark AL, Corn PG, Wen S, Araujo JC, SM T, et al. Platinum-based chemotherapy for variant castrate-resistant prostate cancer. Clin Cancer Res. 2013;19(13):3621–30.
2. Beltran H, Rickman DS, Park K, Chae SS, Sboner A, MacDonald TY, et al. Molecular characterization of neuroendocrine prostate cancer and identification of new drug targets. Cancer Discov. 2011;1(6):487–95.

3. Hirano D, Okada Y, Minei S, Takimoto Y, Nemoto N. Neuroendocrine differentiation in hormone refractory prostate cancer following androgen deprivation therapy. Eur Urol. 2004;45(5):586–92. discussion 92
4. Beltran H, Tagawa ST, Park K, MacDonald T, Milowsky MI, Mosquera JM, et al. Challenges in recognizing treatment-related neuroendocrine prostate cancer. J Clin Oncol. 2012;30(36):e386–9.
5. Aparicio A, Logothetis CJ, Maity SN. Understanding the lethal variant of prostate cancer: power of examining extremes. Cancer Discov. 2011;1(6):466–8.
6. Beltran H, Tomlins S, Aparicio A, Arora V, Rickman D, Ayala G, et al. Aggressive variants of castration-resistant prostate cancer. Clin Cancer Res. 2014;20(11):2846–50.
7. Epstein JI, Amin MB, Beltran H, Lotan TL, Mosquera JM, Reuter VE, et al. Proposed morphologic classification of prostate cancer with neuroendocrine differentiation. Am J Surg Pathol. 2014;38(6):756–67.
8. Sargos P, Ferretti L, Gross-Goupil M, Orre M, Cornelis F, Henriques de Figueiredo B, et al. Characterization of prostate neuroendocrine cancers and therapeutic management: a literature review. Prostate Cancer Prostatic Dis. 2014;17(3):220–6.
9. Jeetle SS, Fisher G, Yang ZH, Stankiewicz E, Møller H, Cooper CS, et al. Neuroendocrine differentiation does not have independent prognostic value in conservatively treated prostate cancer. Virchows Arch. 2012;461(2):103–7.
10. Akamatsu S, Wyatt AW, Lin D, Lysakowski S, Zhang F, Kim S, et al. The placental gene PEG10 promotes progression of neuroendocrine prostate cancer. Cell Rep. 2015;12(6):922–36.
11. Lin D, Wyatt AW, Xue H, Wang Y, Dong X, Haegert A, et al. High fidelity patient-derived xenografts for accelerating prostate cancer discovery and drug development. Cancer Res. 2014;74(4):1272–83.
12. Zou M, Toivanen R, Mitrofanova A, Floch N, Hayati S, Sun Y, et al. Transdifferentiation as a mechanism of treatment resistance in a mouse model of castration-resistant prostate cancer. Cancer Discov. 2017;7:736.
13. Beltran H, Prandi D, Mosquera JM, Benelli M, Puca L, Cyrta J, et al. Divergent clonal evolution of castration-resistant neuroendocrine prostate cancer. Nat Med. 2016;22:298.
14. Mosquera JM, Mehra R, Regan MM, Perner S, Genega EM, Bueti G, et al. Prevalence of TMPRSS2-ERG fusion prostate cancer among men undergoing prostate biopsy in the United States. Clin Cancer Res. 2009;15(14):4706–11.
15. Network CGAR. The molecular taxonomy of primary prostate cancer. Cell. 2015;163(4):1011–25.
16. Lotan TL, Gupta NS, Wang W, Toubaji A, Haffner MC, Chaux A, et al. ERG gene rearrangements are common in prostatic small cell carcinomas. Mod Pathol. 2011;24(6):820–8.
17. Bishop JL, Davies A, Ketola K, Zoubeidi A. Regulation of tumor cell plasticity by the androgen receptor in prostate cancer. Endocr Relat Cancer. 2015;22(3):R165–82.
18. Lee JK, Phillips JW, Smith BA, Park JW, Stoyanova T, McCaffrey EF, et al. N-Myc drives neuroendocrine prostate cancer initiated from human prostate epithelial cells. Cancer Cell. 2016;29(4):536–47.
19. SY K, Rosario S, Wang Y, Mu P, Seshadri M, Goodrich ZW, et al. Rb1 and Trp53 cooperate to suppress prostate cancer lineage plasticity, metastasis, and antiandrogen resistance. Science. 2017;355(6320):78–83.
20. Mu P, Zhang Z, Benelli M, Karthaus WR, Hoover E, Chen CC, et al. SOX2 promotes lineage plasticity and antiandrogen resistance in TP53- and RB1-deficient prostate cancer. Science. 2017;355(6320):84–8.
21. Shen R, Dorai T, Szaboles M, Katz AE, Olsson CA, Buttyan R. Transdifferentiation of cultured human prostate cancer cells to a neuroendocrine cell phenotype in a hormone-depleted medium. Urol Oncol. 1997;3(2):67–75.
22. Zhang XQ, Kondrikov D, Yuan TC, Lin FF, Hansen J, Lin MF. Receptor protein tyrosine phosphatase alpha signaling is involved in androgen depletion-induced neuroendocrine differentiation of androgen-sensitive LNCaP human prostate cancer cells. Oncogene. 2003;22(43):6704–16.

23. Bang YJ, Pirnia F, Fang WG, Kang WK, Sartor O, Whitesell L, et al. Terminal neuroendocrine differentiation of human prostate carcinoma cells in response to increased intracellular cyclic AMP. Proc Natl Acad Sci U S A. 1994;91(12):5330–4.
24. Cox ME, Deeble PD, Lakhani S, Parsons SJ. Acquisition of neuroendocrine characteristics by prostate tumor cells is reversible: implications for prostate cancer progression. Cancer Res. 1999;59(15):3821–30.
25. Cox ME, Deeble PD, Bissonette EA, Parsons SJ. Activated 3′,5′-cyclic AMP-dependent protein kinase is sufficient to induce neuroendocrine-like differentiation of the LNCaP prostate tumor cell line. J Biol Chem. 2000;275(18):13812–8.
26. Qiu Y, Robinson D, Pretlow TG, Kung HJ. Etk/Bmx, a tyrosine kinase with a pleckstrin-homology domain, is an effector of phosphatidylinositol 3′-kinase and is involved in interleukin 6-induced neuroendocrine differentiation of prostate cancer cells. Proc Natl Acad Sci U S A. 1998;95(7):3644–9.
27. Deeble PD, Murphy DJ, Parsons SJ, Cox ME. Interleukin-6- and cyclic AMP-mediated signaling potentiates neuroendocrine differentiation of LNCaP prostate tumor cells. Mol Cell Biol. 2001;21(24):8471–82.
28. Kim J, Adam RM, Freeman MR. Activation of the Erk mitogen-activated protein kinase pathway stimulates neuroendocrine differentiation in LNCaP cells independently of cell cycle withdrawal and STAT3 phosphorylation. Cancer Res. 2002;62(5):1549–54.
29. Mori S, Murakami-Mori K, Bonavida B. Interleukin-6 induces G1 arrest through induction of p27(Kip1), a cyclin-dependent kinase inhibitor, and neuron-like morphology in LNCaP prostate tumor cells. Biochem Biophys Res Commun. 1999;257(2):609–14.
30. Deeble PD, Cox ME, Frierson HF, Sikes RA, Palmer JB, Davidson RJ, et al. Androgen-independent growth and tumorigenesis of prostate cancer cells are enhanced by the presence of PKA-differentiated neuroendocrine cells. Cancer Res. 2007;67(8):3663–72.
31. Ohsaki Y, Yang HK, Le PT, Jensen RT, Johnson BE. Human small cell lung cancer cell lines express functional atrial natriuretic peptide receptors. Cancer Res. 1993;53(13):3165–71.
32. Mertz KD, Setlur SR, Dhanasekaran SM, Demichelis F, Perner S, Tomlins S, et al. Molecular characterization of TMPRSS2-ERG gene fusion in the NCI-H660 prostate cancer cell line: a new perspective for an old model. Neoplasia. 2007;9(3):200–6.
33. Aparicio A, Tzelepi V, Araujo JC, Guo CC, Liang S, Troncoso P, et al. Neuroendocrine prostate cancer xenografts with large-cell and small-cell features derived from a single patient's tumor: morphological, immunohistochemical, and gene expression profiles. Prostate. 2011;71(8):846–56.
34. Lapuk AV, Wu C, Wyatt AW, McPherson A, McConeghy BJ, Brahmbhatt S, et al. From sequence to molecular pathology, and a mechanism driving the neuroendocrine phenotype in prostate cancer. J Pathol. 2012;227(3):286–97.
35. Tzelepi V, Zhang J, JF L, Kleb B, Wu G, Wan X, et al. Modeling a lethal prostate cancer variant with small-cell carcinoma features. Clin Cancer Res. 2012;18(3):666–77.
36. Dardenne E, Beltran H, Benelli M, Gayvert K, Berger A, Puca L, et al. N-Myc induces an EZH2-mediated transcriptional program driving neuroendocrine prostate cancer. Cancer Cell. 2016;30(4):563–77.
37. Gingrich JR, Barrios RJ, Kattan MW, Nahm HS, Finegold MJ, Greenberg NM. Androgen-independent prostate cancer progression in the TRAMP model. Cancer Res. 1997;57(21):4687–91.
38. Qi J, Nakayama K, Cardiff RD, Borowsky AD, Kaul K, Williams R, et al. Siah2-dependent concerted activity of HIF and FoxA2 regulates formation of neuroendocrine phenotype and neuroendocrine prostate tumors. Cancer Cell. 2010;18(1):23–38.
39. Foster BA, Gingrich JR, Kwon ED, Madias C, Greenberg NM. Characterization of prostatic epithelial cell lines derived from transgenic adenocarcinoma of the mouse prostate (TRAMP) model. Cancer Res. 1997;57(16):3325–30.
40. Olivier M, Eeles R, Hollstein M, Khan MA, Harris CC, Hainaut P. The IARC TP53 database: new online mutation analysis and recommendations to users. Hum Mutat. 2002;19(6):607–14.

41. Kaye FJ. RB and cyclin dependent kinase pathways: defining a distinction between RB and p16 loss in lung cancer. Oncogene. 2002;21(45):6908–14.
42. Tan HL, Sood A, Rahimi HA, Wang W, Gupta N, Hicks J, et al. Rb loss is characteristic of prostatic small cell neuroendocrine carcinoma. Clin Cancer Res. 2014;20(4):890–903.
43. Aparicio AM, Shen L, Tapia EL, JF L, Chen HC, Zhang J, et al. Combined tumor suppressor defects characterize clinically defined aggressive variant prostate cancers. Clin Cancer Res. 2016;22(6):1520–30.
44. Tsai H, Morais CL, Alshalalfa M, Tan HL, Haddad Z, Hicks J, et al. Cyclin D1 loss distinguishes prostatic small-cell carcinoma from most prostatic adenocarcinomas. Clin Cancer Res. 2015;21(24):5619–29.
45. Bishop JL, Thaper D, Vahid S, Davies A, Ketola K, Kuruma H, et al. The master neural transcription factor BRN2 is an androgen receptor-suppressed driver of neuroendocrine differentiation in prostate cancer. Cancer Discov. 2017;7(1):54–71.
46. Clark MB, Jänicke M, Gottesbühren U, Kleffmann T, Legge M, Poole ES, et al. Mammalian gene PEG10 expresses two reading frames by high efficiency −1 frameshifting in embryonic-associated tissues. J Biol Chem. 2007;282(52):37359–69.
47. Lux H, Flammann H, Hafner M, Lux A. Genetic and molecular analyses of PEG10 reveal new aspects of genomic organization, transcription and translation. PLoS One. 2010;5(1):e8686.
48. Ono R, Nakamura K, Inoue K, Naruse M, Usami T, Wakisaka-Saito N, et al. Deletion of Peg10, an imprinted gene acquired from a retrotransposon, causes early embryonic lethality. Nat Genet. 2006;38(1):101–6.
49. Okabe H, Satoh S, Furukawa Y, Kato T, Hasegawa S, Nakajima Y, et al. Involvement of PEG10 in human hepatocellular carcinogenesis through interaction with SIAH1. Cancer Res. 2003;63(12):3043–8.
50. Cardno TS, Shimaki Y, Sleebs BE, Lackovic K, Parisot JP, Moss RM, et al. HIV-1 and human PEG10 Frameshift elements are functionally distinct and distinguished by novel small molecule modulators. PLoS One. 2015;10(10):e0139036.

Gene Therapy for Prostate Cancer: Current Status and Future Prospects

40

Yasutomo Nasu and Masami Watanabe

Abstract

Prostate is an ideal target organ for gene therapy as a translational research. It has some advantages as follows: prostate is not a life keeping organ, can be approached easily by ultrasound as a routine clinical practice and PSA is a sensitive and useful tumor marker for the evaluation of clinical response.

Intraprostatic therapeutic gene transduction (in situ gene therapy) is one of the potent therapeutic options for prostate cancer gene therapy aiming at antimetastatic benefits through the generation of immune cell-mediated cytotoxic activities that affect not only the primary tumor but also metastatic lesion. In this chapter, current outcome and future prospect of prostate cancer gene therapy are discussed.

Keywords

Gene therapy · Prostate cancer · Apoptosis · Anti-tumor immunity · Cancer vaccine

40.1 Introduction

Gene therapy involves the introduction, transfer, and expression of genetic material within individual cells to treat certain disorders. The number of cancer gene therapy protocols is 1589 in April 2017 [1]. Although gene therapy is regarded as a potent therapeutic option, many scientific obstacles need to be overcome before it can become a practical form of therapy. The world's first gene therapy for prostate cancer (suicide gene therapy) was initiated in 1996 at Baylor College of Medicine in USA. Since then, the department of Urology at Okayama University has been conducting joint research. Ongoing research and development of gene therapy for castration resistant prostate cancer (CRPC) using adenovirus vector, such as suicide gene therapy (Ad-HSV-*tk*) [2] or the adenovirus-mediated expression of interleukin 12 (Ad-IL-12) and, subsequently, the REIC gene (Ad-REIC), which is an original research development from Okayama University [3], has been making substantial progress. This chapter outlines the current state, clinical development, and prospects of gene therapy for prostate cancer including research outcome at Okayama University.

40.2 Advantages of Prostate Cancer in the Development of Gene Therapy for Solid Tumors

The total number of cancer gene therapy protocols designed worldwide, until April 2017 is 1589. Among them, the number of protocols designed for prostate cancer alone is 144, which was second most to melanoma (Table 40.1). This implicates that prostate cancer can be an ideal target for the clinical development of gene therapy for solid tumors. This aspect is further summarized in Table 40.2. Prostate cancer is one of the most common types of cancers in men, and new innovative treatments are highly anticipated especially for metastatic castration resistant prostate cancer (mCRPC). Prostate is not life keeping organ like brain, liver, lung, and pancreas and functionally is not essential for aged men. Prostate can be easily monitored by ultrasound and needle insertion can be performed safely as a routine clinical practice.

Table 40.1 Current status of gene therapy for cancer: no. of worldwide protocols

Melanoma	221
Prostate cancer	144
Leukemia	135
Lung cancer	105
Brain tumor	93
Breast cancer	87
Head and neck	83
Cancer	76
Ovarian cancer	75
Colon cancer	39
Renal cancer	21
Bladder cancer	510
Others	1589
	(updated Apr. 2017)

http://www.wiley.co.uk/genmed/clinical/

Table 40.2 Prostate cancer is an ideal target for research and development of gene therapy for solid tumors

• Prostate cancer is one of the most common types of cancer
Metastatic, castration resistant prostate cancer eagerly await new treatment
• Prostate is not life keeping nor essential organ for aged men
The therapeutic ablation of the prostate is not life threatening
• Can be easily monitored by ultrasound surveillance
Prostate biopsy and gene transfer can be performed safely and conveniently
• Promoters that control gene expression are available
PSA, PSMA, Probacin, Osteocalcin
• PSA is sensitive tumor marker
Available as an extremely useful indicator of therapeutic evaluation

Specific cancer lesion can also be targeted in combination with ultrasound and MRI. Such less invasiveness has clinical advantage in case of direct injection of therapeutic material into targeted lesion in prostate. Some promoters (PSA, Osteocalcin, PSMA) which control gene expression are highly specific to prostate. PSA is available as an extremely useful tumor marker which indicates therapeutic response.

40.3 Classification of Gene Therapy for Prostate Cancer (Table 40.3)

The method of introducing therapeutic gene can be categorized into ex vivo and in vivo. The treatment strategy involves the selective induction of cancer cell death and activation of anticancer immunity. Prostate cancer is a disease caused by multiple genetic abnormalities. The main genes associated with treatment target are tumor promoting genes or tumor suppressor genes. In reality, treating cancer with complete restoration of the abnormal gene is difficult. The therapeutic effect of p53 gene therapy, which is considered as one of the main anticancer gene therapies, consists of activation of the p53 gene by gene transfer, leading to cell cycle arrest and induction of apoptosis. Suicide gene therapy is another potent choice, which causes direct apoptosis. The therapy involves the combination of herpes simplex virus thymidine kinase (HSV-tk) gene and ganciclovir (GCV)/ valacyclovir (VCV). GCV and VCV are anti-herpetic pro-drugs and can be rapidly phosphorylated into an effective cytotoxic drug by HSV-tk but mammalian thymidine kinase has low affinity with these pro-drugs. The phosphorylated drugs, which are nucleotide analog, are incorporated into DNA during cell division, leading to termination of DNA replication and cell death [2].

In vivo immune gene therapies with modified tumor cells carrying immunomodulatory cytokines such as granulocyte–macrophage colony stimulating factor (GM-CSF), interleukin 2 (IL-2), and interleukin 12 (IL-12) are also being explored.

Table 40.3 Classification of gene therapy for prostate cancer

1. Selective induction of cell death in cancer cells
(a) *Restoration gene therapy*: Apoptosis induced by cancer associated gene repair: *p53, p16, PTEN*, etc.
(b) *Suicide gene therapy*: Apoptosis induction by pro-drug activation gene
• Herpes simplex thymidine kinase (HSV-tk); Ganciclovir (GCV)
• Cytosine deaminase/5-fluroracil (CD/5-FC)
• Double Suicide Gene Therapy: HSV-tk/GCV+ CD/5-FC
(c) *Oncolytic virus therapy*: selective growth of virus using cancer selective promoters
• Oncolytic Adenovirus; Herpes simplex virus
(d) *Combination therapy*
• Gene therapy that incorporates virus growth restriction
• Gene therapy in combination with radiation therapy (synergistic effect)
2. Activation of anticancer immunity: Cytokine gene
(a) *Immune gene therapy (in vivo gene transfer)*: activation of anticancer immunity
• Granulocyte-monocyte colony stimulating factor (GM-CSF), L2, IL12
(b) *Gene tumor vaccine (ex vivo gene transfer)*
• Prostate cancer autologous cell vaccine: GM-CSF vaccine
• Allogenic prostate cancer cell vaccine: *GVAX* (GM-CSF-secreting allogenic cells)
3. Simultaneous activation of cell death and selective cancer immunity
(a) *REIC/Dkk-3 gene therapy*: next generation autologous cancer vaccine therapy
(b) *Armed therapeutic viruses*: Cytokine Gene therapy that incorporates virus growth restriction

The GM-CSF vaccine using surgically extracted autologous prostate cancer cells was originally implemented as an ex vivo gene, but the procedure proved to be too complicated. However, in a large scale clinical trial, the GM-CSF incorporated gene tumor vaccine GVAX® (Cell Genesys) was successfully implemented in cultured human prostate cancer cell lines PC-3 and LNCaP [4].

The new forms of cancer gene therapy, including MDA-7 [5] and REIC/Dkk-3 [3] gene, induce selective cell death and activation of immunity. These are the next generation of autologous cancer vaccines. Among them, REIC/Dkk-3 gene therapy is thought to be very potent. Using a safe technique for local gene vector delivery, significant therapeutic effects at both metastatic and local lesions are anticipated. For the clinical development of novel biologics, proof of concept (POC), as a method of verification in the early stages of clinical trials, is needed. Preoperative neo-adjuvant therapy using new type of therapeutic testing agent followed by prostatectomy can be one of the useful methods to create POC of testing agent [6]. Preoperative PSA response indicates direct clinical reaction and immune and molecular pathological analysis of resected specimens indicate immunological reactions precisely. Neo-adjuvant type of prostate cancer gene therapy produced a paradigm shift in gene therapy methods in exploring POC of the various type of gene therapy [6].

40.4 Ad-REIC/Dkk-3 Gene Therapy for Prostate Cancer, as a New Form of Autologous Cancer Vaccine

40.4.1 REIC/Dkk-3

The REIC/Dkk-3 gene is a tumor suppressor gene, identified independently at Okayama University, whose expression is decreased with the immortalization of normal human fibroblasts [7]. Tsuji et al. performed subtractive hybridization using cobalt irradiation on mRNA of normal fibroblasts which stopped proliferating and mRNA of immortalized fibroblasts which continued to proliferate. They showed that mRNA and protein expression profiling were significantly reduced or absent in immortalized cells. From this unknown mRNA group, the REIC gene had been identified. In addition, REIC is identical to the Dkk-3 gene of the Dkk family. The REIC gene is located on the human chromosome 11p15.1. It contains nine exons spanning over 1050 bp. The cDNA encodes a deduced 38.3 kDa protein with 350 amino acids which possess an N-terminal signal peptide, two cysteine-rich domains, and two coiled-coil domains (identical to the Dkk-3 gene) [8] (Fig. 40.1).

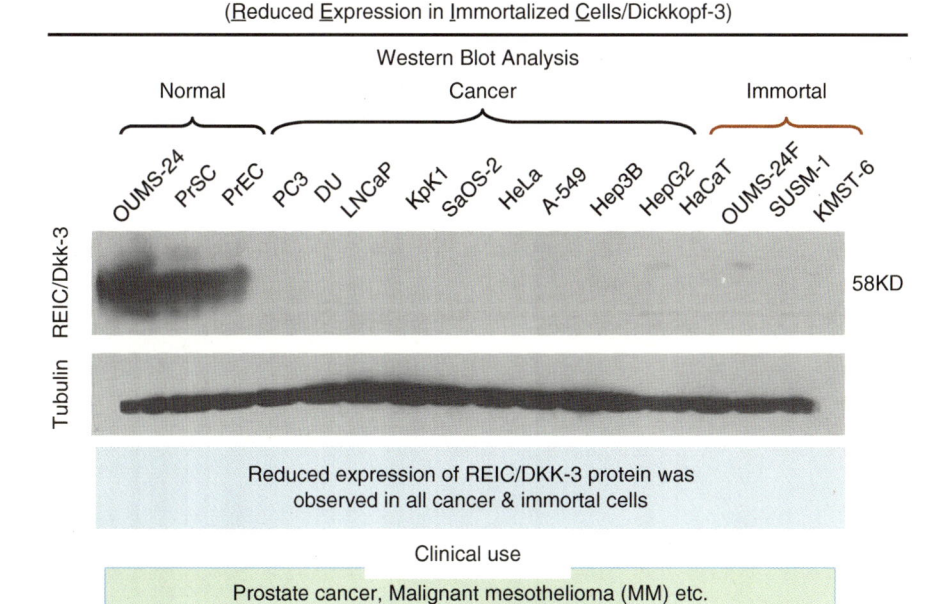

Fig. 40.1 REIC/Dkk-3 (Reduced Expression in Immortalized Cells/Dickkopf-3)

40.4.2 Mechanism of Cancer Gene Therapy by REIC as an Autologous-Cancer Vaccine

Conventionally, in gene therapy for solid tumors, techniques inducing selective apoptosis of cancer cells and activation of anticancer immunity have been studied. By using the Ad-REIC formulation (formulation of REIC gene encodes a full-length in adenovirus vector) to achieve a powerful therapeutic effect based on the strength of REIC gene expression, experiments in tumor-bearing mouse model of prostate cancer, inducing two therapeutic effects, were conducted [9, 10]. The mechanism of this synergistic effect in various cells is shown in Fig. 40.2. Selective cell death in cancer cells is due to direct cell death caused by a failure to accumulate large amounts of REIC protein folding in the lumen of the endoplasmic reticulum of cancer cells, whose REIC gene expression has been suppressed (endoplasmic reticulum stress-induced apoptosis). Mitochondrial transition of Bax and the downregulation of Bcl-2, as a result of c-jun N-terminal Kinase (JNK), have been shown to be directly involved in the molecular mechanism of cell death [11–14].

In addition, the purified REIC protein has the ability to induce differentiation of peripheral blood monocytes into dendritic cell like cells expressing surface antigen specific markers such as CD40 and CD86. Moreover, direct topical administration of REIC protein into experimental tumors showed growth suppressive effects [9]. As shown in Fig. 40.2, dendritic cell like cells for cancer antigen-membrane

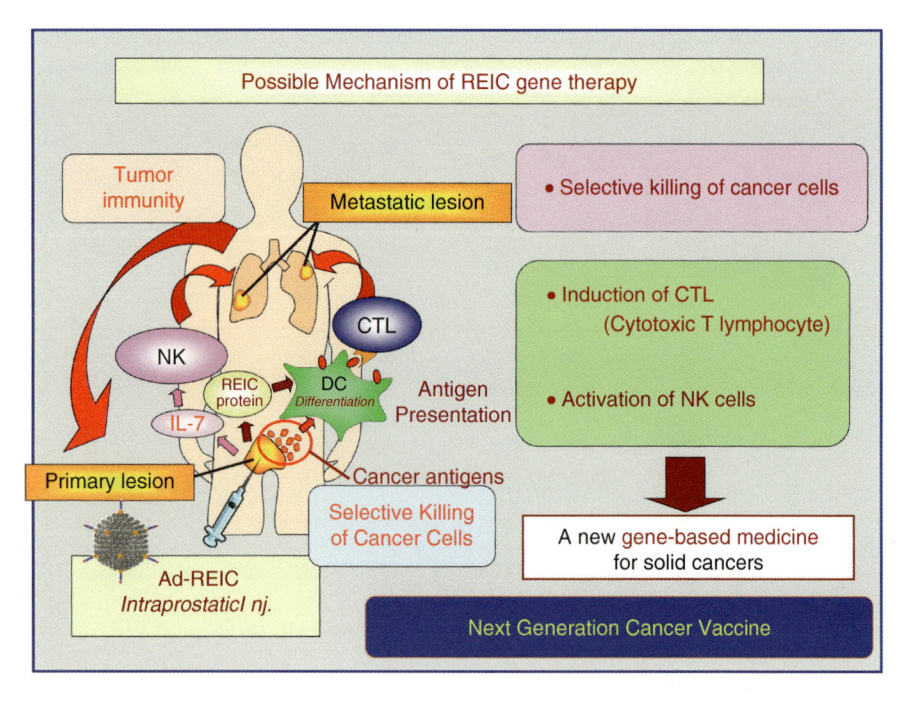

Fig. 40.2 Possible mechanism of REIC gene therapy

fragments arise as a result of selective apoptosis of cancer cells at the tumor site. And systemic activation of cytotoxic T cells is induced and can be considered as an autologous cancer vaccine. On the other hand, it has been proved experimentally that, in normal cells like stromal cells within the tumor, by transfection of Ad-REIC, IL-7 can be produced through the ASK1-p38 kinase system by activation of the stress sensor of endoplasmic reticulum (IRE1). IL-7 is a key molecule to induce anticancer immunity by the activation of NK cells [10]. The enhancing effect of these synergistic antitumor mechanisms (simultaneous T cell and NK cell activation) emphasizes the significance of therapeutic effects not only in local cancer lesions but also in distant metastatic tumors.

40.4.3 Clinical Research on Gene Therapy, Using Ad-REIC Formulation for Prostate Cancer, as an Autologous Cancer Vaccine

Based on the accumulated preclinical studies and production of clinical grade adenovirus vector encoding REIC gene, clinical study protocol was reviewed by local and national review board. After the approval by both review boards, the first-in-human (FIH) clinical study was conducted at Okayama University. Protocol consists of two categories of patient groups (A: neo-adjuvant, B: CRPC with or without metastasis) (Fig. 40.3).

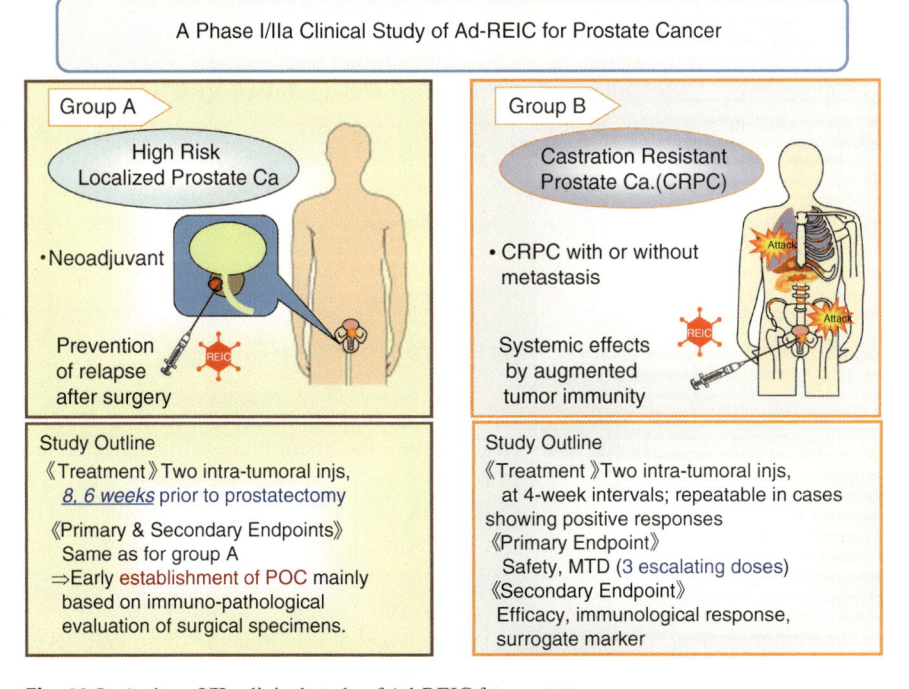

Fig. 40.3 A phase I/IIa clinical study of Ad-REIC for prostate cancer

1. *Group A : High risk localized prostate cancer (neo-adjuvant clinical research)*
   Patients with an indication for radical prostatectomy and having the probability of recurrence rate more than 35%, within 5 years following surgery as calculated by Kattan's nomogram [15], were enrolled. Patients received two ultrasound-guided intratumoral injections at 2-week intervals, followed by radical prostatectomy 6 weeks after the second injection. After confirming the safety of the therapeutic interventions with initially planned three escalating doses of 1.0×10^{10}, 1.0×10^{11}, and 1.0×10^{12} viral particles (vp) in 1.0–1.2 mL ($n = 3, 3,$ and 6), an additional higher dose of 3.0×10^{12} vp in 3.6 mL ($n = 6$) was further studied. All four DL (dose level)s including the additional dose level-4 (DL-4) were feasible with no adverse events, except for grade 1 or 2 transient fever. Laboratory toxicities were grade 1 or 2 elevated aspartate transaminase/alanine transaminase ($n = 4$). Regarding antitumor activities, cytopathic effects (tumor degeneration with cytolysis and pyknosis) and remarkable tumor-infiltrating lymphocytes in the targeted tumor areas were detected in a clear dose-dependent manner [16].
2. *Group B: Castration resistant prostate cancer with or without metastasis*
   Castration resistant prostate cancer patients regardless of the presence or absence of distant metastasis were enrolled. Ad-REIC was injected twice at an interval of 28 days into prostate or metastatic lesion including lymph nodes. After confirming the safety and feasibility of the therapeutic interventions at each escalating doses in conjunction with group A study, clinical effects were also evaluated as secondary endpoints. If clinical effect was observed and if patient desired, treatment was repeated till disease progression. Safety profile as primary endpoint was same as group A study. In addition, we experienced a case which showed dramatic response as follows: A 63-year-old man with mCRPC after docetaxel failure was successfully treated for two years with in situ Ad-REIC gene therapy. Repeated injections of Ad-REIC into metastatic LNs showed remarkable safety profiles and induced potent direct and indirect antitumor effects. Kumon et al. concluded in his case report that these dramatic results have paved the way for a new, future cancer therapeutic vaccine against a variety of intractable solid cancers [17].

40.5 Prospects of Gene Therapy for Prostate Cancer

Recently, it has been studied that blocking immunosuppressive networks and immune checkpoints bring successful immunotherapeutic modalities (so called immune-oncologic drugs: I-O drugs) for the treatment of cancer [18–21]. Theoretically combination of Ad-REIC with I-O drugs may offer a more potent strategy for the cancer immunotherapy. Therefore, in our future study it is important to investigate expression status of the I-O drug related molecules in primary tumor sites, before and after Ad-REIC treatment as well in metastatic tumor sites.

The other strategic direction of the research and development in these fields is to enhance or modify the existing methods. Creation of the next generation of Ad-REIC to enhance the function of original vector or overcome its problems is one of the key methods. Sakaguchi et al. developed a super gene expression (SGE) system and constructed new adenovirus vector (Ad-SGE-REIC) [22]. The SGE system is a new plasmid vector, developed by placing three enhancers in tandem after poly A to realize extremely high expression of the targeted REIC gene [23]. A Phase I/IIa clinical trial of Ad-SGE-REIC for localized prostate cancer is being conducted at two institutions in the United States (https://clinicaltrials.gov/). Similarly, a Phase I/IIa clinical trial for malignant pleural mesothelioma has been initiated in Japan. In addition, preclinical studies of Ad-REIC on various intractable solid cancers including pancreatic cancer [24], lung cancer [25], and malignant glioma [26] have been conducted successfully.

Currently promising clinical outcome of gene therapy including REIC gene therapy has been conducted in Japan from academic site. New innovative "seeds" can be translated to bed side as scientific "fruits" from academia through new research system in Japan. Further innovative development will be anticipated based on the understanding of cancer biology and technology for the treatment of intractable mCRPC.

References

1. http://www.wiley.co.uk/genmed/clinical
2. Nasu Y, et al. Suicide gene therapy with adenoviral delivery of HSV-tK gene for patients with local recurrence of prostate cancer after hormonal therapy. Mol Ther. 2007;15(4): 834–40.
3. Kumon H. Clinical development of gene therapy and gene medicine based on the novel tumor suppressor gene REIC/Dkk-3 (article in Japanese). MOOK 17 (Kawakami Koji). 2010; p. 132–7.
4. Galsky MD, et al. Docetaxel-based combination therapy for castration-resistant prostate cancer. Ann Oncol. 2010;21(15):2135–44.
5. Mitchell E, et al. MDA-7/IL-24: multifunctional cancer killing cytokine. Adv Exp Med Biol. 2014;818(1):127–53.
6. Sonpavde G, et al. Neoadjuvant therapy followed by prostatectomy for clinically localized prostate cancer. Cancer. 2007;110(12):2628–39.
7. Tsuji T, et al. A REIC gene shows down-regulation in human immortalized cells and human tumor-derived cell lines. Biochem Biophys Res Commun. 2000;268(1):20–4.
8. Kobayashi K, et al. Reduced expression of the REIC/Dkk-3 gene by promoter-hypermethylation in human tumor cells. Gene. 2002;282(1):151–8.
9. Watanabe M, et al. Immunological aspects of REIC/Dkk-3 in monocyte differentiation and tumor regression. Int J Oncol. 2009;34(3):657–63.
10. Sakaguchi M, et al. Overexpression of REIC/Dkk-3 in normal fibroblasts suppresses tumor growth via induction of IL-7. J Biol Chem. 2009;284(21):14236–44.
11. Abarzua F, et al. Adenovirus-mediated overexpression of REIC/Dkk-3 selectively induces apoptosis in human prostate cancer cells through activation of c-Jun-NH2-kinase. Cancer Res. 2005;65(21):9617–22.
12. Tanimoto R, et al. REIC/Dkk-3 as a potential gene therapeutic agent against human testicular cancer. Int J Mol Med. 2007;19(3):363–8.
13. Kashiwakura Y, et al. Down-regulation of inhibition of differentiation-1 via activation of activating transcription factor 3 and Smad regulates REIC/Dickkopf-3-induced apoptosis. Cancer Res. 2008;68(20):8333–41.

14. Kawasaki K, et al. REIC/Dkk-3 overexpression down regulates P-glycoprotein in multidrug-resistant MCF7/ADR cells and induces apoptosis in breast cancer. Cancer Gene Ther. 2009;16(1):65–72.
15. Kattan MW, et al. A preoperative nomogram for disease recurrence following radical prostatectomy for prostate cancer. J Natl Cancer Inst. 1998;90(10):766–71.
16. Kumon H, et al. Adenovirus vector carrying REIC/DKK-3 gene: neoadjuvant intraprostatic injection for high-risk localized prostate cancer undergoing radical prostatectomy. Cancer Gene Ther. 2016;23(11):400–9.
17. Kumon H. Ad-REIC gene therapy: promising results in a patient with metastatic CRPC following chemotherapy. Clin Med Insights Oncol. 2015;9(1):31–8.
18. Hodi FS, et al. Improved survival with ipilimumab in patients with metastatic melanoma. N Engl J Med. 2010;363(8):711–23.
19. Topalian SL, et al. Safety, activity, and immune correlates of anti-PD-1 antibody in cancer. N Engl J Med. 2012;366(26):2443–54.
20. Vanneman M, et al. Combining immunotherapy and targeted therapies in cancer treatment. Nat Rev Cancer. 2012;12(4):237–51.
21. Marabelle A, et al. Depleting tumor-specific Tregs at a single site eradicates disseminated tumors. J Clin Invest. 2013;123(6):2447–63.
22. Watanabe M, et al. A novel gene expression system strongly enhances the anticancer effects of REIC/Dkk-3-encoding adenoviral vector. Oncol Rep. 2014;31(3):1089–95.
23. Sakaguchi M, et al. Dramatic increase in expression of a transgene by insertion of promoters downstream of the cargo gene. Mol Biotechnol. 2014;56(7):621–30.
24. Uchida D, et al. Potential of adenovirus-mediated REIC/Dkk-3 gene therapy for use in the treatment of pancreatic cancer. J Gastroenterol Hepatol. 2014;29(7):973–83.
25. Shien K, et al. Anti-cancer effects of REIC/Dkk-3-encoding adenoviral vector for the treatment of non-small cell lung cancer. PLoS One. 2014;9(2):e87900.
26. Shimazu Y, et al. Integrin antagonist augments the therapeutic effect of adenovirus-mediated REIC/Dkk-3 gene therapy for malignant glioma. Gene Ther. 2014;22(2):146–54.

41 Immune Therapy for Castration-Resistant Prostate Cancer

Kazuhiro Yoshimura, Takafumi Minami, Masahiro Nozawa, and Hirotsugu Uemura

Abstract

The standard treatment for advanced metastatic prostate cancer is androgen deprivation therapy. However, for patients with castration-resistant prostate cancer (CRPC), androgen deprivation therapy is ineffective, and subsequent treatment is needed. New agents for the treatment of advanced prostate cancer, such as abiraterone and enzalutamide, have become available; however, these compounds have prolonged survival by only a few months. On the other hand, dramatic and durable treatment responses to immune therapy have been demonstrated in various cancer types. Considering these favorable clinical outcomes, immune therapy has the potential to be one of the available treatment options for patients with CRPC. Immune therapy for the management of prostate cancer consisted mainly of clinical trial investigating therapeutic cancer vaccines and immune checkpoint inhibitors, as manipulation of the immune system has emerged as a new promising strategy for cancer treatment. In this chapter, recent outcomes of these approaches are discussed in the context of future treatments for CRPC.

Keywords

Immune therapy · Prostate cancer · Immune checkpoint blockade · Cancer vaccines

41.1 Introduction

In 1941, Charles Huggins reported that prostate cancer would regress in response to androgen ablation. Since then, primary androgen deprivation still remains as the initial therapy for metastatic prostate cancer. However, the disease becomes lethal when progression occurs despite the low levels of testosterone, and is then referred to as castration-resistant prostate cancer (CRPC). CRPC includes various clinical states ranging from asymptomatic or minimally symptomatic, nonmetastatic disease to symptomatic, metastatic disease (mCRPC), and the time of progression varies for each clinical state in patients. During the past few years, the treatment options for mCRPC have changed drastically. Following docetaxel-based chemotherapy, several new agents have become available to treat men with mCRPC including abiraterone [1], enzalutamide [2], which target androgen receptor axis, cabazitaxel, a new taxane cytotoxic agent [3], sipuleucel-T [4], and radium-223, an alpha-emitting radiopharmaceutical [5]. Despite these advances, median survival for patients with post-chemotherapy mCRPC is about 2 years [1]. Furthermore, there are some patients that show primary resistance against these agents, although mechanism of resistance is not fully understood. Hence, additional treatment strategies are needed to improve survival of patients with CRPC. Immunotherapy with sipuleucel-T is the first therapeutic cancer vaccine demonstrated to improve survival outcomes in an advanced prostate cancer and provides possibilities for further investigation of immunotherapy for mCRPC.

Under these circumstances, multiple immune approaches beyond sipuleucel-T are currently under development, which include antigen-directed immunotherapies as well as monoclonal antibodies against immune checkpoints. Furthermore, combination therapies of immunotherapy and conventional therapies are also being evaluated. In this chapter, we describe the development of immunotherapy for prostate cancer and several strategies currently being investigated.

41.2 Strategies for Immune Therapy of CRPC

Generally, tumor-associated antigen (TAA) peptides derived from the tumor cells are recognized by antigen-presenting cells (APCs, e.g., dendritic cells (DCs)) which in turn present these to CD4+ and CD8+ T cells by the way of major histocompatibility complexes class-I and -II molecules, respectively. This interaction leads to the induction and proliferation of cytotoxic T lymphocyte precursors, and production of antibodies against TAAs which will then establish an antigen-specific population aimed at destroying cancer cells (Fig. 41.1).

Currently, there are two main modalities for cancer immunotherapy (Table 41.1). One is known as active immunotherapy, which includes tumor-specific antigen vaccine therapy. Cancer vaccines are usually provided with adjuvants (e.g., interleukin-2) to enhance the immune response. DC vaccines, vector-based vaccines (using engineered virus or other vectors to carry the immunogen), cell-based vaccines, and peptide vaccines are now being clinically investigated. The other approach is called passive immunotherapy which includes the use of monoclonal antibodies or adoptive transferred T cells. Immune checkpoint inhibitors such as anti-cytotoxic T lymphocyte-associated antigen-4 (CTLA-4) antibody or anti-programmed cell death-1 (PD-1) antibody, anti-PD-1 ligand (PD-L1) antibody, and specific monoclonal antibodies against TAAs are

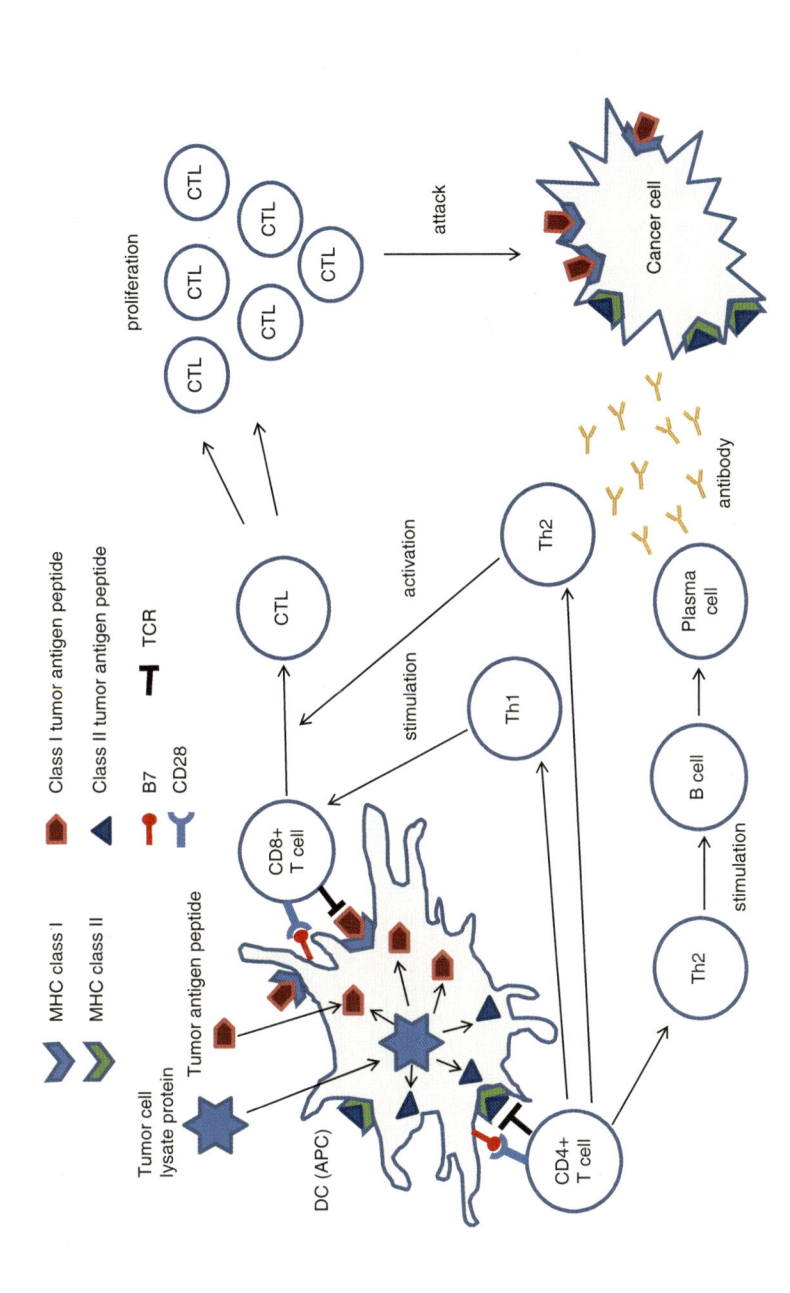

Fig. 41.1 Schematic representation of events in tumor immunotherapy. Tumor peptides presented by MHC class-I complexes are recognized by CD8+ T cells. Tumor peptides presented by MHC class-II complexes on APC activate CD4+ T cells. This interaction leads to the proliferation of cytotoxic T lymphocytes, which will then attack cancer cells. *APC* antigen-presenting cell, *CTL* cytotoxic T lymphocyte, *DC* dendritic cell, *MHC* major histocompatibility complex, *Th1* T helper 1, *Th2* T helper 2, *TCR* T cell receptor

Table 41.1 Characteristics of active and passive immunotherapy

	Active immunotherapy	Passive immunotherapy
Activation of immune system	Stimulation of the host immune system to attack cancer cells (antibodies and T cells)	Use of monoclonal antibodies or adoptively transferred T cells
Duration of response	Persist for a long period of time	Effective only while antibodies present
Specificity of response	Broad response	Prone to relapse if antigen changes
Types of therapy	Cancer vaccine therapy	Immune checkpoint inhibitors
	Dendritic cell vaccine	CTLA-4
	Vector-based vaccine	PD-1, PD-L1
	Cell-based vaccine	Adoptive T cell therapy
	Peptide vaccine	CAR T cell therapy
		Bispecific T cell engager

also being clinically evaluated. Chimeric antigen receptor (CAR) T cells therapy is one of the adoptive T cell transfer therapies, and is being explored in CRPC patients.

41.3 Antigen-Specific Cancer Vaccine Therapies

41.3.1 DC Vaccine Therapy

Sipuleucel-T is the first autologous DC vaccine approved by the US Food and Drug Administration (FDA) in 2010 and by the European Medicines Agency (EMA) in 2013 for the treatment of asymptomatic or minimally symptomatic mCRPC. Autologous APC-containing peripheral blood mononuclear cells (PBMC) of patients are harvested and incubated ex vivo for 36/48 hours with a fusion protein combining prostatic acid phosphatase (PAP) and granulocyte-monocyte colony-stimulating factor (GM-CSF). After washing the fusion protein, the product is reinfused to the patient. Sipuleucel-T contains a minimum of 5×10^7 autologous activated CD54+ DCs and various numbers of T cells, B cells, and natural killer (NK) cells [6]. In a phase III trial known as the Immunotherapy for Prostate Adenocarcinoma Treatment (IMPACT) [4], patients receiving sipuleucel-T had a significant greater median overall survival (OS) of 25.8 months compared to those receiving placebo (21.7 months). At 36 months the survival rate was 31.7% for treated patients (23.0% for those with placebo), although no significant difference was found in progression-free survival (14.6 weeks vs. 14.4 weeks). Recent studies have evaluated the efficacy of sipuleucel-T administered concurrently or sequentially with abiraterone or enzalutamide, and sequential therapy of androgen deprivation therapy following sipuleucel-T treatment (STAMP, STRIDE, and STAND study) [7–9]. In the STAMP study, the authors concluded that sipuleucel-T can be successfully manufactured during concurrent administration of abiraterone acetate plus prednisone without blunting immunologic effects or altering immune parameters that correlate with sipuleucel-T's clinical benefit. A long-term follow-up for OS is ongoing.

Besides sipuleucel-T, there are a few other DC-based immunotherapies being evaluated. Podrazil et al. reported the outcomes of clinical phase I/II clinical trial using DC-based immunotherapy (DCVAC/PCa) combined with chemotherapy in mCRPC [10]. DCs were harvested and pulsed with killed LNCaP (an androgen-sensitive human prostate adenocarcinoma cell line derived from lymph node metastasis). In this phase I/II clinical trial, DCVAC/PCa immunotherapy was demonstrated to be well tolerated and have less severe adverse events. A phase III clinical trial is ongoing to evaluate the efficacy and safety of DCVAC/PCa versus placebo in men with mCRPC in combination with docetaxel chemotherapy.

41.3.2 Vector-Based Vaccine Therapy

In 2014, Gulley et al. reported the clinical outcomes of viral-based vaccine therapy using the poxvirus as a vector [11]. This vaccine is named PROSTVAC (PSA-TRICOM), and is designed to present TRICOM (a triad of T cell costimulatory molecules) protein on APCs. TRICOM protein complex consists of PSA, B7-1 (facilitates T cell activation), LFA-3 (lymphocyte function-associated antigen 3; CD58, enhances signaling through T cell receptor for antigen), and ICAM-1 (intracellular adhesion molecule-1; CD54, cell surface adhesion molecule which plays an important role in regulating migration and activation of both DCs and T cells). In this randomized phase II clinical trial in men with mCRPC, the median OS of the PROSTAVAC treatment group was 25.1 months, whereas that of placebo group was 16.6 months. There was a significant difference of 8 months between the two groups. Furthermore, in patients who had an increase in T cell response and lower regulatory T cell (Treg) activity, a longer survival was observed. In addition, patients with less aggressive or early stage disease had greater clinical benefits in the PROSTVAC treatment group [12]. A randomized, double-blind, phase III efficacy trial of PROSTVAC with/without GM-CSF in men with asymptomatic or minimally symptomatic mCRPC (Prospect trial) is ongoing to determine whether PROSTVAC alone or in combination with GM-CSF is effective in prolonging overall survival (NCT01322490). Other clinical trials of PROSTVAC in combination with flutamide (NCT00450463), enzalutamide (NCT01875250, NCT01867333), docetaxel (NCT02649855), and ipilimumab (NCT02506114) are also ongoing.

41.3.3 Cell-Based Vaccine Therapy

GVAX is a cell-based cancer vaccine that is modified to express GM-CSF using whole autologous or allogeneic tumor cells as a source of immunogens. GVAX is composed of two human prostate cell lines, i.e., LNCaP and PC3 (androgen-insensitive human prostate adenocarcinoma cell line derived from bone metastasis), which are transfected with GM-CSF and thereafter irradiated for safety. After favorable outcomes of phase I/II clinical trial [13], two phase III clinical trials were performed to confirm survival benefits. In the first phase III trial called VITAL-1 (vaccine immunotherapy with allogeneic prostate cancer cell lines-1), comparing GVAX to docetaxel plus prednisone in asymptomatic CRPC, no significant survival benefit was shown in GVAX group (median OS of 20.7 months vs 21.7 months in docetaxel group). The VITAL-2 study, comparing GVAX with docetaxel plus prednisone to docetaxel plus prednisone alone was conducted in symptomatic CRPC patients. This study was terminated early due to increased mortality of 42.6% in the vaccine arm [14, 15]. Despite these results, GVAX is being explored in combination therapies and other tumor types [16].

41.3.4 DNA Vaccine Therapy

McNeel et al. reported that pTVG-HP, which consists of cell-free plasmid DNA encoding PAP, coadministered with GM-CSF, could elicit PAP-specific T cells in 22 patients with early recurrent prostate cancer in 2009 and 2014 [17, 18]. The therapy was well tolerated, and an increase in PSA doubling time was observed in pretreatment compared to on-treatment. Durable antigen-specific T cell responses have been observed with this DNA vaccine therapy and are associated with a greater increase in PSA doubling time (PSADT). A pilot randomized two-arm study of a DNA vaccine encoding prostatic acid phosphatase (PAP) with GM-CSF in patients with nonmetastatic castrate-resistant prostate cancer is currently underway to evaluate the therapy comparing a predetermined dosing schedule versus an adaptive dosing regimen guided by evidence of T cell immune response (NCT00849121). Another phase II clinical trial evaluating metastasis-free survival in biochemically recurrent patients with treatment with DNA vaccine plus GM-CSF versus GM-CSF is also ongoing (NCT01341652).

41.3.5 Peptide Vaccine Therapy

Peptide vaccine therapy has been explored mainly in Japan in recent years. Compared to other vaccine therapies, there are some advantages in peptide vaccine therapy. First, it is easy to manufacture peptide vaccine, and therefore could be accessible to administer to a large number of patients by mass production in clinical practice. Second, it is considerably less expensive compared to other therapies. Third, patients can easily receive personalized medicine since the combination of peptides used can be readily tailored according to clinical evaluation. In 2010, a randomized phase II clinical trial was performed in 57 patients with CRPC. They were randomized in a 1:1 ratio to receive peptide vaccine plus low-dose estramustine phosphate versus estramustine phosphate alone [19]. A significant benefit in the primary endpoint of progression-free survival (PFS) was seen, with a median PFS of 8.5 months in the vaccine group and 2.8 months in the control group. The authors reported another phase II study, in which 20 docetaxel-resistant and 22 docetaxel-naïve CRPC patients were immunized with two to four kinds of peptides selected from 31 available TAAs based on baseline host responses with enzyme-linked immunospot (ELISPOT) assay [20]. In the docetaxel-resistant group, there was a trend towards a survival benefit with vaccination, with median OS of 17.8 months versus 10.8 months in the control group. Furthermore, low levels of interleukin-6 (IL-6) in pretreatment serum were associated with more favorable OS. In 2013, it was also reported that peptide-specific IgG and T cell responses strongly correlated with PSADT and positive IgG responses and the prolongation of PSADT during therapy were significantly associated with OS [21]. A phase III clinical study is now ongoing to evaluate efficacy and safety of peptide vaccine named ITK-1, which includes 12 kinds of peptides.

Yoshimura et al. reported the clinical outcomes of a phase II randomized controlled trial of personalized peptide vaccine immunotherapy with low-dose dexamethasone versus dexamethasone alone in chemotherapy-naive castration-resistant prostate cancer in 2016 [22]. In this study, 37 patients received peptide vaccinations and 35 received dexamethasone alone. The primary endpoint was PSA PFS, which was significantly longer in the vaccination group than in the dexamethasone group (22.0 vs. 7.0 months; $p = 0.0076$). Median OS was also significantly longer in the vaccination group (73.9 vs. 34.9 months; $p = 0.00084$).

41.4 Adoptive T Cell Therapy

To induce an immune response against TAAs, other immunologic treatment strategies, such as adoptive T cell therapy, have been developed using ex vivo isolation and expansion of tumor-reactive T cells, or those engineered to respond to specific TAAs by modifying their T cell receptors (TCRs). Several studies have demonstrated promising antitumor activity using chimeric antigen receptors (CARs) T cell immunotherapy. CAR T cells are based on engineering patient's T cells, which are modified to recognize and destroy cancer cells. CARs consist of an antibody recognition extracellular ligand-binding domain which is fused to TCR intracellular signaling domain of CD3 zeta. Currently, three generations of CARs have been developed. First generation CARs had only T cell CD3 zeta chain and antigen recognition domains, while in subsequent generations, additional costimulatory molecules such as CD28, CD27, 4-1BB, ICOS, or OX40 were added to increase antitumor effects and improve survival of CAR T cells. One of the advantages of CAR T cell immunotherapy is that the recognition of TAAs is not major histocompatibility complex (MHC)-restricted, that is, there is no necessity to present TAAs as a peptide/MHC complex on APCs. Therefore, it can be indicated to all patients irrespective of their human leucocyte antigen (HLA) subtypes.

In prostate cancer, the preliminary results of a phase I dose escalation trial evaluating prostate-specific membrane antigen (PSMA)-specific CAR T cell immunotherapy have been reported [23], and the study is currently still ongoing (NCT01140373). Immune-related adverse events (irAEs) were less than grade 2 in most patients, which could be managed with conservative treatment. Cytokine release syndrome is one of the most severe irAEs also seen in patients treated with CAR T cell immunotherapy.

Bispecific antibodies immunotherapy such as bispecific T cell engagers (BiTEs®) is another promising T cell therapy. These proteins consist of binding domains from two antibodies, one of which is specific for T cells (e.g., CD3), and the other is specific for membrane-associated TAA. These dual antibodies induce the attack to tumor cells by T cells. Currently, clinical trials against solid tumors, including CRPC patients, are underway [24]. Two phase I clinical trials evaluating the safety and efficacy of BiTEs® (CD3 plus PSMA) are ongoing (NCT01723475, NCT02262910).

41.5 Immune Checkpoint Blockade Immunotherapy

Recently, immune checkpoint inhibitors have been available for several cancer types such as melanoma, non-small cell lung cancer, and renal cancer. The most well-investigated immune checkpoints are CTLA-4 and PD-1, inhibitory T cell receptors, which normally allow the immune system to maintain immunological homeostasis by downregulating pathways involved in T cell activation. However, these immune checkpoints also mediate a mechanism of tumor cell escape from immune system. CTLA-4 is expressed on activated T cells and Tregs, and downregulates T cell activation by determining the balance with CD28 signaling. Although both CTLA-4 and CD28 bind the ligand B7-1 (CD80) and B7–2 (CD86), CTLA-4 has a higher affinity to B7-1 and B7-2 compared to CD28. Therefore, anti-CTLA-4 antibodies can remove inhibition signals for effector T cells, deplete Treg activation, and restore immunological response against tumor cells. In 2011, the FDA first approved an anti-CTLA-4 antibody to treat patients with advanced malignant melanoma and several clinical trials are ongoing in several different tumor types including prostate cancer.

The other strategy using immune checkpoint inhibition is the PD-1/PD-L1 signaling axis. PD-1 has two kinds of ligands: PD-L1 (B7-H1) and PD-L2 (B7DC) which are expressed on APCs. PD-1 plays an important role in promoting immune tolerance. Therefore, the interaction of PD-1 and PD-L1 is considered to be principal mediator of immunosuppression. PD-L1 on tumor cells inhibits immune responses against tumor cells, which are associated with tumor progression. The blockade of PD-1/PD-L1 signals could recover immunological function and restore the attack against tumor cells.

It is important to also recognize irAEs when using these immune checkpoint inhibitors. Diarrhea, skin reaction, hepatitis, thyroiditis, adrenal dysfunction, hypophysitis, impaired glucose tolerance, etc. are reported as irAEs (Fig. 41.2). Generally, most irAEs can be managed with discontinuation of the agents and administration of glucocorticoid.

In the field of prostate cancer, ipilimumab, a fully human immunoglobulin G1 (IgG1) monoclonal antibody for CTLA-4, has been most evaluated in patients with mCRPC. A phase I/II clinical trial in patients with mCRPC treated with

Systemic symptoms

symptoms	suggested disorder
Pyrexia Pruritus Rash Hyper/hypotension Dyspnea	Infusion reaction after administration of the agents in 30 minutes
Pruritus Rash Vitiligo Erythema	Skin-related adverse events
Fatigue Pyrexia Chill	Interstitial pneumonia Hypophysitis Hypopituitarism Adrenal insufficiency
Hidrosis Weight loss Insomnia	Hyperthyroidism
Weight loss Thirst Polyposia Polyuria	Diabetes mellitus type 1

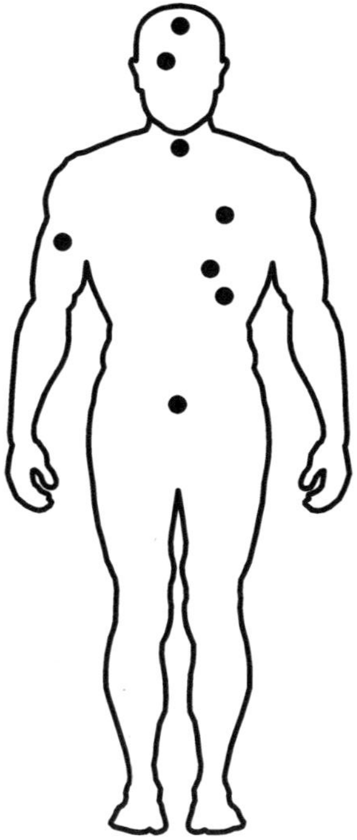

Local symptoms

symptoms	suggested disorder
Headache	Hypophysitis Hypopituitarism
Visual field defect	Hypophysitis
Consciousness disturbance	Diabetes mellitus type 1 Meningitis Encephalitis
Ophthalmalgia Eyesight deterioration Myodesopsia Photalgia	Uveitis
Thyroid swelling Palpitation	Hyperthyroidism
Cough Dyspnea	Interstitial pneumonia
Stomachache Diarrhea Melena	Colitis

Fig. 41.2 Immune-related adverse events

ipilimumab alone or in combination with radiotherapy demonstrated that some patients in combination therapy had a decrease in PSA levels achieving stable disease (SD) with one complete response (CR) [25]. After these favorable clinical outcomes, subsequent phase III randomized trial was performed [26]. In this study, single dose radiotherapy plus ipilimumab given at a dose of 10 mg/kg or placebo every 3 weeks for up to four cycles in mCRPC patients with at least one bone metastasis who progressed after docetaxel treatment were evaluated. Although the primary endpoint objective of OS was not met (11.2 months for ipilimumab and 10.0 months for placebo, HR 0.85: $p = 0.053$), PFS was prolonged in the ipilimumab group (4 months for ipilimumab and 3.1 months for olacebo, HR 0.70, $p < 0.0001$) and PSA response was also favorable in the ipilimumab arm (13.1% versus 5.2%). Moreover, post hoc subgroup analysis suggested that ipilimumab could provide longer OS of 22.7 months versus 15.8 months (HR 0.62, $p = 0.038$) in patients with better prognostic profile, such as no visceral metastases, alkaline phosphatase <1.5 times than normal upper limit, and serum hemoglobin >11 g/dL. Currently, further clinical trials are ongoing including phase III trial in chemotherapy-naïve mCRPC patients (versus placebo, primary endpoint: OS, CA 184-095, NCT01057810) and in a neoadjuvant setting (ipilimumab plus leuprolide acetate, NCT01194271).

Tremelimumab is a fully human IgG2 monoclonal antibody for CTLA-4. In a phase I dose escalation clinical trial, tremelimumab was administered with short-term androgen deprivation therapy in patients with PSA recurrent prostate cancer. A prolongation of PSADT was observed in three of 11 patients several months after completing treatment with tremelimumab. Dose-limiting irAEs including grade 3 diarrhea and skin rash were reported [27].

NIvolumab is a fully human IgG4 monoclonal antibody for PD-1. In a phase I clinical trial evaluating safety and activity of nivolumab in a total of 296 patients with various solid tumors, no objective responses were observed in the subgroup of 17 mCRPC patients, although only one patient had a 28% reduction in measurable lesions. Two of the 17 mCRPC patients involved in this study were available for immunohistochemical analysis of the tissue specimens, both of which were negative for PD-1 expression [28]. To date, clinical outcomes of PD-1 blockade monotherapy have not demonstrated adequate benefits for patients with mCRPC. Therefore, combination therapy of anti-PD-1 antibody with anti-CTLA-4 antibody is under evaluation. In regard to nivolumab, a phase II trial in combination with ipilimumab in patients with AR V7 positive mCRPC is ongoing (NCT02601014). Pembrolizumab is also a fully human IgG4 monoclonal antibody for PD-1, and is now being evaluated in mCRPC patients previously treated with enzalutamide (NCT02312557), and in combination with pTVG-HP DNA vaccine in mCRPC patients (NCT02499835).

Conclusions

Recent advances in the field of cancer immunotherapy, especially in immune checkpoint inhibitors, have led to improved clinical efficacy, even in patients with CRPC. Moving forwards, the rational combination of these checkpoint inhibitors with other agents should be evaluated, as this could potentially lead to further improved clinical outcomes for patients with CRPC. In addition to checkpoint blockade, developments in cancer vaccine immunotherapy and adoptive T cell therapy have progressed remarkably in recent years. We believe that immune therapy for CRPC is a promising therapeutic modality and will become one of the standard treatments for patients with CRPC in the near future.

References

1. Ryan CJ, Smith MR, de Bono JS, Molina A, Logothetis CJ, de Souza P, et al. Abiraterone in metastatic prostate cancer without previous chemotherapy. N Engl J Med. 2013;368:138–48.
2. Scher HI, Fizazi K, Saad F, Taplin ME, Sternberg CN, Miller K, et al. Increased survival with enzalutamide in prostate cancer after chemotherapy. N Engl J Med. 2012;367:1187–97.
3. De Bono JS, Oudard S, Ozguroglu M, Hansen S, Machiels JP, Kocak I, et al. Prednisone plus cabazitaxel or mitoxantrone for metastatic castration-resistant prostate cancer progressing after docetaxel treatment: a randomised open-label trial. Lancet. 2010;376:1147–54.
4. Kantoff PW, Higano CS, Shore ND, Berger ER, Small EJ, Penson DF, et al. Sipuleucel-T immunotherapy for castration-resistant prostate cancer. N Engl J Med. 2010;363:411–22.
5. Parker C, Nilsson S, Heinrich D, Helle SI, O'Sullivan JM, Fosså SD, et al. Alpha emitter radium-223 and survival in metastatic prostate cancer. N Engl J Med. 2013;369:213–23.
6. Small EJ, Schellhammer PF, Higano CS, Redfern CH, Nemunaitis JJ, Valone FH, et al. Placebo-controlled phase III trial of immunotherapy with Sipuleucel-T (APC8015) in patients with metastatic, asymptomatic hormone refractory prostate cancer. J Clin Oncol. 2006;24:3089–94.
7. Small EJ, Lance RS, Gardner TA, Karsh LI, Fong L, McCoy C, et al. Randomized phase II trial of sipuleucel-T with concurrent versus sequential abiraterone acetate plus prednisone in metastatic castration-resistant prostate cancer. Clin Cancer Res. 2015;21:3862–9.
8. Drake CG, Quinn D, Dreicer R, Antonarakis E, Shore N, Corman J, et al. Immune response from STRIDE, a randomized, phase II, open-label study of sipuleucel-T (sip-T) with concurrent vs. sequential enzalutamide (enz) administration in metastatic castration-resistant prostate cancer (mCRPC). J Immunother Cancer. 2015;3:145.
9. Antonarakis ES, Kibel AS, Yu EY, Karsh LI, Elifky A, Shore ND, et al. Sequencing of sipuleucel-T and androgen deprivation therapy in men with hormone sensitive biochemically recurrent prostate cancer: a phase II randomized trial. Clin Cancer Res. 2016. https://doi.org/10.1158/1078-0432.CCR-16-1780.
10. Podrazil M, Horvath R, Becht E, Rozkova D, Bilkova P, Sochorova K, et al. Phase I/II clinical trial of dendritic-cell based immunotherapy (DCVAC/PCa) combined with chemotherapy in patients with metastatic, castration-resistant prostate cancer. Oncotarget. 2015;6:18192–205.
11. Gulley JL, Madan RA, Tsang KY, Jochems C, Marté JL, Farsaci B, et al. Immune impact induced by PROSTVAC (PSA-TRICOM), a therapeutic vaccine for prostate cancer. Cancer Immunol Res. 2014;2:133–41.
12. Gulley JL, Arlen PM, Madan RA, Tsang KY, Pazdur MP, Skarupa L, et al. Immunologic and prognostic factors associated with overall survival employing a poxviral-based PSA vaccine in metastatic castrate-resistant prostate cancer. Cancer Immunol Immunother. 2010;59:663–74.
13. Higano CS, Corman JM, Smith DC, Centeno AS, Steidle CP, Gittleman M, et al. Phase I/II dose escalation study of a GM-CSF-secreting, allogeneic, cellular immunotherapy for metastatic hormone-refractory prostate cancer. Cancer. 2008;113:947–84.
14. Higano C, Saad F, Somer B, et al. A phase III trial of GVAX immunotherapy for prostate cancer vs. docetaxel plus prednisone in asymptomatic, castration-resistant prostate cancer (CRPC) [abstract LBA150]. Proceedings of American Society of Clinical Oncology Genitourinary Cancer Symposium, 2009.

15. Small E, Demkow T, Gerritsen W et al. A phase III trial of GVAX immunotherapy for prostate cancer in combination with docetaxel vs. docetaxel plus prednisone in symptomatic, castration resistant prostate cancer (CRPC) [abstract 7]. Proceedings of American Society of Clinical Oncology Genitourinary Cancer Symposium, 2009.
16. Van den Eertwegh AJ, Verslius J, van den Berg HP, Santegoets SA, van Moorselaar RA, van der Sluis TM, et al. Combined immunotherapy with granulocyte-macrophage colony-stimulating factor-transduced allogeneic prostate cancer cells and ilipimumab in patients with metastatic castration-resistant prostate cancer: a phase 1 dose-escalation trial. Lancet Oncol. 2012;13:509–17.
17. McNeel DG, Dunphy EJ, Davies JG, Frye TP, Johnson LE, Staab MJ, et al. Safety and immunological efficacy of a DNA vaccine encoding prostatic acid phosphatase in patients with stage D0 prostate cancer. J Clin Oncol. 2009;27(25):4047–54.
18. McNeel DG, Becker JT, Eickhoff JC, Johnson LE, Bradley E, Pohlkamp I, et al. Real-time immune monitoring to guide plasmid DNA vaccination schedule targeting prostatic acid phosphatase in patients with castration-resistant prostate cancer. Clin Cancer Res. 2014;20:3692–704.
19. Noguchi M, Kakuma T, Uemura H, Nasu Y, Kumon H, Hirao Y, Moriya F, et al. A randomized phase II trial of personalized peptide vaccine plus low dose estramustine phosphate (EMP) versus standard dose EMP in patients with castration resistant prostate cancer. Cancer Immunol Immunother. 2010;59:1001–9.
20. Noguchi M, Moriya F, Suekane S, Matsuoka K, Arai G, Matsueda S, et al. Phase II study of personalized peptide vaccination for castration-resistant prostate cancer patients who failed in docetaxel-based chemotherapy. Prostate. 2012;72:834–45.
21. Noguchi M, Moriya F, Suekane S, Ohnishi R, Matsueda S, Sasada T, et al. A phase II trial of personalized peptide vaccination in castration-resistant prostate cancer patients: prolongation of prostate-specific antigen doubling time. BMC Cancer. 2013;13:613. https://doi.org/10.1186/1471-2407-13-613.
22. Yoshimura K, Minami T, Nozawa M, Kimura T, Egawa S, Fujimto H, et al. A phase 2 randomized controlled trial of personalized peptide vaccine immunotherapy with low-dose dexamethasone versus dexamethasone alone in chemotherapy-naive castration-resistant prostate cancer. Eur Urol. 2016;70:35–41.
23. Junghans RP, Ma Q, Rathore R, Gomes EM, Bais AJ, Lo AS, et al. Phase I trial of anti-PSMA designer CAR-T cells in prostate cancer: possible role for interacting interleukin 2-T cell pharmacodynamics as a determinant of clinical response. Prostate. 2016;76:1257–70.
24. Klinger M, Benjamin J, Kischel R, Stienen S, Zugmaier G. Harnessing T cells to fight cancer with BiTE® antibody constructs—past developments and future directions. Immunol Rev. 2016;270:193–208.
25. Slovin SF, Higano O, Hamid O, Tejwani S, Harzstark A, Alumkal JJ, et al. Ipilimumab alone or in combination with radiotherapy in metastatic castration-resistant prostatecancer: results from an open-label, multicenter phase I/II study. Ann Oncol. 2013;24:1813–21.
26. Kwon ED, Drake CG, Scher HI, Fizazi K, Bossi A, van der Eartwegh AJ, et al. Ipilimumab versus placebo after radiotherapy in patients with metastatic castration-resistant prostate cancer that had progressed after docetaxel chemotherapy (CA 184-043): a multicenter, randomised, double-blind, phase 3 trial. Lancet Oncol. 2014;15:700–12.
27. McNeel DG, Smith HA, Eickhoff JC, Lang JM, Staab MJ, Wilding G, et al. Phase I trial of tremelimumab in combination with short-term androgen deprivation in patients with PSA-recurrent prostate cancer. Cancer Immunol Immunother. 2012;61:1137–47.
28. Topalian SL, Hodi FS, Brahmer JR, Gettings SN, Smith DC, McDermott DF, et al. Safety, activity, and immune correlates of anti-PD-1 antibody in cancer. N Engl J Med. 2012;366:2443–54.

A New Approach to Castration-Resistant Prostate Cancer Using Inactivated Virus

42

Kazutoshi Fujita, Yasufumi Kaneda, and Norio Nonomura

Abstract

Hemagglutinating virus of Japan (HVJ) is a mouse parainfluenza virus which is not pathogenic for humans, and has a cell fusion activity. Irradiation of HVJ by ultraviolet light causes the RNA genome to fragment into short RNA but still keeps the envelope intact. Resulting HVJ envelope (HVJ -E) has a cell-fusion activity but lacks a replication activity. HVJ-E fused with prostate cancer cells via GD1a, and fragmented RNA genome induced prostate cancer cell apoptosis. HVJ-E also enhanced antitumor response via dendritic cells in vivo. In a phase I/II clinical trial for men with castration-resistant prostate cancer (CRPC), HVJ-E was injected directly into the prostate followed by subcutaneous injections of HVJ-E. HVJ-E treatment for CRPC patients was feasible, and the PSA levels of a subgroup of patients responded. HVJ-E therapy could be an innovative immune therapy for prostate cancer with an acceptable safety profile.

Keywords

Immune therapy · Castration-resistant prostate cancer · HVJ

The number of men with prostate cancer is increasing in Japan, possibly due to the change of lifestyle from the conventional Japanese style to that of western countries. The estimated incidence of prostate cancer ranks first in Japanese men in 2016. Recently, a new generation of hormonal drugs and chemotherapy has begun

K. Fujita (✉) · N. Nonomura
Department of Urology, Osaka University Graduate School of Medicine, Osaka, Japan
e-mail: fujita@uro.med.osaka-u.ac.jp

Y. Kaneda
Division of Gene Therapy Science, Osaka University Medical School, Graduate School of Medicine, Osaka, Japan

to be used in clinical settings, and new drugs with different mechanisms of action are being developed [1]. However, castration-resistant prostate cancer (CRPC) remains a lethal disease, and the development of novel therapeutic approaches is still required.

Sipuleucel-T is a first-in-class immunotherapy drug for prostate cancer approved by the Food and Drug Administration in the United States. Sipuleucel-T delivers active cellular immunotherapy consisting of autologous peripheral blood mononuclear cells including antigen-presenting cells, which have been activated ex vivo with a recombinant fusion protein [2]. The fusion protein consists of a prostate acid phosphatase fused to granulocyte-macrophage colony-stimulating factor. Sipuleucel-T prolonged the overall survival of men with metastatic CRPC but not progression-free survival.

Recently, several immune or oncolytic virus therapies have been developed and evaluated in clinical trials. Immune checkpoint inhibitor therapies (anti-cytotoxic T-lymphocyte antigen-4 [CTLA-4] or anti-programmed cell death-1 [PD-1]) and antigen-specific immunotherapies (dendritic cell-based vaccines or DNA and recombinant protein-based vaccine) were tried in these clinical trials [3]. Oncolytic virus therapy is one of the new mainstream treatments for prostate cancer. The concept behind this therapy is that viruses replicate in cancer cells and kill the cells by direct cytocidal effects [4]. Adenovirus and herpes simplex virus 1 are the major viruses used in oncolytic virus therapy. These viruses were engineered to restrict replication of prostate cancer cells by the inactivation of viral genes and tumor-specific transcriptional control. However, concerns about safety still exist when using live viruses in humans, even if the viruses are engineered not to replicate in the normal cells. It is inevitable that these viruses will remain alive in the targeted cells. Inactivated hemagglutinating virus of Japan (HVJ) has drawn attention to the development of novel anticancer therapy. Inactivated HVJ particles were found to have oncolytic activity and to induce a host immune response against tumor (Fig. 42.1) [5]. Because the HVJ genome is inactivated, no replication or viral gene expression occurs in the cells infected with the HVJ envelope (HVJ-E).

42.1 HVJ-E

Sendai virus, also known as HVJ was discovered in 1953 by Dr. Ishida in Sendai, Japan. HVJ is a mouse parainfluenza virus belonging to the family Paramyxoviridae, which is not pathogenic for humans. HVJ has a negative-sense single-stranded RNA genome. Fusion protein (F) and hemagglutinin neuraminidase (HN) encoded by the HVJ genome are surface proteins of the viral envelope [6]. HN binds to sialic acid on the cellular membrane of the host cells, and then F catalyzes the membrane fusion of the HVJ-E with the host cell membrane. Fused HVJ is then able to introduce a viral genome into the host cell [5]. To exert fusion activity, F needs to be activated by a protease, but humans have no proteases for the activation of F [7]. Thus, HVJ cannot replicate in human cells. Irradiation of HVJ by ultraviolet (UV) light causes the RNA genome to fragment into short RNA but still keeps the envelope intact. The resulting HVJ-E has a cell-fusion activity but lacks a replication

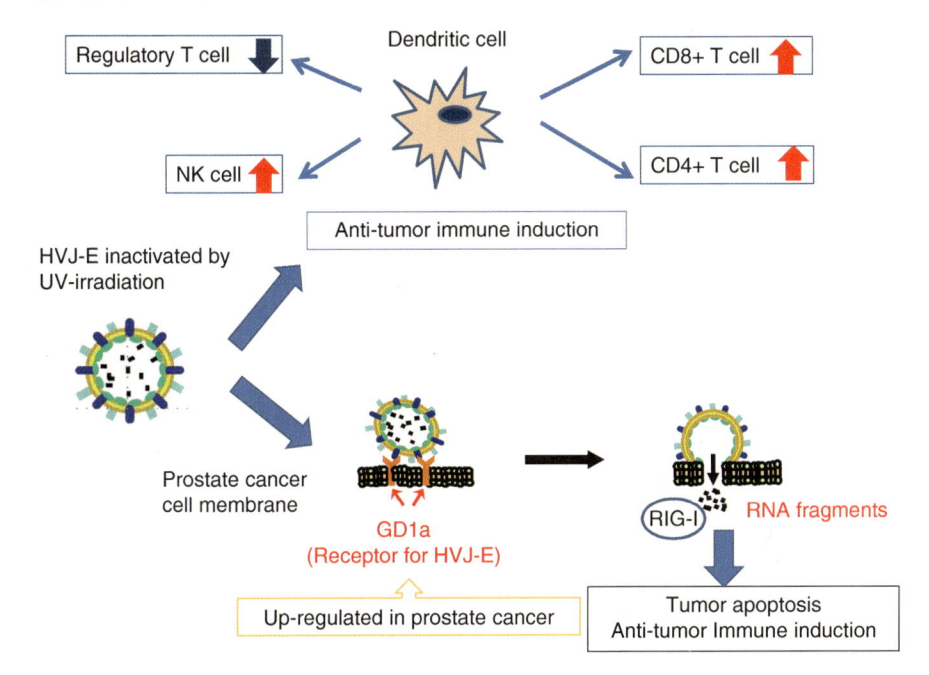

Fig. 42.1 Mechanisms of HVJ-E therapy. HVJ was inactivated by UV irradiation, and the RNA genome was fragmented. HVJ-E enhanced antitumor response via dendritic cells. HVJ-E also fused with prostate cancer cells via GD1a, and fragmented RNAs induced prostate cancer cell apoptosis. NK cell, natural killer cell; RIG-I, retinoic acid-inducible gene-I

activity. Using this fusion activity of HVJ, inactivated HVJ can be used for the delivery of DNA, RNA, proteins, and drugs. An HVJ liposome was constructed by combining a DNA-loaded liposome with inactivated HVJ particles to deliver the DNA in vitro and in vivo [8]. HVJ-E itself without liposomes serves as a vector for gene and drug delivery. Plasmid DNA can also be incorporated into HVJ-E by treatment with mild detergent and centrifugation.

42.2 Antitumor Immune Induction by HVJ-E

Injection of HVJ-E into xenografted murine colon tumor in syngeneic BALB/c mice dramatically eradicated the colon cancer [9]. HVJ-E induced significant infiltration of dendritic cells, CD4+ T cells and CD8+ T cells into the tumor tissues. Cytotoxic T cells were activated in a CD4 + CD25- T-cell-dependent manner. Interleukin 6 (IL-6) produced by HVJ-E-stimulated dendritic cells rescued CD4 + CD25- effector T-cell proliferation suppressed by Foxp3+ CD4+ CD25+ regulatory T cells. Carbohydrate of F protein on the HVJ-E was recognized by the dendritic cells and induced the signal for IL-6 production via NF-κB activation in these cells. HVJ-E alone can eradicate tumors by inducing an antitumor immune response and can simultaneously suppress regulatory T cells [10]. In a mouse model of murine renal cancer (Renca), HVJ-E injection into tumor induced expression of CXCL10 by dendritic cells in the tumor, and CXCL10 promoted the infiltration and activation of natural killer T cells (NK cells). NK cells were also activated by type I interferon released from the HVJ-E-stimulated dendritic cells. In this Renca mouse model, intratumoral injection of HVJ-E suppressed Renca tumor growth in vivo, which was abolished by NK cell depletion [11]. Fragmented RNA genomes of HVJ-E are also recognized by cytoplasmic RNA receptor, retinoic acid-inducible gene-I (*RIG-I*), and induce the production of interferon β [12].

42.3 Tumor Killing by HVJ-E

HVJ-E can also exert a direct killing effect on specific tumors. When HVJ-E was added to the cell culture of PC3, DU145, LNCaP, and PNT2 cells, the viability of PC3 and DU145 was significantly suppressed in a dose-dependent manner, but not that of LNCaP and PNT2. HVJ fused with the cell membrane by attaching with ganglioside GD1a and sialyl paragloboside (SPG) [13]. PC3, DU145, and PNT2 had higher amounts of GD1a and SPG compared with LNCaP. Fusion of PC3 and DU145 with the HVJ-E resulted in apoptosis with the activation of caspase-8 and -9, but HVJ-E could not fuse with LNCaP cells. GD1a is synthesized from GM1 by α2,3 sialyltransferase (ST3Gal) I and mainly by ST3Gal II. The enzyme that synthesizes SPG is ST3Gal VI. The increased expression of GD1a and SPG in CRPC cells was associated with the high expression of ST3Gal II and VI, respectively [14]. NF-κB, mainly RelB, mediates the production of GD1a by the transcriptional control of ST3Gal I and II. GD1a expression was confirmed in prostate cancer cells in specimens from both radical prostatectomy and biopsy of CRPC. One of the mechanisms of inducing the apoptosis of prostate cancer cells is the induction of type I interferon. The fragmented RNA genome of HVJ-E entering into the cytoplasm of PC3 and DU145 is recognized by RIG-I, and then several transcription factors, including IRF3, IRF7, and NF-κB, are activated. These transcription factors induce the expression of type I interferons, which are secreted from the prostate cancer cells and bound to their own surface receptor, resulting in the activation of the Jak-Stat signaling pathway. JAK2/STAT1 signaling activates caspase 8 transcription [15]. PNT2 cells can be fused with HVJ-E via GD1a and SPG, but type I interferons are not secreted from PNT2 cells. When HVJ-E was directly injected into an intradermal tumor of PC3 in SCID mice, a marked reduction in the tumor was observed, and even with the blockade of NK cell function with anti-asialo GM1 antibody, HVJ-E injection could still suppress the intradermal tumor growth.

42.4 Clinical Application of HVJ-E Treatment

Based on the results in vitro and in vivo, a phase I/II clinical trial was performed to assess the safety and efficacy of intratumoral and subcutaneous injection of HVJ-E in CRPC [16]. Seven patients with CRPC who were docetaxel resistant or could not receive docetaxel treatment were enrolled in this study. HVJ was irradiated by treatment with β-propiolactone and UV irradiation, which caused the alkylation and fragmentation of the RNA genome. Clinical-grade HVJ-E was purified by four steps of column chromatography, stabilized by lyophilization, and then stored at 4 °C. The lyophilized HVJ-E was dissolved in distilled water for injection. HVJ-E was injected directly into the prostate on day 1 with the aid of transrectal ultrasound and subcutaneously on days 5, 8, and 12 in two 28-day treatment cycles. The protocol was based on the mechanisms of HVJ-E; HVJ-E injection to the prostate could induce the apoptosis of prostate cancer cells and the antitumor immune response, and subcutaneous injection of HVJ-E could augment the antitumor immune response. Six patients completed the two cycles of HVJ-E treatments. One patient retracted consent after one cycle of HVJ-E treatment due to the progression of disease. The primary endpoints of the safety and feasibility were accomplished. Grade 2 or 3 adverse events (CTCAE Ver. 4.0) were urinary retention and lymphopenia from which the patients recovered spontaneously. Erythema at the injection site (grade 1) was observed in all patients, whereas pyrexia (grade 1) was observed in 57% of them. No grade 4 adverse events were observed. Among the six patients who completed the two cycles of HVJ-E treatment, a decline in the PSA level from 14 ng/mL to 1.9 ng/mL at the end of the two cycles of treatment was found in one patient, the PSA level remained unchanged in one patient, and the other four patients experienced elevation of their PSA levels. The responding patient was 83 years old with bone metastasis and had previously received hormonal therapy, docetaxel treatment, and steroid. The PSA response rate to HVJ-E treatments was 16.6%. Radiographically, four patients had stable disease and two had progressive disease. HVJ-E treatment for CRPC patients was feasible, and the PSA levels of a subgroup of patients responded. Phase I/II clinical trials were also performed for patients with advanced malignant melanoma (UMIN000002376) and patients with chemotherapy-resistant malignant pleural mesothelioma (UMIN000019345).

42.5 Future Directions of HVJ-E Therapy

The recent development of immune checkpoint inhibitors, anti-PD1 antibody or anti-CTLA4 antibody, is opening up new avenues for treating CRPC. The anti-PD-1 antibody nivolumab was administered to 17 patients with CRPC, but no objective responses were observed [17]. The expressions of PD-1 ligand (PD-L1) were immunohistochemically analyzed in 2 of 17 patients with CRPC, and the 2 CRPCs were negative for PD-L1 expression. PD-L1 expression was significantly correlated with an objective clinical response in non-small cell lung cancer and renal cell carcinoma. In contrast, 10 patients with metastatic CRPC who were resistant to enzalutamide were treated with the anti-PD-1 antibody pembrolizumab with enzalutamide, and 3 patients showed a rapid reduction in PSA [18]. Immunohistochemical analysis of baseline biopsy specimens of these responding patients showed the presence of CD3+, CD8+, and DC163+ leukocyte infiltrates and PD-L1 expressions. A phase I/II study of ipilimumab in combination with radiotherapy showed that among 50 patients with metastatic CRPC, 8 patients experienced a decline in PSA of >50%, one had a complete response, and 6 had stable disease [19]. Because the direct injection of HVJ-E into the prostate could induce an antitumor immune response, the combination of HVJ-E treatment with an immune checkpoint inhibitor might be more efficient. Because small anticancer molecules can be loaded inside HVJ-E, it has the potential for combinational immunotherapy with other agents. HVJ-E carrying the IL-2 gene inside the particles (HVJ-E/IL-2) was administered in a mouse model of angiosarcoma by intratumoral injection, which induced the local accumulation of CD8+ T cells and NK cells and reduced regulatory T cells in regional lymph nodes, resulting in inhibition of the growth of angiosarcoma cells [20].

Conclusions

HVJ-E offers a unique mechanism of prostate cancer treatment different from oncolytic virus therapy. Although only a subgroup of patients with CRPC showed a PSA response, HVJ-E therapy could be an innovative immune therapy for prostate cancer with an acceptable safety profile. Further studies to determine the selection of patients who will benefit from HVJ-E therapy and the optimum protocols of HVJ-E administration are necessary.

References

1. Fujimoto N. Novel agents for castration-resistant prostate cancer: early experience and beyond. Int J Urol. 2016;23:114–21.
2. Kantoff PW, Higano CS, Shore ND, Berger ER, Small EJ, Penson DF, et al. Sipuleucel-T immunotherapy for castration-resistant prostate cancer. N Engl J Med. 2010;363:411–22.
3. Drake CG. Prostate cancer as a model for tumour immunotherapy. Nat Rev Immunol. 2010;10:580–93.
4. Taguchi S, Fukuhara H, Homma Y, Todo T. Current status of clinical trials assessing oncolytic virus therapy for urological cancers. Int J Urol. 2017;24:342–51.
5. Saga K, Kaneda Y. Oncolytic Sendai virus-based virotherapy for cancer: recent advances. Oncol Virother. 2015;4:141–7.
6. Curran J, Kolakofsky D. Replication of paramyxoviruses. Adv Virus Res. 1999;54:403–22.
7. Asano A, Asano K. Viral proteins in cell fusion. Tokai J Exp Clin Med. 1982;7(Suppl):193–6.
8. Kaneda Y, Saeki Y, Morishita R. Gene therapy using HVJ-liposomes: the best of both worlds? Mol Med Today. 1999;5:298–303.
9. Suzuki H, Kurooka M, Hiroaki Y, Fujiyoshi Y, Kaneda Y. Sendai virus F glycoprotein induces IL-6 production in dendritic cells in a fusion-independent manner. FEBS Lett. 2008;582(9):1325.
10. Kurooka M, Kaneda Y. Inactivated Sendai virus particles eradicate tumors by inducing immune responses through blocking regulatory T cells. Cancer Res. 2007;67:227–36.
11. Fujihara A, Kurooka M, Miki T, Kaneda Y. Intratumoral injection of inactivated Sendai virus particles elicits strong antitumor activity by enhancing local CXCL10 expression and systemic NK cell activation. Cancer Immunol Immunother. 2008;57:73–84.
12. Kato H, Takeuchi O, Sato S, Yoneyama M, Yamamoto M, Matsui K, et al. Differential roles of MDA5 and RIG-I helicases in the recognition of RNA viruses. Nature. 2006;441:101–5.
13. Sadler AJ, Williams BR. Interferon-inducible antiviral effectors. Nat Rev Immunol. 2008;8:559–68.

14. Hatano K, Miyamoto Y, Nonomura N, Kaneda Y. Expression of gangliosides, GD1a, and sialyl paragloboside is regulated by NF-κB-dependent transcriptional control of α2,3-sialyltransferase I, II, and VI in human castration-resistant prostate cancer cells. Int J Cancer. 2011;129:1838–47.
15. Li L, Zhang J, Jin B, Block ER, Patel JM. Nitric oxide upregulation of caspase-8 mRNA expression in lung endothelial cells: role of JAK2/STAT-1 signaling. Mol Cell Biochem. 2007;305:71–7.
16. Fujita K, Nakai Y, Kawashima A, Ujike T, Nagahara A, Nakajima T, et al. Phase I/II clinical trial to assess safety and efficacy of intratumoral and subcutaneous injection of HVJ-E to castration resistant prostate cancer patients. Cancer Gene Ther. 2017;24(7):277–81.
17. Topalian SL, Hodi FS, Brahmer JR, Gettinger SN, Smith DC, McDermott DF, et al. Safety, activity, and immune correlates of anti-PD-1 antibody in cancer. N Engl J Med. 2012;366:2443–54.
18. Graff JN, Alumkal JJ, Drake CG, Thomas GV, Redmond WL, Farhad M, et al. Early evidence of anti-PD-1 activity in enzalutamide-resistant prostate cancer. Oncotarget. 2016;7:52810–7.
19. Slovin SF, Higano CS, Hamid O, Tejwani S, Harzstark A, Alumkal JJ, et al. Ipilimumab alone or in combination with radiotherapy in metastatic castration-resistant prostate cancer: results from an open-label, multicenter phase I/II study. Ann Oncol. 2013;24:1813–21.
20. Takehara Y, Satoh T, Nishizawa A, Saeki K, Nakamura M, Masuzawa M, et al. Anti-tumor effects of inactivated Sendai virus particles with an IL-2 gene on angiosarcoma. Clin Immunol. 2013;149:1–10.

Patient-Reported Outcome in the Management of CRPC

Nobuaki Matsubara

Abstract

Symptom information is usually collected using patient-reported outcome (PRO) standardized questionnaires. However, there is a discordance between adverse event (AE) and PRO. Because, the current oncology practice for adverse event is based on the implicit assumption that an accurate portrait of patient' subjective experiences can be provided by oncologists' documentation alone. Prostate cancer working group 3 (PCWG3) mentioned the importance of patient-centered drug development and reporting the patient experience on study. Not only clinical trial but also clinical practice, measurement, and collection of PROs are important. Surprising results were presented at ASCO 2017 annual meeting as plenary session. In this study, patients in the PRO study arm were associated with prolonged survival compared with the standard care without these assessments. These results suggested that collecting PROs timely and correctively improves not only QoL but also survival.

Recently, attention is paid in patient preference when treatment decision-making. We also introduce the patient preference study using a discrete-choice experiment method in Japanese patients with metastatic castration-resistant prostate cancer.

Keywords

Patient-reported outcome · Quality of life · patient preference · Castration-resistant prostate cancer

N. Matsubara, M.D.
Department of Breast and Medical Oncology, National Cancer Center Hospital, Chiba, Japan
e-mail: nmatsuba@east.ncc.go.jp

43.1 Introduction

Symptom management is a groundwork of clinical care, especially for incurable, metastatic, and recurrent oncology situations [1]. Almost all oncologists are already aware of the importance of symptom management and are also aware of the difficulty of the systematic collection of symptom information. Symptom information is usually collected using patient-reported outcome (PRO) standardized questionnaires. Collecting PRO itself has been suggested as an approach to improve symptom control [2, 3]. However, several prospective and retrospective investigations reported a discordance between physician-reported outcomes and PROs [4, 5]. In other words, there is a discordance between adverse event (AE) and quality of life (QoL). Because, the current oncology practice for adverse event is based on the implicit assumption that an accurate portrait of patient' subjective experiences can be provided by oncologists' documentation alone.

Results of a recent trial comparing OS in metastatic patients undergoing chemotherapy randomized to the collection of PRO data versus routine care demonstrated surprising data [6]. In this study, patients in the PRO study arm were associated with prolonged survival compared with the standard care without these assessments.

In the area of prostate cancer treatment, several expert reviews, including prostate cancer working group 3 (PCWG3), mentioned the importance of patient-centered drug development and reported the patients' experience on study [7, 8]. Taken together, these data demonstrate the increasing importance and clinical relevance of monitoring PROs.

Patient's voice for treatment decision-making, in other words patient's preference, is also important in the situation of several treatment options existing without randomized trial of head-to-head comparison. For example, abiraterone acetate, enzalutamide, docetaxel, and radium-223 are available and effective treatment option as first-line treatment for patients with metastatic castration-resistant prostate cancer. However, there are no reliable predictive biomarkers and no head-to-head trial of direct comparison between these agents. The decision-making is difficult for physicians and patients.

There are several patterns of decision-making of medical care, such as simple consent, informed consent, and shared decision-making [9]. This review mentioned that physicians need to use them properly at the medical situations, and authors concluded that shared decision-making is most appropriate for incurable oncology practice. In an extensive review of patient preferences and decision-making aids in the context of prostate cancer, Aning and colleagues reiterated the importance of medical care that seeks to adopt shared decision-making and aligns treatment decisions with patient goals and values [10].

In this chapter, we review and discuss the evidences of PRO and patient preference in patients with castration-resistant prostate cancer (CRPC).

43.2 Review of Evidences of PROs in mCRPC

Recently, reflecting an increasing focus on a patient-centric review, PRO to chemotherapy-related toxicity evaluation has been growing [11]. In new agents for mCRPC treatment, PROs have been measured using established QoL scoring system in the registration trials and already reported [12–15]. Table 43.1 shows the

Table 43.1 PROs of recent registration trials

Trial	Agent	Comparator	PRO	Pain
COU-AA-302 [12]	Abiraterone	Prednisone	FACT-P	BPI-SF
PREVAIL [13]	Enzalutamide	Placebo	FACT-P	BPI-SF
			EQ-5D	
ALSYMPCA [14]	Radium-223	Placebo	FACT-P	No measurement
			EQ-5D	
TAX-327 [15]	Docetaxel	Placebo	FACT-P	PPI scale

BPI-SF Brief Pain Inventory Short Form, *FACT-P* Functional Assessment of Cancer Therapy-Prostate, *EQ-5D* EuroQoL 5 Dimension, *PPI* present pain intensity

PRO of the registration trial of new agents. Using PROs and endpoints for evaluations were slightly different between the trials. It makes a little difficult to compare the outcomes between trials.

PCWG3 mentioned the importance of PRO in the clinical trial in order to evaluate value of agents, and several recommendation of selecting PROs. The summary of PCWG3 associated with PRO2 is shown in Table 43.2. Pain is the most established PRO in the population and is associated with inferior survival and diminished quality of life. A baseline assessment uses serial measurements, including pain intensity, pain interference with activities, and opiate intake, over several days before starting treatment, using methods described by the US Food and Drug Administration. PCWG3 supports that pain palliation requires a patient population with clinically meaningful pain at baseline (e.g., ≥ 4 on a 10-point pain intensity scale) and a response at subsequent time point (e.g., a 30% relative or 2-point absolute improvement from baseline at 12 weeks, confirmed at least 2 weeks later, without an overall increase in opiate use).

PCWG3 also recommended that physical function should also be assessed and can be measured at baseline and during treatment using an established multi-item questionnaire, such as the physical function measure of the European Organisation for Research and Treatment of Cancer Quality of Life Questionnaire C30 (EORTC QoL-Q30) or Patient-Reported Outcomes Measurement Information System (PROMIS) instruments. Time to deterioration of physical function and/or QoL scores should also be included, with a priori thresholds defining clinically meaningful deterioration score changes that are based on prior published data for the selected questionnaire.

Not only clinical trial but also clinical practice, measurement, and collection of PROs are important. Recently, surprising results were presented at ASCO 2017 annual meeting as plenary session. Results of a recent trial comparing OS in metastatic patients undergoing chemotherapy, including mCRPC patients, were randomized to the collection of PRO data versus routine care. The concept of this study was to evaluate the outcome of monitoring PRO data that allowed for proactive clinical interventions versus usual care with no PRO collection. In this study, patients in the PRO study arm were associated with prolonged survival compared with the standard care without these assessments (median OS 31.2 months vs. 26.0 months, respectively; $p = 0.03$) [6]. These results suggested that collecting PROs timely and correctively improves not only QoL but also survival. In other words, these data tell oncologists that we have to pay more attention to PROs, "patients' voice," in daily clinical practice.

Table 43.2 The summary of PCWG3 associated with PROs

Standard Baseline Disease Assessments Recommendation
Pain assessment, opiate analgesia consumption, physical functioning (functional status), health-related quality of life; consider fatigue and PRO-CTCAE. Validated PRO instrument strongly recommended
Criteria for Progression at Trial Entry by Disease Manifestation
For pain palliation analysis, presence of clinically meaningful pain at baseline (e.g., ≥4 on a 10-point pain intensity scale) is a prerequisite; for pain progression analysis, patients may have any level of pain at baseline, including no pain
Suggested Frequency of Assessment for Commonly Used Measures in mCRPC Trials
PROs: By cycle (every 3–4 weeks)
Analgesic consumption (opioids/No opioids): By cycle (every 3–4 weeks)
Suggested Outcome Measures for Clinical Trials in mCRPC: Report by Disease Manifestation
Pain palliation assessment required a patient population with clinically meaningful pain at baseline (e.g., ≥4 on a 10-point pain intensity scale) and response defined as a clinically meaningful score improvement at a subsequent time point (e.g., a 30% relative or 2-point absolute improvement from baseline at 12 weeks, confirmed at least 2 weeks later, without an overall increase in opiate use)
For control/relieve/eliminate end points:
Serial (e.g., daily × 7days) assessment at each time point can improve the stability of values. Principles may be extended for any PRO for which a clinically meaningful baseline PRO score has been determined together with a responder definition that is based on a sustained clinically meaningful score improvement
For delay/prevent end points:
Patients with any level of baseline pain, including no pain, are eligible to be evaluated for prevent/delay end points; those without pain are followed for development of pain, whereas those with baseline pain are followed for progression (e.g., a 2-point increase without an overall decrease in opiate use)
Pain assessment should be administered at treatment discontinuation and once again if feasible (e.g., 2–4 weeks later)
Time to deterioration of physical function and/or HRQoL scores should also be included, with a priori thresholds defining clinically meaningful deterioration score changes that are based on prior published data for the selected questionnaire

PRO-CTCAE patient-reported outcomes version of the common terminology criteria for adverse events, *HRQoL* health-related quality of life

43.3 Review of Evidences of Patient Preferences in mCRPC

A recent research has suggested that patient preferences, in the context of breast cancer, possess implications for adherence, persistence, and follow-up care [16]. This research indicated that if patient preferences and prescribed treatment regimens are misaligned, patients could be at an increased risk for discontinuation and nonadherence, which could affect symptom management and survival. In the situation of treatment decision, patient preference is very important, without exception for mCRPC.

Studies from the United States and Europe have been concluded to explore patient preferences among patients with mCRPC having bone metastasis [17,

18]. The results of these studies suggested that patients place substantial value on the delay of bone complications and skeletal-related events. In one study, patients were willing to sacrifice from 3 to 5 months of survival in the interest of avoiding them [17].

These data are surprising for oncologist, because oncologist is usually interested in the prolongation of overall survival. On the other hand, patients do not always focus on overall survival when they have decided treatment decision. Oncologists have to mention patient preference in order to avoid the "silent misdiagnosis."

Last year, we have completed and published patient preference study for treatment of CRPC in Japan [19]. The primary objective of this study was to fill this important gap in the literature by enhancing the understanding of treatment preference among Japanese patients with CRPC using a discrete-choice experiment (DCE). The findings from this study could relate that Japanese patients with CRPC primarily value the risk of fatigue and reduction in the risk of bone pain when considering potential treatment options for their CRPC (Fig. 43.1). These results also suggested that Japanese patients with CRPC place considerable value on their symptom experience when expressing a treatment preference. In other words, Japanese patients with CRPC were more concerned about reduced QoL derived from drug-induced side effects than extension of overall survival, which may impact shared decision-making between patients and oncologists. Our results help to provide insight into the patient experience with CRPC treatments in Japan. Recently, statement paper from American Society of Clinical Oncology reinforced the importance of capturing the patient perspective in defining the value of a treatment option in oncology [20]. Because preference can be unique to each patient, it is important to present the various clinical benefits and risks to ensure patients are kept informed throughout the treatment decision-making process.

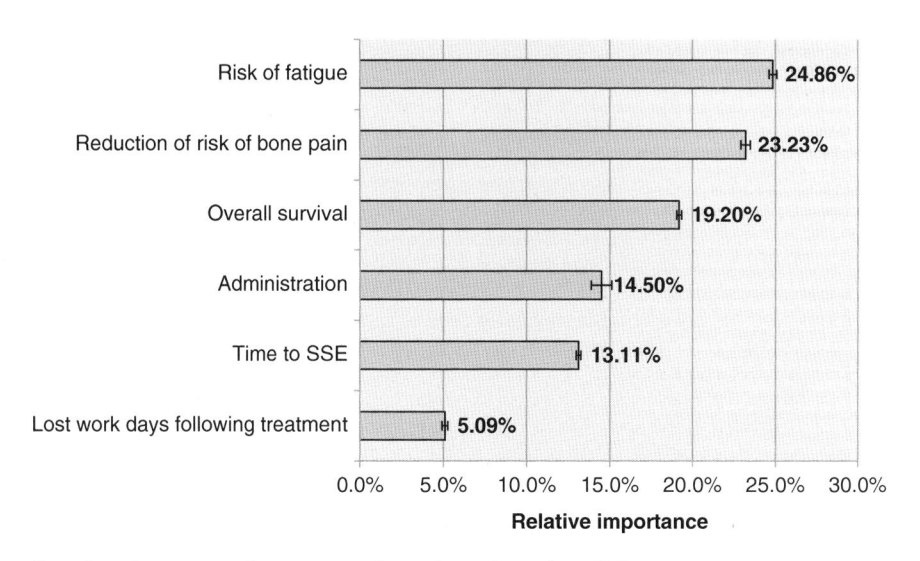

Fig. 43.1 Importance of treatment attributes for patients (from [19])

Conclusion

Now, it is true that PRO and patient preference are hot topics in oncology. At the time of treatment decision-making, in daily practice, oncologists have to pay more attention to and more communication with our patients in order to avoid silent misdiagnosis.

References

1. Reilly CM, Bruner DW, Mitchell SA, Minasian LM, Basch E, Dueck AC, Cella D, Reeve BB. A literature synthesis of symptom prevalence and severity in persons receiving active cancer treatment. Support Care Cancer. 2013;21(6):1525–50. https://doi.org/10.1007/s00520-012-1688-0.
2. Fung CH, Hays RD. Prospects and challenges in using patient-reported outcomes in clinical practice. Qual Life Res. 2008;17(10):1297–302. https://doi.org/10.1007/s11136-008-9379-5.
3. Snyder CF, Aaronson NK, Choucair AK, Elliott TE, Greenhalgh J, Halyard MY, Hess R, Miller DM, Reeve BB, Santana M. Implementing patient-reported outcomes assessment in clinical practice: a review of the options and considerations. Qual Life Res. 2012;21(8):1305–14. https://doi.org/10.1007/s11136-011-0054-x.
4. Fukushi K, Narita T, Hatakeyama S, Yamamoto H, Tobisawa Y, Yoneyama T, Hashimoto Y, Koie T, Ohyama C. Difference in toxicity reporting between patients and clinicians during systemic chemotherapy in patients with urothelial carcinoma. Int J Urol. 2017;24(5):361–6. https://doi.org/10.1111/iju.13318.
5. Basch E. The missing voice of patients in drug-safety reporting. N Engl J Med. 2010;362(10):865–9. https://doi.org/10.1056/NEJMp0911494.
6. Basch EM, Deal AM, Dueck AC, Bennett AV, Atkinson TM, Scher HI, Kris MG, Hudis CA, Sabbatini P, Dulko D. Overall survival results of a randomized trial assessing patient-reported outcomes for symptom monitoring during routine cancer treatment. JAMA. 2017;318(2):197–8.
7. Chen RC, Chang P, Vetter RJ, Lukka H, Stokes WA, Sanda MG, Watkins-Bruner D, Reeve BB, Sandler HM. Recommended patient-reported core set of symptoms to measure in prostate cancer treatment trials. J Natl Cancer Inst. 2014;106(7). https://doi.org/10.1093/jnci/dju132.
8. Scher HI, Morris MJ, Stadler WM, Higano C, Basch E, Fizazi K, Antonarakis ES, Beer TM, Carducci MA, Chi KN, Corn PG, de Bono JS, Dreicer R, George DJ, Heath EI, Hussain M, Kelly WK, Liu G, Logothetis C, Nanus D, Stein MN, Rathkopf DE, Slovin SF, Ryan CJ, Sartor O, Small EJ, Smith MR, Sternberg CN, Taplin ME, Wilding G, Nelson PS, Schwartz LH, Halabi S, Kantoff PW, Armstrong AJ. Trial design and objectives for castration-resistant prostate cancer: updated recommendations from the prostate cancer clinical trials working group 3. J Clin Oncol. 2016;34(12):1402–18. https://doi.org/10.1200/JCO.2015.64.2702.
9. Seibert C, Barbouche E, Fagan J, Myint E, Wetterneck T, Wittemyer M. Prescribing oral contraceptives for women older than 35 years of age. Ann Intern Med. 2003;138(1):54–64.
10. Aning JJ, Wassersug RJ, Goldenberg SL. Patient preference and the impact of decision-making aids on prostate cancer treatment choices and post-intervention regret. Curr Oncol. 2012;19(Suppl 3):S37–44. https://doi.org/10.3747/co.19.1287.
11. Di Maio M, Gallo C, Leighl NB, Piccirillo MC, Daniele G, Nuzzo F, Gridelli C, Gebbia V, Ciardiello F, De Placido S, Ceribelli A, Favaretto AG, de Matteis A, Feld R, Butts C, Bryce J, Signoriello S, Morabito A, Rocco G, Perrone F. Symptomatic toxicities experienced during anticancer treatment: agreement between patient and physician reporting in three randomized trials. J Clin Oncol. 2015;33(8):910–5. https://doi.org/10.1200/JCO.2014.57.9334.
12. Basch E, Autio K, Ryan CJ, Mulders P, Shore N, Kheoh T, Fizazi K, Logothetis CJ, Rathkopf D, Smith MR, Mainwaring PN, Hao Y, Griffin T, Li S, Meyers ML, Molina A, Cleeland C. Abiraterone acetate plus prednisone versus prednisone alone in chemotherapy-naive men with metastatic castration-resistant prostate cancer: patient-reported outcome results

of a randomised phase 3 trial. Lancet Oncol. 2013;14(12):1193–9. https://doi.org/10.1016/S1470-2045(13)70424-8.
13. Loriot Y, Miller K, Sternberg CN, Fizazi K, De Bono JS, Chowdhury S, Higano CS, Noonberg S, Holmstrom S, Mansbach H, Perabo FG, Phung D, Ivanescu C, Skaltsa K, Beer TM, Tombal B. Effect of enzalutamide on health-related quality of life, pain, and skeletal-related events in asymptomatic and minimally symptomatic, chemotherapy-naive patients with metastatic castration-resistant prostate cancer (PREVAIL): results from a randomised, phase 3 trial. Lancet Oncol. 2015;16(5):509–21. https://doi.org/10.1016/S1470-2045(15)70113-0.
14. Nilsson S, Cislo P, Sartor O, Vogelzang NJ, Coleman RE, O'Sullivan JM, Reuning-Scherer J, Shan M, Zhan L, Parker C. Patient-reported quality-of-life analysis of radium-223 dichloride from the phase III ALSYMPCA study. Ann Oncol. 2016;27(5):868–74. https://doi.org/10.1093/annonc/mdw065.
15. Berthold DR, Pond GR, Roessner M, de Wit R, Eisenberger M, Tannock AI. Treatment of hormone-refractory prostate cancer with docetaxel or mitoxantrone: relationships between prostate-specific antigen, pain, and quality of life response and survival in the TAX-327 study. Clin Cancer Res. 2008;14(9):2763–7. https://doi.org/10.1158/1078-0432.CCR-07-0944.
16. Magai C, Consedine N, Neugut AI, Hershman DL. Common psychosocial factors underlying breast cancer screening and breast cancer treatment adherence: a conceptual review and synthesis. J Womens Health (Larchmt). 2007;16(1):11–23. https://doi.org/10.1089/jwh.2006.0024.
17. Hauber AB, Arellano J, Qian Y, Gonzalez JM, Posner JD, Mohamed AF, Gatta F, Tombal B, Body JJ. Patient preferences for treatments to delay bone metastases. Prostate. 2014;74(15):1488–97. https://doi.org/10.1002/pros.22865.
18. Hechmati G, Hauber AB, Arellano J, Mohamed AF, Qian Y, Gatta F, Haynes I, Bahl A, von Moos R, Body JJ. Patients' preferences for bone metastases treatments in France, Germany and the United Kingdom. Support Care Cancer. 2015;23(1):21–8. https://doi.org/10.1007/s00520-014-2309-x.
19. Uemura H, Matsubara N, Kimura G, Yamaguchi A, Ledesma DA, DiBonaventura M, Mohamed AF, Basurto E, McKinnon I, Wang E, Concialdi K, Narimatsu A, Aitoku Y. Patient preferences for treatment of castration-resistant prostate cancer in Japan: a discrete-choice experiment. BMC Urol. 2016;16(1):63. https://doi.org/10.1186/s12894-016-0182-2.
20. Schnipper LE, Davidson NE, Wollins DS, Tyne C, Blayney DW, Blum D, Dicker AP, Ganz PA, Hoverman JR, Langdon R, Lyman GH, Meropol NJ, Mulvey T, Newcomer L, Peppercorn J, Polite B, Raghavan D, Rossi G, Saltz L, Schrag D, Smith TJ, Yu PP, Hudis CA, Schilsky RL, American Society of Clinical Oncology. American Society of Clinical Oncology statement: a conceptual framework to assess the value of cancer treatment options. J Clin Oncol. 2015;33(23):2563–77. https://doi.org/10.1200/JCO.2015.61.6706.

Printed by Printforce, the Netherlands